Essential Notes in Pain Medicine

Essential Notes in Pain Medicine

EDITED BY

Enrique Collantes Celador BSc (Hons), MBChB, FRCA, MSc (Med Ed), FFPMRCA, FANZCA, FFPMANZCA

Consultant in Anaesthetics and Pain Medicine
Clinical Lecturer, Northern Clinical School, Faculty of Medicine and Health, The University of Sydney, Australia
Chris O'Brien Lifehouse Hospital, Sydney, Australia
Royal North Shore Hospital, Sydney, Australia
Concord Hospital, Sydney, Australia
Hornsby Ku-Ring-Gai Hospital, Sydney, Australia
Ryde Hospital, Sydney, Australia
Sydney Adventist Hospital, Sydney, Australia

Jan Rudiger Medical State Exam of University Jena in Germany, MD, FRCA, FFPMRCA

Consultant in Anaesthetics and Pain Management
Clinical Lead in Acute and Chronic Pain Management
Surrey and Sussex Healthcare NHS Trust
Redhill, UK

Alifia Tameem MBBS, MD, DNB, FRCA, FFPMRCA

Consultant in Anaesthetics and Pain Management
Clinical Service Lead in Pain Management
Dudley Group, NHS Foundation Trust
Dudley, UK

OXFORD
UNIVERSITY PRESS

OXFORD
UNIVERSITY PRESS

Great Clarendon Street, Oxford, OX2 6DP,
United Kingdom

Oxford University Press is a department of the University of Oxford. It furthers the University's objective of excellence in research, scholarship, and education by publishing worldwide. Oxford is a registered trade mark of Oxford University Press in the UK and in certain other countries

Topic 14.5 is an extract of a longer expanded article published in Kapur, S., Dunham, R., Balasubramanian, S. (2021). Pain and Placebo. J Pain Relief, 10(4): 370. Distributed under the terms of the Creative Commons Attribution License.

First Edition published in 2022

Impression: 1

Published in the United States of America by Oxford University Press
198 Madison Avenue, New York, NY 10016, United States of America

British Library Cataloguing in Publication Data
Data available

Library of Congress Control Number: 2021941602

ISBN 978–0–19–879944–3

DOI: 10.1093/med/9780198799443.001.0001

Printed in the UK by
Bell & Bain Ltd., Glasgow

Enrique—Dedicated to my wife Alix, our son Henry, and to our family

Alifia—To my husband Mustafa and our boys Zuhair and Zayaan; this could not have been possible without your support

Jan—Dedicated to my wife Tugba and my sons Deniz, Bernhard, and Albrecht

Foreword

The practice of clinical medicine across its various specialties has much in common. It includes at its core patient communication to obtain valid information and to optimize compliance with treatment, consideration of diagnostic probabilities through history, examination, and investigations, and treatment delivery either directly or by referral. These skills are learnt by apprenticeship but, even in the information age, require a substantial body of knowledge to be drawn upon that is wide-ranging. The latter is tested through examination by the governing bodies that regulate postgraduate medical training, and the relatively new specialty of pain medicine has followed suit with fellowship examinations across the world. This book on pain management provides a wide-ranging and detailed overview of topics that would appeal to the examination candidate in need of a summary prior to their sitting of fellowship pain examinations.

The book assumes a background knowledge, but in areas where the reader feels they are limited in this, then references to background sources are provided. The subject is covered in its breadth, ranging from basic sciences underpinning the subject to clinical matters of assessment tools and treatment. Being a book for the trainee sitting examinations, it also includes those rarities oft favoured by examiners to assess clinical acumen and logical thought, but also includes, amongst these, some that will, on occasion, arise in a long career that follows, for example, serotonin syndrome, glossopharyngeal neuralgia, and refractory angina, to name but a few. As such, this book would also appeal to the pain clinician in practice, especially at the start of their career.

In providing such a broad overview, it allows the reader to not only look up matters for reminder of detail such as drug prescription, but also be aware of the treatment options, from which they can consider whether to refer on or obtain further information and apprenticed training to pursue these themselves.

The book provides a summary of pain as a psychophysical phenomenon by including details on physiology and psychology. From this flows the philosophy for assessment and management, and thus this book not only is an aide memoire for examinations, but it also provides an anchor for a clinician's ongoing career with the challenges of new information on current treatments, as well as new treatments to be subsequently appraised in the context of a paradigm for pain management.

The multiauthor book, while drawing predominantly on UK physicians, also includes several from other countries and, in so doing, provides a broad approach. Furthermore, the authorship includes those with excellent and innovative practices, some of whose work is not widely appreciated and whose ideas may offer appealing ways to develop a practice, with some examples being the use of steroid passports, how to write a patient letter, and examination signs of opioid dependence.

Much of pain practice involves the elderly, rheumatological conditions, and psychological problems and all of these are addressed in some depth and will serve the pain physician well.

I congratulate the editors on bringing this broad and skilled authorship together and offering a concise book for the benefit of examination candidates and early career pain physicians.

Jon Raphael
Professor of Pain Science, Birmingham City University

Preface

'Your pain is the breaking of the shell that encloses your understanding' – Khalil Gibran
From *The Prophet* (Knopf, 1923)

Pain is an unpleasant and emotional experience, but it is not just for the person suffering from it, but also for loved ones. It remains underestimated and undertreated, and has a major impact in our society. Treatment for alleviation of pain has been present since the dawn of mankind and has continued to evolve. Various initiatives have been introduced to make pain a priority, as it is one of the most common symptoms with which patients present to general practitioners and hospitals.

In 2012, the Faculty of Pain Medicine of the United Kingdom (UK) introduced the exam for the Fellowship in Pain Medicine (FFPMRCA). We were amongst the first anaesthetists with an interest in pain medicine, sitting this written and oral exam in the UK. With our collective knowledge, skills, and experience, we initially decided to write a book with a collection of relevant questions and answers which would have benefitted mainly the pain fellows and trainees sitting the pain exam. The format of the book was changed to serve as a comprehensive collection of high-quality resources written by various health care professionals, with an interest in pain medicine. It is based on the curriculum of the pain medicine fellowship exam in the UK, including relevant topics, which are vital for pain clinics, interventional procedures, and allied health therapies.

The book will help all pain doctors and medical and allied health care specialists who treat inpatient and outpatient chronic non-cancer and cancer pain patients, as well as pain trainees and fellows who are subspecializing in pain medicine. It will also be an excellent resource for candidates preparing for postgraduate examinations in pain medicine in the UK and/or other countries, as well as for postgraduate examinations of specialist colleges where pain medicine is in the curriculum such as rheumatology, neurology, sports medicine, addiction medicine, general practice, psychiatry, occupational therapy, rehabilitation, surgery, and other specialties.

The chapters have been organized into nine sections, commencing with pain assessment, through physiology, pharmacology, relevant pain interventions, clinical conditions associated with pain, psychological impact, and its multidisciplinary management, along with sections on cancer pain and epidemiology/evidence-based medicine.

We are extremely grateful for the expertise and hard work of our contributors and specialists from all over the world for their continued support and professionalism to make this book a success in providing an excellent and concise overview over the whole spectrum of pain medicine.

We hope that the readers of this book find it useful not only for their exams, but also as a comprehensive and suitable reference guide in their clinical practice, to improve the quality of care we provide to our patients.

Acknowledgements

We are very obliged to have had a fantastic team of authors who have contributed towards this book. Thank you for your precious time, patience, and commitment, while accommodating multiple requests for changes and amendments along the way. It has been a great pleasure working collaboratively with you all.

To write and edit a book is a complex task and has been a great educational experience for us. We could not have achieved this without the invaluable and fantastic support from Rachel Goldsworthy, Geraldine Jeffers, and Fiona Sutherland, from Oxford University Press, and Helen Nicholson from Newgen Publishing UK who have tirelessly helped us through this journey.

Last, but not the least, we are particularly grateful to our families for their constant encouragement, backing, and tolerance during the last few years, thank you!

Contents

Detailed contents

Abbreviations

1st ON	first-order neuron
2nd ON	second-order neuron
3rd ON	third-order neuron
AA	arachidonic acid
AACP	Acupuncture Association of Chartered Physiotherapists
AAGBI	Association of Anaesthetists of Great Britain and Ireland
ACDF	anterior cervical discectomy and fusion
ACEI	angiotensin-converting enzyme inhibitor
acetyl-CoA	acetyl coenzyme A
ACh	acetylcholine
ACJ	acromioclavicular joint
ACPA	anti-citrullinated protein antibodies
ACT	acceptance and commitment therapy
ACTH	adrenocorticotrophic hormone
ADH	antidiuretic hormone
ADL	activities of daily living
ADRB	aberrant drug-related behaviour
AHCPR	Agency for Health Care Policy and Research
AIDS	acquired immunodeficiency syndrome
ALARP	as low as reasonably practical
AMPA	α-amino-3-hydroxy-5-methyl-4-isoxazole propionic acid receptor
ANA	anti-nuclear antibodies
ANCA	anti-neutrophil cytoplasmic antibodies
ANOVA	analysis of variance
ANS	autonomic nervous system
AP	action potential; anteroposterior
ARDS	acute respiratory distress syndrome
ARR	absolute risk reduction
ASA	American Society of Anesthesiologists
ASIS	anterior superior iliac spine
ATLS	Advanced Trauma Life Support
ATP	adenosine triphosphate
AV	atrioventicular
BA	bioavailability
BAcC	British Acupuncture Council
BAI	Beck Anxiety Inventory
BASDAI	Bath Ankylosing Spondylitis Disease Activity Index
BASFI	Bath Ankylosing Spondylitis Functional Index
BBB	blood–brain barrier
BDNF	brain-derived neurotrophic factor
BiPAP	bilevel positive airway pressure
BMAS	British Medical Acupuncture Society
BMD	bone mineral density
BMI	body mass index
BMS	burning mouth syndrome
BNF	British National Formulary
BP	blood pressure
BPI	Brief Pain Inventory
BTX-A	botulinum toxin type A
BTX-B	botulinum toxin type B
BZD	benzodiazepine
Ca^{++}	calcium
CABG	coronary artery bypass grafting
cAMP	cyclic adenosine monophosphate
CBD	cannabidiol
CBG	corticosteroid-binding globulin
CBN	cannabinol

CBR	cannabinoid receptor
CBT	cognitive behavioural therapy
CCP	cyclic citrullinated peptide
CDA	cervical disc arthroplasty
cDMARD	conventional disease-modifying anti-rheumatic medication
CFS	chronic fatigue syndrome
CFT	compassion focused therapy
CGRP	calcitonin gene-related peptide
CHEOPS	Children's Hospital of Eastern Ontario Pain Scale
CI	confidence interval
CINV	chemotherapy-induced nausea and vomiting
CK	creatinine kinase; creatine kinase
Cl	clearance
CMT	Charcot–Marie–Tooth
CMV	cytomegalovirus
CN	cranial nerve
CNCP	chronic non-cancer pain
CNMP	chronic non-malignant pain
CNS	central nervous system
CO_2	carbon dioxide
COMT	catechol-O-methyltransferase
CONSORT	Consolidated Standards of Reporting Trials
COPD	chronic obstructive pulmonary disease
COX	cyclo-oxygenase
CPAP	continuous positive airway pressure
CPAQ	Chronic Pain Acceptance Questionnaire
CPB	coeliac plexus block
CPM	conditioned pain modulation
CPR	cardiopulmonary resuscitation
CPSP	chronic post-surgical pain
CRF	corticotropin-releasing factor
CRH	corticotrophin-releasing hormone
CRP	C-reactive protein
CRPS	complex regional pain syndrome
CSCI	continuous subcutaneous infusion
CSF	cerebrospinal fluid
CSP	Chartered Society of Physiotherapy
CSQ	Coping Strategies Questionnaire
Css	plasma concentration at steady state (mg/mL)
CT	computed tomography
CVS	cardiovascular system
CXR	chest X-ray
CYP	cytochrome peroxidase
CYP450	cytochrome P450 isoenzymes
CYP2C9	cytochrome P450 2C9
CYP3A4	cytochrome P450 3A4
DAG	diacylglycerol
DAP	dose–area product
DASS	Depression, Anxiety, and Stress Scale-21
DBS	deep brain stimulation
DBT	dialectical behaviour therapy
DCT	distal convoluted tubule
DEXA	dual-energy X-ray absorptiometry
DH	dorsal horn
DLPFC	dorsolateral prefrontal cortex
DMSO	dimethylsulfoxide
DMT	disease-modifying therapy
DN4	douleur neuropathique 4
DNA	deoxyribonucleic acid
DOP	delta opioid
DRG	dorsal root ganglion
DSA	digital subtraction angiography
dsDNA	double-stranded DNA
DSM-5	Diagnostic and Statistical Manual of Mental Disorders, fifth edition
DS-SAT	Discomfort Scale-Dementia of Alzheimer Type
DVLA	Driver and Vehicle Licensing Agency
DVT	deep vein thrombosis
EAR	estimated average requirement
EBM	evidence-based medicine
ECG	electrocardiogram
ECSWT	extracorporeal shockwave therapy
ED50	effective dose 50
EDS	Ehlers–Danlos syndrome
EDTA	ethylenediaminetetraacetate
EEG	electroencephalogram
EF	ejection fraction
eGFR	estimated glomerular filtration rate
EMG	electromyography, electromyelogram

EN-PNS	external peripheral nerve stimulation
ENT	ear, nose, and throat
EO	external oblique
EPSP	excitatory post-synaptic potential
EQ-5D	EuroQol-5D
ERCP	endoscopic retrograde pancreaticocholangiography
ESI	epidural steroid injection
ESR	erythrocyte sedimentation rate
EULAR	European League against Rheumatism
FABQ	Fear Avoidance Beliefs Questionnaire
FAIR	flexion, adduction, and internal rotation
FBC	full blood count
FBSS	failed back surgery syndrome
FDA	Food and Drug Administration of the United States
FDG-PET	fluorodeoxyglucose positron emission tomography
FHR	fetal heart rate
FLACC	Face, Legs, Activity, Cry, and Consolability (Scale)
FLAIR	fluid-attenuated inversion recovery
fMRI	functional magnetic resonance imaging
FN	false negative
FP	false positive
FPS-R	Faces Pain Scale-Revised
FRP	functional restoration programme
FSH	follicle-stimulating hormone
G	Gauge
G-6-PD	glucose-6-phosphate dehydrogenase
GABA	gamma aminobutyric acid
GABA-T	GABA-transaminases
GAD	glutamic acid decarboxylase
GAD-7	Generalized Anxiety Disorder-7
GAT	GABA transporter
GC	glucocorticoid; grey commissure
GDNF	glial cell line-derived neurotrophic factor
GDS	Geriatric Depression Scale
GET	graded exercise therapy
GFN	genitofemoral nerve
GFR	glomerular filtration rate
GHQ	General Health Questionnaire
GI	gastrointestinal
GMI	graded motor imagery
GON	greater occipital nerve
GP	general practitioner
GPCR	G-protein coupled receptor
GPM	Geriatric Pain Measure
GWAS	genome-wide association studies
H^+	proton
HADS	Hospital Anxiety and Depression Scale
Hb	haemoglobin
HDU	high dependency unit
5-HIAA	5-hydroxyindoleacetic acid
HIV	human immunodeficiency virus
HLA	human leucocyte antigen
H_2O PET	water-based positron emission tomography
HPA	hypothalamic–pituitary–adrenal
HPPH	5-(p-hydroxyphenyl)-5-phenylhydantoin
HR	heart rate
5-HT	5-hydroxytryptamine (serotonin)
IA	intrinsic activity
IAPT	Improving Access to Psychological Therapies
IASP	International Association for the Study of Pain
IBS	irritable bowel syndrome
ICP	intracranial pressure
ICD-11	International Classification of Diseases, 11th Revision
ICU	intensive care unit
IFN-γ	interferon gamma
Ig	immunoglobulin
IgA	immunoglobulin A
IHD	ischaemic heart disease
IHN	ilio-hypogastric nerve
IIm	internal intercostal membrane
IIN	ilio-inguinal nerve
IL	interleukin
IM	intramuscular
IMMPACT	Initiative on Methods, Measurement, and Pain Assessment in Clinical Trials
IN-PNS	internal peripheral nerve stimulation
INR	international normalized ratio
IO	internal oblique

IP3	inositol triphosphate
IPT	inpatient pain team
IQ	intelligence quotient
IQR	interquartile range
IR	immediate release
IRAS	Integrated Research Application System
IRMER	Ionising Radiation (Medical Exposure) Regulations
ISSVD	International Society for the Study of Vulvovaginal Disease
IT	intrathecal
ITDD	intrathecal drug delivery
IV	intravenous
JIH	joint hypermobility syndrome
K^+	potassium
Ke	elimination rate constant (min^{-1})
KOP	kappa opioid
LA	local anaesthetic(s)
LANSS	Leeds Assessment of Neuropathic Symptoms and Signs
LASER	light amplification by stimulated emission of radiation
LET	linear energy transfer
LFT	liver function test
LH	lateral horn; luteinizing hormone
LLLT	low-level laser therapy
LON	lesser occipital nerve
LSD	lysergic acid diethylamide
LTP	long-term potentiation
MAC	minimum alveolar concentration
MAO	monoamine oxidase
MAOI	monoamine oxidase inhibitors
MAPK	mitogen-activated protein kinases
MBB	medial branch block
MBSR	mindfulness-based stress reduction
MCBT	mindfulness-based CBT
mcg	microgram (μg)
MCP	metacarpophalangeal
MCS	motor cortex stimulation
MD-2	myeloid differentiation protein 2
MDMA	3,4-methylenedioxy-methamphetamine
MDT	multidisciplinary treatment
ME	myalgic encephalomyelitis
MEG	magnetoencephalography
Mg^{++}	magnesium
MHD	monohydroxy derivative
MHRA	Medicines and Healthcare products Regulatory Agency
MI	myocardial infarction; motor imagery
MMPI-2	Minnesota Multiphasic Personality Inventory-2
MOP	mu opioid
MPQ	McGill Pain Questionnaire
MR	modified release
MRI	magnetic resonance imaging
mRNA	messenger ribonucleic acid
MRSA	methicillin-resistant Staphylococcus aureus
MS	multiple sclerosis
MSE	mental state exam
MSK	musculoskeletal
MSU	monosodium urate
MTP	metatarsophalangeal
MTrP	myofascial trigger point
Na^+	sodium
NAPQI	N-acetyl-p-benzo-quinone imine
NASS	National Ankylosing Spondylitis Society
NCS	nerve conduction study
NGF	nerve growth factor
NHS	National Health Service
NICE	National Institute for Health and Care Excellence
NIPS	Neonatal/Infant Pain Scale
NIRS	near infra-red spectroscopy
NK1	neurokinin-1
NK2	neurokinin-2
NLP	neurolinguistic programming
NMDA	N-methyl-D-aspartic acid
NMJ	neuromuscular junction
NNH	number needed to harm
NNT	number needed to treat
NO	nitric oxide
N_2O	nitrous oxide
NOP	nociceptin opioid peptide
NPQ	Neuropathic Pain Questionnaire
NPS	Neuropathic Pain Score
NPV	negative predictive value
nr-ax SpA	non-radiographic axial spondyloarthritis
NRS	Numeric Rating Scale
NRTI	nucleoside reverse transcriptase inhibitor

NSAID non-steroidal anti-inflammatory drug
NSC non-selective cation channel
nsNSAID non-selective NSAID
NT neurotransmitter
OA osteoarthritis
OCD obsessive–compulsive disorder
OCF osteoporotic compression fracture
ODI Oswestry Disability Index
OH hydroxyl group
OIH opioid-induced hyperalgesia
OLP open-label placebo
OMEDD oral morphine equivalent daily dose
ONS occipital nerve stimulation
OR odds ratio
ORT Opioid Risk Tool
OST opioid substitution therapy
OT occupational therapy
OXC oxcarbazepine
PA posteroanterior
$PaCO_2$ Partial pressure of carbon dioxide
PACSLAC Pain Assessment Checklist for Seniors with Limited Ability to Communicate
PACU Post-anaesthesia care unit
PAG periaqueductal grey area
PAINAD Pain Assessment in Advanced Dementia (scale)
PaO_2 Partial pressure of oxygen
PBCL Procedure Behaviour Checklist
PCA patient-controlled analgesia
PCR polymerase chain reaction
PCS Pain Catastrophizing Scale
PCT proximal convoluted tubule
PD personality disorder
PDUQ Prescription Drug Use Questionnaire
PE pulmonary embolus
PEG polyethylene glycol
PENS percutaneous electrical nerve stimulation
PET positron emission tomography
PG prostaglandin
PGI2 prostacyclin
PHN post-herpetic neuralgia
PHQ Patient Health Questionnaire
PIP psychologically informed physiotherapist
PIPP Premature Infant Pain Profile
PMMA polymethylmethacrylate
PMP pain management programme
PNFS peripheral nerve field stimulation
PNS peripheral nerve stimulation
PO per oral
POMS Profile of Mood States
PPV positive predictive value
PRF pulsed radiofrequency
PRN as needed (Latin: pro re nata)
PROSPECT PROcedure-SPECific post-operative pain managemenT
PRP platelet-rich plasma
PSEQ Pain Self-Efficacy Questionnaire
Psi pound per square inch
PSIS posterior superior iliac spine
PTNS percutaneous Posterior Tibial Nerve Stimulation
PTSD post-traumatic stress disorder
QLB quadratus lumborum block
QLM quadratus lumborum muscle
QoL quality of life
QST quantitative sensory testing
RA rheumatoid arthritis; rectus abdominis
rACC rostral anterior cingulate cortex
RAD radiation absorbed dose
RBC red blood cell
RCT randomized controlled trial
RDA recommended daily allowance
Relim rate of drug elimination
REM radiation equivalent in man
RF radiofrequency
RFS Risk Fracture Score
RMP resting membrane potential
RNA ribonucleic acid
RNP ribonucleoprotein
ROM range of movement
RR respiratory rate; risk reduction; relative risk
RS respiratory system
rTMS repetitive transcranial magnetic stimulation
RVM rostroventral medulla
SA sinoatrial
SC subcutaneous
SCI spinal cord injury
SCJ sternoclavicular joint
SCL superior costotransverse ligament

SCS spinal cord stimulation
SD standard deviation
SDS Severity of Dependence Scale
S/E side effect
SEM standard error of the mean
SENS subcutaneous peripheral nerve stimulation
SEP sensory evoked potential
SG substantia gelatinosa
SIADH syndrome of inappropriate antidiuretic hormone
SIGN Scottish Intercollegiate Guidelines Network
SIJ sacroiliac joint
SIS Spine Intervention Society
SISAP Screening Instrument for Substance Abuse Potential
SJS Stevens–Johnson syndrome
SLE systemic lupus erythematosus
SNAP sensory nerve action potential
SNP single nucleotide polymorphism
SNRI serotonin and noradrenaline reuptake inhibitor
SNS sympathetic nervous system
SOAPP Screener and Opioid Assessment for Patients with Pain
SP substance P
SPECT single-photon emission computed tomography
SPG sphenopalatine ganglion
SpO_2 oxygen saturation
SSCS Stress Symptoms Checklist
SSD somatic symptom disorder
SSN suprascapular nerve
SSNRI selective serotonin–noradrenaline reuptake inhibitor
SSRI selective serotonin reuptake inhibitor
STIR short tau inversion recovery
SUA serum uric acid
SUNA short-lasting unilateral neuralgiform headaches with cranial autonomic symptoms
SUNCT short-lasting unilateral neuralgiform headaches with conjunctival tearing
$t^{1/2}$ half-life
TA transverse abdominis
TAC trigeminal autonomic cephalgia
TAP transverse abdominis plane
TB tuberculosis
TC therapeutic community
TCA tricyclic antidepressant
TCM traditional Chinese medicine
TEN toxic epidermal necrolysis
TENS transcutaneous electrical nerve stimulation
TFESI transforaminal epidural steroid injection
TFT thyroid function test
THC delta-9-tetrahydrocannabinol
THCV tetrahydrocannabivarin
TLR Toll-like receptor
TLR4 Toll-like receptor
TMD temporomandibular disorder
TN trigeminal neuralgia; true negative
TNF tumour necrosis factor
TON third occipital nerve
TP transverse process; true positive
TPI trigger point injection
TRP transient receptor potential
TRPV transient receptor potential vanilloid
TSH thyroid-stimulating hormone
TV tidal volume
TXA2 thromboxane
UGT uridine 5′-diphospho-glucurosyltransferase
UMN upper motor neuron
US ultrasound
USS ultrasound scan
UV ultraviolet
VAS Visual Analogue Scale
Vd volume of distribution
VGAT vesicular GABA transporter
VH ventral horn
VMAT vesicular monoamine transporter
VNS vagus nerve stimulation
VRS Verbal Rating Scale
VZV varicella zoster virus
WAD whiplash-associated disorder
WC white commissure
WDR wide dynamic range
WHO World Health Organization
w/v weight by volume

Contributors

Adnan Al-Kaisy, MBChB, FRCA, FPMRCA, FIPP, Consultant in Pain Medicine and Neuromodulation, Clinical Lead, Guy's and St Thomas' Pain Management and Neuromodulation Centre, London, UK *Topic 15.2*

Sabina Bachtold, EDAIC, FRCA, FFPMRCA, Consultant in Anaesthesia and Pain Medicine, Frimley Park Hospital, Camberley, UK *Topics 1.1, 14.1, 30.1, 32.3, 32.4, 24.1*

Shyam Balasubramanian, MBBS, MD, MSc, FRCA, FFPMRCA Consultant in Pain Medicine and Anaesthesia, Associate Medical director, University Hospitals Coventry & Warwickshire NHS Trust, Coventry, UK *Topics 14.5, 17.2, 17.3*

Laura Beard, MBChB, FRCA, PGCME, EDRA, Regional Anaesthesia Reseach Fellow, University Hospital Birmingham, Birmingham, UK *Topics 17.2, 17.3, 17.4*

Hadi Bedran, MD, FCARCSI, FFPMRCA, Consultant in Anaesthetics and Pain Medicine, St George's University Hospital, London, UK *Topics 10.2, 10.5, 11.1, 11.2, 13.1, 22.5, 22.6, 22.7, 22.8*

Sadiq Bhayani, MBBS, FRCA, EDRA, FFPMRCA, CIPS, FIPP, Consultant in Pain Medicine and Anaesthesia, Lead Physician Department of Pain Medicine, University Hospitals Leicester NHS Trust, Leicester General Hospital, Leicester, UK *Topics 14.5, 17.2, 17.3*

Owen Bodycombe, MBChB, FRCA, FFPMRCA, Consultant in Anaesthetics and Pain Medicine, Gloucestershire Hospitals NHS Foundation Trust, Gloucester, UK *Topics 23.1, 24.3*

Simon Braude, BMedSc, MBChB, FRCA, FFPMRCA, Consultant in Anaesthetics and Pain Medicine, Northwick Park Hospital, Harrow, UK *Topics 15.1, 15.3, 15.4*

Caroline Burrow, BSc, PhD, Cpsychol, ClinPsyD, Clinical Psychologist, Northern Meadow Therapy, Cooneen, Brookeborough, Northern Ireland *Topics 30.2, 30.5, 30.9, 30.10, 30.11, 30.12, 30.13, 30.14*

Udaya Chakka, MBBS, MD, FCAI, EDRA, FFPMRCA, Consultant in Anaesthesia and Pain Management, University Hospitals Coventry & Warwickshire NHS Trust, Coventry, UK *Topics 13.2, 13.9, 13.11, 13.16*

Kasia Chmiel, BSc i(Adv), MBBS, FRACP (Med Onc), FAChPM, Head of Palliative Care Department, Chris O'Brien Lifehouse Hospital, Sydney, Australia *Topic 29.7*

Mahesh Choudhari, MBBS, MD, FRCA, FFPMRCA, Consultant in Anaesthesia and Pain Management, Worcester Royal Hospital, Worcester, UK *Topic 29.5*

Bill Clark, FRANZCR, EBIR, Consultant in Radiology, Director Interventional Radiology, Department of Radiology, St George Private Hospital, Sydney, Australia *Topic 22.9*

Enrique Collantes, BSc (Hons), MBChB, FRCA, MSc (Med Ed), FFPMRCA, FANZCA, FFPMANZCA, Consultant in Anaesthesia and Pain Management, Clinical Lecturer, Northern Clinical School, Faculty of Medicine and Health, The University of Sydney, Department of Anaesthesia and Pain Medicine, Royal North Shore Hospital, Sydney, Concord Hospital, Sydney, Hornsby Ku-Ring-Gai Hospital, Ryde Hospital, Sydney Adventist Hospital, Sydney, Australia *Topics 1.6, 2.2, 2.3, 2.5, 2.7, 3.2, 6.1, 6.2, 6.3, 6.4, 6.5, 6.7, 6.8 7.2, 7.13, 8.1, 8.2, 8.3, 8.4, 8.5, 8.6, 10.1, 10.5, 13.3, 13.5, 15.1, 15.3, 15.4, 22.5, 22.6, 22.7, 22.8, 23.5, 23.8, 23.9, 23.14, 24.2, 24.4, 24.7, 24.14, 26.1, 27.1, 27.2, 28.1, 28.8, 28.10*

Sangeeta Das, MBBS, DA, FRCA, FFPMRCA, Assistant Professor Anaesthesia and Pain, Department of Anaesthesia and Pain Management, St John's National Academy of Health Sciences, Bengaluru, India *Topic 20.8*

Mohamed Dorgham, MD, FFPMRCA, FIPP, Consultant in Pain Management and Anaesthesia, University Hospital Birmingham, Birmingham, UK, Lecturer of Anaesthesiology, Critical care and Pain medicine, Ain-Shams University, Egypt *Topics 17.2, 17.3, 23.15*

Alix Dumitrescu, BSc (Med), MBBS, FRACP, FFPMANZCA, FRACP, FAChPM, Consultant in Palliative Care and Pain Management, Department of Pain Medicine and Palliative Care, Royal Prince Alfred Hospital, Sydney, Australia *Topice 29.9*

Rebecca Elijah-Smith, BSc, MSc, PG Cert Pain Management, Lead Physiotherapist in Pain Management, Sandwell and West Birmingham NHS Trust, Birmingham, UK *Topics 31.1, 31.3, 31.4, 31.5, 31.6, 31.7, 31.8*

Bethany Fitzmaurice, MBChB, FRCA, Advance Trainee in Pain Medicine, Sandwell & West Birmingham NHS Trust, Birmingham, UK *Topics 4.5, 12.1, 12.2, 12.3, 12.4, 12.5, 12.6, 13.13, 23.3*

Ann-Katrin Fritz, Medical State Exam Heidelberg University in Germany, FRCA, FFPMRCA, FIPP, CIPS, Consultant in Anaesthetics and Pain Medicine, Norfolk & Norwich University Hospital, Norwich, UK *Topics 16.1, 16.2, 16.3, 16.4, 16.5, 19.2*

Praveen Ganty, MBBS, DA, FRCA, FCARCSI, FFPMRCA, FRCPC, Consultant in Pain Medicine and Anesthesiology, Toronto Rehabilitation Institute, University Health Network, Toronto, Canada *Topics 1.8, 7.13, 13.6*

Sian Griffith, MBChB, MD, MRCP, FRCP, Consultant Rheumatologist, Rheumatology Audit Lead, and Trust Lead for Osteoporosis, Surrey and Sussex Healthcare NHS Trust, Redhill, UK *Topics 25.1, 25.2, 25.3, 25.4, 25.5, 25.6., 25.7*

Anthony Gubbay, MBChB, BSc, FRCA, Consultant in Anaesthesia and Pain Management, Royal Free Hospital, Department of Anaesthesia & Pain Medicine, London, UK *Topic 28.7*

Sumit Gulati, MD, FRCA, FFPMRCA, EDRA, Consultant in Pain Medicine and Anaesthesia, The Walton Centre NHS Foundation Trust, Liverpool, UK *Topics 15.6, 15.7, 24.6, 28.4*

Rajesh Gupta, MBBS, BSc, FRCA, FFPMRCA, Consultant in Pain Medicine and Anaesthesia, Whipps Cross University Hospital, London, UK *Topic 24.4*

Rahul Guru, MBBS, MD, FCARCSI, DPMCAI, Consultant in Pain Medicine and Anaesthesia, University Hospital of Wales, Cardiff, UK *Topic 14.3, 17.1, 19.3, 23.13, 24.12, 30.3*

Sarah Harper, MBChB, FRCA, FFPMRCOA, Consultant in Pain Medicine and Anaesthesia, Gloucestershire Hospitals NHS Foundation Trust, Gloucester, UK *Topics 28.5, 28.9*

Katharine Howells, MBBS, BSc, FRCA, FFPMRCA, Consultant in Anaesthesia and Pain Management, Royal United Hospital Bath NHS Foundation Trust, Bath, UK *Topic 14.2*

James Jack, MBBS, BSc (Hons), Specialty Registrar in Anaesthetics, Surrey and Sussex Healthcare NHS Trust, Redhill, UK *Topics 7.3, 7.4, 7.5, 7.7, 7.8, 7.10, 7.12, 13.10, 14.4*

Senthil Jayaseelan, FRCA, FCARCSI, FFPMRCA, FIPP, Consultant in Anaesthesia and Pain Management, St Helens and Knowsley Teaching Hospitals NHS Trust, Prescot, UK *Topics 4.2, 4.3*

Gustav Jirikowski, Prof Dr phil med habil Professor in Anatomy and Neuroanatomy, Department Vorklinische Medizin, Medical School Hamburg MSH, Hamburg, Germany *Topics 1.4, 2.1, 4.4, 19.1, 20.1, 20.4*

Yehia Kamel, MBBCh, MSc, FRCA, FFPMRCA, FIPP, EDRA, CIPS, Consultant in Anaesthesia and Pain Management, University Hospital of Leicester, Leicester, UK *Topics 1.5, 18.2, 20.12, 23.8, 23.10, 29.4, 29.6, 29.8*

Ilya Kantsedikas, MBBS, BMedSci (Hons), MRCP, FRCA, Specialist Registrar in Anaesthesia, St Mary's Hospital, London, UK *Topics 22.2, 22.1*

Sandeep Kapur, MBBS, MD, FRCA, FFPMRCA, Consultant in Pain Medicine and Anaesthesia, University Hospital Birmingham, Birmingham, UK *Topics 4.6, 14.5, 23.4*

Peter Keogh, MB ChB, FRCA, FANZCA, FFPMANZCA, MAcadMEd, Specialist Pain Medicine Physician and Specislist Anaesthetist, Melbourne, Australia *Topics 8.1, 8.2, 8.3, 8.4, 8.5, 8.6, 10.3, 10.4, 13.5*

Andrzej Krol, MD, DEAA, FRCA, FFPMRCA, EDPM-ESRA, Consultant in Pain Management and Anaesthesia, Pain Clinic, Atkinson Morley Wing, St George's Hospital, London, UK *Topics 22.6, 22.7*

Karen LeMarchand, BSc, MSc, MScDip, CPsychol, AFBPsS, Lead Clinical Psychologist—Pain Management at the Dudley Group of Hospitals, Black Country Partnership Foundation Trust, Dudley, UK *Topics 30.4, 30.6, 30.7, 30.8, 30.15*

Tommy Lwin, MBBS, BSc, Anaesthetic Trainee CT2, Surrey and Sussex Healthcare NHS Trust, Redhill, UK *Topic 28.2*

Deepak Malik, DFPMRCA, EDRA, MRCA, FCARCSI, DA, MBBS, Consultant in Anaesthesia and Pain Management, Queen Elizabeth Hospital Birmingham, Birmingham, UK *Topic 20.9*

Manish Mittal, MBBS, DA, FRCA, EDAIC, FFPMRCA, Consultant Anaesthesia and Chronic Pain, Russell's Hall Hospital, Dudley Foundation trust, Dudley, UK *Topics 4.1, 20.3*

Ramy Mottaleb, MBBS, BSc, FRCA, FFPMRCA, Consultant in Pain Medicine and Anaesthesia, Kingston NHS Foundation Trust, Kingston Upon Thames, UK *Topic 3.3*

Nofil Mulla, MBBS, MD, FRCA, FFPMRCA, NBME (USA), Consultant in Pain Medicine and Anaesthesia, Luton and Dunstable University Hospital, UK *Topics 3.2, 23.2, 23.9, 24.2, 24.7, 24.8, 24.14, 27.1, 28.1*

Yin Yee Ng, BMBS, FRCA, FFPMRCA, Consultant in Anaesthetics and Pain Medicine, North Bristol NHS Trust, Bristol, UK *Topics 18.4, 20.2*

Jonathan Norman, MBBS, MRCP, FRCA, FFPMRCA, Consultant in Pain Medicine and Anaesthetics, DMRC Stanford Hall, Stanford on Soar, UK Topics 7.1, 7.2, 7.6, 7.9, 7.11, 7.13

Paolo Pais, MD, Consultant in Anaesthesia and Pain Medicine, Chivasso Civil Hospital, Chivasso, Italy *Topics 2.5, 23.14, 26.1, 28.8*

Stefano Palmisani, MD, Consultant in Pain Medicine, Guy's and St Thomas' Pain Management and Neuromodulation Centre, London, UK *Topic 20.6*

David Pang, MRCPCH, FRCA, FFPMRCA, FIPP, Consultant in Pain Management, Guy's and St Thomas' Pain Management and Neuromodulation Centre, London, UK *Topics 20.5, 20.7, 20.11, 28.6, 32.1*

Nishi Patel, MBBS, BSc, FRCA, FFPMRCA, Consultant in Pain Medicine and Anaesthesia, Gloucestershire Hospitals NHS Foundation Trust, Gloucester, UK *Topics 5.1, 5.2*

Erlick Pereira, MA(Camb), BM BCh DM(Oxf), FRCS(SN), SFHEA, Reader in Neurosurgery and Consultant Neurosurgeon, Department of Neurosurgery, Atkinson Morley Wing, St George's Hospital, London, UK *Topic 21.1, 21.2, 21.3, 21.4, 24.5*

Arumugam Pitchiah, MBBS, MD, FRCA, FFPMRCA, Consultant in Anaesthesia and Pain Management, Department of Anaesthetics, Royal Preston Hospital, Preston *Topic 13.4, 13.8, 23.6*

Kavita Poply, FRCA, DA, FCA RCSI, FFPMRCA, Consultant in Anaesthesia and Pain Management, Clinical Lecturer, Queen Mary University London, and Consultant in Barts Health NHS Trust, London, UK *Topics 6.1, 6.2, 6.3, 6.4, 6.5, 6.7, 6.8, 13.7, 27.2*

Ashok Puttapa, MD, FCAI, AFRCA, DIFPMCAI, EDPM, MSC, DESRA, Consultant in Anaesthesia and Pain Management, Royal Stoke University Hospital, Stoke-on-Trent, UK *Topics 15.5, 24.1,29.1, 29.2, 29.3*

Bhavesh Raithatha, MBChB, FRCA, FFPMRCA, Consultant in Anaesthesia and Pain Management, Leicester General Hospital, Leicester, UK *Topics 18.3, 19.5*

Subramanian Ramani, MBBS, FRCA, FFPMRCA, PGA-MedEd, Consultant in Anaesthesia and Pain Management, Northampton General Hospital, Northampton, UK *Topic 19.4*

Shankar Ramaswamy, MBBS, MD, FRCA, FFPMRCA, EDRA, Cer Cli res Consultant in Pain Medicine and Anaesthesia, Bart's Health NHS Trust, The Royal London Hospital, London, UK *Topics 23.5, 23.14, 28.10*

Manamohan Rangaiah, MD, DNB, FCAI, FRCA, DIPCAI, EDAIC, EDRA, Consultant in Anaesthesia and Pain Management, Walsall Manor Hospital, Walsall, UK *Topics 13.12, 13.14*

Deepak Ravindran, MD, FRCA, FFPMRCA, FIPP, EDRA, DMSKMed, BSLM Consultant and Clinical Lead for Pain Medicine, Royal Berkshire NHS Foundation Trust, Reading, UK *Topics 1.2, 1.7, 1.9, 1.10, 1.11, 2.1, 2.2, 2.6*

Jan Rudiger, Medical State Exam of University Jena in Germany, PhD, FRCA, FFPMRCA, Consultant in Anaesthetics and Pain Management, Pain Lead, Surrey and Sussex Healthcare NHS Trust, Redhill, UK *Topics 1.2, 1.4, 1.5, 1.7, 1.9, 1.12, 1.13, 1.14, 2.1, 2.2, 6.6, 6.7,7.1, 7.2, 7.6, 7.11, 7.13, 13.6, 13.10, 13.15, 14.4, 15.1, 15.3, 15.4, 16.1, 16.2, 16.3, 16.4, 16.5, 18.1, 19.1, 19.2, 20.1, 23.12, 24.9, 24.11, 24.13, 26.2, 28.2, 28.3*

Mohammed Sajad, MBChB, FRCA, FCAI, PGDip, Consultant in Anaesthesia and Pain Management, Russells Hall Hospital, Dudley Group of Hospitals, Dudley, UK *Topics 9.2, 9.3, 9.4, 9.5, 9.6, 9.7, 9.8, 9.9, 9.10*

Haggai Sharon, MD, PhD, FIPP, Consultant in Pain Management, Institute of Pain Medicine, Tel Aviv Medical Center, Tel Aviv, Israel *Topic 15.2*

Kathleen Shelley, BSc (Hons), BM, FRCA, Specialist Registrar in Anaesthesia, Welsh School of Anaesthesia, Cardiff, Wales, UK *Topics 5.1, 5.2*

Attam Jeet Singh, MBBS, FRCA, FFPMRCA, Consultant in Anaesthesia and Pain Management, West Herfordshire NHS Trust, Watford, UK *Topics 22.1, 22.2*

Thomas E Smith, MBBS, MD, FRCA, FFPMRCA, Consultant in Pain Management and Neuromodulation, Guy's and St Thomas' Pain Management and Neuromodulation Centre, London, UK *Topics 18.1, 23.7, 23.11, 24.10*

Doug Stangoe, BSc, BM, FRCA, Speciality Registrar in Anaesthetics and Intensive Care, Surrey and Sussex Healthcare NHS Trust, Redhill, UK *Topic 17.5*

Maria Stasiowska, MBBS, BSc, FRCA, FFPMRCA, Consultant in Anaesthetics and Pain Medicine, The National Hospital for Neurology and Neurosurgery, London, UK *Topics 2.2, 2.3, 2.4, 2.7, 3.1, 13.3*

Kantharuby Tambirajoo, MB BCh, BAO, BA, Senior Clinical Fellow in Functional Neurosurgery, King's College Hospital, London, UK *Topics 24.6, 28.4*

Alifia Tameem, MBBS, MD, DNB, FRCA, FFPMRCA, Consultant in Anaesthetics and Pain Management, Clinical Service Lead in Pain Management, Russells Hall Hospital, Dudley Group of Hospitals, Dudley, UK *Topics 1.1, 9.1, 9.2, 12.1, 12.4, 13.9, 13.13, 14.1, 15.1, 15.3, 15.4, 15.5, 17.2, 17.3, 24.1, 24.8, 24.12, 29.1, 32.2, 32.3, 32.4, 4.5, 9.10, 12.3, 13.11, 13.12, 13.16, 17.4, 23.1, 23.15, 24.3, 29.2, 29.3, 29.5*

John Tanner, BSc, MBBS, FFSEM, D M-S M DSMSA, Musculoskeletal and Sports Medicine, BASEM Education Committee, Past President of British Institute of Musculoskeletal Medicine, European Faculty of Spine Intervention Society, Hon Lecturer Queen Mary University London, St Bartholomew and Royal London Medical School, External Lecturer MS Ultrasonography Bournemouth University (AECC University College), Registered Osteopath, Oving Clinic, Oving, UK *Topics 1.3, 22.10*

Fiona Thomas, BAppSc, OT Occupational Therapist, The Caulfield Pain Management and Research Centre, Melbourne, Australia *Topic 31.2*

Athmaja Thottungal, MBBS, FRCA, FFPMRCA, EDRA, FIPP, CIPS, Consultant in Pain Medicine and Anaesthesia, Chronic Pain Lead, Kent and Canterbury Hospital, East Kent Hospitals University Foundation NHS Trust, Canterbury, UK *Topic 20.10, 23.12, 24.11, 26.3, 26.4., 26.5, 26.6*

Victoria Winter, BMBCh BA (Hons Oxon), MA (Oxon), FRCA, Specialist Registrar in Anaesthesia, North Central London School of Anaesthesia, Royal Free London NHS, Department of Anaesthesia & Pain Medicine, London, UK *Topic 28.7*

Ivan Wong, MBChB, FRCA, FFPMRCA, Consultant in Pain Medicine and Anaesthesia, The Royal London Hospital, London, UK *Topics 23.5, 28.10*

Matthew Wong, BAppSc, MD, Specialty Registrar in Anaesthesia, Hornsby Ku-Ring-Gai Hospital, Hornsby, NSW, Australia *Topics 3.2, 10.1, 13.1*

SECTION 1

OVERVIEW OF PAIN

CHAPTER 1

Types of Pain and Pain Assessment

Sabina Bachtold, Enrique Collantes, Praveen Ganty, Yehia Kamel, Gustav Jirikowski, Deepak Ravindran, Jan Rudiger, Alifia Tameem, and John Tanner

CONTENTS

1.1 Acute/chronic pain and IASP classification of chronic pain for ICD-11

Definition

Revised (new) definition of pain

'An unpleasant sensory and emotional experience associated with, or resembling that associated with, actual or potential tissue damage'[1]

Previous definition of pain

'An unpleasant sensory and emotional experience associated with actual or potential tissue damage, or described in terms of such damage'[2]

Nociceptive pain

'Pain that arises from actual or threatened damage to non-neural tissue and is due to the activation of nociceptors'[3]

Neuropathic Pain

'Pain caused by a lesion or disease of the somatosensory nervous system'[3]

1. Reproduced with permission from Raja, S., N., *et al. (2020)*. The revised International Association for the Study of Pain definition of pain: concepts, challenges, and compromises, *Pain*. 161(9): 1976–1982. doi: 10.1097/j.pain.0000000000001939.
2. Reproduced with permission from The need of a taxonomy. *Pain*, 6(3). 247–252, 1979. DOI: 10.1016/0304-3959(79)90046-0
3. Reproduced from Kosek E, et al. Do we need a third mechanistic descriptor for chronic pain states?, Pain, 157(7): 1382–1386, copyright 2016, International Association for the Study of Pain.

Table 1.1.1 Difference between acute and chronic pain

Acute pain	Chronic pain
At the same time with an acute illness/injury	Persists beyond the expected time of healing (3 months)
Warning system to alert the body to a problem	Serves no physiological purpose
Predominantly nociceptive	Frequently neuropathic in nature
Usually resolves with complete tissue healing	Persistent
Inadequate treatment can lead to chronic pain states	Negative impact on quality of life. High costs to society

Nociplastic pain

'Pain that arises from altered nociception despite no clear evidence of actual or threatened tissue damage causing the activation of peripheral nociceptors or evidence for disease or lesion of the somatosensory system causing the pain'[3]

The difference between acute and chronic pain

(See Table 1.1.1.)

Transition from acute to chronic pain

- The mechanisms that might underlie the transition are not yet fully understood but may be minimized by early recognition of risk factors (see Table 1.1.2) and early biopsychosocial pain management

Peripherally

- Continuous and prolonged inflammatory reaction releases pro-nociceptive factors, such as cytokines, prostaglandins (PGs), substance P (SP), tumour necrosis factor (TNF) alpha, and interleukins (ILs), resulting in decreased activation thresholds and spontaneous discharge
- **Peripheral sensitization** occurs, causing allodynia and hyperalgesia within an area of inflamed skin

Table 1.1.2 Risk factors for transition from acute to chronic pain

Pre-existing	At the time of injury/surgery	Post-injury/surgery
Pre-existing pain in the area High opioid use Female—higher scores Age (children < elderly < young) Raised BMI Genetic polymorphism Radiation therapy Psychological vulnerability Psychosocial issues Yellow flags Blue flags Black flags Other chronic conditions	Type of surgery (amputation, breast surgery, thoracotomy, hernia repair, coronary artery bypass, Caesarean section) Operations >3 hours Surgical technique Repeat surgery	Severe post-operative pain Poorly treated acute pain Catastrophizing

Spinal cord

- Intense nociceptive activation leads to changes in the dorsal root ganglion (DRG) and dorsal horn (DH) neurons, increasing sodium (Na^+) and transient receptor potential vanilloid (TRPV) 1 receptor and activation of the N-methyl-D-aspartic acid (NMDA) receptor
- There is a phenotypic switch, cross-sprouting with receptive fields on the DH being widened
- **Central sensitization** arises in undamaged tissue away from the site of injury, with secondary allodynia or hyperalgesia. The application of noxious heat and capsaicin has been shown to produce secondary hyperalgesia and reversible changes in the brainstem of human volunteers. This reversible form of central sensitization has been termed 'wind-up'
- **Transcription-dependent central sensitization** is more permanent and occurs if the stimuli triggering central sensitization continue causing new synaptic connections to be made and there may even be death of certain cells. This more permanent form of sensitization may even result in structural changes in the brain that are visible on magnetic resonance imaging (MRI) scanning

Brain

- Functional MRI (fMRI) and positron emission tomography (PET) scans confirmed changes that occur in the pain matrix (thalamus, mid/anterior insula, anterior cingulate and prefrontal cortex, periaqueductal grey area (PAG) and rostroventral medulla (RVM), reticular formation, and amygdala) with increased functional connectivity between the medial prefrontal cortex and nucleus accumbens (the brain's emotion learning circuits) being highly predictive of chronicity
- Strong correlation between mental health of the patient and chronic pain leading to maladaptive coping habits

Further reading

1. Nicholas M, Vlaeyen JWS, Rief W et al. The IASP Taskforce for the Classification of Chronic Pain The IASP classification of chronic pain for ICD-11: chronic primary pain, PAIN. 2019;160(1):28–37
2. Raja SN, Carr DB, Cohen M, et al. The revised International Association for the Study of Pain definition of pain: concepts, challenges, and compromises. Narrative review. Pain 2020;161(9):1976–82 https://journals.lww.com/pain/ https://www.iasp-pain.org/resources/terminology/#pain
3. Feizerfan, A, Sheh, G. Transition from acute to chronic pain. Contin Educ Anaesth Crit Care Pain 2014;15(2):98–102
4. Macrae WA, Davies HTO. Chronic postsurgical pain. In: Crombie IK (ed). Epidemiology of Pain. 1999; pp. 125–42. Seattle, WA: IASP Press
5. Apkarian AV, Baliki MN, Farmer MA. Predicting transition to chronic pain. Curr Opin Neurol. 2013 Aug;26(4):360–7

1.2 History taking in pain medicine

Principles

- A thorough, comprehensive history helps in establishing a good relationship with the patient and to formulate a comprehensive multimodal treatment plan
- Follow the principles of VEMA—Validate their symptoms, Educate the patient, Motivate them, and provide them the tools for Activation
- Screen all patients for pain and perform a comprehensive pain assessment
- Common elements of a thorough, semi-structured interview include:
  - Experience of pain and related symptoms and factors influencing it
  - Treatments received and ongoing

- Current litigation status, if any
- Coping abilities
- Educational/vocational/work/employment status
- Any relevant psychosocial history, including adversity in childhood, if relevant
- Alcohol and any substance misuse
- Ongoing psychological issues, if any
- Concerns and explanations for pain
- Treatment goals

Set the stage

- Reassure patients that you take their pain seriously, and understand its impact and the need for treatment
- Maintain a respectful and professional attitude
- It is important to believe the patient's reports of pain and distress, particularly in the case of patients with chronic non-cancer pain (CNCP) who may have had difficult encounters with previous health care professionals
- Even if psychological issues or addiction are present, respectful validation of the patient's suffering is invaluable to assessment and will lead to more effective treatment planning
- Pain is a multi-dimensional phenomenon that can produce strong emotional reactions that impact on function, quality of life (QoL), emotional state, social and job status, and general well-being
- Pain assessment should also be multi-dimensional: evaluate these various elements during the interview and examination, and include them in the diagnostic formulation
- A thorough history and physical examination are essential for the medical and pain diagnosis and treatment planning
- Careful attention to the patient's reported symptoms will help direct the physical examination and narrow the pain differential diagnosis
- Perform complete neurological and musculoskeletal (MSK) examinations
- Additional testing, such as imaging and laboratory studies or electrophysiological testing (electromyography (EMG)/nerve conduction studies), may be ordered as needed, based on the results of the history and examinations

The RAT model

(See Table 1.2.1.)

Table 1.2.1 The RAT model

Recognize pain	Does the patient have pain? Do other people (carers/family) know that the patient is in pain?
Assess pain	Measure the severity What is the pain score at rest? With movement? How is the pain affecting the patient? What scales would you use? Make a diagnosis Acute or chronic Cancer or non-cancer Nociceptive/neuropathic or mixed or nociplastic Are there other factors? Psychological factors Physical factors (other illnesses)
Treat	Non-drug and drug strategies

Table 1.2.2 Simple steps to make a provisional pain diagnosis

What is the duration of pain?	Acute Chronic Acute-on-chronic
What is the main cause of pain?	Cancer Non-cancer
What is the suspected mechanism?	Nociceptive. Neuropathic Mixed (nociceptive and neuropathic) Nociplastic

- The Faculty of Pain Medicine (UK) advises all health care professionals to consider using the RAT model as a simple framework for patients with pain:
  - R for 'Recognize pain'
  - A for 'Assessment of pain'
  - T for 'Treat the pain using non-drug and drug strategies'
- Another simple way to assess pain is shown in Table 1.2.2

Pain scales

- Pain is a subjective experience with a different meaning to each person
- Changes in pain intensity are valuable when measured for single individuals (e.g. before and after a treatment)
- Pain intensity measures should not be used to compare pain between different individuals. One person's 4/10 might be another's 10/10
- A numeric pain rating scale for most clinical settings. The most common one is the 11-point Likert scale where 0 = no pain and 10 = worst pain imaginable
- For children, consider using the 0–5 Wong-Baker Faces scale (see Table 1.2.3)
- Non-verbal patients (e.g. those in coma or with dementia or other cognitive impairments) must be assessed for pain by the Abbey Pain scale and by other observational means (e.g. body language, movement, autonomic arousal, and non-verbal pain behaviour)

The pain history interview

- A number of mnemonic-based, structured history taking approaches are available such as SOCRATES (see 1.13 Mnemonics for referrals p. 42) or PAIN FRAME
- The mnemonic 'QISS TAPED' is a comprehensive tool to help ensure all information is sought (see Table 1.2.4)

Table 1.2.3 Types of pain assessment tools

Uni-dimensional tools	Verbal Rating Scale Numerical Rating Scale Visual Analogue Scale Faces scale (Wong-Baker scale)
Multi-dimensional tools	McGill Pain Questionnaire Brief Pain Inventory West Haven-Yale Multi-dimensional Pain Inventory (WHYMPI) Medical Outcome Study 36-item Short-form Health Survey (SF-36)
Screening tools for neuropathic pain	Leeds Assessment of Neuropathic Symptoms and Signs (LANSS) Neuropathic Pain Questionnaire (NPQ) DN4 PainDETECT

Table 1.2.4 Pain assessment mnemonic (QISS TAPED)

Q	Quality	What were your first symptoms? What words would you use to describe the pain (aching, sharp, burning, squeezing, dull, icy, etc.)?
I	Impact	How does the pain affect you? What does the pain prevent you from doing? (Depression screen) Do you feel sad or blue? Do you cry often? Is there loss of interest in life? Decreased or increased appetite? (Anxiety screen) Do you feel stressed or nervous? Have you been particularly anxious about anything? Do you startle easily?
S	Site	Show me where you feel the pain. Can you put your finger/hand on it? Or show me on a body map? Does the pain move/radiate anywhere? Has the location changed over time?
S	Severity	On a 0–10 scale, with 0 = no pain and 10 = the worst pain imaginable, how much pain are you in right now? What is the least pain you have had in the past (24 hours, 1 week, 1 month)? What is the worst pain you have had in the past (24 hours, 1 week, 1 month)? How often are you in severe pain (hours in a day, days in a week you have pain)? Consider using Brief Pain Inventory if possible
T	Temporal characteristics	When did the pain start? Was it sudden? Gradual? Was there a clear triggering event? Is the pain constant or intermittent? Does it come spontaneously or is it provoked? Is there a predictable pattern? (e.g. always worst in the morning or in the evening? Does it suddenly flare up?)
A	Aggravating and alleviating factors	What makes the pain better? What makes the pain worse? When do you get the best relief? How much relief do you get? How long does it last?
P	Past response, preferences	How have you managed your pain in the past? (Ask about both drug and non-drug methods) What helped? What did not help? (Be specific about drug trials—how much and for how long?) What medications have you tried? Was the dose increased until you had pain relief or side effects? How long did you take the drug? Are there any pain medicines that have caused you an allergic or other bad reaction? How do you feel about taking medications? Have you tried physical or occupational therapy? What was done? Was it helpful? Have you tried spinal or other injections for pain treatment? What was done? Was it helpful?
E	Expectations, goals, meaning	What do you think is causing the pain? How may we help you? What do you think we should do to treat your pain? What do you hope the treatment will accomplish? What do you want to do that the pain keeps you from doing? What are you most afraid of? (Uncover specific fears, such as fear of cancer, which should be acknowledged and addressed)
D	Diagnostics and physical examination	Examine and inspect the site Perform a systems assessment and examination as indicated Review imaging, laboratory, and/or other test results as indicated

- A pain history should include location, quality, intensity, temporal characteristics, aggravating and alleviating factors, impact of pain on function and QoL, past treatment and response, and patient expectations and goals. Table 1.2.4 summarizes the general categories that should be addressed during a pain assessment, along with examples of questions that may be useful during the interview

Further reading

1. Day MA. Mindfulness-Based Cognitive Therapy for Chronic Pain: A Clinical Manual and Guide. 1st edition, 2017. Chichester, West Sussex: Wiley and Sons
2. Faculty of Pain Medicine (UK). Essential Pain Management UK. Roger Goucke, Wayne Morriss (Australia), Linda Huggins (NZ). 2016
3. Faculty of Pain Medicine ANZCA. How EPM works. 2016. https://www.anzca.edu.au/getattachment/5647be92-3387-4983-807f-06da768f99b1/1-EPM-participant-manual-(English)
4. Gurumoorthi R, Das G, Gupta M, et al. The art of history taking in patient with pain: an ignored but very important component in making diagnosis. Indian J Pain 2013;27:59–66
5. Powell RA, Downing J, Ddungu H, Mwangi-Powell FN. Pain History and Pain Assessment. In: Kopf A, Patel NB (eds). Guide to pain measurement in low-resource settings. 2010. ASP, Seattle https://www.cfpc.ca/CFPC/media/Resources/Pain-Management/Pain-assessment.pdf
6. Medistudents, Other skills – History taking. 2018. London, UK https://www.medistudents.com/osce-skills/patient-history-taking

1.3 Examination in the pain clinic

Introduction

- Pain clinic examination needs to be as broad and deep as the history taking aspect
- Examination is a good opportunity to re-evaluate the entire clinical presentation
- Do not assume that your colleague's referral and examination are correct
- One commonly hears from the patient, after a thorough clinical examination, that 'this is the first time someone has actually taken the trouble to examine me in detail' despite having seen several other clinicians
- Patients appreciate attention to detail, and trust and confidence will be established early
- The history is 80–90% of the diagnosis, but the examination needs to be thorough and detailed to support or refute the diagnostic label (already supplied in most cases) and to provide further specific information regarding the degree of physical impairment, disability, and pain characteristics
- The examination can be divided into *general health and system examination*, and *regional examination*

General health and system examination

- Clinicians are generally good at recognizing unwellness through pallor, breathlessness, flushed skin, unusual discoloration, grey or sallow complexions, and rapid pulse
- The opioid-dependent patient may have a faint layer of sweat, glassy eyes, tremor, and flat affect
- Unexplained features need to be evaluated carefully from a medical point of view, looking at the skin, hands, and nails, with a brief assessment of the cardiovascular system (CVS), abdominal palpation, and other systems, and reviewing medication

- Unexplained rash, itching, or excoriation need to be identified
- Signs of self-harm, whether recent or old, indicate previous mental health problems
- Assessment of posture, gait, and mobility is essential (do not commence the examination on the couch)
- MSK issues: osteoarthritic knees or hips, effusions, muscle wasting, deformities
- Screen all widespread pain patients for hypermobility according to the Brighton criteria
- Obesity and metabolic issues complicate many aspects of management
- General demeanour: affect, responsiveness, ability to communicate (assessment via an interpreter is an unfortunate compromise)
- Pain patients may simply have a nociceptive source such as a specific nerve entrapment
- Peripheral and central sensitization features of neuropathic pain: hyperalgesia or allodynia, cutaneous hyperaesthesia, and possible sensory or motor impairment
- Patients may have a host of psychosocial issues: depression, anxiety, and unhelpful beliefs about the nature of their pain which affect their communication and expression of the pain (identified in their *pain behaviour*)
- Fear of pain and pain avoidance are common (secondary gain factors may drive this)
- Subconscious post-traumatic stress can cause fear and anxiety about their pain condition
- Complex regional pain syndrome (CRPS) in a limb extremity: patients show disaffectation or dissociation from the painful part (lack of voluntary movement is common)
- Faulty movement patterns as a result of inhibition, weakness, or pain avoidance
- Cooperation and consent for a thorough examination of all these aspects must be sought with a statement like 'I would now like to examine you very carefully …'
- Undressing must be sufficient to inspect, assess range of motion, and palpate adequately
- Before any examination, ask the patient to indicate where the pain is or, if absent, at what point the movement provokes it and where
- Depending on the presentation, a neurological examination of the cranial nerves (CNs) and/or peripheral nervous system is needed. Examination of CNs is covered in 16.1 Cranial nerves, p. 299. Upper and lower limb neurological examination includes an assessment of muscle tone, power, reflexes, coordination and sensation (temperature, pinprick, proprioception, light touch, deep touch, brush, sensory mapping) which is covered subsequently in this chapter

Regional examination

Cervical spine for chronic neck pain, arm pain, 'whiplash', and headache

Patient standing or sitting (examiner behind)

- Assess posture (forward head?)
- Muscle wasting or hypertrophy—trapezii muscles
- Active range of motion assesses willingness
- Passive range of motion (to assess end-range feel)
- Foraminal closing test for radicular symptoms (Spurling's test combining extension, ipsilateral rotation, and side-bending sustained, but without axial compression)
- Shoulder: active range of elevation and controlled descent
- Examine upper limbs for referred pain or if neurological deficit for radicular symptoms

Patient supine

- Palpate suboccipital muscles for tender points (localized pain on one side increased by passive flexion may indicate greater occipital nerve entrapment) and other paraspinal muscles (e.g. scalenus muscles)

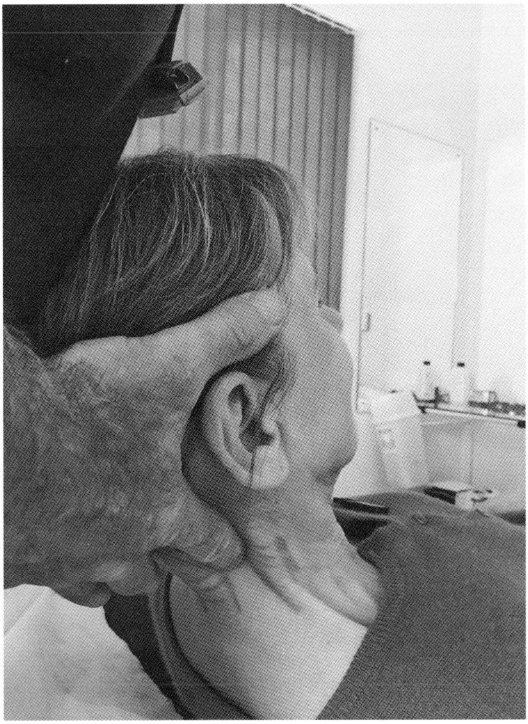

Figure 1.3.1 Palpation points on cervical articular column

- Passive range of nutation at atlanto-occipital joint (usually restricted with cervical extensor muscle shortening or tension)
- Passive rotation at atlanto-axial joints (painful restriction of rotation in one direction indicates C1–2 arthropathy)
- Segmental side gliding for tenderness or localized restriction (fingertips placed at 4 and 8 o'clock over the articular column) identifies dysfunctional level for treatment (see Figs. 1.3.1 and 1.3.2)

Patient prone

- Palpate the medial scapular muscles and trapezii for tender/trigger points and upper thoracic spine segments
- Note: A subroute if thoracic outlet syndrome is suspected: Roos test (hands up), Lindgren's first rib assessment, palpate the supraclavicular fossa and scalenus muscles, neurological assessment of the upper limb

Thoracic spine and chest wall

- Benign pain is common, but referred pain or metastases from malignancy or viscera are not uncommon (in the elderly, compression fractures are often missed)
- Patient stripped to waist (with bra). Note deformities and scoliosis, angular kyphosis on *standing*

Patient sitting

- Observe chest movement with breathing and abnormal pattern (breath holding or hyperventilation)
- Measure chest expansion in suspected ankylosing spondylitis

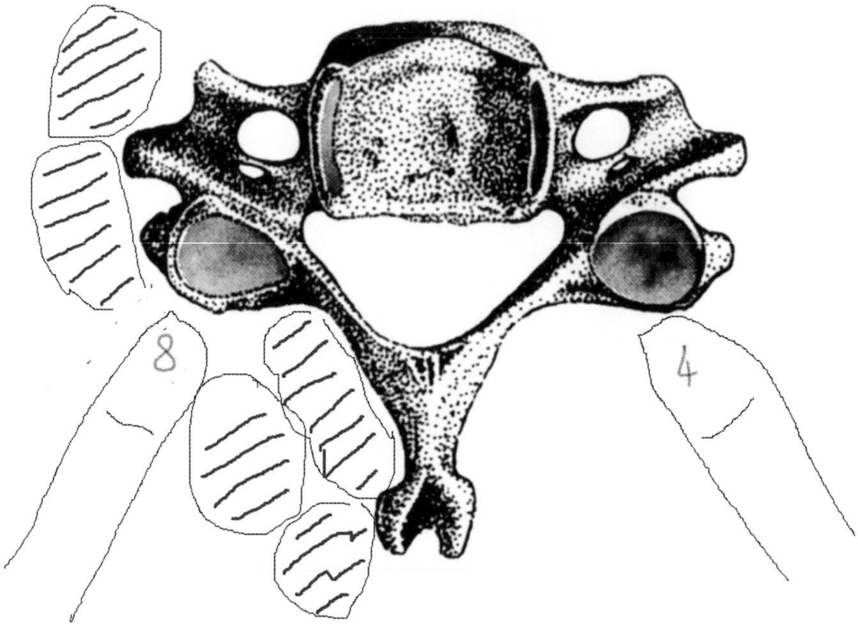

Figure 1.3.2 Fingertips placed at 4 and 8 o'clock over the articular column

- Observe active rotation, side-bending, flexion, and extension in sitting, inspecting from behind (symmetric limitation suggests spondyloarthropathy, whereas asymmetric limitation suggests dysfunction)
- Localized percussion of segments for exquisite pain

Patient prone

- Palpate spinous processes with posterior–anterior and lateral pressures to identify segmental dysfunction
- Repeat localized percussion if indicated
- Palpate paravertebral gutters for muscle tenderness, trigger points, and deeper facet joint tenderness. Palpate costo-transverse joints and rib movements and intercostal muscles with inspiration and expiration

Patient supine

- Palpate costo-chondral junctions for swelling or tenderness

Lumbar spine and sacroiliac joints

Patient standing

- Assess stance from behind—is the pelvis level and the spine straight?
- Is there an antalgic position, e.g. deviation to one side?
- Inspect for scoliosis in full flexion and extension (i.e. rib hump)
- Active side-bending (rotation not necessary unless combined with side-bending for possible facetal pain and stress fracture)
- Extension with side-bending may elicit radicular pain in foraminal stenosis

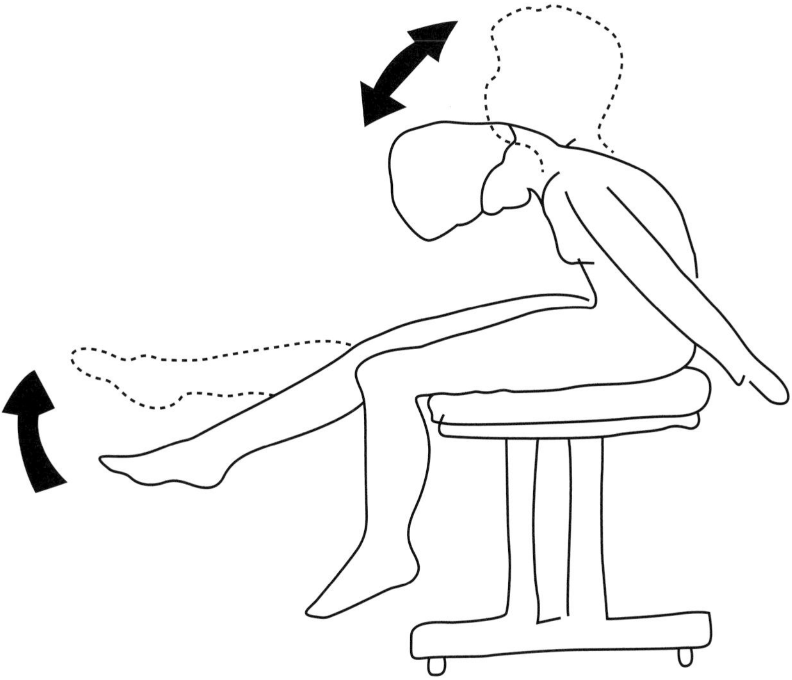

Figure 1.3.3 The slump test identifies dural inflammation usually related to disc herniation

- Forward flexion—is the spine flexing (consider modified Schober's test) or are the hips? Consider fluency and cadence—catch pains and deviatory arcs of movement, as well as fingertip-to-floor distance
- Modified Schober's test: while the patient is in full forward flexion, place your outstretched thumb and index in the midline to span the patient's lumbo-sacral area, with your thumb at the level of the posterior superior iliac spines and your index as high as you can reach on the spine. The span between these digits will be about 15 cm. Ask the patient to extend up to a neutral erect position. The span between your thumb and index should decrease by around 5 cm. Less than 3 cm will indicate significantly decreased lumbar spinal flexion
- Ask to squat: competence of lower limb joints and muscles
- Trendelenburg's test for hip dysfunction
- Ask the patient to raise each heel off the ground as far as possible (supporting them with the hands if necessary) to test S1 myotome
- Ask them to rock back on the heels, looking for signs of a partial foot drop

Patient sitting

- Slump test for dural tension (more sensitive than straight leg raise test) (see Fig. 1.3.3)
- Are iliac crests level? (consider leg length difference or scoliosis)

Patient supine

- Log roll each leg firmly, observing rebound if normal laxity, and whether pain is provoked in the hip at either extreme of internal or external rotation
- Measure leg length (anterior superior iliac spines (ASIS) to medial malleoli)

- Passive knee and hip range of motion testing before straight leg raise test
- Sacroiliac pain provocation tests:
  - Anterior compression and distraction
  - Axial thigh thrust or P4 test (flex one hip to 90° and align the knee vertically over the sacroiliac joint (SIJ); apply firm impulse pressure through the axis of the femur to provoke pain in the posterior SIJ region. Compare both sides. Caution: lumbar pain may also be provoked by this test if lordosis is not supported (use the patient's hand). The same false positive may occur with anterior compression or distraction tests.
  - Gaenslen's test (move the patient to one side of the couch and bring one hip and knee into full flexion; then drop the other hip and knee into full extension off the side of the couch to provoke pain in either joint. Repeat on other side)
  - Faber's test (**F**lexion—**Ab**duction—**E**xternal **R**otation) of one hip—apply overpressure to the ipsilateral knee (pain must be provoked in the posterior SIJ region. Test is not valid with any associated hip or adductor/symphysis problem)
- Perform sensory, reflex, and motor tests for lumbar radiculopathy, including plantar responses for upper motor neuron (UMN) lesion

Patient prone

- Femoral nerve stretch test
- Post-sacral spring test (for SIJ)
- Buttock clench test for S1 myotome
- Spring in a postero-anterior direction the lumbar spinous processes, first gently, then deeply for segmental pain
- Palpate the SIJ sulcus and paravertebral muscles and facetal areas for tenderness

Patient side-lying or in decubitus position

- Lateral compression (for SIJ)
- Palpate the trochanteric area for tenderness over the trochanter or gluteus medius/minimus tendons and piriformis and hip external rotators
- Palpation over the sciatic foramen is unreliable for piriformis syndrome diagnosis. Test shortening of external hip rotators in supine position by laterally rotating the hip; maintain while slowly bringing towards greater flexion. Pain and reproduction of symptoms occur earlier than on the normal side

Further reading

1. Hutson M, Ward A. Textbook of Musculoskeletal Medicine. 2nd edition, 2015. Oxford: Oxford University Press

1.4 Dermatomes and myotomes

Definitions

Dermatomes

- Areas of skin that receive sensory innervation from a specific cranial or spinal nerve
- Sensory neurons are located either in the DRGs or in the trigeminal ganglia (ganglion Gasseri or nucleus spinalis V)

- Each of these nerves relays sensations (including pain) from a particular skin region to the dorsal horn of the spinal cord or to the brain

Myotomes

- Groups of skeletal muscles that receive motor innervation from the ventral root of a single cranial or spinal nerve
- Motor neurons are located in the motor nuclei of the brainstem or in the ventral horn of the spinal cord

Anatomy

Dermatomes

(See Fig. 1.4.1.)

Trigeminal nerve:

V1: forehead, eye
V2: upper face, nose
V3: lower face, chin

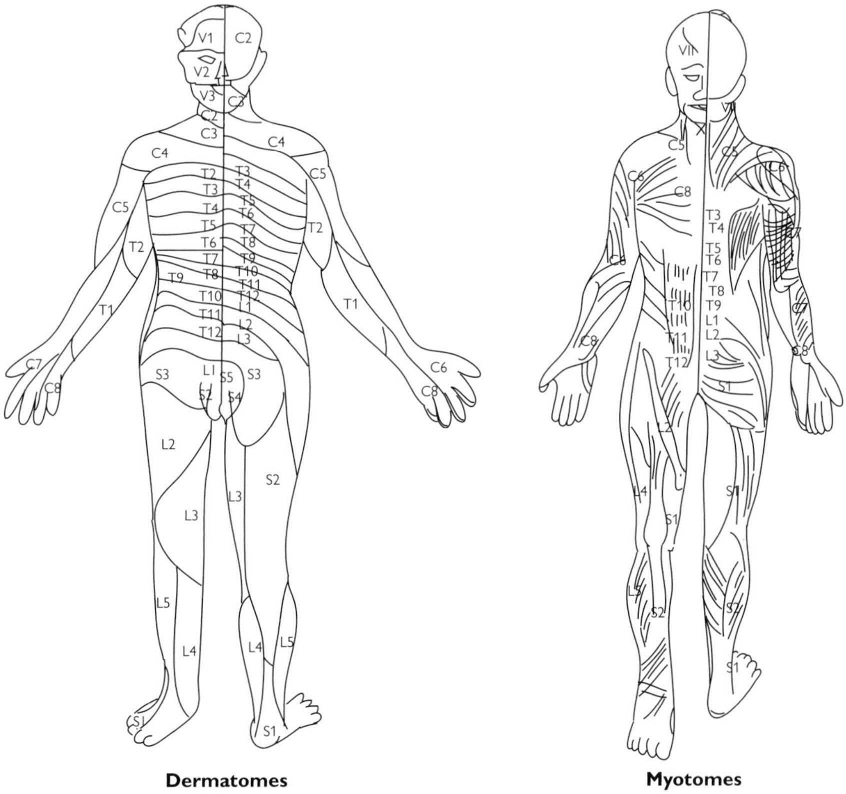

Figure 1.4.1 Human dermatomes and myotomes, and innervation of bones and other skeletal tissues (sclerotomes)

Cervical nerves:

- C2: base of the skull
- C3: supraclavicular and mid-clavicular line
- C4: acromion
- C5: cubital fossa and elbow
- C6, C7, C8: upper arm, forearm, and hands

Thoracic nerves:

- T1: medial aspect of the forearms
- T2: axilla and medial aspect of upper arms
- T3–T8: corresponding intercostal spaces
- T9: area between xiphoid process and umbilicus
- T10: umbilical region
- T11: lower abdomen
- T12: inguinal region

Lumbar nerves:

- L1: inguinal region and upper anterior thigh above L2
- L2: antero-medial thigh
- L3: antero-medial aspect of the knee
- L4: medial aspect of the lower leg and medial ankle
- L5: lateral aspect of the leg, dorsal aspect of the foot and heel

Sacral segments:

- S1: postero-lateral leg, lateral aspect of the foot and sole of the foot ± heel
- S2: postero-medial leg, popliteal fossa
- S3: ischium and infra-gluteal fold
- S4–S5: perianal area

Myotomes

(See Fig. 1.4.2.)

Trigeminal nerve: V1: jaw muscles, tensor tympani

Facial nerve: mimics muscles, M. stapedius

Vagus nerve: larynx

Cervical segments:

- C1/2/3: neck flexion/extension
- C4: shoulder elevation, diaphragm (phrenic nerve)
- C5: shoulder abduction (axillary nerve)
- C6/7/8: shoulder adduction
- C5: elbow flexion (musculocutaneous nerve)
- C7: elbow extension (radial nerve)
- C6/7: wrist flexion and extension
- C7: finger extension (radial nerve)
- C8: finger flexion (median nerve)

Thoracic segments:

- T1: finger abduction (ulnar nerve), thumb abduction (median nerve)
- T1–T12: intercostal muscles, abdominal muscles, paravertebral back muscles

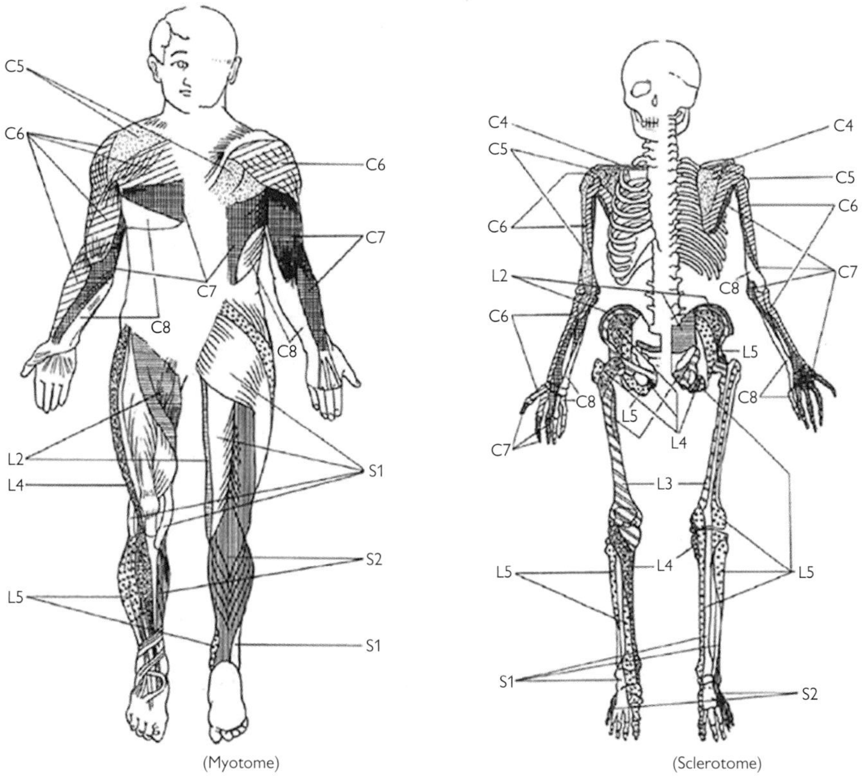

Figure 1.4.2 Myotomes, innervation of bones and other skeletal tissues (sclerotomes)

Lumbar segments:

L2: hip flexion (femoral nerve); L5: hip extension (inferior gluteal nerve)

L3/4: knee extension (femoral nerve)

L4: ankle dorsiflexion (deep peroneal nerve)

L5: big toe dorsiflexion (deep peroneal nerve)

Sacral segments:

S1: ankle plantarflexion, foot eversion, hip extension

S2: knee flexion

S3–S4: perineal region and anal sphincter

Clinical relevance

- Dermatome testing assesses distribution of pain symptoms and reduced sensation to determine the level of a spinal nerve lesion (e.g. after disc prolapse). However, there can be overlapping supply of spinal nerves to dermatomes
- Visceral sensations can map to specific dermatomes. Some sensations are felt locally, whereas others are perceived over areas that are more distant from the involved organ ('referred pain'). Pain in the left shoulder can indicate angina pectoris. These dermatomes are referred to as 'head zones'

- Viral infections of ganglia (e.g. varicella zoster virus (VZV)) can cause either pain or rash, or both, in a pattern defined by a dermatome or part of it (zosteriform pattern)
- Testing of myotomes is more reliable than dermatomal testing in determining the level of a spinal nerve root lesion or irritation. Isometric resisted muscle strength is tested. Assessment of muscle weakness in a particular region could indicate a lesion of the spinal cord, nerve root, or an intervertebral disc herniation/prolapse

Further reading

1. Magee DJ. Orthopaedic Physical Assessment. 4th edition, 2006. St Louis, Missouri, USA: Elsevier
2. Marieb EN, Mallatt JB, Wilhem PB. Human Anatomy. 5th international edition, 2008; pp. 450–2. London: Pearson
3. Sounders P. Dorland's Illustrated Medical Dictionary. 32nd edition, 2011; p. 1226. Amsterdam: Elsevier

1.5 Flags in pain medicine

- Different colour flags are used to identify a serious pathology or an underlying concern, and to help triaging patients within the pain service and to other health care professionals and to consider further investigations
- Many of these presentations can be transferred to other pain conditions

Red flags (organic pathology)

- History, signs, and symptoms that could denote a serious medical condition with an underlying pathology such as:
  - Age of onset <20 years or >55 years
  - History of serious pathology (e.g. carcinoma)
  - Ill health (acutely unwell) or presence of other medical illness or infection (e.g. human immunodeficiency virus (HIV), spinal tuberculosis (TB), ischaemia)
  - Thoracic pain
  - Severe unremitting night pain, night fever
  - Progressive neurological deficit (weakness ± sensory deficit)
  - Disturbed gait, saddle anaesthesia
  - Vertebral fracture or deformity (e.g. traumatic or osteoporotic)
  - Unexplained weight loss (e.g. >10% body weight in last 3–6 months)
  - Bladder or bowel dysfunction (e.g. in cauda equina)
  - Immunosuppression
  - History of corticosteroid use
  - History of intravenous (IV) drug use
- Although there has been recent controversy about its utility, red flags still remain integral to many guidelines for triaging patients
- The recommendation is to pursue further investigations and refer to a specialist

Yellow flags (psychological and behavioural)

- These refer to psychosocial and environmental factors that could interfere with assessment and management plans, in addition to long-term pain and associated disability
- They tend to be in the domains of patients' beliefs, judgements, appraisals, emotional responses, pain behaviour, and coping strategies:
    - A negative belief that their pain is damaging or potentially severely disabling
    - A belief in the lack of benefit from treatment
    - Fear avoidance behaviour
    - Lack of acceptance
    - Poor coping, reduced self-efficacy
    - Maladaptive behaviour/cognition
    - Diminished activity levels/activity pattern that aggravate pain
    - A reliance on passive treatment modalities (analgesia, interventions, cold packs, hot packs)
    - A tendency to depression, worries, fears, and anxiety
    - Social withdrawal
    - Social or financial problems
    - Increased drug use, reliance on aids (smoking)
    - Secondary gain (e.g. overprotective family)
    - Litigation, compensation
- Managed by strategies to tackle the maladaptive beliefs through education and psychological approach

Orange flags (referral to mental health team if not optimized)

- Psychiatric illness
- Major personality disorder
- Post-traumatic stress syndrome
- Psychosis
- Addiction
- Increased levels of distress
- Suicidal ideations

Blue flags (work perception)

- An individual's perception of work (if accurate or not) about the relationship between the employment or the nature of the work performed and the state of health, with a belief that it may negatively impact their pain
- Patients could also encompass a belief that their superiors and colleagues are unsupportive
- Unemployment, poor job satisfaction
- Fear of (re-)injury at work, stress at work

Black flags (work conditions)

- Actual contextual work place or insurance obstacles that could delay a return to work and perpetuate the condition
- May include legislation that restricts the options of those attempting return to work

- It may also include objective work demands or conditions such as heavy, physically demanding duties that have not been modified
- Unsociable hours

Further reading

1. Nicholas M, Linton S, Watson P, Main C. Early identification and management of psychological risk factors ('yellow flags') in patients with low back pain: a reappraisal. Phys Ther 2011;91:737–53
2. Samanta J, Kendall J, Samanta A. 10-minute consultation: chronic low back pain. BMJ 2003;326:535
3. Shaw W, van der Windt D, Main C, et al. Early patient screening and intervention to address individual-level occupational factors ('blue flags') in back disability. J Occup Rehabil 2009;19:64–80
4. Underwood M, Buchbinder R. Red flags for back pain. BMJ 2013;347:f7432

1.6 Mental state exam

Introduction

- Mental state exam (MSE) is essential for the biopsychosocial assessment of pain patients, especially in patients that also have mental health conditions
- Involves a systematic assessment of the appearance, behaviour, speech, mood, affect, mental functioning, and overall demeanour of a person
- Provides a snapshot of the psychological function of a person which helps to understand the factors that influence experience, behaviours, distress, and suffering of patients
- MSE enables the detection of conditions which need to be treated simultaneously with pain to achieve a good outcome. These conditions can include mood disorders, panic disorders, post-traumatic stress disorder (PTSD), disorders of cognitive impairment (e.g. stroke, dementia, head injury), personality disorders (PDs), substance use disorders, and other psychiatric conditions
- Every time clinicians interact with patients, they intuitively perform many parts of the MSE

Domains of a mental state exam

Appearance

- Can provide clues of patients' lifestyle, well-being, health, nutrition, and functioning on a daily basis
- Components normally evaluated include body posture, body built, nutritional features, clothing, grooming, skin (colour, tattoos, marks, scratches), fingers/hands, distinctive features, ethnicity, cosmetics, jewellery, evidence of physical deconditioning, malnourishment, and sequelae of having chronic diseases

Behaviour

- Verbal and non-verbal behaviours provide a picture of the emotional state, attitude, appropriateness, activity levels, and response of the patient to the clinician (e.g. cooperative, willing to disclose information)
- The following are evaluated: body language (calm, agitated, restless, withdrawn), rapport, facial expressions, mannerism, eye contact, interactive style, movements (repetitive, slowed, involuntary, tremors), and hallucinatory behaviours

Affect and mood

- Affect describes the immediate expressions which describe a patient's current emotional state. Affect can be described in terms of its appropriateness (inappropriate or appropriate), range (blunted, flat, restricted, expansive, labile), and stability (non-stable or stable). Affect is sometimes described as 'how the patient's emotional state is perceived by the clinician conducting the consultation'
- Mood describes a patient's emotional state over days/weeks/months. A patient's mood can be depressed, neutral, irritable, anxious, angry, or apprehensive. Mood can be stable or labile. Mood can also be described as 'how the patient describes their emotional state over a period of time of days/weeks'

Speech

- Certain speech patterns can be found in some conditions such as anxiety, depression, schizophrenia, and organic diseases
- The aspects of speech normally evaluated include the rate, amplitude, modulation, and ease of conversation

Thought form

- This describes how patients generate, organize, process, and express their thoughts
- Examples of disorders: circumstantial thinking (excessive vagueness), flight of ideas (topics are frequently changed), word salad (nonsense words), derailment (irrelevant comments), thought racing or blocking (pressured or halted speech)

Thought content

- The detail of the conversation or content of patients' thoughts, including preoccupations, obsessions, psychotic phenomena, and homicidal or suicidal ideation
- Some pain patients have thoughts of self-harm. Risk factors include PD, major psychiatric/medical comorbidities, previous attempts, substance used (alcohol, illicit drugs), and poor social and emotional support, single/widowed, or unemployed
- Patients with thoughts of self-harm should be assessed by mental health

Cognition

- Describes the ability of patients to process information
- A common cause of cognitive dysfunction is impaired conscious state from underlying medical conditions and adverse reactions from drugs (prescribed, not prescribed, and/or illegal)
- One of the most common assessment tools to assess cognitive function is the Mini-Mental State Examination which evaluates concentration, memory, and orientation. A score of 25–30 points is normal. Results indicative of cognitive impairment can be mild (21–24 points), moderate (12–20 points), and severe (<12 points).

Perceptual disturbances

- It is important to assess for disturbances in perception such as dissociative symptoms (depersonalization, derealization), delusions, hallucinations, and the associated distress
- Delusion is an irrational belief that someone has, even sometimes when there is no evidence that the belief is real (e.g. grandiose, passivity, somatic, nihilistic, persecutory, jealousy)
- Hallucination is a distortion in a person's perception of reality which is normally accompanied by a powerful sense of reality (e.g. visual, auditory, olfactory, somatic, gustatory)

Insight and judgement

- Insight is the ability of a patient to acknowledge that he/she has a mental health problem, their level of understanding of the treatments available, and the locus of control (internal or external). Also reflects the ability of patients to identify hallucinations, thoughts of self-harm, or other pathological events
- Judgement describes the ability to problem-solve, decision-making, and behaviour in that particular context
- Insight and judgement can reflect the ability of a patient to manage difficulties. This is influenced by multiple factors such as personal, environmental, cultural, family history, and previous history which can influence a patient's compliance, rapport, and outcomes

Features of mental state examination associated with psychopathologies in pain patients

- Anxiety disorder: apprehensive, fidgety, hard to sit still, anxious, irritable
- Chronicity: patient looks older than their stated age, poor dentition, poor hygiene, deconditioned physical appearance from the chronic condition
- Depression: poorly groomed, unkempt, delusions, poverty of ideas, slow speech, depressed mood, irritable, depressed affect, withdrawn
- Delirium: poorly groomed, unkempt, not cooperative, delusions, thoughts formed in a disordered manner, hallucinations, withdrawn, threatening, unusual behaviour
- Dementia: poorly groomed, unkempt, poverty of ideas, cognitive impairment
- Mania: agitation, cannot sit down, bright make-up, colourful, strange appearance, disinhibited, delusions, flight of ideas, thoughts formed in a disordered manner, speech rate fast, seductive towards the clinician, threatening
- PD: bizarre appearance, scarred wrists, tattoos of not very good quality, not cooperative, seductive towards the clinician, threatening
- Psychotic disorder: poorly kempt, staring/bizarre appearance, not cooperative, unusual behaviour
- Schizophrenia: unkempt, poorly groomed, delusions, flight of ideas, thoughts formed in a disordered manner, poverty of ideas, hallucinations, blunted affect, inappropriate behaviour
- Substance intoxication or withdrawal: not cooperative, hallucinations, threatening, unusual behaviour, tremors, needle marks in skin

Further reading

1. Mental state examination, 2018 https://www.rch.org.au/clinicalguide/guideline_index/Mental_state_examination/
2. Talley N, O'Connor S. Clinical Examination: A Systematic Guide to Physical Diagnosis. 7th edition, 2013. Sydney: Churchill Livingstone

1.7 Investigations in pain medicine

Introduction

- Investigations form the last, but important part of a triad (history, examination, investigations) to formulate a diagnosis

- Medical technology has advanced considerably, such that it is easy to evaluate and identify structural abnormalities
- However, it is often difficult to correlate the anatomical changes with the patient's symptoms and the degree of functional impairment reported
- Functional imaging is the most exciting and rapidly evolving technology to understand the cortical activity for many cognitive processes

Blood tests

- Blood tests are often useful for ruling out inflammatory arthritis as a cause for MSK pain
- C-reactive protein (CRP) and erythrocyte sedimentation rate (ESR) are often evaluated and found elevated in patients with a strong inflammatory component (see Chapter 25)
- Low levels of vitamin D are associated with widespread pain symptoms such as fibromyalgia
- Other blood tests include thyroid function tests (TFTs), early morning cortisol, and levels of testosterone
- In patients who are on long-term opioids (>100 mg oral morphine equivalent dose per day), consider testing for total testosterone and early morning cortisol levels, in addition to other tests, to assess the endocrine system

Imaging techniques

(See Table 1.7.1.)

- Objective quantification is difficult/impossible for a cognitive phenomenon such as pain
- Therefore, imaging should only be used in:
  - Presence of red flags
  - Severe or traumatic injury
  - Suspicion of serious pathology
  - Unusual clinical presentations
  - Unknown diagnosis following examination
  - Injuries that are unresponsive to treatment
- Investigations are usually only indicated if the outcome is likely to change treatment and should be discussed on an individual basis
- It is often unnecessary to perform expensive investigations to confirm an already obvious clinical diagnosis

Table 1.7.1 Imaging modalities in pain medicine

Electrical activity (increased/decreased excitatory or inhibitory activity, increased/decreased action potentials)	EEG (electroencephalography) EMG (electromyography) MEG (magnetoencephalography)
Metabolic activity (glucose and oxygen consumption)	FDG-PET (fluorodeoxyglucose positron emission tomography) Autoradiography
Haemodynamic response (blood flow, blood volume, and blood oxygenation)	H_2O PET (water-based positron emission tomography) NIRS (near infra-red spectroscopy) Optical imaging and fMRI (functional MRI)

X-ray scan

- Simple X-rays are useful in acute injury and help in guiding treatment
- It uses electromagnetic radiation to produce images of dense tissues such as bone

Computed tomography (CT) scanning

- Uses X-ray beams and a computer to produce cross-sectional images of bone and soft tissues
- CT uses a significant amount of radiation; therefore, MRI is often preferred
- CT scans show the bone cortex distinctly, and fractures, loose bodies, and spine changes are better seen
- Choice of investigation when patients are fitted with a spinal cord stimulator

Magnetic resonance imaging scan

- MRI is the most frequently used investigation in pain patients (no radiation is involved)
- Fine resolution is achieved in multiple planes; therefore, diagnostic accuracy is excellent
- Useful in neuraxial investigations to recognize spinal stenosis, disc prolapse, and nerve root compromise
- MRI is commonly used to assess for bone abnormalities, joint abnormalities, soft tissue abnormalities, and nerve root compression, as well as various medical conditions (such as tumours or diseases of internal organs)
- Gadolinium enhancement, in addition to MRI, gives better resolution
- T1-weighted images: water dark, fat bright (e.g. to assess cortex, fatty tissue, liver lesions) (shorter relaxation time); low signal (dark, e.g. in bone marrow) indicates increased water content and loss of fatty tissue; abnormally low signal indicates pathology (e.g. trauma, infection, cancer)
- T2-weighted images: water and fat are bright (e.g. oedema, inflammation, white cortex); abnormally high signal (bright) indicates pathology (e.g. trauma, infection, cancer)
- Short tau inversion recovery (STIR) sequence: signal suppression for fat; only water is bright (e.g. in discitis)
- If T1 and STIR are compared: abnormally low signal (dark) on T1 and abnormally high signal (bright) on STIR indicates abnormal fluid
- Fluid-attenuated inversion recovery (FLAIR) images: signal suppression for fluid (e.g. cerebrospinal fluid (CSF)), used in brain imaging—high signal (bright) shows pathology (e.g. infection, tumour, demyelination)
- Few contraindications to MRI: certain brain aneurysm clips, neurostimulators, cardiac pacemakers

Radionucleotide bone scan

- Radio-isotopic bone scan or bone scintigraphy is a nuclear scanning test used to detect areas of increased bone turnover such as bone growth or damage (e.g. stress fractures)
- It involves injection of a radioactive substance into the body, followed by taking of a series of images using a special camera to detect the radioactive substance (which concentrates in areas where there is increased blood flow and bone turnover such as at fracture sites)
- A bone scan is particularly useful for identifying:
  - Bone stress reactions
  - Bone stress fractures (e.g. navicular, pelvic, pars interarticularis)
  - Osteochondral lesions (e.g. osteochondral fracture of the talar dome)
  - Other medical conditions affecting bones (such as bone cancers or bone infections)
- Isotopic bone scan is the investigation of choice for evaluating skeletal metastasis

Bone density scan (DEXA scan = Dual-Energy X-ray Absorptiometry)

- Used to assess the density (strength) of bones
- Indications can be:
  - To assess the risk/stage of osteoporosis in patients over 50 years of age
  - To assess the risk/stage of osteoporosis in patients aged under 50 years with other risk factors (smoking, drinking, family history of hip fracture, body mass index (BMI) <21)
  - Previous bone fracture after minor injury or fall
  - Postmenopausal women or after removal of ovaries in women under the age of 45 years (decreased oestrogen levels result in decreased bone density)
  - In arthritis or with steroid intake (>3 months)
  - May be used to confirm fracture risk to initiate medical treatment
- Radiation exposure is much lower than with standard X-rays (however, not recommended in pregnancy)
- The scanner is open, and the scan takes 10–20 minutes; the hip, spine, or forearm are scanned
- A special type of X-ray is used (DEXA) to measure how much radiation passes through the bones and then compared to a healthy young adult (T-score) or a healthy adult of the same age (Z-score), gender, and ethnicity
- The difference is calculated as a standard deviation (SD)
- T-score: above −1 SD is normal; between −1 and −2.5 indicates mildly reduced bone mineral density (BMD); above −2.5 is defined as osteoporosis
- Z-score: below −2 SD indicates that the BMD is lower than expected at a certain age

Ultrasonography

- An ultrasound scan (USS) is a painless method of imaging that uses high-frequency sound waves (2–15 MHz)
- A probe is usually applied to the skin with the help of a conductive medium (ultrasound (US) gel) to transmit sound waves and assess soft tissues underneath the skin
- US is a safe imaging technique as it does not expose the patient to any radiation
- Investigation of choice for superficial soft tissue pathology for both diagnosis and treatment
- Changes in water content that occur with inflammation and malignant or degenerative processes in muscles, tendons, or tendon sheaths can be detected with USS
- One major disadvantage of ultrasound is that it is dependent on the skills and expertise of the operator in question
- Unfortunately, US does not provide information on the deeper structures such as joints or bones

Neurophysiology

- Neurophysiological tests can be beneficial to investigate some peripheral nerve and root lesions. Also frequently used when there is no clear-cut diagnosis
- In subclinical abnormalities, it is important that the results correlate with the clinical picture

Nerve conduction tests and electromyography

- Diagnostic tests of the peripheral nervous system; especially useful in evaluating diseases/disorders of the muscles, nerves, and nerve roots (e.g. peripheral nerve palsy)
- They record electrical activity of the muscles and the passage of these along nerves in the limbs
- Pathological changes and associated disorders can either be acute or have a slow-developing nature

Sensory evoked potential (SEP)

- Diagnostic test that evaluates sensory tracts of the central and peripheral nervous systems by recording the electrical responses of the brain and spinal cord to sensory stimulation

Functional biomarkers and network analysis

- Biomarkers for pain are actively being researched and will be the future to bring in personalized treatments for patients
- Biomarkers can be blood-based or imaging-based around network analysis, fMRI, or magnetoencephalography (MEG)/EEG. This is a fast-evolving field and of great topical interest

Further reading

1. Gunn J, Hill MM, Cotten BM, Deer TR. An analysis of biomarkers in patients with chronic pain. Pain Physician 2020;23(1):E41–9
2. Health A to Z. Bone Density Scan (DEXA scan). 2019 https://www.nhs.uk/conditions/dexa-scan/
3. Sutherland S. Pain research leaders convene to chart a path to pain biomarkers. An objective measure of chronic pain could improve treatment and translation. 2019 https://www.painresearchforum.org/news/114200-pain-research-leaders-convene-chart-path-pain-biomarkers
4. Lloyd-Jones G. MRI interpretation. 2017 https://www.radiologymasterclass.co.uk/tutorials/mri/mri_scan
5. Knott D. Clinical examination. In: Hutson M, Ward A (eds). Oxford Textbook of Musculoskeletal Medicine. 2nd edition, 2016; pp. 219–228. Oxford, UK: Oxford University Press
6. Knott D. Investigative techniques. In: Hutson M, Ward A (eds). Oxford Textbook of Musculoskeletal Medicine. 2nd edition, 2016; pp. 228–235. Oxford, UK: Oxford University Press
7. Tracey I. Imaging pain. Br J Anaesth 2008;101(1):32–9

1.8 Quantitative sensory testing

Introduction

- Quantitative sensory testing (QST) is an investigation modality to document the function of smaller nerve fibres (in comparison, nerve conduction studies only test large nerve fibres, whereas QST could be used to test both large and small nerve fibres)
- It tests for temperature (small, unmyelinated nerve fibres), cold (A- δ fibres), warmth (C-fibres), vibration (large, myelinated A-α and β nerve fibres), and touch (A-α and β fibres)
- The posterior columns and lateral spinothalamic tract are tested during QST
- QST is time-consuming and used more commonly in research trials and longitudinal studies
- QST has been used to diagnose diabetic neuropathy, small fibre neuropathy, and chemotherapy-induced neuropathy

QST measurement parameters

- Allodynia—dynamic mechanical allodynia, punctate mechanical allodynia, pressure-evoked mechanical allodynia, cold allodynia (warmth allodynia is optional)
- Hyperalgesia—punctate hyperalgesia
- Hyperpathia—this is the clinical equivalent to the 'wind-up' phenomenon
- Two-point discrimination

- Vibration threshold
- Sensory area mapping
- To resolve inter-observer variability, the Neuropathic Special Interest Group of the International Society for the Study of Pain (IASP) formulated guidelines in 2013

QST reports

- Certain QST findings may relate to specific pathophysiologic mechanisms associated with neuropathic pain: heat hyperalgesia to peripheral sensitization, and static mechanical hyperalgesia or dynamic mechanical allodynia to central sensitization
- Thus, it may be useful in differentiating between central and peripheral sensitization
- QST has also been used to predict histological small fibre neuropathy in postural tachycardia syndrome

Advantages of QST

- Sensory area mapping is possible if the tests are done accurately
- QST has shown to be relatively consistent in normal subjects (controls)

Disadvantages of QST

- It is a psychophysical test (results will vary, depending on the patient's mood, level of engagement with the test, and the patient's mental condition, including fatigue and drowsiness)
- It has large inter-observer variability in patients with neuropathic symptoms (hence, it is not easily reproducible)
- Results could vary, depending on the manufacturer of the kit (there is no standardization)
- QST cannot differentiate between a peripheral nerve lesion and a central cause since the whole pathway from the peripheral receptor, through the peripheral nerve, to the thalamus, is tested
- It has not been used to differentiate between neuropathic and non-neuropathic pain

Additional information

- QST has recently been used to differentiate between completers and non-completers of an interdisciplinary pain programme, with maximum differentiation in the temperature thresholds

Further reading

1. Backonja MM, Attal N, Baron R, et al. Value of quantitative sensory testing in neurological and pain disorders: NeuPSIG consensus. Pain 2013;154(9):1807–19
2. Billig SCI, Schauermann JC, Roman R, et al. Quantitative sensory testing predicts histological small fiber neuropathy in postural tachycardia syndrome. Neurol Clin Pract Nov 2020;10(5):428–34
3. Horowitz S. Neuropathic pain: Is the emperor wearing clothes? In: Smith HS (ed). Current Therapy in Pain. 2009; pp. 9–13. Philadelphia, PA: Saunders-Elsevier
4. Siao P, Didier P. Quantitative sensory testing. Phys Med Rehabil Clin N Am 2003;14(2):261–86

1.9 Measurement of pain

Introduction

- Pain is a complex, multi-dimensional biopsychosocial phenomenon and its subjective nature makes it challenging to assess and measure

- When measuring pain, it is important to consider which aspects of pain information is needed
- Scientifically valid tools are essential to determine the intensity of pain, choose treatment, and assess outcome after treatment
- Measurement tools are needed in clinical and research settings to evaluate outcomes after therapy and in pain research

Clinimetrics (= the measurement of clinical phenomena)

1. Scale of pain measurement:
   i. Dichotomous scale (Yes or No)
   ii. Ordinal scale (Mild, Moderate, Severe)
   iii. Interval scale (Visual Analogue Scale (VAS) score)

2. Choice between objective and subjective measurements in pain:
   i. Pain is typically subjective
   ii. Objective measures are not necessarily better than subjective measures
   iii. The scale of measurement is not related to the subjectivity of the measurement

Clinimetric properties

Validity

(= measure of how well a tool measures the construct that it is supposed to measure)

1. *Criterion validity*
   - This is the most powerful form of validity (the tool is compared to the 'gold standard')

2. *Construct validity*
   - Next best option when a gold standard is not available (e.g. one measure of pain intensity is compared to another measure with a previously defined hypothesis)

3. *Content validity*
   - It is the degree to which the test measures all relevant items in a given condition

4. *Face validity*
   - A test appears to measure the construct without paying close attention to the component parts (e.g. VAS pain score has a high face validity)

Reproducibility

- Whether the measurement tool provides the same answers when repeated either in time or by different observers
- There are two types:
    - Agreement (= lack of measurement error—how close the value of two different measurements is in absolute terms)
    - Reliability (= relative measure, based on the consistency of the measure across different conditions and time points, e.g. test–retest reliability, internal consistency, and interrater reliability)

Responsiveness

- Parameter for tools that measure change over time, e.g. outcome measures in studies on effects of a pain treatment

Interpretability

- Meaning of a specific score on a tool, e.g. what a score of 10 on the McGill Pain Questionnaire (MPQ) means

Sensitivity of a measure

- Ability to correctly identify the presence of a condition where it exists

Specificity of a measure

- Ability to correctly identify the absence of a condition where it does not exist

Choice of outcome measures in research and clinical trials

Depends on three questions

1. What does one want to know about pain (dimensions and time frame)?
2. Why measure pain?
3. Which instrument is the most appropriate?

Four core outcome domains are recommended by The Initiative on Methods, Measurement, and Pain Assessment in Clinical Trials (IMMPACT)

1. Pain intensity—Numeric Rating Scale (NRS)
2. Physical functioning—Brief Pain Inventory (BPI) or Multidimensional Pain Inventory
3. Emotional functioning—Beck Depression Inventory and Profile of Mood States
4. Patient rating of improvement—Patient Global Impression of Change scale

Choice of outcome measures in clinical practice

- The Faculty of Pain Medicine (UK) and the British Pain Society released a publication in January 2019, highlighting the most useful outcome measures presently in use in pain clinics in the UK
- For each measure, they provide a sense of its validity and reliability, conditions for use, and advantages and disadvantages

Measurements in acute pain

- Measurement scales in acute pain are uni-dimensional and designed for the assessment of intensity and degree of pain relief, and the trend is more important than the number (useful in routine post-operative care and in hospital acute surgical or medical care)
- Commonly used scales: (0 = no pain; 10 or 100 = worst pain imaginable)
    - VAS (usually 0–10 or 0–100)
    - NRS (usually 0–10)
    - Verbal Rating Scale (VRS: none, mild, moderate, severe)
    - Correlation between VRS and NRS: none = 0, mild = 1–3, moderate = 4–6, severe = 7–10
- These are reliable, valid measures of intensity of pain and easy to use
- NRS is clinically preferred due to its simplicity, while VAS is used in research. VRS is a quick and simple tool, with high validity as an indicator of pain intensity
- Acute post-surgical neuropathic pain occurs in 3% of all patients and needs a multi-dimensional tool, e.g. LANSS (Leeds Assessment of Neuropathic Symptoms and Signs), DN4 (Douleur Neuropathique 4), and PainDETECT

Measurements in chronic pain (multi-dimensional scales required)

Brief Pain Inventory

- A 17-item scale, along with 11-point NRS, to assess pain intensity in the preceding 24 hours and 11-point NRS of interference in seven domains of usual activities/functions and mood (site, severity, impact of pain on physical function, mood, sleep, social aspects)

McGill Pain Questionnaire and its Short Form

- Twenty subgroups of words describing sensory, affective, evaluative, and miscellaneous components of pain

SF36-version 2 and abbreviated SF12-version 2

- Eight domains assessing mental and physical functioning and overall health-related QoL (mean score = 50%; >50% is better physical and mental health than mean; <50% worse than mean)

Measurements in neuropathic pain

LANSS (Leeds Assessment of Neuropathic Symptoms and Signs)

- Seven weighted items:
  - Five sensory items and two clinical examination findings.

DN4 (Douleur Neuropathique 4)

- Nine items:
  - Six items related to symptoms
  - Three physical examination findings identifying pain components

PainDETECT

- Ten items:
  - Self-reported tool
  - Originally distinguished neuropathic lower back pain from mechanical low back pain

Neuropathic Pain Score (NPS)

- Eleven items:
  - First scale to measure severity of neuropathic pain based on 11 descriptors

Measurements of mood and affect—anxiety and depression scores

Hospital Anxiety and Depression Scale (HADS)

- Fourteen items:
  - Seven items for anxiety and seven for depression

Depression, Anxiety, and Stress Scale-21 (DASS-21)

- Twenty-one items:
  - Graded as normal, mild, moderate, severe, and very severe

Generalized Anxiety Disorder-7 (GAD-7)

- Seven items:
  - Score of 0–3 per item (5–9 mild, 10–14 moderate, 15–21 severe)
  - A score of >10 warrants further assessment ± referral to mental health professional

Patient Health Questionnaire—9 items (PHQ-9)

- Nine items:
  - Score of 0–3 per item to assess severity of depression (0–4 none to minimal, 5–9 mild, 10–14 moderate, 15–19 moderate to severe, 20–27 severe)

Patient Health Questionnaire–2 (PHQ-2)

- Two items:
  - Score of 0–6, with 3 being the cut-off
  - Only two items from the PHQ-9 scale, and serves as a screening tool

Measurements of other parameters

Pain belief and coping

- Pain Catastrophizing Scale (PCS)—a 13-item scale

Pain beliefs and attitudes

- Include **Pain Self-Efficacy Questionnaire (PSEQ)**:
  - Assesses confidence in performing daily activities (ten statements relate to daily life on a 7-point scale)

Fear Avoidance Beliefs (FABQ)

- Sixteen items

Pain Catastrophizing Scale (PCS)

- Thirteen items:
  - Correlates with development of chronic pain

Health-Related Quality of Life assessment

- Measure of QoL; can reflect the overall impact of the condition on the patient's life and the effect of treatment

EuroQol-5D (EQ-5D)

- Measures five domains (mobility/self-care/usual activity, pain, and mood) against a 5-point descriptor scale of symptoms/impact intensity

Pain-related functional assessment

- Measures disability level and pain interference with daily activity

Pain Disability Index (PDI)—seven domains

- Brief self-assessment of function
- It has seven domains which are all assessed on 11-point NRS

Oswestry Disability Index (ODI), version 2.1a

- Measure of degree of disability and determines the QoL (minimal, moderate, severe, crippled, bedbound); self-administered

Roland–Morris Disability Index—24-point assessment

- Used exclusively for low back pain
- Used for assessment of disability; free and easy to use

Pain Self-Efficacy Questionnaire (PSEQ)—ten items

- Assesses confidence of patients to perform activities while in pain (e.g. for return to work, functional gain)

Patient Global Impression of Change (PGIC)

- Assesses all aspects of a patient's health and if there has been an improvement or a decline in clinical status (after treatment or intervention)

Other areas

Cancer pain

- **Memorial Symptom Assessment Scale (MSAS)** and its **Short Form (MSAS-SF)**

Paediatric pain

(See 1.11 Pain assessment in children, p. 36.)

- Piece of **Hurt scale** for children aged 3–4 years
- Faces Pain Scale for 4- to 12-year olds and VAS (older than 8 years)
- Behavioural scales such as **FLACC** (face, leg, activity, cry, and consolability) for post-operative pain
- **COMFORT Scale** for intensive care patients

Geriatric pain

(See 1.10 Pain assessment in the elderly, p. 32 and 28.7 Pain in the elderly, p. 574.)

- NRS and facial pain scales are associated with high completion rate, good concurrence, and acceptable reliability
- **MOBID-2** can be used for dementia patients

Further reading

1. De Vet H. Choice of pain outcome measures from a clinimetric point of view. In: Wittink H, Carr D (eds). Pain Management: Evidence, Outcomes and Quality of Life. 1st edition, 2008; pp. 21–5. New York: Elsevier
2. Dworkin RH, Turk DC, Farrar JT, et al. Core outcome measures for chronic pain clinical trials: IMMPACT recommendations. Pain 2005;113(1):9–19
3. Husebo BS, Ostelo R, Strand LI. The MOBID-2 pain scale: reliability and responsiveness to pain in patients with dementia. Eur J Pain 2014;18(10):1419–30
4. Jensen MP. Pain assessment in clinical trials. In: Wittink H, Carr D (eds). Pain Management: Evidence, Outcomes and Quality of Life. 1st edition, 2008; pp. 57–82. New York: Elsevier

1.10 Pain assessment in the elderly

Introduction

- People over 65 years account for 65% of admissions to hospital, with 40% of the budget of primary care
- Prevalence of chronic pain in older people living in the community ranges from 25% to 76%, with those in residential care being higher, ranging from 83% to 93%
- Most common sites of pain in older people: back, legs, knees, or hips and 'other' joints
- Multidisciplinary approach is essential, but the process can become quite complex due to various challenges
- Loneliness and social isolation are strongly associated with increased risk of pain

- Signs and symptoms of mood disturbance (depression) and social isolation are strongly associated with pre-existing pain or are a predictor of future pain onset
- Pain in the elderly is also covered in 1.9 Measurement of pain—pain scales, p. 27, and in 28.7 Pain in the elderly, p. 574

Challenges in assessment

- Attitudes and beliefs influence all aspects of the pain experience in this age group
- Stoicism appears to be more evident in current generations of older people and may contribute to the underreporting of pain (this may not be the case for future generations)
- Spouse beliefs can have a negative impact on the development of adaptive responses to chronic pain
- Professionals may share or inculcate patients' maladaptive beliefs that hurt equals harm, and consequently recommend or reinforce behaviours such as activity avoidance
- Differences in both patterns and sites have been noted in men and women

Communication

- There is a paucity of research regarding the best way of communicating pain information
- The level of cognitive impairment should be considered in the assessment of pain
- Patients with severe cognitive impairment are unable to self-report pain information

Principles of assessment

1. Assessment of pain information should be multi-dimensional and include eliciting pain treatment information, as well as location and sensory aspects of pain
2. Use of open-ended, rather than closed-ended, questions
3. Do not interrupt when patients are conveying pain information, as this disrupts the amount and nature of pain information conveyed
4. Information regarding prognosis is vital for the elderly (usually only provided in 30%)
5. Assessment of pain can be complicated if the patient has severe cognitive impairment, with communication difficulties or language and cultural barriers (observational assessment is required, in addition)
6. Scales that can be used for older patients: **VAS**, **NRS**, **verbal descriptor scale** (presented in large, clear letters/numbers and in good lighting)
7. Patient observation is vitally important to note features such as facial expressions, physical reactions (e.g. guarding, bracing, rubbing the painful area), and negative reactions (e.g. agitation)
8. Pain behaviours are based on individual and clinical judgements, and familiarity with the older person is important in interpreting behaviour
9. Consider including carers in any pain assessment process as they are often more familiar with the subtle changes in the patient's behaviour that indicate pain
10. Self-reporting is the most reliable and valid indicator of pain, even if it is subjective
11. It may be necessary to ask the question in a variety of ways to elicit a consistent response
12. While self-reporting scales are good, they fail to capture fluctuations in capacity and pain

Suggested guidance for assessment of pain

1. Assessing for the presence of pain:
   - Screening, history, observation, involving families and carers
2. Establish the cause (check for red flags)
3. Multi-dimensional assessment:

- **Location** (self-pointing in cognitively intact older people; pain maps to help locate the site and extent of pain)
- **Intensity** (verbal rating/descriptor scales and NRS for intensity of pain in older people with no cognitive impairment and with mild to moderate cognitive impairment)
- **Impact of pain** and tools for assessment (impact on mood, sleep, mobility, function, and QoL)
- **Mood** (HADS and Geriatric Depression Scale (GDS)—30 items)
- **Mobility** (standardized measure, e.g. Timed-Up-and-Go)
- **Functional ability** (Nottingham Extended Activities of Daily Living Scale or Barthel Index)

Pain assessment tools

- No evidence that any one multi-dimensional assessment tool is better than another
- All older people in whom pain is detected should have a clinical assessment of the multi-dimensional aspects of pain, including:
  - A sensory dimension which describes the intensity and nature of pain, e.g. crushing, sharp
  - An affective/evaluative dimension which describes the emotional component of pain and how pain is perceived (e.g. dangerous, exhausting, frustrating, frightening)
  - The impact on life, including physical, functional, and psychosocial effects
- Health care professionals should familiarize themselves with relevant assessment tools and use them routinely
- Assessors should consider the use of one tool, or a combination of tools, to assess the differing dimensions of pain

Verbal descriptor scale

- Pain thermometer = pictorial modification of a verbal descriptor scale
- No pain (0), slight (1), mild (1–3), moderate (3–5), severe (5–7), very severe (7–9), worst possible pain (10)

Geriatric Pain Measure (GPM) 73

- A 24-item multi-dimensional pain assessment tool designed for older people

Brief Pain Inventory (BPI)

- Considered as part of a multi-dimensional assessment of pain in older people
- The short form has 15 items that assess severity of pain, interference of daily activities due to pain, and impact of pain on mood and enjoyment of life

McGill Pain Questionnaire (MPQ)

- Standardized scale for the assessment of pain in cognitively intact adults
- Assessment of sensory, affective, and evaluative dimensions of pain

Pain in older adults with cognitive impairment

- A number of behavioural scales have been developed to assess pain in older adults with cognitive impairment (no single instrument can be recommended for general use)
- Seven indicators: physiological observation, facial expressions, body movements, verbalizations, changes in interpersonal interactions, activity/routines, and mental status

- A hierarchical pain assessment algorithm was proposed that can be utilized either for patients who are self-reporting or for cognitively impaired patients:
    - Self-report from patient (or reason for not doing it)
    - Behavioural assessment tools to observe pain behaviours during clinical assessment
    - Assessment report by the patient's caregivers
    - List of analgesic trials and non-pharmacologic interventions and their outcomes

Tools for patients with cognitive impairment

- In older people with cognitive impairment or with difficulty in communication, observational assessment becomes essential for assessing for the presence of pain
- Carers familiar with older people with cognitive impairment should be included in the assessment of their pain

Discomfort Scale-Dementia of Alzheimer Type (DS-SAT)

- Developed and evaluated in nursing home residents in whom the tool had reasonable reliability and validity

The Abbey Pain Scale

- Developed for end-stage dementia; was built based on the DS-DAT
- Even though widely used, there has not been adequate critical evaluation

Doloplus-2

- French tool developed for multi-dimensional assessment of pain
- Includes ten items covering somatic (five), psychomotor (two), and psychosocial (three) reactions to pain
- Most promising tool in terms of evidence

The Pain Assessment in Advanced Dementia (PAINAD) Scale

- Simple 5-item observational tool, developed and validated in residents with advanced dementia

The Pain Assessment Checklist for Seniors with Limited Ability to Communicate (PACSLAC)

- A 60-item tool covering subtle, as well as common, pain behaviours

The NOPAIN tool

- Observation of patients' pain behaviours (verbalization, vocalization, face, bracing, rubbing, and restlessness) during activities of daily living (ADL) such as bathing and dressing

Advantages of pain assessment in the elderly

- Uncontrolled pain impacts upon the physical health of the older adult and QoL
- Therefore, assessment and management of pain are important in all clinical settings

Formal record

- Documentation of our pain management practice
- From a professional and legal perspective, we have a duty of care to our patients, regardless of age

- In these days of litigation, we could easily become victim of such lawsuits if pain is not recognized and treated appropriately

Faster recovery

- Research has demonstrated that if pain is assessed appropriately, it can be treated more effectively and subsequently patients would recover more quickly

Improved understanding

- Identification of treatments that are not working, to raise awareness of effective and ineffective treatment strategies

Summary

- **Assessment of pain** in older adults can be carried out using the NRS or verbal descriptors, even in the presence of mild to moderate cognitive impairment
- There are a number of **behavioural scales** available with high consistency (the most promising in terms of evidence are the Doloplus-2 and PAINAD scales, but the PACSLAC and Abbey Pain Scale are promising in terms of clinical utility)
- **Observation** is an important skill in identifying pain amongst the older population
- **Staff and caregivers** must familiarize with the locally used tools for assessing pain (this will improve the effectiveness of the assessment tool)
- All providers must have structured training in assessment and management of pain in the elderly according to their experience

Further reading

1. Abdulla A, Adams N, Bone M, et al. Guidance on the management of pain in older people. Age Ageing 2013;42 Suppl 1:i1–57.
2. Molton IR, Terrill AL. Overview of persistent pain in older adults. Am Psychol 2014;69(2): 197–207
3. Rastogi R, Meek BD. Management of chronic pain in elderly, frail patients: finding a suitable, personalized method of control. Clin Interv Aging 2013;8:37–46
4. Schofield PA. Assessment and management of pain in older adults: current perspectives and future directions. Scottish Universities Medical Journal 2014;Epub 3:03. http://sumj.dundee.ac.uk/data/uploads/epub-article/3003-sumj.epub.pdf
5. Schofield PA. The assessment and management of peri-operative pain in older adults. Anaesthesia 2014;69(Suppl 1):54–60
6. Schofield PA. The assessment of pain in older people: UK national guidelines. Age Ageing 2018;47:i1–22

1.11 Pain assessment in children

Introduction

- Children's pain perception should be an integral part of their pain assessment
- This supports Meinhart and McCaffery's statement that 'pain is whatever the person says it is'
- It is important to listen to, and understand, the child to create a "child-centred focus"

Challenges in assessment

- Previous erroneous assumptions have hampered efforts to assess and manage pain effectively in children
- Prevalent myths supported by the following assumptions:
    - Young children are unable to sense pain neurologically
    - They do not interpret noxious stimuli as pain
    - They do not experience the deleterious consequences of severe pain in the same way as adults
- It is now well accepted that anatomical, physiological, and biochemical mechanics needed for pain perception are present early in intrauterine life
- In fact, preterm infants can perceive pain in a way comparable to older children

ABCs of pain management

A—Ask about pain regularly. Assess pain systematically

B—Believe the patient and family in their reports of pain and what relieves pain

C—Choose pain control options appropriate for the patient, family, and setting

D—Deliver interventions in a timely, logical, and coordinated fashion

E—Empower patients and their families. Enable patients to control their course

Pain assessment in preverbal population

- Recommendations focus on multi-dimensional aspects that are characterized by behavioural and physiological indicators of pain

Neonates—Neonatal Pain Assessment Tool

- Developed for post-operative pain, but useful for other pain
- Variables to a maximum of 20 points looking at physical and physiological parameters (posture/tone, sleep, expression, cry, colour, respiration, heart rate (HR), saturation, blood pressure (BP), perception of nurses)
- <5: nursing comfort, >5: + paracetamol, >10: + opioid

Premature Infant Pain Profile (PIPP)

- Three behavioural indicators (facial actions for 30 seconds: brow bulge, eye squeeze, and nasolabial furrow), two physiological indicators (HR and oxygen saturation), and two contextual variables (gestational age and behavioural state) that modify pain (each of the seven domains scores 0–3)
- 0–6: no or minimal discomfort (no action); 7–12: slight–moderate pain (nursing comfort, paracetamol); >12: severe pain (pharmacological measures, e.g. narcotics)

Pain assessment in young infants

Face, Legs, Activity, Cry, and Consolability (FLACC) Scale

- Five pain behaviours that make up the scale's name: facial expression, leg movement, activity, cry, and consolability (each behaviour is scored from 0 to 2)
- 0: comfortable; 1–3: mild discomfort; 4–6: moderate pain; 7–10: severe discomfort/pain

Neonatal/Infant Pain Scale (NIPS)—under 1 year old

- Crying (0–2), facial expression, breathing pattern, arms, legs, state of arousal (all 0–1)
- Total score of >3 indicates pain

Pain assessment in school-aged children and adolescents (4–12 years of age)

- Several tools are available
- In younger children, developmental capabilities may hinder the use of purely numeric scales, and therefore, pictorial-based pain scales, such as the Faces Pain Scale, may be more suitable (e.g. Wong-Baker Faces)
- For older children (>8 years of age) who are able to understand abstract concepts, the VAS and 0–10 NRS can be used

Methods to aid the assessment of pain

QUESTT

- **Q**uestion the child (appropriate language, use dolls/toys)
- **U**se a pain rating scale (faces, numeric, behavioural, behavioural/physiological)
- **E**valuate behaviour and physiological changes (e.g. FLACC scale)
- **S**ecure parents' involvement
- **T**ake cause of pain into account
- **T**ake action and evaluate results

Assessing pain in non-verbal disabled children

- No speech
- Limited or absent communication
- May have cognitive impairment
- Altered body movement
- Other pre-existing conditions
- Ask carers' opinion

Common problems for disabled children

- Spasm/spasticity
- Positioning issues
- Pressure areas
- Bowels
- Reflux/gastritis
- Surgical complications/late diagnosis
- Fear/anxiety/sadness
- Environment

Self-report assessment tools

Visual analogue scale (VAS)—age 3 years to adult

- Self-reported tool for pain intensity
- Horizontal line, with 'no pain' at one end to 'worst possible pain' at the other
- Patient draws a line that intersects to indicate intensity

Wong-Baker Faces Pain Rating Scale—age 3–18 years

- Self-reported faces scale for acute pain
- Six line-drawn faces, ranging from no pain to worst pain, with a numerical value assigned to each face
- It also adds word descriptors to each face (no hurt, hurts a little, hurts a whole lot, etc.)

Faces Pain Scale-Revised (FPS-R)—age 4–16 years

- Self-reported faces scale for acute pain
- Six cartoon faces ranging from neutral to high pain expression (numbered 0, 2, 4, 6, 8, and 10)

Poker chip tool—age 4–7 years

- Self-reported poker chips are used to represent pain intensity
- Child chooses which chips represent the pain they experience, with one chip indicating a little hurt and all four chips indicating the most hurt a child could have

Observational assessment tools

FLACC Pain Assessment Tool

(See 1.11 Face, Legs, Activity, Cry, and Consolability (FLACC) Scale, p. 37.)

- Five categories of pain behaviours
- Simple framework for quantifying pain behaviours in children who may not be able to verbalize the presence or severity of pain

Procedure Behaviour Checklist (PBCL)—age 3–8 years

- Observational measure of pain and anxiety during invasive medical procedures
- Eight defined behaviours are assessed: muscle tension, screaming, crying, restraint used, pain verbalized, anxiety verbalized, verbal stalling, and physical resistance (scale 1–5)

Children's Hospital of Eastern Ontario Pain Scale (CHEOPS)—age 1–12 years

- Observational measure of post-operative pain in children
- Six behaviours that include cry, facial, child verbal, torso, touch, and legs (scale of 0–3, based on intensity)

COMFORT Scale—age 0–18 years

- Observer-rated measure for use in intensive care environments
- Eight domains thought to be indicative of pain and distress (alertness, calmness/agitation, respiratory response, physical movement, mean arterial BP, HR, muscle tone, and facial tension)
- Each domain is scored between 1 and 5, and the scores are added to yield a measure of sedation

Further reading

1. Nair S, Neil MJE. Paediatric pain: physiology, assessment and pharmacology. Anaesthesia tutorial of the week 289. 2013 http://www.frca.co.uk/Documents/289%20Paediatric%20Pain%20-%20Physiology,%20Assessment%20and%20Pharmacology.pdf
2. Manocha S, Taneja N. Assessment of paediatric pain: a critical review. J Basic Clin Physiol Pharmacol 2016;27(4):323–31
3. Wong C, Lau E, Palozzi L, Campbell F. Pain management in children: Part 1—Pain assessment tools and a brief review of non-pharmacological and pharmacological treatment options. Can Pharm J (Ott) 2012;145(5):222–5
4. Children's pain management service, Royal Children's Hospital. Melbourne https://www.rch.org.au/uploadedfiles/main/content/anaes/pain_assessment.pdf

1.12 Pain letter template

Box 1.12.1 shows an example of a structured patient letter.

Box 1.12.1 Structured patient letter

Thank you for referring this ... year old gentleman/lady ... to the pain clinic. He/she is suffering from ...
Referred by ...
Patient has been reviewed by the spine surgeon ... who does/does not recommend a surgical intervention ...
Furthermore, has been seen by ... for duodenal ulcer, etc.

Impression

Non-specific low back pain
Right leg radiculopathy into L5 dermatome (MRI with right L5 foraminal narrowing)

Medication

Pain meds (for how long, how effective, side effects)
Other
Allergies/sensitivities

Past medical history

Cardiovascular, respiratory, gastrointestinal, endocrinological (e.g. diabetes), neurological, kidney, or liver comorbidities/problems
Operations (disc, back, joints)
Trauma
Osteoporosis, osteopenia
Vitamin deficiencies (vitamins D and B, folic acid)

Presenting complaint

How long for, sudden or gradual onset (what happened then)
Site/side of pain
Is pain constant, intermittent
Pain intensity (e.g. 0–10/10 on average, range on a good and bad day)
Referred to .../radiating to ... (legs, arms), which dermatomes
Pain quality (nociceptive, neuropathic symptoms)
Pain is worse with ...
Pain is better with ...
Red flags (bladder or bowel problems, recent infection, falls, fractures, night sweats, unexpected weight loss)

Imaging/investigations

X-rays
Ultrasound
MRI scans
CT scans
DEXA scan (bone scan)

PET scan
Other investigations (e.g. gastroscopy, colonoscopy, diagnostic laparoscopy)

Social history

Living with partner/spouse/children/other people
Children (how many and how old)
Profession/employment
Sleep pattern (how many hours per night, waking in pain?)
Impact of pain on daily activities and quality of life (e.g. what does it stop you from doing?)
Previous abuse (physical, sexual, emotional, torture, etc.) if patient happy to disclose

Previous treatments

Physiotherapy (hydrotherapy), massage
Gym/exercises
Warm/cold applications
TENS
Injections
Chiropractor/osteopath
Acupuncture

On examination (chaperone: …), e.g. for lower limb

Lumbar flexion, extension, side flexion (aggravating pain symptoms?)
Toe and heel walking
(Weakness, numbness)
Power—hip, knee, and ankle flexion/extension (myotomes)
Sensory supply (dermatomes)

Supine

Hip internal/external rotation
Faber's/SIJ stretch tests (supine, lateral, prone)
Piriformis test (if applicable)
Straight leg raise

Prone

Femoral nerve stretch
Palpation of hips, paravertebral lumbar areas, SIJ, iliac crest (cluneal nerves), piriformis muscle

Plan

(Clear and easy to follow, for example:)

1. Continue regular exercising and stretching. Useful exercises may be swimming, cycling, walking, yoga, pilates …/referral to physiotherapy (e.g. for core exercises)
2. As flare-up medication, try … up to four times per day, but not regularly
3. Wean amitriptyline by 10 mg per day at weekly intervals
4. Try nortriptyline, instead of amitriptyline, to be started at 10 mg at night and gradually increased by 10 mg every week, up to a daily maximum as tolerated and needed
5. Lumbar MRI scan ordered
6. Referred to orthopaedics for review
7. Patient may benefit from the attendance of a pain management programme, and referred to …

If you disagree with the content of this letter, or you feel that I have misunderstood you or misrepresented your position, please contact me as soon as possible so that I can issue a correction.
(Copy of the letter supplied to the patient)

Kind regards
Yours sincerely
Dr J Rudiger
Consultant in Pain Medicine

1.13 Mnemonics for referrals

These mnemonics can be useful to request more information from the referrer when a patient is referred to a pain service:

Thank you for referring this patient. Unfortunately, I am unable to accept this patient since your referral letter does not provide enough details about the underlying problem/the reason of the referral.

I would recommend the mnemonic SOCRATES to be able to triage your referral appropriately.

SOCRATES

S—Site/side of symptoms

O—Onset (sudden/gradual, when, constant/intermittent)

C—Character of the pain symptoms (neuropathic, nociceptive, mixed)

R—Radiation (arms, hands, legs, feet) or referral of symptoms (e.g. buttock, shoulder)

A—Associated symptoms (tiredness, fatigue, depression, impact on QoL)

T—Time course/pattern (at rest, with activity)

E—Exacerbating/relieving factors (e.g. lifting, driving, sitting)

S—Severity of pain (e.g. VAS, mild–moderate–severe)

Additional information

Psychosocial background (family, relationship, dependants, employment, stress)

Previous treatments (e.g. injections, physiotherapy, osteopath, chiropractor)

Mental health and addiction medicine

OLD CARTS

O—Onset

L—Location

D—Duration

C—Character

A—Alleviating and Aggravating factors

R—Radiation

T—Treatments

S—Severity

PQRST

P—Provoking factors

Q—Quality

R—Region and Radiation

S—Severity

T—Time

Further reading

1. Nursejanx. Old Carts, Socrates, PQRST – Nursing mnemonics for pain & symptoms. Richmond, VA, USA. 2018 https://forum.nursejanx.com/t/old-carts-socrates-pqrst-nursing-mnemonics-for-pain-symptoms/550

1.14 Waddell's signs

- Waddell's signs are a number of physical signs that were first described by Gordon Waddell in 1980
- Intensity of chronic pain is a subjective finding
- Pain has been known to be associated with atypical or unexpected symptoms and clinical signs on examination
- In the absence of clear diagnostic criteria and a possibility of litigations and secondary gains, it makes it even more complex to diagnose
- Neurologists in the late nineteenth century identified a group of eight neurological signs which they thought were of non-organic origin, and thus suggestive of malingering
- Professor Gordon Waddell, a Scottish orthopaedic surgeon in the 1980s, grouped these eight signs into five categories:
    1. Tenderness (widespread superficial tenderness to light pinch or deep tenderness in non-anatomical distribution)
    2. Simulation (based on movements which produce pain, without actually stressing anatomical structures, e.g. lumbar pain with axial loading from the head or pain on simulated rotation)
    3. Distraction (rechecking of positive tests when the patient's attention is distracted; for example, a straight leg raise might cause pain when lying down, but a much greater range of pain-free movement may be possible with the same test when sitting)
    4. Regional (lower extremity weakness or sensory changes not corresponding to accepted neuroanatomy, e.g. nerve root distribution)
    5. Overreaction (subjective signs, such as grimacing, pleading to stop, and tremor, that seem out of proportion to the actual examination)
- Waddell suggested that chronic pain patients who are positive in three out of five categories should have an evaluation for underlying psychological problems
- These signs were quite popular and were often used by clinicians on behalf of insurance companies to diagnose malingering
- A rigorous evidence-based review suggested that Waddell's signs were organic phenomena, and that they were not associated with secondary gain or psychological distress. This review also suggested that patients with positive Waddell's signs had a higher intensity of pain, displayed reduced functional performance, and had poor outcomes after surgery

- There are two important components (regional) of Waddell's signs: the presence of non-dermatomal sensory abnormalities and limb weakness, rather than localized changes
- In studies on rodents, it was found that peripheral neuropathies can lead to non-dermatomal sensory abnormalities, while control of pain in humans showed improved hypoaesthesia in limbs. Researchers also suggest that the motor unit firing rates are painful and their synergistic pain-free muscles are inversely proportional to the pain reported by the patient
- Waddell's signs are now considered to be of neurophysiological, rather than behavioural, origin and should not be considered to be diagnostic of malingering

Further reading

1. D'Souza RS, Dowling TJ, Law L. Wadell Sign. 2021: Treasure Island, Florida, USA: StatPearls Publishing LLC https://www.ncbi.nlm.nih.gov/books/NBK519492/
2. Waddell G, McCulloch J, Kummel E, Venner R. Nonorganic physical signs in low-back pain. Spine 1980;5(2):117–25

1.15 IASP classification of chronic pain for ICD-11

- Chronic pain has been recognised as a new diagnosis (disease in its own right)
- Chronic primary pain (pain has persisted for more than 3 months and is associated with significant emotional distress and/or functional disability, and the pain is not better accounted for by another condition)
- Secondary chronic pain (another diagnosis accounts for the presenting symptoms, pain may at least initially be conceived as a symptom secondary to an underlying disease)[4]

Further reading

1. Nicholas M, Vlaeyen JWS, Rief W et al. The IASP Taskforce for the Classification of Chronic Pain The IASP classification of chronic pain for ICD-11: chronic primary pain, PAIN. 2019;160(1):28–37

4. Reproduced from Nicholas M, et al. The IASP classification of chronic pain for ICD-11: chronic primary pain, *PAIN*, 160(1):28–37, copyright 2019, International Association for the Study of Pain.

SECTION 2

PAIN PHYSIOLOGY

CHAPTER 2

Pain Pathways

Enrique Collantes, Gustav Jirikowski, Paolo Pais, Deepak Ravindran, Jan Rudiger, and Maria Stasiowska

CONTENTS

2.1 Peripheral nociceptors

Definitions and introduction

- Nociceptors are specialized peripheral dendritic receptors of pseudo-unipolar neurons that encode and transduce noxious stimuli
- Nociceptors are sensory receptors of the peripheral somatosensory nervous system
- The cell bodies of these pseudo-unipolar neurons are located in specific ganglia: DRGs, nerve plexuses, CN ganglia (trigeminal ganglion), and nucleus spinalis of the brainstem
- Nociceptors are exclusively associated with the extracellular matrix of connective tissues (subcutaneous, fasciae, tendons, organ capsules, periosteum, perineurium, perimysium, periodontium, dura mater, etc.)
- No nociceptors are found in the central nervous system (CNS)
- Nociceptors develop from neural crest stem cells and are formed during neurogenesis

Anatomy

- Nociceptive axons terminate in non-specialized 'free nerve endings'
- Nociceptive nerve endings are devoid of myelin sheaths; they branch widely into their target region
- A single peripheral axon emanates from the cell body in neural ganglia (DRG, trigeminal ganglion) to innervate the skin and a central axon synapses with second-order neurons (2nd ONs) in the DH of the spinal cord or the trigeminal subnucleus caudalis, respectively
- The different types of nociceptors are morphologically indistinguishable
- The axons associated with nociceptors are A-delta (myelinated, fast, sharper and better localized sensation) and C-fibres (unmyelinated, slow, poorly localized sensation)
- In the spinal cord, the spinothalamic tract constitutes the major ascending nociceptive pathway

Types of nociceptors

- Nociceptors are not uniformly sensitive
- They are categorized according to their responses to mechanical, thermal (>40–45°C or <15°C), and/or chemical stimuli liberated by tissue damage, tumour, and/or inflammation
- Location: external areas (e.g. skin, cornea, mucosa) and internal areas (e.g. digestive tract, joints, muscle, ligaments)

Skin nociceptors

- Four different types of nociceptors have been identified based on their response to different stimuli:
  - High-threshold mechanical nociceptors, only responding to intense mechanical stimulation (e.g. pinching, cutting, stretching, pressure)—via A-delta fibres
  - Thermal nociceptors for cold and heat, also responding to above mechanical stimuli—via A-delta fibres
  - Chemical nociceptors responding to chemical substances (e.g. cytokines, acids, electricity)—via A-delta fibres
  - Polymodal nociceptors responding to a variety of high-intensity stimuli (e.g. mechanical, thermal, and chemical substances like the previous three types)—via C-fibres

Joint nociceptors

- The joint capsules and ligaments contain high-threshold mechanoreceptors, polymodal nociceptors, and 'silent' nociceptors
- Many of the fibres innervating these nerve endings in the joint capsule contain neuropeptides such as SP and calcitonin gene-related peptide (CGRP)

Visceral nociceptors

- Visceral organs contain mechanical pressure, temperature, chemical, and silent nociceptors (many are silent)
- The noxious information from visceral organs and skin are carried to the CNS in different pathways

Silent nociceptors

- In skin and deep tissues, there are additional nociceptors called 'silent' or 'sleep' nociceptors
- These receptors are normally unresponsive to noxious mechanical stimulation but become 'awakened' (responsive) to mechanical stimulation during inflammation and after tissue injury
- Awakening occurs with continuous stimulation from damaged tissue that reduces the threshold of these nociceptors and causes them to respond
- The activation of silent nociceptors may contribute to the induction of hyperalgesia, central sensitization, and allodynia

Physiology

- Nociceptors respond to noxious stimuli (extremes in temperature and pressure)
- The presence of injured tissue or inflammatory mediators transduces these stimuli into long-ranging electrical signals that are relayed to the brain (the perception of pain is confined to the brain)
- Nociceptors stay sensitized by prolonged stimulation (making them responsive to other sensations as well)

- Speed of transmission depends on dendritic diameters and on their extent of myelination: A-delta fibres, 2–30 m/s (fast); C-fibres: 0.25–1.5 m/s (slow)
- It is still unclear whether a single nociceptive neuron can extend neurites equipped with several different nociceptors
- Nociceptive neurons release a variety of chemical substances from their central terminals to stimulate 2nd ONs

Molecular basis of nociception

- Nociceptors are excitatory neurons and release glutamate as their primary NT (as well as SP, CGRP, and somatostatin)
- The following substances (inflammatory mediators) are released with tissue damage and can cause nociceptor activation:
  - Globulin and protein kinases, arachidonic acid, bradykinin, cytokines, histamine, nerve growth factor (NGF), SP and CGRP, protons (H^+) (low pH), potassium (K^+), PGs, serotonin (5-hydroxytryptamine (5-HT)), acetylcholine (ACh), lactic acid, and adenosine triphosphate (ATP) (subcutaneous (SC) injections of minute quantities of these products excite nociceptors)
- Sensation of noxious cold is facilitated by the menthol-activated non-selective cation channel (NSC) TRPM8. Temperature changes activate nociceptors through the cation channel TRPA1
- Noxious heat is thought to activate nociceptor membranes through NSC TRPV1
- Mechanical and chemical nociceptors are stimulated by various factors, including SP, NGF, CGRP, sodium (Na^+) channels, and transient receptor potential (TRP)-family channels that may become novel targets for therapies
- Synapses of nociceptors in DH nuclei show remarkable plasticity, probably important for the development of adaptation and chronic pain

Clinical significance

- Most nociceptors can be simultaneously stimulated by capsaicin
- Local anaesthetics (LAs) aim to block signal transduction in interstitial spaces of connective tissue (e.g. injections of procaine, lidocaine, etc.)
- Non-steroidal anti-inflammatory drugs (NSAIDs) act on nociceptors
- Anti-nociceptive properties have been described for numerous substances (including cannabinoids). Although they most likely interact with the above-mentioned ion channels, their mode of action is largely unknown
- Peripheral neuropathic pain is the result of hyperexcitability of nociceptors after trauma or chronic inflammation
- Acupuncture stimulates liberation of opioid peptides from clusters of dermal and interstitial cells (= acupuncture points) to achieve temporary blockade of nociceptors
- Naloxone prevents anti-nociceptive effects of acupuncture

Further reading

1. Bannister K, Kucharczyk M, Dickenson AH. Hopes for the future of pain control. Pain Ther 2017;6(2):117–28
2. Dubin AE, Patapoutian A. Nociceptors: the sensors of the pain pathway. J Clin Invest 2010;120(11):3760–72

3. Dafny N. Chapter 6: Pain principles. In: Neuroscience online. 2020. McGovern Medial School at UTHealth, Department of Neurobiology and Anatomy https://nba.uth.tmc.edu/neuroscience/s2/chapter06.html
4. Kim PS, Fishman MA. Cannabis for pain and headaches: primer. Curr Pain Headache Rep 2017;21(4):19
5. Purves D, Augustine GJ, Fitzpatrick D, et al. Chapter 8: The Somatic Sensory System - Cutaneous and Subcutaneous Somatic Sensory Receptors. Neuroscience. 3rd edition. 2001; pp. 189–192. Sunderland, MA: Sinauer Associates, Inc. https://www.hse.ru/data/2011/06/22/1215686482/Neuroscience.pdf

2.2 Ascending pain pathways

Introduction

- There are ascending and descending pain pathways
- Nociception is the neural mechanism by which a person detects a noxious stimulus to the periphery
- Peripheral nociceptive stimuli are transduced into action potentials (APs), transmitted and modulated along first-, second-, and third-order neurons to higher brain centres where the information is processed and perceived

Nociceptive pathways—transduction, transmission, processing, and perception

Transduction

- Physiological process whereby a potentially harmful noxious stimulus (thermal, chemical, or mechanical) is converted into an electrical impulse (AP) by a peripheral nociceptor (see 2.1 Peripheral nociceptors, p. 47)
- Peripheral nociceptors are free nerve endings of primary afferent A-beta, A-delta, and C-fibres located in the skin, tissues, or organs

Transmission

First-order neurons (1st ONs)

- 1st ONs conduct APs from the periphery in a saltatory manner via A-beta, A-delta, and C-fibres (see Table 2.2.1) to the DH of the spinal cord or the medulla oblongata where they terminate and synapse with 2nd ONs (the DRG contains the cell bodies of 1st ONs)

Table 2.2.1 Type of peripheral nerves

Nerve type	Properties	Velocity (m/s)	Function
A-beta (large)	Myelinated	30–70	Touch Pressure Vibration
A-delta (small)	Myelinated	3–30	Pain (pinprick) Temperature (cold threshold)
C (small)	Unmyelinated	0.5–2	Pain (heat/cold/pressure) Temperature (heat threshold)

- First-order nociceptive afferents terminate predominantly in superficial layers of the DH (rexed laminae 1 and 2), while non-nociceptive afferents terminate in the deeper layers (lamina 5)
- Cell bodies of 1st ONs from the head, mouth, and neck are found in the trigeminal ganglion and transfer APs to the trigeminal nucleus of the brainstem

Second-order neurons

- The cell bodies of 2nd ONs are located in the DH of the spinal cord (substantia gelatinosa (SG) or nucleus proprius) and medulla oblongata, and transmit APs to the thalamus, PAG, and RVM by the spinothalamic, spinoreticular, and spinomesencephalic pathways (see Table 2.2.2). (Also see Fig. 20.1.2 in 20.1 Anatomy of the spinal cord, p. 368)
- Types of 2nd ONs in the DH:
  - Nociceptive-specific
  - Wide dynamic range (WDR) neurons transmit noxious and non-noxious stimuli. Their activity is proportional to the signal intensity and frequency, and they are involved in wind-up and referred pain mechanisms
  - Local interneurons (modulate the activity of 1st and 2nd ONs, e.g. inhibitory local interneurons decrease transmission of nociceptive signals from periphery to brain)
  - Short projection neurons

Table 2.2.2 Ascending pain pathways

Tract	Location of third-order neuron cell body	Function and final destination
Lateral spinothalamic	Ventromedial posterior nucleus, medial dorsal nucleus, and ventral post-lateral nucleus of thalamus	Primary somatosensory cortex: sensory and discriminative aspects of pain (intensity, quality, location) Insular and cingulate cortex: memories, emotions, mannerism Hypothalamus: temperature
Anterior spinothalamic	Intralaminar nuclei of the thalamus and reticular formation in the brainstem	Primary somatosensory cortex: crude touch, pressure Hypothalamus, amygdala: affective aspects such as unpleasantness or fear of pain
Spinoreticular	Medullary-pontine nuclei of the reticular formation	Reticular formation has projections to the thalamus and cerebral cortex which regulate arousal and neural activity influencing the affective, emotional, and motivational aspects of pain
Spinomesencephalic	Midbrain tectum and periaqueductal grey area	Midbrain: integration of somatic stimuli with audiovisual information, and emotional and affective components of pain Periaqueductal grey area: modulation and descending inhibition of painful stimuli
Spinocerebellar	Not present	Cerebellar cortex: proprioception
Fasciculus gracilis and cuneatus	Thalamic ventral posterolateral nucleus	Primary somatosensory cortex: fine touch, pressure, and vibration from levels above T6 by fasciculus cuneatus and below T6 by fasciculus gracilis

- Transmission of noxious stimuli from the DH to higher brain centres via ascending pathways is determined by multiple mechanisms and mediators at the pre- and post-synaptic terminals of the spinal cord such as:
  - Excitatory mechanisms:
    - Chemicals: CGRP, cholecystokinin, SP, somatostatin, glutamate, aspartate
    - Receptors: α-amino-3-hydroxy-5-methyl-4-isoxazole propionic acid receptor (AMPA), NMDA, glutamate, neurokinin-1 (NK1)
    - Immune system (glia) which secrete chemokines, brain-derived neurotrophic factor (BDNF), IL-1 beta, interferon gamma (IFN-γ), reactive oxygen species, TNF alpha, intracellular pathways (p38, cyclic adenosine monophosphate (cAMP) response binding element), mitogen-activated protein kinases, SRC family kinases
  - Inhibitory mechanisms:
    - Chemicals: gamma aminobutyric acid (GABA), glycine, endogenous opioids, noradrenaline, serotonin
    - Receptors: cannabinoids, opioid, GABA, glycine, serotonin, noradrenaline
    - Local inhibitory interneurons and descending inhibitory pathways activate inhibitory mechanisms which reduce the transmission of noxious stimuli to the brain

Notes on ascending pathways

- 1st ON cell bodies are located in the DRGs
- 2nd ON cell bodies are located in the DH (posterior grey horn) of the spinal cord, except for the fasciculus gracilis and cuneatus which are located in the nucleus gracilis and nucleus cuneatus, respectively
- Ascending tracts which cross over to the other side of the spinal cord:
  - Spinothalamic tracts at the level they enter the spinal cord
  - Fasciculus gracilis and cuneatus tracts before joining the medial lemniscus
  - Anterior spinocerebellar tracts before entering the spinal cord and then cross again in the cerebellum

Third-order neurons (3rd ONs)

- 3rd ONs transmit the signals from the nuclei of the thalamus to terminate in higher brain centres (primary somatosensory cortex, cerebellum, anterior cingulate cortex, prefrontal cortex, basal ganglia, amygdala, insular cortex)
- There are also projections to the PAG

Pain processing in the brain

- Imaging techniques, such as fMRI, have demonstrated that a large brain network is activated during the acute pain experience (cerebral signature for pain, traditionally called the 'pain matrix')
- The **'Pain Matrix'** is used to describe areas of the brain activated when someone experiences pain (3rd ONs terminate in the pain matrix):
  - Primary somatosensory cortex: conscious information about pain (**intensity, quality, location**) from contralateral aspect of the body
  - Prefrontal cortex: integration of sensory messages, memory retrieval, decision-making, and attention processing
  - Insular cortex: behavioural and autonomic responses to pain (**memories, emotions, unpleasantness, and mannerisms** associated with pain, leading to negative behavioural and emotional responses)

- Anterior cingulate cortex: anxiety, anticipation, attention, and motor responses
- Hippocampus, amygdala, and other parts of the limbic system: development and storage of memories related to affect, emotional events, pain experiences, and the process of learning from these events

- The most common areas activated include the primary and secondary somatosensory cortices (S1 and S2), insula, anterior cingulate cortex, prefrontal cortex, thalamus, and limbic system (important areas of pain perception)
- Other regions such as the basal ganglia, cerebellum, amygdala, hippocampus, and areas within the parietal and temporal cortices can also be active, dependent upon the individual
- In chronic pain, processing mostly involves the limbic circuits, especially the hippocampus, amygdala, and nucleus accumbens, indicating an emotional component involvement

Pain perception

- Refers to the process by which a noxious event is recognized as pain by a conscious person
- This is complex, and there is no one place within the brain where pain perception occurs
- The receptive fields of all pain-sensitive neurons are relatively large, particularly at the level of the thalamus and cortex, because the detection of pain is more important than its precise localization
- Treatments used in pain management work by inhibiting the excitatory mechanisms or enhancing the inhibitory mechanisms that modulate the perception of pain

Further reading

1. Basbaum AI, Jessel TM. The perception of pain. In: Kandel XX, Schwartz JH, Jessel TM (eds). Principles of Neural Science. 4th edition, 2000; pp. 473–7. New York, NY; McGraw Hill
2. Yang H, Bie B, Naguhib MA. Chapter 6: Pain physiology ascending pathway for pain transmission. In: Flood P, Rathmell JP, Urman RD (eds). Stoelting's pharmacology and physiology in anaesthetic practice. 6th edition. 2021. Philadelphia, USA: Wolter, Kluwer
3. Cioffi CL. Modulation of glycine-mediated spinal neurotransmission for the treatment of chronic pain. J Med Chem 2018;61(7):2652–79
4. Patestas MA, Gartner LP. Ascending sensory pathways. In: Patestas MA, Gartner LP (eds). A Textbook of Neuroanatomy. 2nd edition, 2016; pp. 187–227. Philadelphia, PA: John Wiley & Sons
5. Yaksh TL, Luo ZD. Anatomy of the pain processing system. In: Waldman SD (ed). Pain Management. 2007, Vol 1; pp. 11–20. Philadelphia, PA: Elsevier
6. Dafny N. Chapter 7: Pain tracts and sources. In: Neuroscience online. 2020. McGovern Medical School at UTHealth, Department of Neurobiology and Anatomy https://nba.uth.tmc.edu/neuroscience/s2/chapter07.html

2.3 Descending pain pathways

Introduction

- Ascending nociceptive signals are modulated by the descending pathways
- Descending modulation originates in the cortex, midbrain, pons, and medulla. These complex pathways have many interconnections and feedback loops

- Descending inhibitory and facilitatory projections travel down the dorsolateral and ventrolateral funiculi of the spinal cord, and terminate in the DH. They facilitate or inhibit nociceptive signal transmission between primary and secondary afferents by modulating:
  - Release of neurotransmitters (NTs) and chemicals causing direct pre- or post-synaptic inhibition or excitation, e.g. noradrenaline, serotonin, dopamine, glycine, GABA, endogenous opioids (enkephalins, dynorphins, beta-endorphin), cannabinoids, neurotensin, cholecystokinin, ACh
  - Stimulation or inhibition of local interneurons, to inhibit or excite primary and secondary afferents
  - Regulate the activity of glia and immune-related mechanisms

Areas in the brain associated with descending modulation

- Cortex—somatosensory, cingulate, and insular
- Amygdala—located in the temporal lobes, part of the limbic system
- Parabrachial nucleus—part of the reticular formation between the midbrain and the pons
- Nucleus tractus solitarius—sensory nuclei in the medulla
- Rostroventral hypothalamus
- Thalamus
- Nucleus raphe magnus, RVM—located in the brainstem
- Locus coeruleus—located in the pons
- PAG—grey matter in the midbrain around the cerebral aqueduct

Pathways associated with descending modulation

Noradrenergic pathways

- Originate in the **locus coeruleus and pontine nuclei**
- Project to laminae 1, 2, 4, 5, and 10 of the spinal cord DH
- Directly stimulate alpha 1 and 2 receptors on pre- and post-ganglionic neurons, and excitatory/inhibitory interneurons
- Alpha 1 receptors increase calcium (Ca^{2+}) and reduce K^+ influx, causing excitation. Alpha 2 receptors have the opposite effect
- Cause inhibition and excitation at the DH

Dopaminergic pathways

- Originate from the **periventricular and posterior parts of the hypothalamus**
- Affect first-order afferents and interneurons at the DH
- Dopaminergic type 1 and 2 receptors are located on the superficial (1 and 2) and deep (X) laminae of the DH
- Cause inhibition and excitation at the DH

Serotonergic pathways

- Originate in the dorsal **raphe nucleus, nucleus raphe magnus, and RVM**
- Project directly to excitatory and inhibitory interneurons of laminae 2 in the DH
- Cause inhibition and excitation at the DH

Periaqueductal grey area

- PAG is the grey matter located around the cerebral aqueduct within the tegmentum of the midbrain

- Critical structure coordinating descending modulation from supraspinal centres
- Receives nociceptive information directly from the DH and indirectly from the thalamus, cortex, limbic system, hypothalamus, nucleus tractus solitarius, and parabrachial nucleus
- Main effect is via activation/inhibition of the RVM and locus coeruleus serotonergic and noradrenergic pathways
- It is the main site for action of endorphins and analgesics (opiates and cannabinoids)

Other factors involved in pain modulation

- Attention, hypervigilance, observation, empathy
- Cognitions (catastrophizing, expectations)
- Mood (anxiety, stress)
- Genetic factors
- Placebo response

Conditioned pain modulation (CPM)

- CPM is a psychophysical experimental measure of the endogenous pain inhibitory pathways
- CPM is believed to measure the mechanism by which a painful stimulus inhibits/reduces the intensity of further painful stimuli (i.e. the 'pain inhibits pain' phenomenon)
- CPM represents the human behavioural correlate of diffuse noxious inhibitory control which was initially described in rat experimental models
- Dysfunctional CPM is common in chronic pain and associated with:
  - Decreased central inhibition
  - Lower pain threshold
  - Development and maintenance of chronic pain

Further reading

1. Lewis GN, Rice DA, McNair PJ. Conditioned pain modulation in populations with chronic pain: a systematic review and meta-analysis. J Pain 2012;13(10):936–44
2. Ren K, Dubner R. Descending control mechanisms. In: Basbaum A, Bushnell M, Smith D, et al. (eds). The Senses: A Comprehensive Review. 2007, Vol 5; pp. 723–62. New York, NY: Academic Press Books, Elsevier

2.4 Theories of pain

Theories of mechanisms of pain

Theories about pain physiology and its perception have been developing since ancient Greek times. The most famous pain models include the following.

Descartes model

- Describes pain as a sensation in the brain resulting from a nociceptive signal being transduced and transported via specific neural pathways

Specificity theory

- Each sensation modality has its own receptor and pathway from the periphery to the CNS

Intensity theory

- Any type of stimulus that is sufficiently intense can produce a painful signal

Pattern theory

- All somatosensory sensations travel via the same type of peripheral receptor and nerve fibre, but the rate and intensity of the resulting signal encodes the stimulus type

Gate control theory of pain

- Described in 1965 by Ronald Melzack and Patrick Wall
- The central idea of the 'gate theory' is the action of interneurons which modulate signal conduction between primary and secondary afferent neurons
- Interneurons are inhibitory cells in the SG (grey matter structure of the dorsal spinal cord) which release GABA and glycine to hyperpolarize secondary afferent neurons and reduce or prevent signal transmission to the brain
- Theory postulated that the 'gating effect' of interneurons could be controlled by large myelinated and small unmyelinated fibres, which increase or decrease the activity of interneurons, respectively
- Non-painful signals transmitted via large A-beta fibres stimulate inhibitory interneurons which 'close the gate' to nociceptive signals from C-fibres. This prevents conduction of painful signals from primary to secondary afferents and further along to the brain
- When nociceptive signals exceed a threshold, large-fibre inhibition is overridden by small-diameter fibres that reduce interneuron inhibition and 'open' the gate to nociceptive signal transmission to the brain
- The 'gate theory' is used to explain the effects of transcutaneous electrical nerve stimulation (TENS), which stimulates superficial non-nociceptive fibres and produces analgesia over the affected area, as well as using counterstimulation, such as rubbing a painful area, to reduce pain intensity

Integrated models

Neuromatrix model

- Incoming sensory information is modified by the activity of certain specific regions of the central nervous system which are collectively called the neuromatrix (brain stem, thalamus, limbic system, prefrontal cortex)
- The output from the interaction of the sensory information with these regions results in a "signature of pain" which then defines the patients pain experience

Biopsychosocial model

- Contribution of the psychological and social elements to the experience of pain
- First attempt to move away from the previous biological models and theories of pain

Mature organism model

- Suggesting that incoming nociceptive signals travel to the brain and are simultaneously compared to a number of other information such as proprioception, interoception, exteroception and cognition
- The total sum of the scrutiny of this information results in an output which in a feedback loop influences further input thus dynamically changing the organisms response to future stimuli and modulating pain.

Bayesian probability theory

- Most recent theory that takes into account the concept of predictive processing (Bayesian approach to sensory perception)
- This theory helps in accounting for the phenomena of medically unexplained symptoms and the success of placebo treatments
- The top down flow of previous brain predictions is met by a bottom up incoming input from any of the senses, and the mismatch between the predicted input and the actual input results in a prediction error which helps the system to revise its initial predictions
- A central tenet is that we perceive the world not as it is but our brains best guess, and this is constantly refined by our senses, both internal and external.

Further reading

1. Melzack R. From the gate to the neuromatrix. Pain Suppl 1999;6:S121–6
2. Melzack R, Wall PD. Pain mechanisms: a new theory. Science 1965;150:971–9
3. Gifford L. Pain, the Tissues and the Nervous System: A conceptual model. Physiotherapy 1998;84(1):27–36
4. Ongaro G, Kaptchuk TJ. Symptom perception, placebo effects, and the Bayesian brain. PAIN 2019;160(1):1–4

2.5 Pathophysiology of nociceptive, visceral, and neuropathic pain

Introduction

Nociceptive pain

- Pain that arises from actual or threatened damage to non-neural tissue and is due to the activation of nociceptors

Visceral pain

- Pain from the activation of nociceptors of the thoracic, pelvic, or abdominal viscera

Neuropathic pain

- Pain caused by a lesion or disease of the somatosensory nervous system. It can be further categorized as peripheral or central

Similarities in the pathophysiology of nociceptive, visceral, and neuropathic pain

- Some experts believe they are similar entities as they involve similar processes that control signalling of noxious stimuli in the somatosensory nervous system such as:
  - Genetic, immune, chemicals, enzymes, and receptors
  - Primary afferent nerve—peripheral sensitization
  - DH—central sensitization
  - Brainstem—dysregulation of the descending pathways that modulate spinal signalling
  - Higher brain centres—increased activity of similar mechanisms/areas of the pain matrix
- There is an overlap in the response to treatments for different types of pain
- Low treatment success from lack of specific pathophysiological mechanisms in different conditions

Pathophysiology of nociceptive pain

- Involves the transduction of a non-electrical signal to an electrochemical signal
- Well localized
- Also referred as somatic pain which can be further subclassified as:
  - Superficial somatic pain—derived from superficial structures
  - Deep somatic pain—derived from deeper structures such as muscles, tendons, and joints

Peripheral pathways

- High-density innervation
- Highly developed thermal and mechanical nociceptors with discrete receptor fields
- Mostly via fast A-delta fibres which synapse with 2nd ONs at laminae 1 and 5 of the SG of the DH of the spinal cord. Less conduction by C-fibres (slower, less myelinated) which finish at lamina 2 of the SG
- Small number of collateral neural fibres

Central pathways

- Fast conduction of nociceptive messages in the CNS
- Most travel via the lateral ascending pathways (spinothalamic tract) which transmit well-localized noxious stimuli. A very small number travel by the medial ascending pathways
- High topographic representation in the somatosensory cortex and spinal cord
- Dominance of the lateral pain system neuromatrix characterized with less emotional responses and better localization of nociceptive messages

Pathophysiology of neuropathic pain

- Damage to the nerve pathways at any point from the terminals of the peripheral nociceptors to the cortical neurons in the brain:
  - Peripheral: small fibres, nerve, plexus, nerve root
  - Central: spinal cord, brainstem, thalamus, cortex
- Common causes: trauma, ischaemia, haemorrhage, inflammation, neurodegeneration, neurotoxicity, cancer, paraneoplastic, vitamin deficiency, metabolic, autoimmune, hereditary, infection, demyelination, surgery, idiopathic
- Development of persistent pain is more common after an injury to a major nerve than after an injury to a non-nervous tissue

Mechanisms of the pathophysiology of neuropathic pain

- Injury to a nerve, spinal cord, or brain leads to disinhibition, ectopic discharges, and hyperexcitability
- Oedema, increased vascular permeability, and production of inflammatory mediators such as:
  - PGs, bradykinin, SP, and CGRP
  - Pro-inflammatory cytokines as IL-1B, IL-6, and TNF
  - Intracellular phosphorylating mechanisms such as cAMP and protein kinase C
- Changes in the structure and function of nerves:
  - Ephaptic transmission: adjacent nerve fibres are excited by 'non-synaptic cross-talk'. This also happens between somatosensory nerves and nerves of the autonomic nervous system (ANS)
  - Expansion of the receptive fields of injured nerves
  - Sensory denervation and sprouting of collateral nerve fibres
  - Upregulation of ion channels (e.g. Na^+, Ca^{2+}, NMDA, glutamate, etc.)
  - Phenotypic switch of nerve fibres: expression pro-nociceptive mediators (e.g. SP, CGRP) in nerve fibres that do not normally transfer painful stimuli such beta fibres

- In sympathetically mediated pain, there can be vasoconstriction reducing oxygen cell supply, alpha-2 adrenoreceptors expression in afferent sensory fibres, denervation, and sprouting of sympathetic fibres in the spinal cord
- In the CNS, important mechanisms include:
  - Increased glutamatergic activity
  - Glial activation
  - Cortical reorganization as in, for example, phantom limb pain
  - Dysfunction of the descending brainstem inhibitory controls, inhibitory neurons at the spinal cord, and production of inhibitory neuropeptides, NTs, receptors, and enzymes

Pathophysiology of visceral pain

- Mechanisms in visceral pain, visceral hyperalgesia/allodynia, and referred pain overlap and coexist

Classification of visceral pain

- *True visceral pain (tissue insult):* nociception arising from neural sources in deep organs of the body
- *Visceral hyperalgesia (visceral allodynia):* non-noxious stimuli are interpreted as pain due to alterations in nerves carrying visceral sensations at the peripheral and/or central level
- *Referred pain:*
  - Viscero-visceral referral: one sensitized organ causes sensitization of another visceral organ
  - Viscero-somatic referral: visceral pain causes referred somatic pain
  - Somatic-visceral referral: somatic pain causes referred visceral pain

Visceral pain—tissue insult

- Poorly localized, diffuse, and poorly defined sensation
- Visceral fibres are not homogenous and transmit painful and non-painful stimuli. For example, vagal fibres transmit painful and non-painful sensations (e.g. nausea, hunger, thirst, defecation)
- Normally cutting and burning of a visceral structure does not cause visceral pain. Visceral pain can be caused by distension, spasm, traction, ischaemia, and inflammation affecting the internal organs
- Neurohumoral system influences function and pain from visceral structures—interplay between the ANS, innate and adaptive immune cells, and localized nerve cells
- Can be accompanied with motor and autonomic reflexes (e.g. nausea, vomiting, sweating, reflex muscle spasm, changes in heart rate and blood pressure)

Peripheral pathways

- Wide and overlapping receptive fields
- Lower-density innervation as compared to somatic innervation and multiple collateral neural fibres
- One nerve innervates two visceral organs/structures
- Mostly C-fibre conduction (slow) and minority by A-delta fibres (faster)
- Visceral innervation:
  - Extrinsic innervation by the ANS via sympathetic fibres (sympathetic chain, splanchnic nerves, coeliac, mesenteric, hypogastric plexuses, ganglion impar) and parasympathetic fibres (vagal, sacral, and pelvic nerves, and their branches)
  - Intrinsic innervation which regulates blood flow, secretions, motility, etc.
  - The interaction between extrinsic and intrinsic innervation of visceral structures is not well understood

- Poorly developed nociceptors: mechanoreceptors, thermoreceptors, and silent nociceptors. Low-threshold nociceptors are more common than high-threshold nociceptors (3:1)

Central pathways

- Afferent fibres enter the spine via the dorsal root, mostly to superficial lamina 1 and deeper laminae 5–7
- Travel in ipsilateral (dorsal columns) and contralateral (spinothalamic) ascending pathways to the brain
- Extensive arborization and spread of afferent visceral fibres within the spinal cord
- Poor representation in the somatosensory cortex—scattered cortical afferent inputs
- Dominance of the medial pain system neuromatrix characterized by emotional responses

Visceral hyperalgesia (visceral allodynia)

- Normally associated with peripheral and central sensitization
- Noxious stimuli in childhood can lead to visceral hyperalgesia later in life
- Can develop after and/or coexist with:
  - Inflammatory conditions (e.g. cystitis, colitis)
  - Trauma/stressful situations (e.g. maternal separation, violence, torture)
- Stress has an important effect on the immune system which can lead to visceral inflammation, enhancing visceral permeability and mechanisms involved in visceral hypersensitivity
- Autonomic system has an important role; for example, in irritable bowel syndrome (IBS), the enteric nervous system in the abdominal viscera forms the 'second brain'
- Some of the pathophysiology mechanisms include:
  - Dysregulation of the hypothalamic–pituitary–adrenal axis and raised levels of corticotrophin-releasing factor secretion. This is one of the mechanisms that can lead to visceral hyperalgesia in the absence of a tissue injury in situations such as emotional trauma (e.g. witnessing torture)
  - Hyperexcitability and increased responsiveness of the visceral pathways; for example, in studies where the bowel is distended, patients with IBS have higher discomfort than controls
  - Neuroplastic changes in the response from visceral afferent pathways and enhanced brain responses to expectations of visceral pain; for example, in pelvic pain, there can be a change in the sensitivity of the mechanosensitive nociceptors in the bladder, afferent and efferent pathways resulting in increased urinary frequency, voiding with a lower threshold, and non-noxious stimuli in the bladder perceived as painful
  - Increased sensitivity of the reflex pathways of visceral organs (e.g. defecation reflex after a bowel infection and urinary micturition reflex after a urinary tract infection)
  - Neuroimmune mechanisms:
    - Increased activity of glia which produce pro-inflammatory mediators (e.g. TNF alpha and multiple pro-nociceptive mediators)
    - Upregulation of ions, channels, and receptors (e.g. NMDA, glutamate, TRPV1, serotonin)
    - Visceral inflammation promotes visceral hypersensitivity and epithelial permeability. In IBS, mast cells have been found to secrete NGF, serotonin, proteases, and cytokines which excite/promote visceral hypersensitivity.

Referred visceral pain

- Viscero-viscero, viscero-somatic, and somato-visceral referral can occur because of:
  - Sharing common aspects of their afferent pathways
  - Cross-talk between visceral and/or somatic afferent fibres

- Referred pain can present:
  - Without hyperalgesia/allodynia. This can occur by visceral somatic convergence (i.e. noxious stimuli travelling from internal organs connect with sensory pathway of somatic organs which are close by). For example, some patients with angina experience referred localized sharp pain radiating down the left arm
  - With features of hyperalgesia/allodynia, most likely the result of central sensitization resulting from mechanisms such as convergence facilitation and other mechanisms described. For example, in patients who have passed a renal stone, palpation of the superficial skin/muscles flank can make them feel the visceral pain caused by the renal calculus

Further reading

1. Cohen SP, Mao J. Neuropathic pain: mechanisms and their clinical implications. BMJ 2014;348:f7656
2. Giamberardino MA. Visceral pain. IASP Pain: Clinical Updates 2005;XIII(6):1–6
3. Haanpää M, Treede RD. Diagnosis and classification of neuropathic pain. IASP Pain: Clinical Updates 2010;XVIII(7):1–5
4. Sikandar S, Dickenson AH. Visceral pain: the ins and outs, the ups and downs. Curr Opin Support Palliat Care 2012;6(17):17–26
5. Steeds CE. The anatomy and physiology of pain. Surgery (Oxford) 2013;31(2):49–53

2.6 Peripheral sensitization

Introduction

- Nociception refers to the perception of noxious stimuli
- It is often a protective response and can prevent injury by generating both a reflex withdrawal and enabling behavioural strategies to avoid such stimuli in the future
- One such strategy is the sensitization of the nociceptive system such that the threshold for its activation falls and responses to subsequent inputs are amplified

Peripheral sensitization

- Results in increased/amplified nociceptive signals and subsequent input to the spinal cord following persisting inflammation at the peripheral nociceptors either in the viscera or in the skin
- If there is no tissue injury, the increased sensitivity usually returns to the normal baseline over time
- Nociceptor-induced sensitization of the somatosensory system is adaptive by making the system hyperalert
- Sensitization is the expression of different forms of functional, chemical, and structural alterations in the nervous system that are mediated by the nociceptor input
- The excitation threshold of polymodal nociceptors is reduced to an extent that pain can be elicited by innocuous (normally non-painful) stimuli (allodynia), and pain can be exaggerated and prolonged in response to noxious stimuli (primary hyperalgesia), and it may spread beyond the site of injury (secondary hyperalgesia)
- Triggering factors for peripheral sensitization include exposure to **inflammatory mediators** and **damaged tissue**, which change the response of ion channels through the activation of second messenger systems (see Fig. 2.6.1)

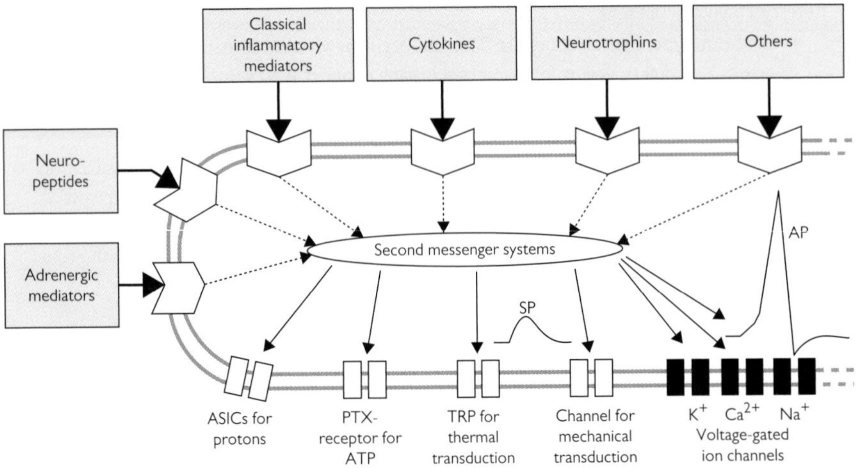

Figure 2.6.1 Schematic drawing of a sensory ending of a nociceptor in the tissue

The membrane at the bottom shows ion channels for transduction (which produce a sensor potential, SP), a voltage-gated Na^+ channel for the generation of action potentials (APs), and voltage-gated K^+ and Ca^{2+} channels that control excitability. Classical inflammatory mediators are bradykinin, prostaglandin E2, 5-hydroxytryptamine, and histamine

ASIC = acid-sensing ion channel; PTX = purinergic ion channel; TRP = transient receptor potential.

Reproduced with permission from Schaible, H-G., Ebersberger, A., Natura, G. (2011). Update on peripheral mechanisms of pain: beyond prostaglandins and cytokines. *Arthritis Research & Therapy*, 13(210). https://doi.org/10.1186/ar3305

Differences between peripheral and central sensitization

- Peripheral and central mechanisms differ in terms of the underlying molecular mechanisms
- Peripheral sensitization causes sensitization of the nociceptive system and causes inflammatory painful hypersensitivity, and this generally requires ongoing peripheral pathology for maintenance
- Peripheral sensitization appears to play a major role in altered heat sensitivity; mechanical sensitivity is a major feature of central sensitization
- Silent nociceptors are recruited and this adds significantly to the inflammatory nociceptive input to the spinal cord. Resting discharges may be induced or increased in nociceptors because of inflammation, providing continuous afferent signals to the spinal cord maintaining peripheral sensitization
- Once peripheral sensitization has occurred, normally non-painful stimuli can cause pain (allodynia)
- Peripheral sensitization often leads to central sensitization
- Central sensitization does not require ongoing peripheral pathology
- In central sensitization, nociceptive neurons in the DHs of the spinal cord are sensitized by peripheral tissue damage or inflammation with subsequent neuroplastic changes, leading to enhanced facilitation and amplification of pain signals, which are responsible for the spatial, temporal, and threshold changes in acute and chronic pain states (possible causative mechanism for chronic pain conditions, including allodynia and hyperalgesia)

Further reading

1. Cioffi CL. Modulation of glycine-mediated spinal neurotransmission for the treatment of chronic pain. J Med Chem 2018;61(7):2652–79

2. Latremoliere A, Woolf CJ. Central sensitization: a generator of pain hypersensitivity by central neural plasticity. J Pain 2009;10(9):895–926
3. Schaible HG. Peripheral and central mechanisms of pain generation. Handb Exp Pharmacol 2007;177:3–28
4. Schaible HG, Ebersberger A, Natura G. Update on peripheral mechanisms of pain: beyond prostaglandins and cytokines. Arthritis Res Ther 2011;13:210

2.7 Central sensitization

Introduction

- Definition: 'Increased responsiveness of nociceptive neurons in the central nervous system to normal or sub-threshold afferent input'
- Central sensitization is an umbrella term used to described changes in the CNS which lead to increased pain perception, due to both increased neuronal excitation and ineffective inhibition
- The most commonly described phenomena related to generating central sensitization are long-term potentiation (LTP) and wind-up at the DH:
  - Wind-up results from progressive, low-frequency (>0.5 Hz) C-fibre stimulation and causes activation of NMDA receptors which increases post-synaptic AP frequency at the DH
  - LTP is elicited by high-frequency stimulation and can lead to longer-lasting changes in the DH synapse. The magnitude of LTP is directly proportional to the magnitude of post-synaptic intracellular Ca^{2+} rise
  - LTP describes a cellular model of synaptic plasticity, where changes in pre- and post-synaptic neuron structure and function increase the synaptic strength. Practically, this is observed as a rise in post-synaptic current for any given pre-synaptic AP
- Central sensitization is likely to occur in the context of an ongoing pain condition. Most patients also commonly experience a host of other symptoms such as fatigue, memory difficulties, mood disturbances, appetite changes, and sleep disturbance (no common underlying mechanism has been identified to explain the associated symptoms)
- Allodynia, hyperalgesia, hyperpathia, hyperaesthesia, or dysaesthesia are clinical features that accompany central sensitization

Aetiology

- The mechanisms that lead to the development and persistence of central sensitization are not clearly understood
- Patients can develop central sensitization after prolonged and/or repeated noxious stimulation of the DH from ongoing nociceptive, visceral, or neuropathic input (e.g. peripheral conditions such as rheumatoid arthritis (RA) and sickle cell disease, or central conditions such as spinal cord injury (SCI) and malignancy)
- In many cases, there is no clear noxious input driving the sensitization process
- Many patients with chronic overlapping pain conditions, which include fibromyalgia, IBS, temporomandibular joint disorder, chronic low back pain, chronic pelvic pain, tension-type headaches, and migraines, do not have a clear demonstrable physical injury to account for their symptoms. Possible aetiologies of central sensitization in these patients include:
  - Single or repetitive stressful events have been linked to acquired or innate changes in nociceptive signal modulation in the spinal cord and the brain
  - Genetic susceptibility to central sensitization
  - Altered function of the immune, chemical, and electrophysiological systems involved in the perception of pain

- Stress, emotions, motivation, cognitions, vigilance, attention, and mood influence the development, persistence, and experience of pain in patients with central sensitization

Long-term potentiation in central sensitization

- LTP is a Ca^{2+}-dependent process which leads to increased excitability in second-order nociceptive neurons at the DH
- LTP affects synapses of A-delta and C-fibres stimulated at 100 Hz
- Changes in both pre- and post-synaptic neurons, such as increase in NTs and numbers/activity of receptors, contribute to the overall increase in synaptic strength
- LTP process is facilitated by NMDA (inotropic glutamate channel receptors) and non-NMDA components (NK1 and 2, group 1 metabotropic glutamate receptors, and voltage T-type Ca^{2+} channels)
- Rises in post-synaptic intracellular Ca^{2+} activate Ca^{2+}-dependent signal transduction pathways (activation of protein kinase A and C, Ca^{2+}–calmodulin-dependent protein kinase A, phospholipase C, inositol triphosphate (IP3) receptors, nitric oxide (NO) synthase), ultimately leading to:
  - Phosphorylation of AMPA receptors and voltage-gated T-type Ca^{2+} channels to lower activation threshold
  - Trafficking and insertion of new AMPA receptors onto post-synaptic membrane
  - Facilitation of Ca^{2+} release from existing intracellular Ca^{2+} stores
- LTP has an early phase, which is independent of *de novo* synthesis and lasts up to 3 hours, and a late phase which involves new protein synthesis and structural synapse changes lasting over 3 hours

Role of wind-up in central sensitization

- AP wind-up results from temporal summation of slow synaptic potentials, which leaves insufficient time for 2nd ONs to come back to the resting potential in between stimuli (>0.2 Hz)
- The slow (0.5 Hz), repetitive, high-threshold noxious stimulation of C-fibres releases the pro-nociceptive peptides SP and CGRP from primary terminals, which activate NK1 and CGRP receptors on 2nd ONs in the DH
- This facilitates activation of NMDA and AMPA receptors by removing the voltage-dependent magnesium (Mg^{2+}) block, boosting post-synaptic AP in a non-linear fashion
- Wind-up is reversible and disappears after seconds at the end of a stimulus train (e.g. 30 seconds of stimulation at 2 Hz)

Role of NMDA receptors in central sensitization

- Glutamate receptors include:
  - Ionotropic receptors: NMDA, AMPA, kainate, and delta
  - Metabotropic receptors: group I (coupled with intracellular Ca^{2+} signalling), and groups II and III (negatively coupled to adenylyl cyclase)
- The binding of glutamate and glycine to their respective NMDA binding sites allows the displacement of Mg^{2+} from the central ion pore, opening the receptor complex to intracellular Ca^{2+} and Na^{+} influx
- The resulting post-synaptic AP activates T-type voltage-gated Ca^{2+} channel opening and activation of multiple Ca^{2+}-dependent pathways (described above in the section of long-term potentiation in central sensitization)
- Glutamate also stimulates the release of other pro-nociceptive substances (SP, CGRP, BDNF in the CNS), which decrease synaptic excitability threshold, sensitize 2nd ONs, and activate

wide-dynamic neurons in the DH by non-nociceptive afferent impulses. Other glutamate-mediated changes of the DH synapse architecture and function include:

- Activation of protein kinase enzymes such as JUN N-terminal kinase, mitogen-activated protein kinases (extracellular signal-regulated kinase, tyrosine kinases such as SRC, LYN, and FYN), and p38, which cause:
  - Recruitment of pro-nociceptive receptors (AMPA, glutamate, kainate, NK1, mGlu)
  - Activation of cyclo-oxygenase (COX)-2 and NO synthase generates prostaglandin E2 (PGE2) and NO which promote the release of glutamate and other nociceptive neuropeptides such as SP
  - Activation of protein kinase G1-mediated phosphorylation of IP3 receptors which recruit glutamate-filled synaptic vesicles close to the cell membrane
- Activation of multiple cell nuclear transcription pathways, e.g. c-fos, cAMP response binding element
- Decreased activity of local inhibitory mechanisms:
  - Ca^{2+}-mediated NO synthase-interacting protein and metabotropic glutamate receptor disassembling post-synaptic complexes
  - GABA and glycine as important inhibitory interneurons. Their function is inhibited by:
    - PGE2-driven inhibition of glycine receptor phosphorylation
    - Nerve injury-induced loss of GABA-mediated post-synaptic currents, with loss of potassium chloride channel function

Role of the immune system in central sensitization

Glial cells

- Constitute 70% of the CNS
- Have a crucial role in maintenance and homeostasis of the CNS
- Injury and/or high-threshold activation of 1st ONs release ATP, chemokines (e.g. CC-chemokine ligand), cytokines, and endogenous danger signals (also called damage-associated molecular patterns) which activate glia
- Activated glial cells like astrocytes produce pro-nociceptive factors, such as excitatory amino acids (e.g. glutamate), cytokines, and PGs, and reduce the availability of inhibitory NTs (GABA, glycine)

Microglial cells

- Under normal conditions, microglia constitute <20% of all spinal glial cells. Nerve injury induces rapid microglia proliferation in the DRGs and spinal cord
- Activated microglia are associated with spinal excitation by several mechanisms:
  - Increased release of pro-nociceptive substances such as chemokines, cytokines, and cytotoxic substances (NO and free radicals)
  - Increased activity of pro-nociceptive receptors (e.g. glutamate receptors such as NMDA)
  - Increased activity of excitatory protein kinase enzymes and transcription pathways
- Studies have identified an immunological mediated 'fear memory' where pro-inflammatory cytokines (IL-1B) secreted by microglia trigger conditioned fear-related memories with associated behavioural responses
- Immuno-modulating therapies, such as minocycline and pentoxifylline, decrease the activity of microglia, with positive results in neuropathic pain pre-clinical models (to date, clinical human studies have not been satisfactory)

Role of endogenous pain modulatory systems in central sensitization

- Neuroimaging studies (fMRI, PET, proton spectroscopy) have identified several potential changes in descending inhibitory pathways, which could be responsible for central sensitization
- Structural and functional changes in the anterior cingulate cortex, prefrontal cortex, primary somatosensory cortex, secondary somatosensory cortex, thalamus, and insula have been identified in patients displaying features of central sensitization
- Dysregulation in the connectivity of different structures of the 'pain matrix' include:
  - Increased connectivity between the insula and other pain-processing regions not usually involved in pain signalling
  - Decreased connectivity between anti-nociceptive regions such as the brainstem, the origin of most descending inhibition pathways
  - Decreased activity of the dorsolateral funiculus—the preferred descending inhibition pathway
  - Increased activity of descending facilitatory pathways
  - Improved connectivity and activity of anti-nociceptive regions, such as PAG, have been found in patients who responded well to to antidepressants that work by serotonin and noradrenaline reuptake inhibition
- In the pain matrix and spinal cord:
  - Reduced activity of inhibitory NTs (GABA, serotonin, dopamine) and inhibitory receptors (e.g. mu-opioid binding and activity). Clinical studies have shown patients who responded to gabapentinoids decreased their central glutaminergic activity
  - Increased activity and concentrations of excitatory NTs like glutamate have been found after noxious and non-noxious stimulation

Role of the endocrine system and autonomic nervous system in central sensitization

- Elevated levels of salivary cortisol and CSF corticotropin-releasing factor point to a dysfunction in hypothalamic–pituitary–adrenal (HPA) axis and the ANS
- Stress modulation has been shown to normalize cortisol and corticotropin-releasing factor levels in patients who underwent non-pharmacological psychological interventions, as part of their pain management

Further reading

1. Harte SE, Harris RE, Clauw DJ. The neurobiology of central sensitisation. J Appl Behav Res 2018;23:e12137. https://doi.org/10.1111/jabr.12137
2. International Association for the Study of Pain. IASP terminology. Pain terms. Central sensitization. 2017. https://www.iasp-pain.org/Education/Content.aspx?ItemNumber=1698#Centralsensitisation

Neurotransmitters and Receptors

Ramy Mottaleb, Nofil Mulla, Maria Stasiowska, and Matthew Wong

CONTENTS

3.1 Neurotransmitters

Introduction

- NTs facilitate signal transmission between nerve cells and non-neuronal targets such as muscle cells and glands
- NTs are released from pre-synaptic terminals into a synaptic cleft to interact with corresponding receptors on pre-/post-synaptic membranes
- Termination of transmission occurs when the NT is removed from the cleft by enzymatic breakdown or uptake into pre-/post-synaptic cells
- NTs are synthesized in pre-synaptic terminals, and packaged and stored in vesicles concentrated at the nerve terminal. APs stimulate Ca^{2+} influx and cause vesicles to move and release their contents into the synaptic cleft by exocytosis

Acetylcholine (ACh)

Synthesis

- From choline and acetyl coenzyme A (acetyl-CoA) by choline acetyltransferase

Metabolism

- By acetylcholinesterase enzyme into the inactive metabolites choline and acetate at the neuromuscular junction (NMJ) and cholinergic synaptic clefts

Distribution

- In pre-synaptic terminals of motor neurons, pre- and post-ganglionic nerve fibres of the parasympathetic nervous system, and preganglionic nerve fibres of the sympathetic nervous system (SNS) and brain (mesopontine tegmentum, basal ganglia, neocortex, and hippocampus)

Receptors

- Nicotinic receptors are ligand-gated ion channels permeable to Na^+, K^+, and Ca^{2+}, located at the NMJ and CNS. Activation cause Ca^{2+} influx which leads to myocyte contraction or a post-synaptic AP, respectively
- Muscarinic receptors are G-protein coupled receptors (GPCRs) in the CNS and ANS supplying the heart, lungs, gastrointestinal (GI) tract, and sweat glands:
  - M1, M3, and M5 receptors (G-q) stimulate phospholipase C to generate IP3 and diacylglycerol (DAG), increasing intracellular Ca^{2+} and causing cell excitation
  - M2 and M4 receptors (G-i) inhibit adenylyl cyclase and reduce intracellular cAMP and Ca^{2+}

Effects

- NMJ: contraction of smooth and striated muscles
- Parasympathetic nervous system: lacrimation, salivation, digestion, urination, defecation, and sexual arousal
- SNS: activation of sweat glands
- CNS: arousal, attention, and memory formation
- Other: endothelial muscarinic receptors stimulate production of NO, causing vasodilation

Endorphins

Synthesis

- Neuropeptides produced from pro-opiomelanocortin

Metabolism

- Metabolized by peptidase enzymes (aminopeptidases, angiotensin-converting enzymes, and serine proteases)

Distribution

- Produced primarily in the anterior pituitary gland; however, the precursor pro-opiomelanocortin is extensively distributed in the CNS

Receptors

- Mu-opioid receptor agonists activate G-inhibitory proteins, reducing intracellular cAMP and decreasing intracellular Ca^{2+}

Mechanism of action

- Produced in the pituitary gland in times of stress, released into the bloodstream, and distributed throughout the body, causing:
  - Parasympathetic nervous system—reduction of pain signal transmission at the DH
  - CNS—activation of descending inhibition from the amygdala, PAG, reticular formation, and RVM. Also works by increasing dopamine levels in the Mesolimbic Reward System, causing pleasure and reward

Gamma-aminobutyric acid (GABA)

Synthesis

- Formed in pre-synaptic terminals of the CNS
- The precursor glutamine, stored in glial cells, is converted to glutamate and GABA by glutamic acid decarboxylase (GAD) and pyridoxal phosphate (cofactor)

- GABA is packaged into vesicles by vesicular GABA transporter (VGAT) and stored in inhibitory nerve terminals
- Excess GABA is broken down in nerve terminals by GABA transaminases (GABA-T) into succinic semialdehyde and glutamate

Metabolism

- Removed from the synaptic cleft by transporter proteins into pre-synaptic terminals of inhibitory neurons and adjoining astrocytes
  - Reuptake into a GABA terminal via GABA transporter (GAT) type 1 (GAT-1) repackages GABA into vesicles using VGAT or breaks it down via GABA-T
  - Reuptake into a glial cell via GAT-1 or GAT-3 transporters causes intracellular breakdown via GABA-T and conversion to glutamate

Distribution

- Throughout the CNS

Receptors

- GABA-A: fast-acting ligand-gated ion channel on post-synaptic nerve terminals. Activation causes influx of chloride and efflux of K^+ ions and hyperpolarizes cell membranes, reducing AP transmission
- GABA-A rho (also known as GABA-C): ligand-gated chloride channel and a subtype of GABA-A receptors in the retina
- GABA-B: inhibitory G-protein reduces intracellular Ca^{2+} by inhibiting adenylyl cyclase and promoting K^+ efflux. Slower than ligand-gated GABA-A, mediates both post-synaptic and pre-synaptic transmission

Mechanism of action

- Principal inhibitory NT in the CNS; reduces neural tone and regulates muscle tension

Serotonin

Synthesis

- Serotonin, or 5-HT (5-hydroxytryptamine), is a monoamine produced in the enterochromaffin cells of the GI tract where it acts locally facilitating peristalsis, or systemically causing platelet aggregation and vasoconstriction
- In the CNS, 5-HT is produced from L-tryptophan (amino acid) transported from the blood to the brain by facilitated transport. L-tryptophan is converted to 5-hydroxytryptophan in serotonergic cells by tryptophan hydroxylase, and finally to 5-HT via L-amino acid decarboxylase

Metabolism

- Serotonin is removed from the synaptic cleft by serotonin transporters. Once in the pre-synaptic nerve terminal, 5-HT is metabolized by monoamine oxidase (MAO) and aldehyde dehydrogenase into 5-hydroxyindoleacetic acid (5-HIAA), and is then excreted in the urine

Distribution

- CNS: 5-HT is produced in the raphe nuclei and reticular formation, the cell bodies of which project into the spinal cord, cerebellum, and most areas of the brain
- Gut: food stimulates enterochromaffin cells in the gut lumen to release 5-HT, which stimulates peristalsis
- 5-HT stimulates the chemoreceptor trigger zone, causing emesis

Receptors

- 5-HT1 and 5-HT5 are inhibitory GPCRs and reduce intracellular levels of cAMP and Ca^{2+} in post-synaptic neurons
- 5-HT2, 5-HT4, 5-HT6, and 5-HT7 are excitatory GPCRs and increase the levels of intracellular cAMP and Ca^{2+} in post-synaptic neurons
- 5-HT3 are ligand-gated cation channels, causing cell depolarization and excitation

Mechanism of action

- CNS: controls mood, memory processing, sleep, and cognition. 5-HT3 causes vomiting, anxiety, and seizures
- 5-HT also mediates gut motility, emesis, vascular smooth muscle tone, and bone metabolism

Noradrenaline

Synthesis

- L-tyrosine is actively transported into post-ganglionic sympathetic axons and converted to DOPA by tyrosine hydroxylase (rate-limiting step). DOPA is converted to dopamine by DOPA decarboxylase and transported into vesicles by vesicular monoamine transporter (VMAT). Inside vesicles, dopamine is converted to noradrenaline by dopamine-β hydroxylase
- Adrenaline is synthesized in cells of the adrenal medulla. The synthesis process is the same as for noradrenaline, with the added final conversion of noradrenaline to adrenaline via phenylethanolamine-N-methyltransferase

Metabolism

- Noradrenaline is removed from the synaptic cleft via pre-synaptic transporter reuptake (UPTAKE 1). Some diffuses into the bloodstream and is taken up by extraneural cells (UPTAKE 2) such as the myocardium and smooth muscles
- Inside the cells, noradrenaline is either repackaged into vesicles by VMAT or broken down by MAO and catechol-O-methyltransferase (COMT) into metanephrine, dihydroxymandelic acid, and finally vanillylmandelic acid

Distribution

- SNS: noradrenaline is the primary NT of post-ganglionic sympathetic nerve fibres. It is also released from the adrenal medulla into the systemic circulation, acting like a sympathetic hormone rather than like a NT
- CNS: the locus coeruleus contains noradrenergic neurons and projects throughout the brain (brainstem, cerebellum, hypothalamus, thalamus, amygdala, neocortex) and spinal cord

Receptors

- GCPRs on cell membranes of the CNS, ANS, and target organs
  - α-2 receptors reduce intracellular cAMP and Ca^{2+}. Located on pre-synaptic terminals of the CNS and ANS, they reduce pre-synaptic NT release
  - α-1 and β-1, -2, and -3 receptors increase intracellular Ca^{2+} by activating phospholipase C, increasing levels of DAG and IP3 (α-1 receptors) or cAMP (β-1, -2, and -3 receptors)

Mechanism of action

- Stimulates the CNS to maintain alertness, arousal, and memory. Mediates descending inhibition via α-2 receptors in the pre- and post-synaptic neurons at the DH

- Outside of the CNS, noradrenaline mediates sympathetic nerve function. α-1 receptors on smooth muscles stimulate vascular, sphincter, and visceral contraction. β-receptors are widely distributed and mediate chronotropy, inotropy, bronchodilation, and lipolysis

Prostaglandins

Synthesis

- Produced by most nucleated cells in the body from essential fatty acids
- The main precursor arachidonic acid (AA) is synthesized from diglycerols and phospholipids found in cell membranes, by phospholipase C and A2
- AA is processed via the lipoxygenase pathway into leukotrienes, or the COX pathway into PGs
- Enzymes in the COX pathway include tonically produced cyclo-oxygenase 1 (COX1) to maintain normal baseline PG production, and cyclo-oxygenase 2 (COX2) induced by stress and inflammation
- AA is converted to prostaglandin H2 (PH2) and then into PGD2, PGE2 (dinoprostone), PGF2, PGI2 (prostacyclin), and TXA2 (thromboxane)

Metabolism

- Taken into cells by specific carrier proteins and inactivated in the cytoplasm by 15-hydroxyprostaglandin dehydrogenase

Distribution

- Produced throughout the body
- Final conversion into specific PG is at the effector site:
  - PGD2: mast cells and brain
  - PGE2: smooth muscle, brain, platelets
  - PGF2: smooth muscle
  - PGI2: smooth muscle, platelets, CNS, parasympathetic nervous system
  - TXA2: platelets

Receptors

- GCPRs located on target cell membranes
- Receptor activation can cause either cell stimulation or inhibition, depending on the receptor type (Gs/Gq or Gi):
  - TXA2, PGD2, and PGE2 have inhibitory and excitatory receptors
  - PGI2 and PGF2 have only excitatory receptors

Mechanism of action

- Contribute to pain and inflammation; control systemic blood vessel and smooth muscle tone (uterus, GI tract, bronchi, gut, renal vessels), GI secretion, renal function, platelet aggregation, adipogenesis, and protein synthesis
- In the parasympathetic nervous system and spinal cord, PGs facilitate peripheral and central sensitization:
  - Reduce nociceptor activation threshold
  - Increase nociceptor availability on cell membranes
  - Increase sensory nerve ending growth and sprouting
  - Reduce inhibitory interneuron activity

- In the brain, PGs modulate pre-synaptic release and post-synaptic effects of other NTs (dopamine, serotonin, and noradrenaline)
- PGE2 has a direct effect on the hypothalamus to enhance sympathetic outflow and causes fever

Further reading

1. Neurotransmitters and neuromodulators. In: Barrett KE, Barman SM, Boitano S, Brooks H (eds). Ganong's Review of Medical Physiology. 23rd edition, 2010; pp. 129–47. London: McGraw-Hill.
2. Ricciotti E, FitzGerald GA. Prostaglandins and inflammation. Arterioscler Thromb Vasc Biol 2011;31:986–1000

3.2 Opioid receptors

Introduction

- Opioid receptors are inhibitory GPCRs
- The term 'opiate' refers to all naturally occurring substances with morphine-like properties derived from the natural alkaloid *Papaver somniferum* (examples are morphine, codeine, and thebaine)
- The term 'opioid' is a general term used for synthetic and natural substances that have an affinity for opioid receptors. These include all endogenous neuropeptides (endorphins, enkephalins, and dynorphins), as well as exogenous substances (fentanyl, alfentanil, pethidine, etc.)

Structure of opioid receptors

- Glycoproteins found in cell membranes at multiple sites
- Highest concentrations are found in the PAG (brain) and SG (spinal cord)
- Lower concentrations are found in other areas such as the digestive tract and joints
- Members of a large superfamily of GPCRs with:
  - Seven-transmembrane receptors
  - Extracellular N-terminus
  - Intracellular C-terminus
  - Heterotrimeric complexes with $\alpha/\beta/\gamma$ subunits
  - Activated by endogenous peptides, as well as exogenous agonists

Molecular mechanism of opioid receptors

- Endogenous or exogenous opioids bind to the opioid receptor, producing:
  - Pre-synaptic terminal: inhibitory effect (Gi) closes voltage-gated Ca^{2+} channels and stimulation of K^+ efflux, causing hyperpolarization. Adenylyl cyclase is inhibited, reducing cAMP and preventing the release of pro-nociceptive NTs (noradrenaline, ACh, dopamine) and other mediators such as SP, CGRP, etc.
  - Post-synaptic terminal: K^+ channels open and hyperpolarize post-synaptic neurons, inhibiting neural transmission
- GABA inhibition pre-synaptically increases dopamine in the nucleus accumbens, initially leading to pleasure/reward. After repeated exogenous opioid exposure, the symptoms of pleasure

diminish and exogenous opioid administration prevents opioid withdrawal symptoms (see 4.5 Tolerance, dependence, addiction, and pseudoaddiction, p. 87)
- NMDA antagonism activates serotonin/noradrenergic pathways

Intrinsic receptor activity of opioid receptors

- Opioids can be classified according to their intrinsic activity at that receptor site:
  - Full agonists interact with the receptor to produce a maximal response, e.g. morphine
  - Partial agonists bind to receptors to produce a partial response, irrespective of the dose administered, e.g. buprenorphine
  - Antagonists bind to the receptor but produce no response, e.g. naloxone
  - Mixed agonists/antagonists act as agonists on one or more receptor subtypes and as antagonists at one or more subtypes, e.g. nalbuphine, butorphanol

Opioid receptor subtypes

- There are at least 12 pharmacologically defined opioid receptor subtypes classified
- Only four opioid receptors have been cloned. Opioid receptors were named based upon their original discovery by the International Union of Pharmacology. Various nomenclatures have been devised since the discovery to name these receptors, some based upon the discovery of 'new' opioid receptors
- The three primary receptors that are antagonized by naloxone are named as mu for morphine, delta for vas deferens, and kappa for ketocyclazocine. They have 65–70% sequence homology

Mu opioid receptor

- Other names: MOR, OP3, MOP
- Endogenous ligand: met-enkephalin, leu-enkephalin, β-endorphin
- Prototype agonist: morphine
- Subtypes: μ1, μ2, μ3
- Effects of receptor activation:
  - μ1 causes supraspinal and spinal analgesia, immune euphoria, urinary retention, locomotion, memory/learning, hypothermia, and hormone secretion
  - μ2 produces supraspinal and spinal analgesia, respiratory depression, tolerance, constipation, nausea, vomiting, urinary retention, pruritus, miosis, anorexia, euphoria, and dependence
  - μ3: several roles, including NO release

Kappa opioid receptor

- Other names: KOR, OP2, KOP
- Endogenous ligand: β-endorphin, dynorphin
- Prototype agonist: ketocyclazocine
- Subtypes: κ_1, κ_2, κ_3
- Effects of receptor activation: spinal analgesia, hallucinations, dysphoria, sedation, oliguria, tolerance, dependence, hyperalgesia, neuroendocrine, slowing of GI transit, less respiratory depression compared to mu receptors, oliguria (inhibits antidiuretic hormone (ADH) secretion), and immunological (see 7.1 Overview of opioids, p. 119)

Delta opioid receptor

- Other names: DOR, OP1, DOP
- Endogenous ligand: leu-enkephalin, met-enkephalin, β-endorphin
- Prototype agonist: ala-leu-enkephalin
- Subtypes: δ_1, δ_2
- Effects of receptor activation: supraspinal > spinal analgesia without respiratory depression, facilitates the activity of mu receptor, *thermoregulation,* mood, seizures, dysphoria, psychomimetic effects, and physical dependence

Orphanin FQ (nociceptin) receptor

- Other names: NOR, OP4, NOP
- Endogenous ligand: orphanin FQ peptide
- Effects of receptor activation: analgesia, associated with less analgesic tolerance, drug reward. Also involved in modulation of pain, behaviour, learning, and memory
- Not antagonized by naloxone

Changes in opioid receptors with prolonged exposure to opioids

- Decreased receptor activation (desensitization)
- Increased receptor phosphorylation
- Receptor internalization via endocytosis
- Activation of intracellular pro-nociceptive regulatory proteins/enzymes:
  - Examples: GPCR kinases, β-arrestin-2, mitogen-activated phosphorylation pathways
  - β-arrestin-2 knockout mice have been found to have less opioid receptor desensitization, decreased activity of opioid GCPR kinases, enhanced analgesia, and less anti-nociceptive tolerance by opioids. Buprenorphine is associated with less tolerance than other opioids and has been found not to bind/recruit β-arrestin-2 receptors
- Reduction/inhibition of intracellular regulatory proteins/enzymes:
  - Example: opioids cause analgesia by inhibiting adenylyl cyclase which inhibits cAMP (cAMP promotes the release of pro-nociceptive NTs and mediators). With prolonged exposure to opioids, inhibition caused by opioids on adenylyl cyclase decreases
- Activation of glial cells (astrocytes) by opioids binding to Toll-like receptors (TLRs), mu, and kappa receptors activates/increases neuronal signalling and secretion of pro-inflammatory cytokines (TNF/IL1, IL6)
- Prolonged exposure to opioids has effects on other receptors, with inhibitory actions as NMDA–$\alpha 2\delta$-1 receptors. Animal studies blocking the NMDA–$\alpha 2\delta$-1 interaction has reduced opioid-induced hyperalgesia (OIH) and opioid tolerance receptor activation
- The above mechanisms are involved in opioid tolerance and OIH (see 2.5 Pathophysiology of nociceptive, visceral, and neuropathic pain, p. 57; 2.6 Peripheral sensitization, p. 61; 4.1 Immunology, inflammation, glia, and pain, p. 79; 4.5 Tolerance, dependence, addiction, and pseudoaddiction, p. 87)

Further reading

1. Fine PG, Portenoy RK. A Clinical Guide to Opioid Analgesia. 2004. New York: McGraw Hill
2. Trescot AM, Datta S, Lee M, Hansen H. Opioid pharmacology. Pain Physician 2008;11(2 Suppl):S133–53

3.3 Non-opioid receptors

Introduction

- Receptors are proteins found throughout the peripheral and central nervous systems
- Activation of receptors causes changes within the cell or tissue
- By targeting key receptors involved in the transmission of the pain pathways, we are able to potentially offer patients better pain management

Transient receptor potential vanilloid receptor 1 (TRPV1)

- Structure: non-selective cation channel
- Location: predominantly in the periphery in nociceptors but can also be found centrally
- Activators of TRPV1 receptor: heat, physical and chemical stimulation (Ca^{2+} and Mg^{2+}). Initially, upon stimulation, there is increased sensitization with hyperalgesia. Prolonged exposure typically causes desensitization of TRPV1
- Function: regulation of body temperature and detection of scalding heat
- Drugs acting on the TRPV1 receptor: capsaicin

GABA (γ-aminobutyric acid) receptor

- Structure: there are two main classes. $GABA_A$ are ligand-gated ion channels and $GABA_B$ are GCPRs
- Location: CNS, particularly the brain. Approximately 20–50% of all synaptic connections in the brain contain $GABA_A$ receptors
- Activators of the GABA receptor: GABA is the endogenous ligand
- Function: GABA is the chief inhibitory NT within the CNS, and inhibits neurons to which it binds
- Drugs acting on the GABA receptor:
  - $GABA_A$: benzodiazepines (BZDs), ethanol, anaesthetic agents, e.g. barbiturates, volatile agents
  - $GABA_B$: baclofen
- GABAPENTINOIDS DO NOT DIRECTLY ACT ON THE GABA RECEPTOR!

N-methyl-D-aspartate (NMDA) receptor

- Structure: glutamate receptor and ion channel protein
- Location: pre-synaptic terminals and post-synaptic excitatory neurons
- Activators of the NMDA receptor: glutamate, glycine, or serine binds to the receptor, allowing positively charged ions to flow through the membrane
- Function: Ca^{2+} flux through the NMDA receptor is important for synaptic plasticity. It plays a role in wind-up and central sensitization
- Drugs acting on the NMDA receptor: ketamine, nitrous oxide (N_2O), phencyclidine, Mg^{2+}

Cannabinoid receptor (CBR)

- Structure: GCPR with two subtypes (CB-1 and CB-2)
- Location:
  - CB-1: one of the most common GPCRs in the brain (particularly in the basal ganglia and limbic system). Also found in the lungs, liver, and kidneys
  - CB-2: located predominantly peripherally in the immune system, haematopoietic cells, spleen, and peripheral nerve terminals

- Activators of the CBR: can be synthetic, plant-based, or endocannabinoids
    - Tetrahydrocannabinol (THC): primary psychoactive component and acts by binding to CB-1
    - Cannabidiol (CBD): non-psychotropic, little affinity to CB-1 or 2 receptors, has neuroprotective and anti-inflammatory effects, modulates ascending and descending pathways
- Function:
    - CB-1: appetite, nausea and vomiting, mood, pain, memory
    - CB-2: inflammation, pain modulation
- Drugs acting on CBRs: nabilone, Sativex®, CBD oil

Alpha-2 receptor

- Structure: GCPRs with three subtypes (α-2A, α-2B, and α-2C)
- Location: α-2A and 2C subtypes are found mainly in the CNS. α-2B receptors are found mainly on vascular smooth muscle, but also in the CNS
- Activators of α-2 receptors: endogenous agonists include noradrenaline and adrenaline as part of a feedback loop. All three subtypes have been shown to inhibit adenylyl cyclase, which decreases cAMP, causing hyperpolarization of noradrenergic neurons. This leads to neuronal suppression and inhibition of noradrenaline release, reducing ascending noradrenergic pathways
- Function:
    - Suppression of ascending noradrenergic pathways causes sedation and hypnosis
    - Stimulation of α-2 receptors in the DH inhibits nociceptors and the release of SP
    - The negative feedback loop may cause reductions in HR and BP, and attenuation of the sympathetic stress response
- Drugs acting on α-2 receptor: clonidine, tizanidine, dexmedetomidine

Serotonin (or 5-HT) receptors

- Structure: seven receptor subtypes. All are GCPRs, except 5-HT3 which is a ligand-gated ion channel
- Location: blood vessels, central and peripheral nervous system, platelets, smooth muscle, and GI tract
- Activators of serotonin receptor: serotonin
- Function:
    - Pain modulation: has a role in both excitatory and inhibitory pain pathways, as well as contributes to hyperalgesia
    - Receptor activation modulates the release of SP and NTs such as glutamate, GABA, dopamine, noradrenaline, and ACh. 5-HT1A, 5-HT2A, 5-HT3, and 5-HT7 receptors are implicated in most with pain states
- Other functions include mood regulation, emesis, cardiovascular and respiratory autoregulation, addiction, appetite, and sexual behaviour
- Drugs acting on serotonin receptors:
    - Atypical antipsychotics: olanzapine, risperidone
    - Tricyclic antidepressants (TCAs): amitriptyline, nortriptyline
    - Selective serotonin reuptake inhibitors (SSRIs) and selective serotonin and noradrenaline reuptake inhibitor antidepressants: citalopram, duloxetine, fluoxetine
    - Opioids: tramadol

Glycine receptor

- Structure: ligand-gated ion channels
- Location: CNS, including the brainstem and spinal cord. Predominantly post-synaptic
- Activators of the glycine receptor: glycine opens the glycine receptor, causing an influx of chloride ions, which hyperpolarizes the post-synaptic cell, inhibiting neuronal firing
- Function:
    - Mediates fast inhibitory neurotransmission
    - Controls a variety of motor and sensory functions, including vision and hearing
    - In laminae 1 and 2 of the DH, it inhibits the propagation of nociceptive signals to higher brain regions
- Drugs acting on the glycine receptor: cannabinoids

Further reading

1. Steeds CE. The anatomy and physiology of pain. Surgery 2009;27(12):507–51
2. Yam MF, Loh YC, Tan CS, et al. General pathways of pain sensation and the major neurotransmitters involved in pain regulation. Int J Mol Sci 2018;19:2164

CHAPTER 4

Neurobiology of Pain

Bethany Fitzmaurice, Senthil Jayaseelan, Gustav Jirikowski, Sandeep Kapur, Manish Mittal, and Alifia Tameem

CONTENTS

4.1 Immunology, inflammation, glia, and pain

Definitions

- **Glial cells:** most abundant cells in the CNS, providing support to neurons, but not conducting electrical impulses, e.g. oligodendrocytes, astrocytes, ependymal cells, Schwann cells, microglia, satellite cells
- **Microglia:** these are quiescent immune cells of the CNS; when activated, can phagocytose, present antigen to T cells, and produce cytokines
- **Astrocytes:** specialized glial cells of the nervous system that perform multiple homeostatic functions for the survival and maintenance of the neurovascular unit. Astrocytes have neuroprotective, angiogenic, immunomodulatory, neurogenic, antioxidant properties, and modulate synaptic function
- **Neuropathic pain:** pain due to lesion or disease of the somatosensory nervous system

Common causes of neuropathic pain

- Post-herpetic neuralgia (PHN) after a herpes zoster infection, painful diabetic polyneuropathy, trigeminal neuralgia, post-amputation pain, persistent post-operative or post-traumatic pain, pain in cancer patients and HIV patients

Association between activation of microglial cells in response to nerve injury and development and maintenance of neuropathic pain

- Multiple studies have suggested that the immune system is involved not only in neuropathic pain conditions, but also in most chronic pain conditions, and drives the acute to chronic pain transition
- Opioids activate glia, which are involved in opioid tolerance and OIH. Mu-opioid agonists activate innate immune receptors, and not the classic opioid receptors, creating neuroinflammation by binding to myeloid differentiation protein 2 (MD-2), an accessory

protein of Toll-like receptor 4 (TLR4). This induces TLR4 oligomerization and triggers pro-inflammation

What happens then?

At site of nerve injury

1. Nerve injury results in recruitment of resident and blood macrophages with the chemokines CCL2 and 3
2. Activated macrophages and denervated Schwann cells secrete metalloproteases, which attack the basal lamina of endoneural blood vessels, causing interruption of the blood–nerve barrier
3. Nerve injury causes the release of vasoactive mediators from injured axons, i.e. SP, CGRP, bradykinin, and NO, causing **hyperaemia and swelling of neurons**
4. These processes further support the invasion of macrophages, T lymphocytes, and mast cells at the lesion site and DRG, and in the ventral and dorsal roots of the spinal cord
5. Within minutes of injury, neuregulin, a growth and differentiation factor on the axonal membrane, induces activation of ERBB2 (a tyrosine kinase receptor), which helps in **Schwann cell proliferation**
6. Schwann cells release the chemical signals NGF and glial cell line-derived neurotrophic factor (GDNF), which promote axonal growth and remyelination, and also **sensitize nociceptors**, initiating pain in response to nerve injury
7. Schwann cells, macrophages, mast cells, and neutrophils release pro-inflammatory cytokines ILs (1β, 6, 12, 18), TNF, and interferon gamma (IFN-γ), which cause **axonal damage and modulate nociceptor sensitivity**

At dorsal root ganglion

1. Peripheral nerve injury triggers the release of the chemokines CCL1 (fractalkine) and CCL2, which further **triggers the invasion of macrophages**, supported by locally present macrophages and T cells
2. The density of macrophages increases in the DRG 1 week after injury and remains elevated for at least 3 months, after which macrophages then turn into active phagocytes, removing debris from injured sensory neurons
3. This persistence of the immune response in the DRG contrasts with the peripheral reaction which ends with removal of myelin debris during Wallerian degeneration
4. The signalling pathway that modulates neuronal and macrophage function in the DRG involves purinergic (P2) receptors, activated by ATP release from injured nerves and surrounding tissue. Nociceptors predominantly express P2X and P2Y receptors in macrophages
5. These P2 receptors are responsible for increasing nociceptor sensitivity and activity, **causing hypersensitivity to mechanical and thermal stimuli**, also mediated by voltage-gated Na^+ channels, which are activated by cytokines (TNF, IL1, IL6) released by macrophage activation
6. The cytokine IL6, in association with NGF and neurotrophin-3 from satellite cells, is also responsible for **triggering sprouting of sympathetic fibres** around large-diameter sensory neurons (A-beta)

In spinal cord

1. Microglial cells are key in the inflammatory response to direct injury of the CNS inflicted by trauma, ischaemia, autoimmune disorders (multiple sclerosis (MS)), and neurodegenerative disorders

2. Microglia form dense clusters around the dorsal and ventral horns after neuronal injury. The process involves **recruitment and activation** of microglia by different pathways, leading to neural inflammation
3. Three signalling pathways mediate **recruitment of microglia and circulating macrophages** at the spinal cord level:
   - Chemokine fractalkine, a neuronal transmembrane glycoprotein
   - CCL2
   - Mammalian Toll-like receptors (TLRs) involved in initiation of innate immunity against invading pathogens
4. Activation of microglia involves binding of ATP, released from injured primary and DH neurons, to the purinergic receptor P2RX4
5. Activation of microglia initiates the process involved in **central sensitization**:
   - Release of BDNF which prompts reversal of inhibitory GABA currents, causing **mechanical allodynia**
   - Enhanced spontaneous and evoked excitatory post-synaptic potential (EPSP)
   - Glutamate release in the DH, **activating NMDA receptors**
   - Increased synthesis of lysosomal proteases, ILs, and TNF, which cause direct modulation of the DH in the spinal cord
   - Proliferation and activation of astrocytes, which are responsible for **prolonged or sustained sensitization of the DH**

New treatment opportunities

1. Currently, most anti-neuropathic drugs aim to reduce the excitability of neurons in the peripheral nervous system or CNS, without affecting glial plasticity, which is responsible for initiation of the cascade, leading to the development of established neuropathic pain
2. Current therapy targeting glial cells mainly involves anti-inflammatory (propentophylline, pentoxyfylline, methotrexate, minocycline) or anti-metabolic (fluorocitrate, fluoroacetate), which can be counterproductive as it may affect normal glial cells, which have vital housekeeping and surveillance functions
3. More targeted interventions aimed at purinergic receptors and CBRs, mitogen-activated protein kinase (MAPK), TNF, and ILs
4. CBR2 receptors are expressed primarily by immune cells, including microglia and astrocytes, and may be the target to avoid glial plasticity

Conclusion

- Contribution of immune and glial cells to the development of acute and persistent neuropathic pain challenges the concept of neuronal involvement only in the development of neuropathic pain
- Animal studies direct us towards the concept of neuronal inflammation, and further studies are required to correlate the inflammatory markers in the periphery, DRG, and DH with the incidence of acute and chronic neuropathic pain
- Therapies directed at prevention of neuropathic pain after injury by modulating neuroglial plasticity may be the target for future treatment strategy

Further reading

1. Gosselin R-D, Suter MR, Ji R-R, et al. Glial cells and chronic pain. Neuroscientist 2010;16(5):519–31
2. Scholz J, Woolf CJ. The neuropathic pain triad: neurons, immune cells and glia. Nature Neurosci 2007;10(11):1361–8

4.2 Genetics and pain

Background

- Pain is a very subjective experience, and everyone is unique in their perception and response to pain
- As a complex trait, pain is polygenic and shaped by environmental pressures
- Genetic contribution to pain perception is about 50%

Basic overview

What is a gene?

- Genes are parts of deoxyribonucleic acid (DNA) molecules that contain the information used by cells to construct protein molecules. They code for proteins and it is these proteins that carry out work of the cell such as enzymatic action, motility, and electrical impulse generation

What is a pain gene?

- A 'pain gene' is a gene for which there are one or more polymorphisms, i.e. variations in the sequence of DNA base pairs that affect the expression or functioning of its protein product in a way that affects pain response

How do DNA polymorphisms affect pain?

- In the human genome, at least 99.9% of a base pair sequence is identical from one person to the next. The remaining 0.1% represents about 3 000 000 base pairs that might differ amongst individuals
- DNA polymorphisms can be in the form of single nucleotide polymorphism (SNP) or sequence polymorphism occurring in the sequence of DNA base pairs that actually encodes the protein, i.e. in exons, which might destroy the protein's function completely or alter it in more subtle ways, including enhancing its function
- Sequence polymorphisms can also occur in nearby regions of the DNA molecule that regulate the 'expression' of a pain gene
- Such variants might affect how much of the gene product is synthesized without having any effect on the structure or function of the protein product itself
- A DNA sequence polymorphism can also affect the 'bar code' address of a gene's protein product, the part of the sequence that tells the cell where specifically to send this particular protein molecule
- If the protein molecule is not sent to the correct part of the cell ('trafficking error'), pain processing may not work properly

Examples

$Na_v1.7$ Na^+ channel (*SCN9A*)—protein with direct relevance to excitability of sensory neurons

- Erythromelalgia—gain-of-function mutation
- Paroxysmal extreme pain disorder—gain-of-function mutation
- Congenital insensitivity to pain—loss-of-function mutation

Fibromyalgia

- Specific genetic polymorphisms involving the serotonin 5-HT2A receptor, serotonin transporter, dopamine 4 receptor, and COMT have been reported more frequently in patients with fibromyalgia

Finding the pain genes

Linkage analysis

- Useful in large families where some individuals develop the painful condition and others do not
- Useful in single-gene mutation of major effect ('Mendelian gene')—Charcot–Marie–Tooth (CMT) neuropathy, erythromelalgia
- Limited to diseases that arise spontaneously and not well suited to painful conditions that arise following injury or disease such as low back pain, diabetic neuropathy, or phantom limb pain

Association studies

- Comparing the genomes of large cohorts that differ in the trait of interest but are as similar as possible with regard to other parameters such as environment and ethnic background
- Two alternative strategies: (1) testing for allelic differences in a small number of 'candidate genes' selected on the basis of prior hypotheses on where the differences might lie; (2) searching for potential differences in all genes and regulatory regions in a hypothesis-free manner (genome-wide association studies (GWAS))

Use of genetics

- Diagnostic and prognostic information—a genetic polymorphism may indicate that a particular individual is prone to post-surgical pain and this information can be useful to perioperative physicians and surgeons
- Pharmacogenetics—study of genetic differences in response to analgesic drugs can help in individualizing pain treatment to specific patients
- Contribution to patient–clinician relationship—since pain is very subjective, genetics may help in better understanding without labelling people as malingerers or complainers
- Understanding of pain mechanisms

Further reading

1. Devor M, Tracey I. Pain 2012 refresher courses. 14th World Congress on Pain, 2012. Seattle, WA: IASP Press
2. LaCroix-Fralish ML, Mogil JS. Progress in genetic studies of pain and analgesia. Annu Rev Pharmacol Toxicol 2009;49:97–121
3. Neilsen CS, Stubhaug A, Price DD, et al. Individual differences in pain sensitivity: genetic and environmental contributions. Pain 2008;136:21–9

4.3 Gender and pain

Background

- Women and men differ in their responses to pain, with increased pain sensitivity and risk of clinical pain commonly observed amongst women
- The differences in clinical and experimental pain are attributed to several biopsychosocial mechanisms

Gender differences in clinical pain and experimentally induced pain

- Women report pain more frequently than men
- The population prevalence of several common chronic pain conditions is greater in women than in men, including fibromyalgia, migraine, chronic tension-type headache, IBS, temporomandibular disorders, and interstitial cystitis
- Regarding pain severity, the findings are less consistent and are likely influenced by multiple methodological factors, including selection biases in clinical studies and the potential for sex differences in the effects of pain treatments
- The direction of sex differences in pain responses across multiple experimental stimulus modalities and pain measures is highly consistent, with women showing greater sensitivity than men
- However, the magnitude (and statistical significance) of sex differences varies across measures, as it does across published studies

Gender differences in response to pain interventions

- Greater 'analgesic' effects were observed for women using patient-controlled analgesia (PCA) with morphine
- In clinical studies, women exhibit greater analgesia than men in response to mixed action opioids, e.g. butorphanol, nalbuphine, pentazocine
- Several studies suggest that differences in pain treatment between women and men are influenced by both patient and provider characteristics, an effect which may lead to disparities in pain management
- Responses to non-pharmacological treatments may differ for men and women; for example, when patients were asked to focus on the sensory components of pain, men reported less pain than women, whereas when they focused on the affective components of pain, women reported more pain than men

Mechanisms of gender differences in pain

- Interaction among biological, psychological, and socio-cultural factors probably contributes to these differences

Biological factors

- Influence of sex hormones represents an important source of pain-related variability
- There is evidence suggesting sex-related cortical differences during the processing of pain-related stimuli, thus potentially implicating the influence of sex hormones on differential brain activation
- There are also findings which suggest that the interactive effects of the opioidergic system with gonadal hormones may be an important determinant of sex-based differences in pain sensitivity
- Testosterone appears to be more anti-nociceptive and protective in nature, especially given the association between decreased androgen concentrations and chronic pain
- The effects of oestradiol and progesterone on pain sensitivity are relatively complex as both exert pro-nociceptive and anti-nociceptive effects on pain
- Pain perception varies according to the menstrual cycle phases in women with chronic pain perception, with patients rating pain significantly higher in some phases of menstrual cycle than in others

- Fibromyalgia symptoms are associated with the luteal phase, when both oestrogen and progesterone levels are high

Psychological factors

- Increased prevalence of depression and anxiety in females, compared to males, is a likely contributor to the gender difference in pain perception
- Women are known to catastrophize more than men, and this involves magnification and self-rumination of pain-related information
- Pain coping strategies are different between men and women:
    - Men tend to use behavioural distraction and problem-focused tactics to manage pain
    - Women tend to use a range of coping techniques, including social support, positive self-statements, emotion-focused techniques, cognitive reinterpretation, and attentional focus

Socio-cultural factors

- Social factors, such as gender role expectations, stereotypes, and cultural differences in pain-related beliefs, play an important role in gender difference in pain across various cultural and ethnic backgrounds

Further reading

1. Bartley EJ, Fillingim RB. Sex differences in pain: a brief review of clinical and experimental findings. Br J Anaesth 2013;111(1):52–8
2. Packiasabapathy S, Sadhasivam S. Gender, genetics and analgesia: understanding the differences in response to pain relief. J Pain Res 2018;11:2729–39

4.4 Stress and pain

Definition

- Stress response is amongst the functional properties of the limbic system
- The axis of central (hypothalamic) and systemic (pituitary and adrenal) stress response is a physiological cascade, essential for survival (HPA axis)
- Systemic stress response includes increased serum levels of adrenal gland hormones
- Perception and cognition of pain is a brain function (neuropathic pain), not necessarily linked to activation of peripheral and central nociceptors (nociceptive pain)
- Pain is a potent stressor
- Chronic stress and depression are closely linked

Endocrine basis

- Glucocorticoids (GCs) are released from the adrenal cortex in response to pituitary adrenocorticotrophic hormone (ACTH), which is released in response to corticotropin-releasing hormone (CRH) from the hypothalamus
- GCs are steroid hormones that have multiple genomic effects through nuclear receptors
- GCs have anti-inflammatory, and therefore indirect, analgesic effects due to their ability to block cytokine release and to control oedema

- GCs are likely to have direct inhibitory actions on nociceptors via membrane receptors
- In response to stress, adrenal medullary monoamines (adrenaline, noradrenaline) are released, which modulate the sympathetic nervous system

Neuroanatomy of the stress–pain axis

- Nociceptors in the DRG and their ascending fibre tracts reach specific nuclei of the posterior thalamus. Their projections terminate in the post-central gyrus
- Thalamo-cortical projections are the basis of cognition
- The cingulate cortex is the port of entry of nociceptive inputs into the limbic system, which is the activator of central stress response
- GCs cross the blood–brain barrier (BBB) to modulate the central pathways of pain
- The reticular formation (RF) in the brain and spinal cord is part of the pain modulatory system. It is activated upon stress response
- The dorsal portion of the RF enhances nociceptive responses
- The ventrolateral part of the RF has anti-nociceptive properties
- Neuroplasticity is thought to be the cause of adaptation to pain and its link to stress response

Inflammation

- Inflammation is caused by the liberation of cytokines that can be blocked by GCs
- Cytokines can induce changes in neurotransmitter metabolism, neuroendocrine function, and neuroplasticity
- Inflammatory stress activates the HPA axis

Clinical relevance

- Intense acute stress has analgesic effects: perception of pain seems to be impaired in patients under shock
- Chronic stress and chronic depression are frequently linked to chronic pain. These three symptoms seem to potentiate each other. The underlying mechanisms are still largely unclear
- Sensation of pain is increased (altered) in depressed patients
- Cytokines activate nociceptors
- Central and peripheral nociceptive pathways express opioid receptors. Their ligands play an important role in therapy of both depression and chronic pain
- Monoamine transmitters (e.g. serotonin) and their receptors in the limbic system are pharmacological targets for treatment of both chronic pain and depression

Further reading

1. Martins I, Tavares I. Reticular formation and pain: the past and the future. Front Neuroanat 2017;11:1–14
2. Sheng J, Liu S, Wang Y, et al. The link between depression and chronic pain: neural mechanisms in the brain. Neural Plast 2017;2017:9724371
3. Steinthorsdottir KJ, Kehlet H, Aasvang EK. The surgical stress response and the potential role of preoperative glucocorticoids on post-anesthesia care unit recovery. Minerva Anestesiol 2017;83:1324–31

4.5 Tolerance, dependence, addiction, and pseudoaddiction

Tolerance

- Predictable physiological phenomenon where drug exposure → diminution of effect, or where higher doses are required to produce the same effect

Innate tolerance

- Genetically determined

Acquired tolerance

- Pharmacokinetic tolerance: due to changes in drug metabolism and distribution after repeated administration, i.e. enzyme induction and receptor desensitization
- Pharmacodynamic tolerance: drug-induced changes in receptor density

Specific to opioid tolerance

- Functional decoupling of opioid receptors from G protein-regulated cellular mechanisms (see 3.2 Opioid receptors, p. 72)
- Downregulation of endogenous opioids or opioid receptors
- Behavioural changes

Selective tolerance

- Tolerance to different opioid side effects develops at different rates
- Tolerance to euphoria, respiratory depression, sedation, nausea, and vomiting develops rapidly
- Tolerance to constipation and miosis is minimal

Cross-tolerance

- Tolerance to other drugs within the same class
- Opioids have incomplete cross-tolerance due to differing opioid receptor subtype affinity
- NMDA antagonists may block the anti-nociceptive tolerance to morphine

Dependence

- Predictable physiological phenomenon where repeated exposure produces changes in gene expression

Physical dependence

- Seen with chronic drug use where reduction/discontinuation results in drug-specific withdrawal symptoms

Psychological dependence

- A lot of drugs can produce it, but not all will produce dysfunctional behavioural patterns

Opioid dependence

- Neuroplastic changes not fully reversible, contributing to susceptibility to relapse upon opioid re-exposure
- Unpleasant withdrawal symptoms usually occurring at 2–5 days, making patients unwilling to discontinue opioids

- The International Classification of Diseases, 11th Revision (ICD-11) diagnostic criteria: '*The features of dependence are usually evident over a period of at least 12 months but the diagnosis may be made if opioid use is continuous (daily or almost daily) for at least 1 month*'

Addiction

- Unpredictable phenomenon complicated by genetic, environmental, and psychosocial factors
- Maladaptive behaviours: impaired control, craving, continued and compulsive use despite physical, social, and psychological harm
- Quick to relapse into addiction after a period of abstinence

Risk factors

- Family history of drug dependence, lack of employment, lack of stable social and family relationships

Implicated neurobiological mechanisms

- Homeostasis theory (disequilibrium between positive reward of drug and subsequent negative reinforcement)
- Incentive salience theory (sensitization of dopaminergic mesolimbic reward system and dysfunction of modulating systems → craving)
- Habit theory (learnt behaviour)

Pseudoaddiction

- Iatrogenic syndrome of behavioural changes that may occur when pain is undertreated—patients may request or seek additional medications (legally or illegally) due to being prescribed insufficient drug doses
- Patient demonstrates similar drug-seeking behaviours:
    - Drug hoarding
    - Attempts to obtain extra supplies
    - Doctor-shopping
    - Requests for early prescriptions and increased dosages
    - May even resort to illicit drug use
- Common occurrence is switching from parenteral to oral dose of opioid—where dose is thought to be equivalent but is insufficient
- Main distinguisher between addiction and pseudoaddiction: in pseudoaddiction, the inappropriate behaviour ceases once pain has been treated

Additional information

- Confusion between dependence and addiction:
    - Dependence = requiring drug to prevent physical withdrawal syndrome
    - Addiction = continued use of a drug despite harmful effects
- Opiophobia is the phenomenon of failure to administer opioids due to fear of addiction developing

Further reading

1. Bell J. 10_01_03 Drug Addiction, Dependency and Pain – Introduction. 2015. https://portal.e-lfh.org.uk/Component/Details/409079

2. Bell J. 10_01_04 Drug Addiction, Dependency and Pain – Management. 2015. https://portal.e-lfh.org.uk/Component/Details/409083
3. Tordoff SG, Ganty P. Chronic pain and prescription opioid misuse. Contin Educ Anaesth Crit Care Pain 2010;10(5):158–61

4.6 Neurobiological and physiological changes in response to drug misuse

Substance misuse disorders were once viewed as a character failing but are now considered to be chronic illnesses, associated with comorbidity, social dysfunction, impaired voluntary control, poor compliance, and behavioural issues.

Risk factors for addiction

- Genetic factors may account for up to 70% of individual differences. Genes involved in strengthening neuronal connections, as well as those involved in alcohol and nicotine metabolism, have been associated with addiction risk
- Psychological make-up
- Environmental and socio-cultural factors
- Mental health problems
- Poverty and poor support network

Three-stage vicious addiction cycle

Binge/intoxication stage

- Mediated at the basal ganglia level, specifically the nucleus accumbens (pleasure/reward effect: dopamine-/endogenous opioid-mediated) and the dorsal striatum (habit formation: dopamine-/glutamate-mediated)

Withdrawal/negative affect stage

- Mediated by activation of 'stress systems' in the extended amygdala (NTs: corticotropin-releasing factor (CRF), noradrenaline, and dynorphin), accompanied by diminished activation of the basal ganglia's dopamine reward systems
- The individual then tries to alleviate the negative emotional state by compulsive drug use

Third stage (preoccupation/anticipation)

- Deterioration in judgement and executive control ('stop' and 'go' systems) caused by a compromised prefrontal cortex
- It is driven by glutamate overactivity and promotes impulsive and compulsive drug-seeking behaviour

Opioids

- Attach to specific opioid receptors in the brain, causing the release of dopamine in the nucleus accumbens, which leads to euphoria, respiratory depression, analgesia, and sedation
- Chronic exposure causes a cycle of intoxication, tolerance, escalating use, and finally withdrawal
- Opioid withdrawal manifests as physical and psychological features: body aches, increased pain, sweating, abdominal cramps and diarrhoea associated with profound agitation, emotional distress, tearfulness, anxiety, and low mood
- Result in intense cravings

Alcohol

- Interacts with GABA and glutamate NT pathways, leading to euphoria, sedation, reduced anxiety, and motor impairment, including cravings, negative emotions, and withdrawal symptoms

Cannabis

- Causes increased dopamine release in the basal ganglia
- Due to the longer half-life of THC, cannabis users typically do not smoke it as frequently as tobacco
- The interaction of cannabis with endogenous cannabinoid NTs results in distortion of motor coordination and time perception

Stimulants (cocaine, amphetamines)

- Increase dopamine levels in the brain's reward centres, resulting in a euphoric 'high' and increased focus on tasks, which is why stimulants are prescribed for attention-deficit hyperactivity disorder (methylphenidate, dextroamphetamine)
- The release of noradrenaline results in sympathetic stimulation
- Results in binge intoxication, followed by a crash and then intense cravings

Synthetic drugs

- They work through the above NT systems as well but are more potent and therefore result in more intense cravings and withdrawals
- Some, such as MDMA (*3,4-methylenedioxy-methamphetamine*) and LSD (lysergic acid diethylamide) also work through serotonin pathways to produce changes in perception ('trips')
- MDMA also alters mood and perception, and increases the activity of dopamine and noradrenaline
- LSD is hallucinogenic, causes anxiety and depression, and activates the CVS

Mental illness and addiction

- Over 40% of individuals have a concurrent mental illness
- Schizophrenia is associated with a high incidence of smoking, and PTSD with alcohol overuse
- Drug use provides individuals with mental illness a temporary 'escape'

Further reading

1. American Psychiatric Association. Diagnostic and Statistical Manual of Mental Disorders (DSM-5). 5th edition, 2013. Arlington, VA: American Psychiatric Publishing
2. US Department of Health and Human Services (HHS), Office of the Surgeon General. Facing Addiction in America: The Surgeon General's Report on Alcohol, Drugs, and Health. 2016. Washington, DC: HHS

SECTION 3

PHARMACOLOGY

CHAPTER 5

Basic Principles of Pharmacology

Nishi Patel and Kathleen Shelley

CONTENTS

5.1 Agonists and antagonists

Basic terminology

Ligands

- Any substance which binds to a receptor is known as a *ligand*
- Ligands that activate a receptor to produce a biological response are called *agonists*
- Ligands that block agonist-mediated responses are called *antagonists*

Drug-receptor interaction

- Affinity and intrinsic activity (IA) determine the pharmacological effect of a drug
- Affinity—describes how avidly a drug binds to a receptor
- IA—refers to the magnitude of response once the drug is bound:
    - IA value of 1 = 100% response
    - IA value of 0 = 0% response
    - IA value of −1 = 100% opposite response to agonist (inverse agonist)

Agonists

Characteristics

- High affinity to the receptor
- Full IA

Classification

- *Endogenous agonist*—naturally present in the body, and binds to and activates a receptor
- *Full agonist*—activates the receptor and produces full efficacy equal to that of the endogenous ligand (IA = 1) (see Fig. 5.1.1)
- *Super agonist*—produces a greater response than the endogenous agonist (IA >1)
- *Partial agonist*—binds to and activates the receptor, but only with partial efficacy relative to a full agonist (IA <1). Can act as an antagonist if it prevents full agonist binding to the receptor
- *Inverse agonist*—binds to the receptor, inhibits normal activity, and exerts the opposite pharmacological activity (IA = −1)

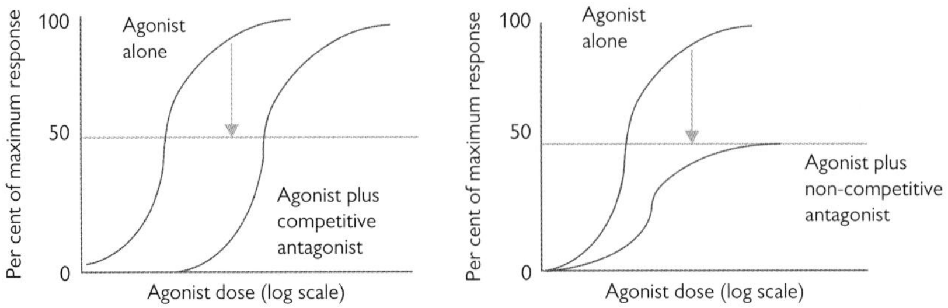

Figure 5.1.1 Dose–response curve: effect of antagonists on agonists

Antagonists

Characteristics

- High affinity to the receptor
- No IA = 0

Classification

- *Competitive antagonist:*
  - Binds to the receptor in a reversible way without activating the effector system for that receptor
  - In the presence of a competitive antagonist, the log dose–response curve is shifted to the right (i.e. higher dose of agonist required to produce the same maximal effect)
- *Non-competitive antagonist:*
  - Binds to a different site on the receptor and causes a conformational change to prevent agonist binding
  - Cannot be overcome by increasing the concentration of agonists

Examples

- Receptor = mu-opioid receptor
  - Full agonist = morphine, fentanyl, codeine
  - Partial agonist = buprenorphine, butorphanol
  - Mixed agonist = pentazocine
  - Antagonist = naloxone, naltrexone

Further reading

1. Peck TE, Hill SA. Pharmacology for Anaesthesia and Intensive Care. 3rd edition, 2008. Cambridge: Cambridge University Press

5.2 Pharmacokinetics

- Pharmacokinetics describes the absorption, distribution, metabolism, and elimination of drugs

Basic principles

Drug passage across the cell membrane

- Drugs need to pass through one or more cell membranes to reach their site of action:
    - Cell membrane = 10 nm bilipid layer
    - Contains glycoproteins which act as ion channels, receptors, intermediate messengers (G proteins), or enzymes

Crossing mechanisms

- Passive diffusion—most common; drug diffuses down a concentration gradient
- Facilitated diffusion—rate of diffusion is enhanced by transport proteins
- Active transport—requires energy and pumps against the concentration gradient
- Pinocytosis—invagination of drug in membrane

Determinants of diffusion

- Surface area
- Molecular weight
- Concentration
- Ionization: unionized form will cross the bilipid layer
    - pKa is the pH at which a drug is 50% unionized and 50% ionized
    - pH = pKa + log (proton acceptor (alkali))/(proton donor (acid))
    - pH = pKa + log (aH)/(a^-)
    - Acid environments shift the equation to the left
    - Alkaline environments shift the equation to the right
    - A weak acid in an acidic environment will remain mainly in its unionized form, therefore greater membrane crossing
    - In an alkaline solution, a weak acid will remain trapped as it is ionized
    - Acidic drugs—if pH < pKa = greater unionized concentration and greater absorption, e.g. aspirin in the stomach
    - If pH > pKa, then a greater degree is ionized
    - A weak base in an alkaline solution—a greater concentration is unionized
    - A weak base in an acidic solution—a greater concentration is ionized

Protein binding

- Affects the duration of effect
- Only unbound drugs have an effect—therefore, caution in states of low protein concentration

Absorption

- Absorption is passage of a drug from the site of drug administration into plasma
- The rate and extent of drug absorption depend on the route of administration

Routes of administration

Enteral

- Oral:
    - Drug is absorbed in the stomach or small bowel (mainly passive transfer), then enters the portal venous system and passes through the liver, before gaining access into the systemic circulation
    - Affected by:

    - Drug factors:
        - Drug particle size and formulation, e.g. slow release
        - Physicochemical, i.e. interaction with another compound; for example, tetracycline precipitates with Ca^{2+}
    - Patient factors:
        - Relation to a meal—slower absorption of drug post-meal
        - GI motility, e.g. gastric stasis
        - GI pH, e.g. strong bases poorly absorbed in acidic stomach and GI tract
        - Splanchnic blood flow
        - First-pass metabolism—the drug passes into the portal circulation from the gut and is metabolized by the liver, therefore reducing the concentration available systemically
- Buccal/sublingual/rectal:
    - Some drugs introduced into the alimentary tract are absorbed directly into the systemic circulation without passing through the liver, thereby avoiding metabolism by gut wall or liver enzymes (first-pass metabolism):
        - Rectal:
            - If drug is inserted lower down in the rectal passage, it enters the inferior rectal vein, to the pudendal vein and the inferior vena cava, and avoids first-pass metabolism
            - If drug is inserted higher up, it enters the middle and superior rectal veins which lead to the portal veins, and undergoes first-pass metabolism
            - Absorption is affected by the proximity to faeces
            - Contraindicated if recent bowel surgery, rectal pain, diarrhoea, or immunocompromised

Parenteral

- This includes any route that avoids absorption via the GI tract such as administration by injection or inhalation or by application to the skin
    - IV:
        - Fastest and most certain route of administration
        - Peak concentration depends on the rate of administration
    - Intramuscular (IM)/SC:
        - Depends on perfusion to injection site—heat can increase perfusion by 30%
        - Overdose risk in shocked patients with poor perfusion—often given repeated doses, which risks a high drug load when perfusion improves
    - Intranasal:
        - Avoids first-pass metabolism, except for any fraction that is swallowed
        - Particle size needs to be <1 micrometre in order to enter the alveoli and bloodstream
    - Transdermal:
        - Advantages:
            - Controlled absorption
            - Constant concentration
            - Avoids first-pass metabolism
            - Can improve compliance
        - Disadvantages:
            - Not all drugs suitable
            - Reduced absorption if shocked
            - Affected by temperature
            - Expensive

        - Skin irritation
        - Slower onset of action and titration—this is not a desirable property for medications used in acute pain management
    - Drug:
        - Needs to be low molecular weight (<500 Da)
        - Low melting point (liquid on the skin)
        - Unionized
        - Potent—low volume
        - Hydrophilic and lipophilic
        - Short half-life (t1/2)
- Epidural/intrathecal:
    - Delivers drug close to the spinal cord at low doses
    - Single shot or infusion

Bioavailability

- Bioavailability (BA) = the fraction of a drug dose which reaches systemic circulation, compared with the IV dose (see Fig. 5.2.1)
- This is, in turn, affected by:
    - Preparation
    - Ionization—highly ionized molecules have low BA
    - First-pass metabolism

Distribution

Influences

- Lipid solubility:
    - pK
    - pH
    - Protein binding—affects free concentration of the drug
    - Regional blood flow
    - Specific property of the drug

Volume of distribution (Vd)

- The theoretical volume into which a drug distributes following its administration

$$Vd = D/C_0$$

where D = dose, C0 = concentration at time 0

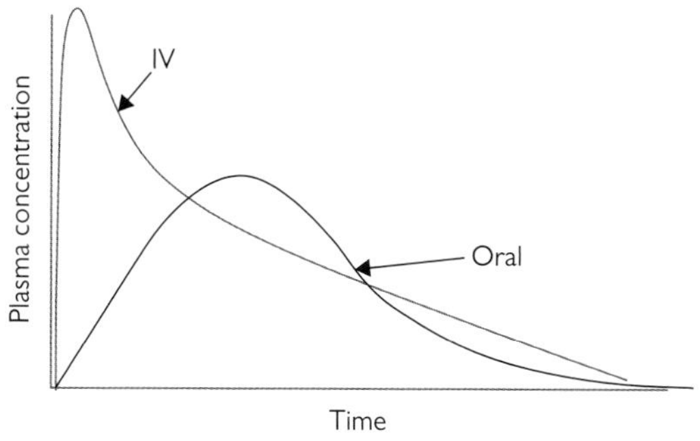

Figure 5.2.1 Bioavailability of drugs

- Vd = volume of water in which an injected dose would have to be diluted in order to give the measured plasma concentration
- Vd = blood volume for a drug confined to plasma, e.g. warfarin
- Vd = total body water volume for a drug that distributes throughout the body, e.g. theophylline
- Vd > total body water for a drug that is concentrated in the tissues, e.g. chloroquine
- In general, drugs with high polarity and those that are highly protein-bound and highly ionized have lower Vd
- Vd may be altered in disease states such as renal failure (fluid retention) and liver failure (altered body fluid and protein binding)
- Compartment modelling have been devised to further explain the distribution of drugs in the body

Metabolism

- Process by which drugs are chemically transformed (usually in the liver) from a lipid-soluble form, suitable for absorption and distribution, to a more water-soluble form that is suitable for excretion (usually by the kidneys)
- Usually reduces drug activity unless it is a prodrug, e.g. diamorphine
- Non-liver sites of metabolism include the lungs, kidneys, and GI tract
- Performed by zero- and first-order kinetics (see Fig. 5.2.2)

Metabolism—phase I

- Non-synthetic/functional reactions:
  - Oxidation (mostly)
  - Reduction
  - Hydrolysis
- Mainly in the endoplasmic reticulum of the liver by cytochrome P450 (see below)
- Also in the lungs, GI tract, brain, and kidneys
- Metabolism—cytochrome P450:
  - Superfamily of iron-containing enzymes
  - >70 isoforms
  - Pigmented pink, hence 'P', and peak absorption of light is at 450 nm in the presence of carbon monoxide

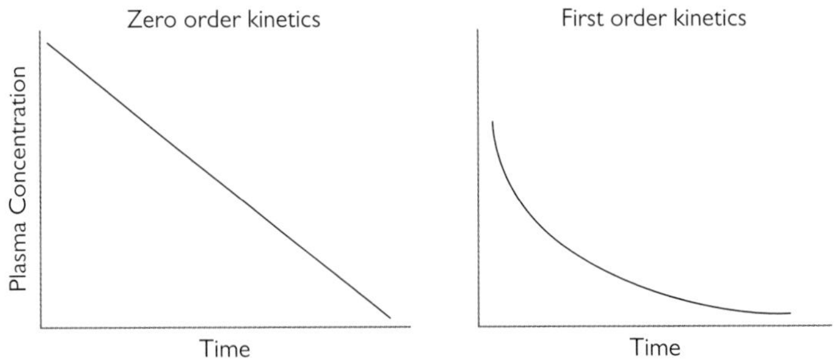

Figure 5.2.2 Zero- and first-order kinetics

- Important in metabolism of a number of endogenous and exogenous compounds
- Mediates the majority of phase I reactions
- Predominantly found in the smooth endoplasmic reticulum of the liver and small intestine
- Divided into families according to structure, e.g. CYP1, CYP2
- Clinically important—CYP2D6 and CYP3A4:
  - Enzyme induction, e.g. anticonvulsants, barbiturates, alcohol, smoking
  - Enzyme inhibition, e.g. amiodarone, cimetidine, fluoxetine

Metabolism—phase II

- Synthetic reactions
- Molecules of phase I metabolites (or, in some cases, unchanged drug) combine with an endogenous substrate to form an inactive conjugate that is much more water-soluble than the phase I metabolite:
  - Glucuronidation
  - Methylation
  - Sulphation
  - Acetylation
- Also in plasma, e.g. by plasma cholinesterases (ester LAs) and by non-specific esterases (remifentanil)
- Genetic polymorphisms affect metabolism (e.g. codeine)

Excretion

- Process by which drugs are removed from the body, the route of which is largely determined by the molecular weight and structure of the drug
- Most common routes of excretion:
  - Urine—particularly for low-molecular weight drugs (depends on glomerular filtration rate (GFR)/water solubility)
  - Bile
  - Also via:
    - Saliva and sweat
    - Faeces (larger-molecular weight drugs)
    - Expired air
    - Breast milk

Renal excretion

- Mechanisms of renal excretion:
  - Glomerular filtration of drugs which are:
    - Small
    - Ionized
    - Free (not protein-bound)
  - Active transport and secretion in proximal convoluted tubules (PCTs)
  - Diffusion into distal convoluted tubules (DCTs):
    - Can be increased by alkalinizing urine, e.g. TCA overdose
- Renal failure:
  - Risk of drug accumulation due to impaired excretion
  - Drug dose = dose × (impaired clearance/normal clearance)

Biliary excretion

- These are often larger-molecular weight compounds (>30 000 Da) and are actively excreted from hepatocytes into the biliary canaliculus against a concentration gradient
- May re-enter enterohepatic circulation
- Bile > small bowel > reabsorbed into the portal circulation > liver > re-excreted into bile or back into systemic circulation
- Presence of small bowel bacterial glucuronidase can render some conjugates lipid-soluble and hence reabsorbed
- Liver failure:
  - Complex pharmacokinetic implications, including:
    - Reduced protein binding (from decreased protein synthesis)
    - Decreased metabolism (phase I and II reactions)
    - Increased Vd (ascites)
    - Reduced hepatic clearance and increased BA (from porto-systemic shunts)
  - Care with BZDs and opioids in encephalopathy

Elimination

- Relationship between rate of drug elimination (R_{elim}) and plasma drug concentration
- Limited by enzymes and carrier-mediated processes which can become saturated at supratherapeutic doses
  - First-order kinetics:
    - R_{elim} is dependent and proportional to plasma drug concentration (simple exponential process)
    - System exhibits excess capacity
    - Most drugs eliminated in this way
  - Zero-order kinetics:
    - R_{elim} occurs at a constant rate and is independent of plasma drug concentration
    - First-order kinetics may become zero-order when the elimination system is at saturated capacity, e.g. aspirin, phenytoin, ethanol

Clearance (Cl) and rate of elimination (R_{elim})

- Clearance = *volume of plasma* cleared of a drug per unit time (mL/min)
  - $Cl = K_e \times Vd$
  - Cl = elimination rate constant (min^{-1}) × Vd (mL)
  - Used to measure drug elimination by metabolism ± excretion
  - Also used to determine the rate of elimination below
- Rate of elimination = *amount of drug* removed per unit time (mg/min)
  - $R_{elim} = Cl \times Css$
  - R_{elim} = Cl (mL/min) × plasma concentration at steady state (mg/mL)
  - Used to determine the rate of drug administration

Further reading

1. Peck TE, Hill SA. Pharmacology for Anaesthesia and Intensive Care. 3rd edition, 2008. Cambridge: Cambridge University Press

CHAPTER 6

Local Anaesthetics

Enrique Collantes, Kavita Poply, and Jan Rudiger

CONTENTS

6.1 Local anaesthetics

Introduction

- LAs cause reversible blockage of Na^+ channels, blocking the transmission of APs across nerve cells
- The function of sensory and motor nerve fibres are affected to different degrees by LA, depending on the:
  - Anatomy of the nerve fibres
  - LA properties (concentration, pKa, volume), route of delivery, pH balance, and use of other agents that alter the duration and onset of action of LAs

Classification

- LAs are broadly divided into two categories, based on the linkage between the aromatic (lipophilic) and amine (hydrophilic) groups:
  - Esters (O-C-O), e.g. procaine, tetracaine, cocaine
  - Amides (CO-NH), e.g. lidocaine, prilocaine, bupivacaine, ropivacaine, dibucaine

Mechanism of action

- A resting membrane potential (RMP) of −80 mV is maintained across the neuronal cell membranes by:
  - Na^+/K^+ ATPase activity which keeps a 30-fold K^+ concentration gradient inside, and a 10-fold Na^+ concentration gradient outside, the cell membrane
  - Intracellular anionic proteins preventing leakage of K^+ outside the cell membrane
- In the resting state, nerve cell membranes are impermeable to Na^+ ions
- An AP is generated as follows:
  - A chemical/electrical trigger alters the permeability of Na^+ channels
  - When the intracellular cell membrane reaches −55mV, voltage-sensitive Na^+ channels open. The AP is conducted across the cell and the membrane potential across the neuronal cell membranes reaches +30mV
  - Finally, Na^+ channels close, with K^+ efflux restoring a RMP of −80 mV

- LAs block Na^+ channels, stopping the transmission of AP across nerve cells as follows:
  - Unionized form (lipid-soluble) of LAs passes through the membrane. The ionized form of LAs binds to the internal surface of Na^+ channels, resulting in prevention of Na^+ entry inside the cell, causing hyperpolarization
  - An alternative theory describes that LAs dissolve in the cell membrane, causing expansion and inactivation of Na^+ channels

Physiochemical characteristics

- Weak bases
- Water-soluble hydrochloric salts containing sodium metabisulphite and fungicide preservatives
- Only subarachnoid preparations are preservative-free
- At physiological pH, LAs remain in ionized forms as their pKa is higher than the pH:
  - Lidocaine has a pKa of 7.9 and a neutral pH of 7.4
  - $pH = pKa + \log[B/BH^+]$
  - $7.4 = 7.9 + \log[B/BH^+]$
  - $-0.5 = \log[B/BH^+]$
  - $0.3 = [B/BH^+]$
  - Therefore, at physiological pH, lidocaine is 25% unionized (B) and 75% ionized (BH^+)

Onset of action, duration, and potency

- These factors are dependent on individual LA chemical structure (see Table 6.1.1)
- Potency is related to:
  - Lipid solubility—the more lipid-soluble, the higher the potency
  - Intrinsic vasodilator properties—affect the amount of available LA at the site
- Duration of action has a direct relationship with the protein-binding capacity

Table 6.1.1 Doses, onset, and duration of action of local anaesthetics

	Lidocaine	Prilocaine	Bupivacaine	Levobupivacaine	Ropivacaine
Description	Amide	Amide	Amide	Amide	Amide
Relative potency	2	2	8	8	6
Onset	5–10 minutes	5–10 minutes	10–15 minutes	10–15 minutes	10–15 minutes
Duration (without adrenaline)	1–2 hours	1–2 hours	3–12 hours	3–12 hours	3–12 hours
Duration (with adrenaline)	2–4 hours	2–4 hours	4–12 hours	4–12 hours	4–12 hours
Maximum dose (without adrenaline)	3 mg/kg	6 mg/kg	2 mg/kg	2.5 mg/kg	3 mg/kg
Maximum dose (with adrenaline)	7 mg/kg	9 mg/kg	2.5 mg/kg	3 mg/kg	4 mg/kg

- Onset of action has an inverse relationship with the pKa. At physiological pH, the higher the LA's pKa, the more ionized form of the LA is present and the less ability to penetrate the cell membrane to act upon the ion channel, leading to a slower onset of action, while the converse is true with low pKa. In an acidic environment (e.g. infected abscess), LAs work less, as a greater ionized fraction is present, not allowing penetration of the LA across the cell membrane
- Other agents can be added to some LAs:
  - Adrenaline or felypressin slows down the absorption from the site of injection, hence prolonging the duration of action
  - Bicarbonate alkalinizes the pH, resulting in a higher proportion of LA in the unionized preparation, hence increasing the onset of action

Pharmacodynamics

Cardiovascular system

- Lidocaine can be used to treat cardiac arrhythmias. It blocks cardiac Na^+ channels, hence decreasing the maximum rate of increase of phase 0 of the cardiac AP
- PR and QRS intervals are prolonged
- Direct myocardial depressant activity (bupivacaine > lidocaine), with the potential to develop re-entrant arrhythmias and ventricular fibrillation due to prolonged binding to Na^+ channels
- Tachycardia further potentiates frequency-dependent blockade by bupivacaine, hence resulting in cardiac toxicity. Ropivacaine (propyl substitution for the butyl group of bupivacaine) S-enantiomer is less cardiotoxic due to rapid dissociation from the cardiac channels. However, ropivacaine is less potent and has a shorter duration of action than bupivacaine

Central nervous system

- LAs cause reversible neural blockade. Administration of LA to the CNS (e.g. in LA toxicity) leads to a biphasic effect:
  - Initially, there is rapid onset of an excitatory phase due to blockage of inhibitory interneurons. This leads to circumoral tingling, visual disturbances, tremors, and dizziness
  - Later, complete CNS depression occurs, which culminates in convulsions, apnoea, and coma

Pharmacokinetics

Absorption

- It depends on the individual agent, the site of injection (intercostal > caudal > epidural > brachial plexus > SC) and the addition of a vasoconstrictor ± bicarbonate
- Less than 10 mg of lidocaine injected in the vertebral/carotid artery can cause coma and convulsions

Distribution

- LAs have higher affinity to α1-acid glycoprotein, although albumin binds to more LAs due to its relative abundance
- The higher the protein binding, the less available the proportion of the active unbound fraction
- Amide LAs are more extensively bound than esters
- In certain situations where protein binding is increased, less free drug is available to work, e.g. in renal failure, infants, myocardial infarction (MI), and post-operatively

- The higher the protein binding, the lower the degree of placental transfer. There is more placental transfer of lidocaine (70% protein-bound) than of bupivacaine (95% protein-bound)
- Esters have rapid metabolism, and therefore, large amounts do not cross the placenta

Metabolism and elimination

- Esters are hydrolysed to inactive metabolites by plasma cholinesterases and other esterases. Para-aminobenzoate is one of the inactive metabolites associated with hypersensitivity reactions
- Amides are metabolized by amidases in the liver at a rate that is slower than that of plasma hydrolysis; hence, they are more prone to accumulation with continuous infusion
- In hepatic ischaemia or inflammation, due to reduced enzyme activity, LA metabolism may be affected and toxicity can occur

Further reading

1. Peck TE, Hill SA. Local anaesthetics. In: Peck TE, Hill SA (eds). Pharmacology for Anaesthesia and Intensive Care. 4th edition, 2008; pp. 163–74. New York, NY: Cambridge University Press
2. AnaesthesiaUK. https://www.frca.co.uk

6.2 Lidocaine

Class of drug

- Amide LA

Indications

- Ventricular tachyarrhythmias—class Ib antiarrhythmic activity (level 1 evidence)
- Chronic neuropathic pain (level 1 evidence)
- Acute neuropathic pain: no level 1 evidence, but widely used based on the evidence for chronic neuropathic pain
- Acute perioperative pain (level 1 evidence). A systematic review of 45 randomized controlled trials (RCTs) (2802 post-surgery patients) showed the following:
    - Pain scores (numerical rating score) at 1–4 hours reduced by 0.8, at 24 hours reduced by 0.3, and no effect at 48 hours
    - Effective only in open abdominal and laparoscopic surgery
    - Trials were heterogenous and small
    - Limited evidence of positive effects on post-operative GI recovery, opioid requirements, post-operative nausea and vomiting, and length of hospital stay
- Headaches: migraine, medication overuse headaches (level 1 evidence with variable efficacy)

Contraindications

- Known allergy to amide local anaesthetics. Use with caution in patients with myasthenia gravis, severe shock, or impaired cardiac concuction

Preparations

- Liquid solutions:

    - Concentrations: 0.5%, 1%, 2%, 4%, 10%
    - With or without adrenaline at different concentrations
    - Viscous preparations for mucous membranes (e.g. for urinary catheterization, mouthwashes)
- Sprays:
    - Concentrations: 2%, 4%, 10%
    - With or without a vasoconstrictor such as phenylephrine
- Creams:
    - Concentrations: 0.5%, 1%, 2%, 4%
    - Eutectic mixtures such as EMLA™ (2.5% lidocaine and 2.5% prilocaine)
    - Liposomal lidocaine 4% or 5% (liposomal preparations facilitate the rate and extent of drug absorption and prevent rapid lidocaine metabolism)
- Patches:
    - 5% lidocaine (Versatis®): soft, stretchy, adhesive hydrogel plaster, 14 × 10 cm size with 5% lidocaine equivalent to a total of 700 mg. Applied on unbroken, clean, dry skin, and the plasters can be cut to fit the painful area being treated. Up to three plasters can be used in each application to cover the area of pain. The plasters are worn 12 hours on and 12 hours off
    - Lidocaine 7% and tetracaine 7% patch (Synera®, Pliaglis®)
- Other preparations: throat lozenges, ointments, eye drops, gel with or without antiseptics such as chlorhexidine

Dosage

- Dose varies, depending on the indication (anaesthesia, analgesia for acute/cancer/chronic pain syndromes) and route of delivery:
    - CNS—intrathecal/epidural
    - Peripheral nervous system—nerve blocks, local infiltration, catheter infusions, patches
    - CNS and/or peripheral nervous system—IV infusions
    - Mucosal surfaces—gel/cream, inhaled, drops, liquid preparations
- Doses normally used:
    - Ventricular tachyarrhythmias: 50–100 mg IV under electrocardiogram (ECG) monitoring at a rate of 25–50 mg/min. Further doses if no response. No more than 200–300 mg over 60 minutes
    - Anaesthesia without adrenaline 3 mg/kg, and with adrenaline 7 mg/kg
    - Topical use in awake fibreoptic intubations—up to 9 mg/kg
    - Pain management:
        - Topical use: up to 4 mg/kg
        - IV/SC use (different doses in different institutions)
    - Doses used range from 1–3 mg/kg/hour
    - In the LOLIPOPS trial (The Long-term Outcomes of Lidocaine Infusions for persistent PostOperative Pain in patients undergoing breast cancer surgery). Dose regime used in the trial (trial has not been published yet):
        - 2.5 mg/kg lean body weight IV as a bolus, after induction of anaesthesia and prior to surgical incision
        - 3.33 mg/kg/hour IV intraoperatively
        - 2.22 mg/kg/hour SC for 24 hours post-surgery

Duration and onset of action

- Onset of action: 1–5 minutes
- Duration of action: 30 minutes to 2 hours. Addition of adrenaline (concentrations of 1:100000 or 1:200000) may extend the duration up to 3 hours

Mode of action

- Na^+ channel blockage (see 6.1 Local anaesthetics, p. 101)
- At sub-anaesthetic doses, decreased hyperexcitability and spontaneous neural activity
- Other postulated mechanisms which can explain its analgesic effects include:
  - Anti-hyperalgesic: increased release of inhibitory NTs (e.g. glycine), less protein phosphorylating pathways (e.g. protein kinase c), and less activity of NMDA receptors and Ca^{2+}-mediated central nociceptive neural excitability
  - Stimulation of descending inhibitory pathways by its anticholinergic activity
  - Anti-inflammatory: inhibits the release of lysosomal enzymes, activity of granulocytes, and activity of toll-like receptor 4 (a pain-related receptor in glial cells, macrophages, fibroblasts, T cells, and B cells), resulting in a decreased production of inflammatory cytokines, ILs. Also decreases the activation of phosphorylating cellular pathways, and development of memory of pain (see 2.7 Central sensitization p. 63 & 4.1 Immunology, inflammation, glia and pain p. 79)
  - Reduction of transmission of nociceptive signals: monoethylglycinexylidide, a metabolite of lidocaine, increases glycine levels by inhibiting the glycine transporter
- 5% lidocaine plaster has an additional mechanical action (hydrogel plaster protecting the hypersensitive area)

Side effects

- Similar to other amide LAs
- Topical use is sometimes associated with mild sensation of burning, itching, or warmth at the application site
- Lidocaine toxicity at >5 mcg/mL serum levels (see 6.8 Local anaesthetic toxicity, p. 116)

Pharmacokinetics

- Absorption:
  - After topical use, only 3% of lidocaine is systemically available
  - Systemic absorption with 5% lidocaine plaster is very low (3%). Plasma concentration with a 3-day application is 130 ng/mL, as compared to 5000 ng/mL required for cardiotoxicity
- Distribution: 60–80% protein-bound. A continuous infusion (without a bolus) will take 4–8 hours to achieve a steady-state plasma concentration
- Metabolism: N-dealkylation compounds, which are less active than lidocaine and available in low concentrations. Lidocaine has a high hepatic extraction ratio and its metabolism depends not only on hepatic metabolic capacity, but also on hepatic blood flow
- Excretion: renal system. Elimination t1/2 is 100 minutes. Context-sensitive t1/2 after a 3-day lidocaine infusion is approximately 20–40 minutes, and there is no accumulation over time in healthy individuals

Pharmacodynamics

- CVS: slight increase in peripheral vascular resistance and APs (decreased phase 4 depolarization, conduction velocity, and refractory period). The ED50 (the dose that produces

a specified effect ("response") in 50% of the population under study) of IV lidocaine is 21 mg/kg (95% confidence interval (CI): 19.0–23.4 mg/kg) for ECG evidence of cardiac toxicity
- CNS: as other LAs. The ED50 of IV lidocaine for CNS toxicity is approximately 19.5 mg/kg (95% CI: 17.7–21.3 mg/kg)

Special circumstances

- Pregnancy: crosses the placental barrier. Despite possible absorption by fetal tissues, no specific incidence of malformations or other harmful effects on the fetus have been reported
- Breastfeeding: probably excreted in breast milk in very small quantities and generally poses no risk to the child at therapeutic dose levels
- Elderly: may require dose reduction

Additional information

- Lidocaine is the 'recommended international non-proprietary name', also known as lignocaine

Cost

- Lidocaine hydrochloride 0.5% 10 mL (10 ampoules, £7.00)
- Lidocaine hydrochloride 1% 10 mL (20 ampoules, £11.21)
- Lidocaine hydrochloride 2% 5 mL (10 ampoules, £12.00)
- Lidocaine medical plaster 700 mg (30 plasters, £72.40)
- Lidocaine ointment 5% (15 g, £6.18)

Further reading

1. Joint Formulary Committee. British National Formulary. 2020. London: BMJ Group and Pharmaceutical Press. https://www.bnf.org
2. Cheung HM, Lee SM, MacLeod BA, et al. A comparison of the systemic toxicity of lidocaine versus its quaternary derivative QX-314 in mice. Can J Anaesth 2011;58:443–50
3. Peck TE, Hill SA. Local anaesthetics. In: Peck TE, Hill SA (eds). Pharmacology for Anaesthesia and Intensive Care. 4th edition, 2008; pp. 163–74. New York, NY: Cambridge University Press
4. Weibel S, Jokinen J, Pace NL, et al. Efficacy and safety of intravenous lidocaine for postoperative analgesia and recovery after surgery: a systematic review with trial sequential analysis. Br J Anaesth 2016;116(6):770–83

6.3 Bupivacaine

Presentation and properties

- Amide LA
- Clear, colourless solution
- Concentration 0.1%, 0.25% and 0.5% (with or without adrenaline 1:200 000)
- 0.5% (heavy) solution with 80 mg/mL glucose (specific gravity 1.026) for intrathecal use

Indications

- Surgical anaesthesia and acute, chronic, and cancer pain responsive to:
    - Neuraxial block (intrathecal or epidural)

- Peripheral major or minor nerve and fascial plane blocks (single shot or infusions)
- SC infiltration (single shot or infusions)
- Mostly used in acute pain management (perioperatively, labour)

Contraindications

- More cardiotoxic than other LAs such as ropivacaine and levobupivacaine
- Contraindicated for IV regional anaesthesia

Dose

- Maximum dose 2 mg/kg. A 70-kg adult can tolerate well up to 400 mg/24 hours
- Can be given topically, intrathecal, epidural, and SC

Mode of action

- Block Na^+ channels. The lipid-soluble (unionized) drug permeates through the phospholipid membrane where it is ionized. It then binds to the internal surface of the Na^+ channel and inactivates it
- LA dissolves into the phospholipid membrane and may cause swelling and inactivation of Na^+ channels

Side effects and toxicity

- Adverse reactions are rare when there is no overdosage or intravascular administration
- CNS: restlessness, anxiety, incoherent speech, light-headedness, numbness and tingling of the mouth and lips, metallic taste, tinnitus, dizziness, blurred vision, tremors, twitching, depression, and drowsiness may be early warning signs of CNS toxicity
- CVS:
  - Decreases the slope of the rise in phase 0 of the AP, hence causing direct myocardial depression
  - Increases the PR and QRS intervals and the refractory period, which can result in cardiac dysrhythmias
  - Intrathecal/epidural bupivacaine should be used with caution in patients with severe disturbances of cardiac rhythm, shock, heart block, and haemodynamic instability. It is markedly cardiotoxic and can cause myocardial depression
  - In severe toxicity, there is major CVS and CNS instability (see 6.8 Local anaesthetic toxicity, p. 116)

Pharmacokinetics

- Duration of action: long-acting
  - Dose, route of delivery, vascularity at the injection site, and addition of vasoconstrictors affect the duration of action
  - A single epidural injection of 0.5% concentration normally provides a motor block for 2–5 hours. When used at 0.25% or lower concentrations, the duration of action is shorter, with reduced effects on motor nerves, which can be advantageous post-operatively or during labour
  - Repeat doses increase the degree of motor block
- Absorption: pKa of bupivacaine is 8.1; only 15% is unionized at physiological pH to penetrate phospholipid membranes. Therefore, the onset of action is intermediate- or slow-acting at 10–20 minutes, with peak plasma levels reached within 30–45 minutes
- Distribution: very highly protein-bound (95%), hence long duration of action

- Metabolism: in the liver by N-dealkylation to pipecolylxylidine and pipecolic acid
- Elimination: via urine. Elimination t1/2 160 minutes

Interactions

- Increases myocardial depression when given with antiarrhythmics
- Risk of cardiac toxicity increases with propranolol

Special circumstances

- Safe to use in pregnancy, breastfeeding, paediatric patients, and the elderly

Additional information

- When levobupivacaine (S-enantiomer of bupivacaine) is administered via the epidural route, it has a shorter duration of motor blockade and longer sensory blockade, and causes less CVS and/or CNS toxicity than bupivacaine

Cost

- Bupivacaine hydrochloride 0.25% 10 mL (20 ampoules, £17.50)
- Bupivacaine hydrochloride 0.5% 10 mL (20 ampoules, £18.30)

Further reading

1. Joint Formulary Committee. British National Formulary. 2020. London: BMJ Group and Pharmaceutical Press. https://www.bnf.org
2. Peck TE, Hill SA. Local anaesthetics. In: Peck TE, Hill SA (eds). Pharmacology for Anaesthesia and Intensive Care. 4th edition, 2008; pp. 163–74. New York, NY: Cambridge University Press

6.4 Ametop®

Class of drugs

- 4% tetracaine gel, stored at between 2°C and 8°C

Indications

- Dermal anaesthesia (e.g. venepuncture, lumbar puncture, vaccination, and minor superficial surgical procedures such as skin grafting)
- Topical skin anaesthesia (e.g. superficial cleaning, debridement of ulcers or burns)

Contraindications

- Premature infants or full-term infants under 1 month old
- Ester LA allergy
- Concomitant use of sulphonamides and/or anticholinesterases
- Do not apply on mucous membranes or broken skin

Dose

- Available in 1.5 g tubes that delivers 1 g of the drug when squeezed

- Apply one tube content in appropriate proportions for venepuncture (30 minutes) and venous cannulation (45 minutes) under occlusive dressing
- Children (aged 5 years and above) and adults—maximum five tubes can be applied at separate sites at a single time
- Onset of LA action 30–45 minutes
- Duration of action 4–6 hours

Mode of action

- (See 6.1 Local anaesthetics, p. 101)

Side effects

- A single application does not generally cause systemic side effects (S/Es)
- Minor S/Es: burning, itching, swelling, or rash at the application site

Pharmacokinetics and pharmacodynamics

- Systemic absorption is minimal
- Metabolized by enzymatic hydrolysis in blood
- Normally causes tetracaine-induced capillary vasodilatation which can help during cannulation

Interactions

- As explained in contraindications

Special circumstances

- Paediatrics: not recommended in infants under 1 month of age
- Pregnancy: can be used
- Lactation: not recommended as not known if tetracaine or its metabolites are secreted in breast milk

Cost

- Ametop® 4% gel (1 g, £1.08)

Further reading

1. Joint Formulary Committee. British National Formulary. 2020. London: BMJ Group and Pharmaceutical Press. https://www.bnf.org
2. Peck TE, Hill SA. Local anaesthetics. In: Peck TE, Hill SA (eds). Pharmacology for Anaesthesia and Intensive Care. 4th edition, 2008; pp. 163–74. New York, NY: Cambridge University Press

6.5 EMLA™

Class of drug

- Eutectic mixture of lidocaine 2.5% and prilocaine 2.5% (amide LAs)
- Combining lidocaine and prilocaine results in a eutectic mixture which has a lower melting point than its individual components, forming an oil above 16°C

Indications

- Dermal anaesthesia (e.g. venepuncture, lumbar puncture, vaccination, and minor superficial surgical procedures such as laceration repair and skin grafting)
- Topical skin anaesthesia (e.g. superficial cleaning and debridement of ulcers)

Contraindications

- Known sensitivity to prilocaine, lidocaine, or other amide LA
- Methaemoglobinaemia: congenital or idiopathic
- Glucose-6-phosphate dehydrogenase (G-6-PD) deficiency
- Caution if used with class I antiarrhythmic drugs (e.g. tocainide, mexiletine), as toxic effects are additive and potentially synergistic
- Should be avoided on mucous membranes due to its rapid systemic absorption

Dose, onset, and duration of action

- Available in 5 g and 30 g tubes
- EMLA™ 5% cream contains lidocaine 25 mg/g and prilocaine 25 mg/g
- Apply under occlusive dressing
- LA onset of action in 30–60 minutes (60 minutes is recommended)
- Duration of anaesthesia after removing EMLA™ dressing at least 2 hours
- Dose is 1.5–2 g/10 cm^2 for 1–5 hours, maximum dose 60 g, and maximum treatment area 600 cm^2
- Children—maximum dose and maximum treatment area:
  - 0–3 months: 1 g/24 hours and 10 cm^2
  - 3–12 months: 2 g/24 hours and 20 cm^2
  - 1–6 years: 10 g/24 hours and 100 cm^2
  - 6–12 years: 20 g/24 hours and 200 cm^2
- EMLA™ patches 5%:
  - One patch covers approximately 10 cm^2 and contains 1 g of EMLA™
  - Apply at least 1 hour before procedure
  - Children: <3 months old, one patch; 3–12 months, 1–2 patches; and 1–12 years old, up to five patches

Mode of action

- (See 6.1 Local anaesthetics, p. 101)

Side effects

- A single application does not generally cause systemic S/Es
- Minor S/Es: burning, itching, swelling, or rash at the application site
- Methaemoglobinaemia (<1/1000) has been reported with prolonged use

Pharmacokinetics and pharmacodynamics

- Systemic absorption is minimal
- Metabolized primarily in the liver
- Lidocaine and prilocaine both have rapid onset of action, toxic blood level >5 mcg/mL, and elimination t1/2 100 minutes

Interactions

- As explained in contraindications

Special circumstances

- Pregnancy: lidocaine and prilocaine cross the placental barrier. Despite possible absorption by fetal tissues, no specific incidence of malformations or other harmful effects on the fetus have been reported
- Breastfeeding: lidocaine and probably prilocaine are excreted in breast milk in very small quantities and generally pose no risk to the child at therapeutic dose levels
- Paediatric: avoid in infants <12 months old at risk of developing methaemoglobinaemia (G-6-PD deficiency, gestational age <37 weeks, and receiving methaemoglobin-inducing drugs such as sulphonamides and phenytoin)

Cost

- EMLA™ 5% cream (5 g, £2.25–2.99; 25 g, £11.70; 30 g, £12.30)

Further reading

1. Joint Formulary Committee. British National Formulary. 2020. London: BMJ Group and Pharmaceutical Press. https://www.bnf.org
2. Peck TE, Hill SA. Local anaesthetics. In: Peck TE, Hill SA (eds). Pharmacology for Anaesthesia and Intensive Care. 4th edition, 2008; pp. 163–74. New York, NY: Cambridge University Press

6.6 Cocaine

Physiochemical properties and presentations

- Ester LA made from *Erythroxylum coca*
- Cocaine hydrochloride solution 1–10%
- Cocaine paste 1–4%
- Moffatt's solution (2 mL 8% cocaine, 2 mL 1% sodium bicarbonate, 1 mL 1:1000 adrenaline)

Indications

- Local anaesthesia and vasoconstriction of mucous membranes (e.g. oral, laryngeal, and nasal cavities). Vasoconstriction helps in preventing excessive blood loss and reduces obstruction of the operative field during surgery

Contraindications

- *Not for oral, SC, IV, neuraxial, or peripheral nerve infusions*
- Largely metabolized by cholinesterase inhibitors. Therefore, avoid its use in patients with pseudocholinesterase deficiency or those on cholinesterase inhibitors (e.g. echothiopate eye drops for glaucoma, neostigmine for myasthenia gravis) due to the risk of higher blood levels and drug toxicity
- Adrenaline increases catecholamine levels and can enhance cocaine toxicity. Thus, avoid sympathomimetic and α-modifying drugs such as guanethidine sulphate, reserpine, TCAs, etc.
- Epilepsy—lowers the seizure threshold
- Can exacerbate porphyria

Dose

- Only for topical use on mucosal membranes

- Duration of action 20–30 minutes
- Maximum total dose 1.5 mg/kg or 100 mg
- Toxic dose 3 mg/kg
- Aerosol/spray delivery: available in 2.5 mL solution at a concentration of 10% (100 mg/mL). One spray contains 130 microlitres/13 mg of cocaine. Maximum dose for 70-kg adult is equivalent to approximately 8–9 sprays

Mode of action

- Inhibits reuptake of serotonin, noradrenaline, and dopamine in the brain, causing cortical stimulation, and may result in restlessness, excitement, euphoria, garrulousness, and increased motor activity
- Central sympathetic stimulation
- Can exert direct pyrogenic effect on thermoregulatory centres in the hypothalamus
- Blocks Na^+ ions during depolarization, thus blocking initiation and conduction of electrical impulses in nerve cells

Monitoring

- Monitoring is always recommended for any signs or symptoms of toxicity
- CNS stimulant and used as an illegal recreational drug for its euphoric properties. It is a very frequently used illegal drug

Side effects and toxicity

- Restlessness, excitement, euphoria, increased motor activity, confusion, paranoia, hallucinations, altered tactile sensations, and psychosis
- Migraine-like headache may appear as a result of cocaine-induced vascular changes
- Reduction of rapid eye movement sleep and total sleep
- Anorexic effect in low doses
- Easily crosses the BBB and may lead to breakdown of the barrier
- When used above therapeutic doses or in high-risk patients, it can precipitate seizures, hyperpyrexia, pulmonary oedema, gut/myocardial infarction, disseminated intravascular coagulation, rhabdomyolysis, and life-threatening cardiac arrhythmias

Pharmacodynamics

- CNS: cortical stimulation, and may result in restlessness, excitement, euphoria, garrulousness, and increased motor activity
- CVS: tachycardia and hypertension (causes vasoconstriction). At large doses, can cause ventricular fibrillation and myocardial depression
- Respiratory system: at therapeutic concentrations, increases minute ventilation
- Abdominal system: nausea and vomiting
- Metabolic: increased body temperature

Pharmacokinetics

- Absorption: oral bioavailability 30%, and intranasal bioavailability 50%
- Distribution: 98% plasma protein-bound
- Metabolism: mostly (90%) by hydrolysis by serum and liver cholinesterases to ecgonine methyl ester, benzoylecgonine, and ecgonine. Also metabolized by oxidation (minor pathway) to produce norcocaine nitroxide, which is responsible for hepatotoxicity when used above recommended doses

- Excretion: in urine; 10% excreted unchanged

Interactions

- (See in section Contraindications, p. 112)

Special circumstances

- Not recommended in paediatric populations, the elderly, pregnancy, and lactation
- If used during pregnancy, can cause neonatal dependence
- Impairs cognitive function, and can affect a person's ability to drive safely and operate machinery. Cocaine is on the list of drugs included in regulations under Section 5A of the Road Traffic Act 1988

Cost

- Price not found in the British National Formulary (BNF)

Further reading

1. Joint Formulary Committee. British National Formulary. 2020. London: BMJ Group and Pharmaceutical Press. https://www.bnf.org
2. Pomara C, Cassano T, D'Errico S, et al. Data available on the extent of cocaine use and dependence: biochemistry, pharmacologic effects and global burden of disease of cocaine abusers. Curr Med Chem 2012;19(33):5647–57
3. Sharma HS, Muresanu D, Sharma A, Patnaik R. Cocaine-induced breakdown of the blood–brain barrier and neurotoxicity. Int Rev Neurobiol 2009;88:297–334

6.7 Mexiletine

Class of drug and name

- Na^+ channel blocker (reduces delay of muscle relaxation/decreases muscle stiffness)
- Namuscla®: 167 mg capsules

Indications

- Symptomatic myotonia (muscle pain, stiffness, weakness, dysphagia) in non-dystrophic myotonic disorders (only indication in the BNF)
- Pain in peripheral neuropathy, refractory pain disorders (successful treatment with IV lidocaine may predict response to mexiletine)
- Intractable headache
- Cardiac arrhythmias

Contraindications

- Heart failure (ejection fraction (EF) <50%), cardiogenic shock
- Second- or third-degree atrioventricular (AV) block, sinus node dysfunction
- Atrial and ventricular tachyarrhythmias, atrial fibrillation or flutter
- Abnormal Q waves, previous MI, angina symptoms
- Caution in epilepsy (increased seizure risk)
- Severe renal and liver impairment

Dose

- Starting with 167 mg/day (for at least 1 week), can be increased to 2 × 167 mg/day (for at least 1 week), then further to 3 × 167 mg/day (maximum daily dose 500 mg, as per the BNF)
- If tolerated and needed, careful titration (check serum levels) up to 400–1200 mg/day
- Take with food to reduce S/Es

Mode of action

- Class Ib antiarrhythmic (oral analogue of lidocaine)
- Actions on surface and membranes of skeletal muscle
- Blocks neuronal Na^+ channels
- May take days or weeks to titrate and to achieve pain relief in chronic pain or myotonia

Monitoring

- Obtain baseline ECG (before starting treatment) and when new symptoms occur
- Check ECG within 48 hours of starting treatment and during treatment
- Check electrolytes before starting and during treatment
- Liver enzymes and full blood count (FBC) during therapy (leukopenia is rare)
- Check serum mexiletine levels to guide therapy and in cases of S/Es

Side effects

(Check serum level and ECG. If severe, e.g. arrhythmias, stop drug.)

- Stop if new or worsening arrhythmias (AV block)
- Common: GI (nausea, vomiting, heartburn, abdominal pain) CVS (arrhythmias, chest discomfort, vasodilation, hypotension), CNS (drowsiness, headache, insomnia, tremor, coordination problems, paraesthesia, malaise, extremity pain, blurred vision, vertigo), skin reactions—more common with serum levels above 2 mcg/mL
- Uncommon: seizure, slurred speech
- Sedation can happen
- Weight gain unusual

Pharmacokinetics

- Metabolized in liver by CYP2D6 and 1A2 to less potent metabolite
- Half-life: 10–12 hours
- Protein binding: 50–60%
- Renal impairment: no effect on dose
- Caution in hepatic impairment
- Caution in underlying arrhythmias and cardiac failure (possible life-threatening arrhythmias)

Interactions

(Multiple; also check the BNF.)

- Caffeine, cimetidine, atropine, opioids, and Mg^{2+} may slow absorption
- Metoclopramide increases absorption and levels
- CYP2D6 inhibition (propafenone, fluoxetine, duloxetine), and CYP1A2 inhibitors (fluvoxamine) may increase levels

Pregnancy

- Not recommended in pregnancy and breastfeeding (excreted in breast milk)

Additional information

- Has been used in the past after successful trial of IV lidocaine
- May require individual funding request if used for chronic pain

Cost

- Capsule 167 mg: £50 per capsule (£1600–5000 per month)

Further reading

1. Joint Formulary Committee. British National Formulary. 2020. London: BMJ Group and Pharmaceutical Press. https://www.bnf.org

6.8 Local anaesthetic toxicity

Introduction

- Maximum LA doses cannot be applied universally, as many factors are important (e.g. body habitus, genetic, gender, pharmacokinetic and pharmacodynamic factors) (see Table 6.8.1)
- Bupivacaine appears to be the most toxic LA. Toxic effects are due to effects on the excitable plasma membranes of the CNS and CVS

Type of adverse reactions and toxicity to local anaesthetics

Allergic reactions

- True allergy is rare
- Hypersensitivity to ester LAs is not uncommon. It happens due to para-aminobenzoic acid which is produced when ester LAs are metabolized. It does not cause cross-sensitivity to amides

Additive toxicity

- Due to vasopressors and preservatives, e.g. inadvertent vasoconstriction due to cocaine in the presence of other vasoconstricting drugs such as monoamine oxidase inhibitors (MAOIs)
- Simultaneous use of other medications which block ion channels (e.g. Na^+, Ca^{2+}, K^+) such as antiarrhythmics, antiepileptics, and antipsychotics

Table 6.8.1 Doses of local anaesthetics

	Lidocaine	Prilocaine	Bupivacaine	Levobupivacaine	Ropivacaine
Maximum dose (without adrenaline)	3 mg/kg	6 mg/kg	2 mg/kg	2.5 mg/kg	3 mg/kg
Maximum dose (with adrenaline)	7 mg/kg	9 mg/kg	2.5 mg/kg	3 mg/kg	4 mg/kg

Local (neuronal) toxicity

- Intraneural injection, neuronal ischaemia due to high pressure, and nerve irritation

Methaemoglobinaemia

- Iron in haemoglobin (Hb) is altered, reducing oxygen-carrying capacity of Hb. As a result, cyanosis and hypoxia occur
- Benzocaine, lidocaine, and prilocaine due to its metabolite O-toluidine cause this effect

Systemic toxicity

- Occurs when plasma concentration reaches beyond toxic levels

Local anaesthetic toxicity—pharmacodynamics

Cardiovascular system

- Lidocaine and bupivacaine:
  - Block cardiac Na^+ channels, decreasing the slope of the rise of phase 0 of the AP. This leads to direct myocardial depression
  - Increased PR and QRS intervals and refractory period (risk of cardiac dysrhythmias)
- Bupivacaine has a slow dissociation from cardiac Na^+ channels, hence leading to prolonged myocardial depression and subsequent ventricular dysrhythmias and re-entry arrhythmias
- Ropivacaine is a single S-enantiomer of bupivacaine and has a propyl group substitution for the butyl group. This enables its relatively quick dissociation from Na^+ channels; hence, it is less cardiotoxic. Ropivacaine is required in larger doses due to its short duration of action and lower potency than bupivacaine

Central nervous system

- LAs penetrate the brain tissue very rapidly and exert a biphasic effect:
  - First phase: inhibit inhibitory interneurons, resulting in an excitatory phenomenon, i.e. perioral twitching/tingling, visual disturbances, tremors, and fits
  - Second phase: there is CNS depression, resulting in coma and apnoea

Local anaesthetic toxicity—pharmacokinetics

Absorption

- Absorption depends upon specific character of the agent used, concentration, volume, site of injection, addition of alkaline solutions (e.g. bicarbonate), and vasoconstrictors (e.g. adrenaline)
- Risk of toxicity is higher from injection into certain places where the absorption rate is higher than at other sites, i.e. intercostal > caudal > epidural > brachial plexus > SC
- Inadvertent intravascular injection can lead to rapid systemic toxicity, e.g. 10 mg of lidocaine injected in the vertebral artery can lead to immediate CNS toxicity

Distribution

- α1-acid glycoprotein and albumin are the main proteins bound to LAs. Amides (bupivacaine > ropivacaine > lidocaine > prilocaine) are more extensively bound to these proteins than esters. α1-acid glycoprotein binds with greater efficacy; yet albumin, due to its relative abundance, binds more extensively
- In conditions where there is increased protein binding (pregnancy, renal failure, post-operatively, and infancy), the free fraction of the LA is reduced, hence less likelihood of toxicity

- The degree of protein binding affects the extent of placental transfer. Bupivacaine, being more bound to protein, crosses the placenta less

Metabolism

- Unexpected LA toxicity can occur in cardiac or hepatic failure where drug metabolism is reduced or alterations in plasma protein binding can occur

Treatment of local anaesthetic toxicity

- Treatment depends on the severity, following guidelines from the Association of Anaesthetists of Great Britain and Ireland on the management of LA toxicity
- Mild toxicity normally presents with a simple rash and improves by stopping further LA injection, giving antihistamines, and observation
- In severe toxicity, with CVS and/or CNS instability:
    - Stop further LA injection
    - Cardiopulmonary resuscitation (CPR), oxygenation, organ support, call for help
    - Intralipid® 20% infusion:
        - Mechanism of action is not well understood; seemingly, a pool of lipid in the blood acts as a sink and removes lipophilic LA molecules from cardiac and nervous system tissue reducing neural blockade, seizures and improving cardiac contractility, conduction and coronary blood flow
        - Initial bolus 1.5 mL/kg, and start 15 mL/kg/hour infusion
        - Second bolus 1.5 mL/kg at 5 minutes, and double infusion rate to 30 mL/kg/hour
        - Third bolus 1.5 mL/kg at 10 minutes, and continue infusion
        - Maximum cumulative dose of 12 mL/kg
- Critical care support and subsequent monitoring of amylase/lipase for 48 hours
- Report/investigate/discuss as per local clinical governance

Further reading

1. Association of Anaesthetists of Great Britain and Ireland. Management of severe local anaesthetic toxicity. 2010. https://anaesthetists.org/Home/Resources-publications/Guidelines/Management-of-severe-local-anaesthetic-toxicity
2. Litz RJ, Popp M, Stehr SN, et al. Successful resuscitation of a patient with ropivacaine-induced asystole after axillary plexus block using lipid infusion. Anaesthesia 2006;61(8):800–1
3. Rosenblatt MA, Abel M, Fischer GW, et al. Successful use of a 20% lipid emulsion to resuscitate a patient after a presumed bupivacaine-related cardiac arrest. Anaesthesiology 2006;105(1):217–18

CHAPTER 7

Opioids

Enrique Collantes, Praveen Ganty, James Jack, Jonathan Norman, and Jan Rudiger

CONTENTS

7.1 Overview of opioids

Introduction

- Opiate use dates from as far back as early Egyptian times, initially as mixed alkaloids from poppies
- It was not until the 1970s that opiate receptors and their natural analogues were discovered
- All strong opioids are classed as controlled (known as scheduled in the USA) drugs
- If opioids are used, doses must be titrated to response (start low and go slow)

Classification of opioids

1. Opiates (naturally occurring opioids) = morphine, codeine, and papaverine
2. Semi-synthetic opioids = diamorphine, buprenorphine, and oxycodone
3. Synthetic opioids = fentanyl and its derivatives, methadone, pethidine, tramadol, and tapentadol

Chemical classification (four subtypes)

1. Phenanthrenes (morphine, codeine, oxycodone, buprenorphine)
2. Phenylpiperidines (fentanyl derivatives, pethidine)
3. Diphenylheptanes (methadone)
4. Benzomorphans (pentazocine)

→ Tramadol and tapentadol do not fit into this classification.

Opioid receptors

(See 3.2 Opioid receptors, p. 72.)

- Most opioids used in clinical practice work by binding at the mu opioid (MOP) (or mu) receptors, inducing G-protein-mediated hyperpolarization of the cell
- There are several subtypes of the MOP receptor; the difference is mainly at the external binding site of the receptor, and some of these variants may have an effect on clinical practice, although this is not fully understood
- The other main receptor types are kappa opioid (KOP) (or kappa) and delta opioid (DOP) (or delta) receptors

Mechanism of action

- Clinically, opioids act as pure opioid receptor agonists such as morphine, partial agonists (or agonist/antagonist) such as buprenorphine, or agonists at >1 opioid receptor such as oxycodone, codeine, methadone, and pethidine
- Some opioids such as tramadol, tapentadol, and methadone also have pharmacological activity at non-opioid receptors (there is some contention as to how useful this is clinically)
- The most potent opioid analgesics tend to be pure mu receptor agonists

Metabolism

- Metabolism occurs by two pathways:
- Glucuronidation (for morphine, hydromorphone, and oxymorphone)
- Oxidation (almost all other opioids) via the cytochrome P450 system (for drugs that are oxidized, there is the potential for significant drug interactions)
- Most opioids produce active metabolites which are clinically relevant
- Methadone and fentanyl do not produce clinically relevant active metabolites
- Oxycodone, buprenorphine, hydromorphone, and tapentadol produce active metabolites of limited clinical relevance
- The pharmacokinetics of opioids varies according to age, sex, and race, and for those opioids metabolized by oxidation by significant genetic variability in the cytochrome P450 enzymatic system

Hepatic impairment

- Metabolism by glucuronidation and oxidation occurs in the liver. There are multiple changes in the metabolism of opioids in liver impairment. Some of the key changes include:
  - Higher oral bioavailability of some opioids because there is less first-pass metabolism
  - Prolonged effects as opioids are metabolized for clearance more slowly
- **All opioids need to be used with caution in hepatic impairment.** Generally, the doses of opioids and choice of opioids recommended in hepatic impairment include the following:
  - No change of dose generally needed: oxycodone, alfentanil, fentanyl, buprenorphine, morphine (reduce dose if morphine being used orally)
  - Reduce dose in significant hepatic impairment: tramadol, tapentadol, hydromorphone, methadone
  - Avoid: pethidine

Renal impairment

- Renal impairment has a very important effect on the doses and choice of opioids selected. Some of the key changes that occur from renal impairment include:
  - Decreased excretion of opioids that are excreted by the kidney
  - Decreased excretion of active metabolites of opioids
  - These patients tend to be on other drugs which are nephrotoxic (e.g. furosemide, angiotensin-converting enzyme inhibitors (ACEIs), gentamicin) and can further worsen the renal function, further limiting the use of most analgesics
- **All opioids need to be used with caution in renal impairment.** Although some have a better profile, this does not necessarily mean they are completely safe. The choice of opioids recommended include:
  - No change of dose needed, as have no active metabolites: fentanyl (first line), methadone (lower doses in severe impairment)
  - No dose changes generally needed, has weakly active metabolites: buprenorphine (excretion of metabolites mostly by biliary metabolism, so the pharmacokinetics of the drug is not majorly affected)
  - No dose changes generally needed in mild to moderate renal impairment, as have low amount of, or weakly active, metabolites: alfentanil, oxycodone, tapentadol
  - Ideally another agent should be used, as these have active metabolites: codeine (morphine), tramadol (O-desmethyltramadol), morphine (morphine-6-glucuronide), hydromorphone (hydromorphone-3-glucuronide)
  - Contraindicated: pethidine (norpethidine)

Side effects

(See Table 7.1.1.)

- Wide and similar S/E profile of opioids between individual drugs
- Reported rate by patients of at least one S/E is 80%, and 50% for two or more

Table 7.1.1 Opioid side effects according to systems

System	Side effects
Neurological	Hallucinations, confusion, vertigo, euphoria, dysphoria, mood changes, dizziness, drowsiness, sleep disturbance, headache, miosis, nightmares, visual disturbances, weakness, anxiety, agitation, tremor, brain fog, memory problems, balance problems, mydriasis
Respiratory	Cough, rhinitis, pharyngitis, respiratory depression, dyspnoea, worsening of asthma
Cardiovascular	Bradycardia, tachycardia, palpitations, postural hypotension
Gastrointestinal	Nausea and vomiting, constipation, diarrhoea, stomach pain, flatulence, poor appetite
Endocrine	Adrenal insufficiency, dysmenorrhoea, lymphadenopathy, decreased libido (sexual dysfunction), ureteric spasms
Others	Dry mouth, biliary spasm, peripheral oedema, difficulty in passing water, urinary retention, ureteric spasm, sweating, flushing, rash, urticaria, itching Serotonin syndrome, rigors, back pain, fatigue (weakness), muscle cramps, sense of body temperature change

- Most commonly of **gastrointestinal** origin (including nausea, constipation, and dry mouth) and **neurological** origin (drowsiness, fatigue, poor concentration, and dizziness commonly)
- **Itching and sweating** are also common
- Adverse effects are more common when opioids are used in conjunction with other centrally acting drugs, particularly with benzodiazepines (BZDs)
- There is a correlation between serum levels of an opioid and the frequency of S/Es
- With chronic use, tolerance may develop to many of the S/Es, with the exceptions of constipation and excess sweating
- Opioids have wide-ranging effects on the **endocrine system**, stimulating the release of insulin and glucagon from the pancreas, as well as growth hormone and prolactin. They inhibit the secretion of adrenocorticotrophic hormone (ACTH) and luteinizing hormone (LH), leading to hypogonadism, decreased libido, impotence, amenorrhoea, and infertility
- Opioids appear to have a wide range of possible effects on the **immune system**, probably with a pro-inflammatory effect with increased production of TNF-α, IL1 and IL6
- Opioids have been associated with cases of **serotonin syndrome** either on their own or more often in combination with other serotonergic drugs (tramadol, tapentadol, and methadone are seen as higher risk)
- Increasingly, studies looking at **tolerance and hyperalgesia** with opioid use suggest that hyperalgesia tends to occur mostly at higher opioid doses. The mechanisms, while not fully understood, appear to involve both reduced expression and sensitivity of MOP receptors and upregulation of NMDA receptors. The effects may occur acutely with potent short- acting opioids (e.g. remifentanil), and there is evidence of persistence after cessation of opioid treatment

Contraindications/caution

- Patients with, or at risk of, significant respiratory depression and/or obstructive airways
- Acute intoxication with alcohol, prescribed and not prescribed drugs
- Comatose patients, head injury, raised intracranial pressure (ICP)
- Severe liver and renal disease
- Known allergy or hypersensitivity to opioids

Caution

- Children, elderly, pregnancy, drug misuse
- Acute abdomen, delayed gastric emptying, heart failure, chronic lung disease, phaeochromocytoma, cardiac arrhythmias, pancreatitis, cor pulmonale, risk of paralytic ileus, acute ulcerative colitis, diarrhoea, antibiotic-associated colitis (e.g. pseudomembranous colitis)
- Patients on polypharmacy

Use of opioids for acute pain

- Many initiatives and guidelines have been developed to reduce opioid-related harm. It has been recommended to use immediate-release opioids and to avoid slow-release opioids for the management of patients with acute pain, to decrease the risk of respiratory depression
- The use of opioid-sparing techniques is recommended (non-steroidal anti-inflammatory drugs (NSAIDs), paracetamol, regional techniques, and other adjuvants)

Long-term use of opioids for chronic non-cancer pain

- The benefits of taking opioids long-term are primarily decreased in pain, although this appears modest at around 20%

- Sleep may be improved (worsened in some cases), but there is no convincing evidence that long-term opioids improve function and there is some controversy on how important this is as a primary outcome factor
- Evidence for the use of long-acting opioids in chronic non-cancer pain (CNCP) is limited to short-term studies (trials often demonstrate a high rate of dropout due to the lack of efficacy or problems with S/Es)
- There is limited evidence demonstrating better outcomes when two or more different opioid preparations are used simultaneously
- **Not all pain is opioid-responsive!**

The opioid crisis

- The introduction of long-acting formulations in the 1980s led to a rapid rise in the use of opioids for the management of chronic pain from late twentieth century to the present day
- During this period, the wish to relieve suffering overcame fears of addiction, which was thought to be as low as 2–3%
- More recent studies suggest problem behaviours in at least 10% of patients. It is now clear that long-term use of opioids is also associated with an increased risk of overdose, death, falls, fractures, and accidents, including association with impaired driving, as well as changes to the immune system that may alter response to disease (there is increasing evidence of problem behaviours reported with long-term use, particularly in North America)
- There are now guidelines in many countries on how to use and limit strong opioids in chronic pain
- These guidelines usually recommend dose limitation (in the UK 120 mg, and in Australia 60–80 mg, of oral morphine equivalent dose per day). This limitation is primarily due to the lack of studies on high-dose opioids, rather than a known lack of effect

Driving and opioids

- The recently updated laws on drugs and driving still allow patients to drive while using opioids in the UK, if they are being used on prescription appropriately and not causing an impairment of judgement
- Avoid driving for a few days when commencing a new pain medication (including opioids), increasing or decreasing the dose, or adding another drug (e.g. sedatives) that may affect driving
- In the UK, it is the patient's duty to determine if they are fit to drive or not
- However, it is against the law to drive if they have been advised not to by a medical professional (May 2020)

Further reading

1. Babalonis S, Walsh SL. Warnings unheeded: the risks of co-prescribing opioids and benzodiazepines. Pain Clin Updates 2015;23(6):1–7
2. Faculty of Pain Medicine of The Royal College of Anaesthetists. Driving and Pain. London, UK. 2019. https://fpm.ac.uk/sites/fpm/files/documents/2019-07/FPM-Driving-and-Pain-members-information.pdf
3. Faculty of Pain Medicine of The Royal College of Anaesthetists. Controlled drugs and the law. London, UK. 2021. https://fpm.ac.uk/opioids-aware-best-professional-practice/controlled-drugs-and-law
4. UK Government. Drugs and driving: the law. https://www.gov.uk/drug-driving-law

5. Manchikanti L, Helm S, Fellows B, et al. Opioid epidemic in the United States. Pain Physician 2012;15:ES9–38
6. Faculty of Pain Medicine of The Royal College of Anaesthetists. Opioids Aware. London, UK. https://fpm.ac.uk/opioids-aware
7. Trescot A, Datta S, Lee M, Hansen H. Opioid special issue. Pain Physician 2008;11:S133–53
8. Wersocki E, Bedson J, Ying C, et al. Comprehensive systematic review of long-term opioids in women with chronic noncancer pain and associated reproductive dysfunction (hypothalamic–pituitary–gonadal axis disruption). Pain 2017;158(1):8–16

7.2 Buprenorphine

Class of drugs

- Buprenorphine is a strong opioid, a thebaine derivative (classified as a narcotic, controlled drug)
- Buprenorphine is an atypical opioid with a different mode of action (partial agonist) and a better safety profile than conventional opioids
- Buprenorphine-patch to oral morphine equivalence is 1:60–1:100

Preparations

- Sublingual tablets:
  - Temgesic®: 200 and 400 mcg; Subutex®: 2 and 8 mg
  - Suboxone® (buprenorphine + naloxone in 4:1 ratio): 2 and 8 mg
- Oral tablets:
  - Espranor® 2 and 8 mg (oral lyophilisate)
- Transdermal patches:
  - Butrans®, Bunov®, Butec®, Norspan® in doses of 5, 10, 15, 20, 30, 40 mcg/hour
  - Bupeaze®, Hapoctasin®, Transtec® in doses of 35, 52.5, 70 mcg/hour
- Modified-release liquid solution for SC injection (weekly or monthly):
  - Buvidal® as 8 mg/0.16 mL, 16 mg/0.32 mL, 24 mg/0.48 mL, 32 mg/0.64 mL, 64 mg/0.18 mL, 96 mg/0.27 mL, 128 mg/0.36 mL
- Liquid solution for IV use:
  - Temgesic®: 300 mcg/mL

Indications

- Acute pain:
  - Sublingual (Temgesic®: 200–400 mcg)
  - IM injection of 300–600 mcg (300 mcg/1 mL)
- Chronic non-cancer pain (CNCP) and cancer pain (moderate to severe):
  - Sublingual (Temgesic®: 200–400 mcg 3–4 times per day)
  - Transdermal patches:
    - Butrans®, Butec®, Norspan®: 5–20 mcg/hour every 7 days, assess effect after 72 hours)
    - Norspan®, Transtec®, Bupeaze®: 35–50–70 mcg/hour every 4 days, assess effect after 24 hours
  - For CNCP, buprenorphine doses should be titrated to a maximum of oral morphine equivalent daily dose (OMEDD) of 80 mg (as recommended by the Faculty of Pain Medicine)

- Opioid replacement therapy programme:
  - Sublingual tablets (Subutex®, Suboxone® = buprenorphine + naloxone), 0.8–4 mg initially, with 4–24 mg/day as maintenance (for opioid substance use and dependence)
  - Oral tablets (Espranor®)
  - Modified-release SC injection (Buvidal® given weekly or monthly, Sublocade® given monthly)
- Premedication (sublingual 400 mcg, IM 300 mcg)
- Intraoperative analgesia (slowly IV: 300–450 mcg)

Contraindications

- (See opioid contraindications in 7.1 Overview of opioids, p. 119)

Mode of action (partial mu agonist, weak kappa and delta antagonist)

- Partial MOP receptor agonist (with high affinity for mu receptors, but low intrinsic activity)
- Weak KOP receptor and DOP receptor antagonist
- Nociceptin or opioid-receptor-like 1 receptor agonist—most likely explains the specific advantageous effects of buprenorphine
- As a partial agonist, its maximal opioid effects are less than effects of full agonists, and higher doses of buprenorphine can be administered with fewer adverse effects (e.g. respiratory depression) than seen with higher doses of full mu agonist opioids
- At low doses, it is more potent/efficacious than morphine. Opioid-naïve patients can have a very good analgesic effect when they receive a low dose of buprenorphine (e.g. in rib fractures)
- At lower doses, buprenorphine appears to behave as a full agonist, with partial agonist effect only at higher doses seen in drug dependence programmes
- Analgesic effects reach a ceiling where higher doses of buprenorphine do not result in greater pain relief, but higher doses increase the duration of withdrawal suppression and opioid blockade
- Animal studies have shown that when buprenorphine is used with other MOP receptor full agonists (e.g. morphine, oxycodone, fentanyl), buprenorphine displaces and prevents them from acting on the mu receptors, due to high affinity of buprenorphine to mu receptors
- This effect is dose-related, as shown in a study demonstrating that the 16 mg dose of the sublingual buprenorphine-alone tablet was more effective than the 8 mg dose in blocking the reinforcing effects of heroin
- Therefore, some centres continue buprenorphine in hospitalized patients with acute pain (surgical and non-surgical) and use multimodal analgesia with other MOP receptor agonists
- It is difficult for opioid antagonists (e.g. naloxone) to displace buprenorphine and precipitate withdrawal (higher than usual doses of naloxone may be needed in a buprenorphine overdose)
- Buprenorphine has a slow dissociation rate from the MOP receptor, which gives rise to its prolonged suppression of opioid withdrawal and blockade of exogenous opioids
- This enables buprenorphine dosing to occur on a less frequent basis than full opioid agonists (buprenorphine can be given as infrequently as three times per week)

Monitoring of treatment

- Regular liver function tests (LFTs) in patients with hepatic deficiency
- Regular clinical supervision as part of a drug maintenance programme
- Monitoring of neonates (drowsiness, weight gain, development) recommended in breastfeeding mothers

- Androgen deficiency testing is advised only if issues are clinically suspected

Clinical advantages of buprenorphine over conventional opioids (full MOP receptor agonists)

- Clinically buprenorphine behaves like a full MOP receptor agonist with similar efficacy and causes fewer adverse effects
- Less respiratory depression with ceiling effects on respiratory function has been reported at a daily dose of buprenorphine of 16 mg
- Can be used in patients with mild-moderate renal failure as there is no build up of active metabolites. In patients with severe renal failure may need to change the doses used
- Less opioid-induced androgen dysfunction (due to its partial agonist effect versus full agonists)
- Less opioid-induced hyperalgesia (OIH) due to less activation of glia
- Lower rate of sedation and cognitive dysfunction
- Less opioid-induced constipation
- Long duration of action, enabling dosing to occur on a less frequent basis for the treatment of opioid addiction/dependence, in contrast to other shorter-acting opioids
- Other: less itching, safer in the elderly, and milder withdrawal than with other opioids

Clinical disadvantages of buprenorphine over conventional opioids (full MOP receptor agonists)

- In overdose, buprenorphine is only partially reversed by naloxone
- Buprenorphine can precipitate withdrawal when used acutely in opioid-dependent patients (due to its high affinity and low efficacy at mu receptors). Despite the partial agonist effect, buprenorphine can cause drug dependence at a lower dose than morphine. Gradual dose reduction is recommended to avoid withdrawal after long-term treatment
- When titrating upwards with buprenorphine patches, it is not recommended to increase straight to 35 mcg/hour from 20 mcg/hour. However, some preparations do not allow small dose titrations (Transtec® patches are only available in 35, 52.5, and 70 mcg/hour)
- Stigma
- Transdermal patches can cause skin erythema (20%)

Pharmacokinetics

- Oral bioavailability: poor, only 6% (extensive first-pass metabolism), making it ineffective when taken orally (Espranor® is a lyophilized (rapidly disintegrating) buprenorphine tablet, which is placed on top of the tongue, with a bioavailability of 25–30%)
- Lipid solubility: high (leading to higher bioavailability when administered sublingually)
- Protein binding: high (low plasma concentrations, but no obvious correlation between plasma level and clinical effect)
- Vd: >5000 L
- Metabolism: hepatic, mainly via dealkylation (CYP450 3A4), but also via glucuronidation (no active metabolites)
- Distribution half-life: 2–3 hours (initially)
- Elimination half-life: 24–36 hours
- Excretion: in urine and faeces

Transdermal patches

- The transdermal buprenorphine to oral morphine equianalgesic ratio is about 1:60-1:100 (multiply patch dose in micrograms by 2 to obtain the OMEDD in milligrams), e.g. patch 10 mcg/hour (240 mcg/24 hours) ≈ 20 mg of oral morphine/24 hours

- Peak plasma levels: 48–80 hours
- Time to steady concentration: 72 hours
- Half-life after removal of patch: 10–24 hours
- Change of patch: every 7 days (5–40 mcg patches)
- Suitable for cancer pain and CNCP (not appropriate in acute pain when rapid dose titration is needed)

Sublingual preparations

- Forty times more potent than oral morphine (0.4 mg sublingual buprenorphine = 16 mg oral morphine = 5 mg IV morphine)
- Bioavailability 50% (due to high lipid solubility)
- Peak plasma levels after 90 minutes
- Doses for acute pain management in opioid-naïve patients: 0.2–0.6 mg 3–4 times per day (suitable for patients who are nil by mouth)
- When used for opioid replacement therapy programmes:
  - Doses vary enormously (it can be used in high doses, e.g. 2–32 mg/day)
  - Suboxone® contains naloxone to deter the abuse of tablets by crushing and IV injection

Intravenous and intramuscular preparations

- Peak plasma levels: IV after 2 minutes and IM after 5 minutes
- Dose: 0.3–0.6 mg 3–4 times/day (IV 0.3 mg buprenorphine have produced a greater analgesic effect than 10 mg IV morphine in double-blind studies in major surgery)
- Buprenorphine PCA (demand dose 80 mcg) has been found as effective as fentanyl PCA in major surgery (this might be useful for acute pain management of patients already on high doses of buprenorphine)

Modified-release subcutaneous preparation

- Used for the treatment of opioid dependence following stabilization on sublingual buprenorphine/naloxone for >7 days
- The available modified-release preparations last for 1 and 3 months
- To switch from sublingual buprenorphine to the monthly Buvidal® depot preparation:
  - Patients on sublingual buprenorphine 8–10 mg/day—can be switched to SC Buvidal® 64 mg/month
  - Patients on sublingual buprenorphine 12–16 mg/day—can be switched to SC Buvidal® 96 mg/month
  - Patients on sublingual buprenorphine 18–24 mg/day—can be switched to SC Buvidal® 128 mg/month

Interactions

- CYP3A4 inhibitors (e.g. azole antifungals, protease inhibitors for HIV) increase the plasma concentrations of buprenorphine and nor-buprenorphine
- CYP3A4 inducers (carbamazepine, phenytoin, and rifampicin) have not been investigated but seem likely to reduce the plasma concentrations of buprenorphine

Special circumstances

- Not recommended in children under 16 years of age
- Unlicensed oral use in children under 6 years
- Unlicensed IM and IV use in children under 6 months

- In pregnancy, there are insufficient data:
  - Neonatal respiratory depression and withdrawal syndrome reported
  - There are insufficient data on the safety of naloxone in the fetus (Suboxone® is not used in pregnant women on a buprenorphine maintenance programme)
  - Women who are already on Suboxone® and become pregnant normally stop it and rotate to a mono-buprenorphine regime such as Subutex® (this may require more supervision as there is a higher risk of injection abuse of a mono-buprenorphine regime, compared to a Suboxone® regime which contains buprenorphine and naloxone, to decrease the risk of injection abuse)
- To be used with caution in sleep apnoea, asthma, simultaneous use of other sedatives/respiratory depressants, and moderate to severe renal and liver impairment

Sublingual tablets

- 200–400 mcg every 6–8 hours: £0.10–0.20 per tablet (£9–24 per month)
- Buprenorphine 2–8 mg tablets sublingual (indicated for management of addiction): £1–3 per tablet (£60–260 per month)

Buprenorphine patches

- Lower dose (Butrans® 5–20 mcg/hour): £1.40–14.00 per patch (£5.50–57.00 per month)
- Higher dose (Transtec® 35–70 mcg/hour): £2.50–8.00 per patch (£20–63 per month)

Intramuscular or slow intravenous injection

- 300–600 mcg every 6–8 hours: £0.49–0.98 per injection

Subcutaneous injection

- Buvidal® (SC injection) 8–128 mg (£56–240 per month)

Oral lyophilisate

- Espranor® 2–8 mg: £6–19 for seven tablets (£25–80 per month)

Cost

- (Large variability)

Further reading

1. Joint Formulary Committee. British National Formulary. 2020. London: BMJ Group and Pharmaceutical Press. https://www.bnf.org
2. Electronic Medicines Compendium (eMC). Buprenorphine drug data sheet. https://www.medicines.org.uk
3. The National Alliance of Advocates for Buprenorphine Treatment. Pharmacology of Buprenorphine. http://www.naabt.org/education/pharmacoloy_of_buprenorphine.cfm
4. Schug SA, Palmer GM, Scott DA, et al. Acute Pain Management: Scientific Evidence. 4th edition, 2015. Melbourne: Australian and New Zealand College of Anaesthetists and Faculty of Pain Medicine
5. US Food and Drug Administration. Buprenorphine. https://www.accessdata.fda.gov/drugsatfda_docs/label/2019/018401s025lbl.pdf
6. UpToDate. Buprenorphine. https://www.uptodate.com

7.3 Codeine

Class of drugs, names

- Weak opioid (analgesic, controlled drug)
- Codeine phosphate 15 mg, 30 mg, 60 mg
- Tablet, oral solution (Galcodine®), as solution for injection
- With paracetamol: co-dydramol (8/500), co-codamol (10/500), co-codamol (30/500)
- With ibuprofen: Nurofen® Plus (12.8/200)

Indications

- Licensed: mild to moderate pain
- Unlicensed: diarrhoea, cough suppression

Codeine-specific contraindications

(For general opioid contraindications, see 7.1 Overview of opioids, p. 119.)

- Acute ulcerative colitis, antibiotic-associated colitis
- All children under 12 years, children under 18 years undergoing removal of the tonsils or adenoids for the treatment of sleep apnoea. Codeine has been implicated in the deaths of children (ultrafast metabolizers produce higher morphine levels, causing respiratory depression). These children normally had other risk factors for respiratory depression
- Conditions where abdominal distension develops, conditions where inhibition of peristalsis should be avoided
- Known ultra-rapid codeine metabolizers (CYP2D6 variant)—increased risk of respiratory depression, especially if taking other sedatives, sleep apnoea, or other comorbidities that can affect respiratory function (higher risk of 'euphoria' that can lead to misuse and dependence)
- Avoid in renal impairment—accumulation of metabolites of codeine glucuronide and morphine
- **Caution:** acute abdomen, cardiac arrhythmias, gallstones, adolescents aged 12–18 years with breathing problems

Dose

- PO/IM 15–60 mg every 4 hours PRN (titrated to effect), maximum daily dose = 240 mg
- Hepatic impairment: may precipitate coma. Avoid or reduce dose
- Renal impairment: increased cerebral sensitivity, effects increased and prolonged. Avoid use or reduce dose

Equivalence and conversion

- Oral morphine equivalence 1:8 (oral morphine 30 mg ≈ oral codeine 240 mg)

Mode of action

- Prodrug converted to the active metabolites codeine 3-glucuronide, codeine 6-glucuronide, norcodeine, and morphine
- Principle analgesic effect (MOP receptor): codeine-6-glucuronide and morphine

Monitoring of treatment

- No specific long-term monitoring required

Codeine—specific side effects

(For general opioid side effects, see 7.1 Overview of opioids, p. 119.)

- Abdominal pain and constipation are common
- Minimal pain relief in slow CYP2D6 metabolizers (see pharmacokinetics of codeine)

Pharmacodynamics

- Respiratory: antitussive. Respiratory depression, ↓ ventilatory response to hypoxia and hypercapnia
- Cardiovascular: ≈ 10% potency of morphine
- GI: constipation secondary to ↓ GI motility

Pharmacokinetics

- Oral bioavailability: approximately 90%
- Metabolism: hepatic metabolism to 3- and 6-glucuronides of codeine (UGT2B7), norcodeine (CYP3A4), and morphine (CYP2D6)
  - 0.5–2.0% of population are ultra-rapid metabolizers: ↑ CYP2D6 activity, very sensitive
  - 5–10% poor metabolizers: codeine is ineffective and these patients can experience codeine-related S/Es
- Onset of action: 15–30 minutes
- Biological half life: 2.5–3 hours
- Duration of action: 4–6 hours
- Excretion: codeine metabolites excreted renally as conjugates with glucuronic acid

Interactions

- Anti-muscarinics: possible increased risk of anti-muscarinic S/Es when given concomitantly
- Rifampicin and phenytoin: accelerated metabolism of codeine
- Alcohol, antipsychotics: enhanced hypotensive and sedative effects
- Anaesthetic agents: possibly enhance effects of IV and volatile general anaesthetics
- TCAs, sedating antihistamines: sedative effects possibly increased
- Anxiolytics and hypnotics: increased sedative effects
- Cimetidine and some SSRIs: metabolism inhibited
- Domperidone: antagonism of domperidone-mediated GI activity

Special circumstances

- Pregnancy: neonatal respiratory depression and withdrawal symptoms, and maternal gastric stasis and aspiration pneumonia reported if used peri-partum
- Breastfeeding: contraindicated. Secreted into breast milk in small quantities. Higher production of morphine in ultra-rapid metabolizers, with potentially serious respiratory risks to infants from respiratory failure (deaths of newborns have been reported during breastfeeding)
- Elderly: possible confusion, oversedation, risk of falls, constipation

Additional information

- In acute pain: codeine 60 mg = NNT 7; codeine 60 mg/paracetamol 1 g = NNT 2.2 (paracetamol 1 g with ibuprofen 400 mg = NNT 1.5)
- Codeine alone for acute pain has low efficacy. It works better when combined with paracetamol and NSAIDs. Low doses of codeine (8/10/15 mg) used alone are unlikely to produce better analgesic effect than using paracetamol and NSAIDs

- Low-dose over-the-counter codeine preparations, combined with paracetamol and/or NSAID, are easily accessible. Misuse of these preparations commonly lead to patient harm from GI ulceration and bleeding, renal failure (renal tubular acidosis with hypokalaemia), protein-losing enteropathy, and hepatic impairment (toxic paracetamol metabolite)
- Studies have shown that low doses of codeine cause neuroimmune changes via the activation of glia, TLRs, and other changes associated with OIH/tolerance. It is hypothesized that this explains higher opioid use after surgery in some patients who were on codeine preoperatively

Cost

- Tablets: 15 mg: £0.04/tablet; 30 mg: £0.05/tablet; 60 mg: £0.09/tablet (£ 4.80–10.80 per month, depending on dose)
- Syrup: 25 mg/5 mL: £0.05/25 mg
- Oral solution: 15 mg/5 mL: £9.90
- Injection: 60 mg/mL 1 mL: £2.37

Further reading

1. Joint Formulary Committee. British National Formulary. 2020. London: BMJ Group and Pharmaceutical Press. https://www.bnf.org
2. American Society of Health-System Pharmacists. Codeine. In: Drug Information. 2016; p. 2868. Bethesda, MD: American Society of Health-System Pharmacists
3. Electronic Medicines Compendium (emc). Codeine phosphate tablets 30mg. 2020. http://www.medicines.org.uk/emc/medicine/23910
4. Shen H, He MM, Liu H, et al. Comparative metabolic capabilities and inhibitory profiles of CYP2D6.1, CYP2D6.10, and CYP2D6.17. Drug Metab Dispos 2007;35(8):1292–300

7.4 Dihydrocodeine

Class of drugs, names

- Dihydrocodeine tartrate
- Semi-synthetic opioid analgesic
- DF 118, DHC contus

Indications

- Licensed uses: moderate to severe pain, chronic severe pain, antitussive
- Unlicensed use: not licensed for children under 4 years

Dihydrocodeine-specific contraindications

(For general opioid contraindications, see 7.1 Overview of opioids, p. 119.)

- Acute ulcerative colitis, antibiotic-associated colitis
- All children under 12 years, children under 18 years undergoing removal of the tonsils or adenoids for the treatment of sleep apnoea. Codeine has been implicated in children's death (ultrafast metabolizers produce higher morphine levels, causing respiratory depression). These children normally had other risk factors for respiratory depression
- Conditions where abdominal distension develops, conditions where inhibition of peristalsis should be avoided

- Known ultra-rapid codeine metabolizers (CYP2D6 variant)—increased risk of respiratory depression, especially if also on other sedatives, sleep apnoea, or other comorbidities that can affect respiratory function (higher risk of 'euphoria' which can lead to misuse and dependence)
- Avoid in renal and hepatic impairment
- **Caution:** acute abdomen, cardiac arrhythmias, gallstones, adolescents aged 12–18years with breathing problems

Dose

Moderate to severe pain

- PO 30–60 mg 4- to 6-hourly as needed (PRN) (up to 240 mg/day)
- SC/IM: up to 50 mg 4- to 6-hourly PRN

Chronic severe pain

- PO 60–120 mg 12-hourly (modified-release) (max 240 mg/day)

Equivalence and conversion

- Oral morphine equivalence 1:8 (oral morphine 30 mg ≈ oral codeine 240 mg)

Renal impairment

- Avoid or reduce dose; opioid effects increased and prolonged; increased cerebral sensitivity occurs

Mode of action

- The active metabolite dihydromorphine is a highly selective MOP receptor agonist

Monitoring of treatment

- No specific long-term monitoring required

Specific side effects

(For general opioid S/Es, see 7.1 Overview of opioids, p. 119.)

- Abdominal pain and constipation are common
- Minimal pain relief in slow CYP2D6 metabolizers

Pharmacodynamics

- Limited data, similar to codeine

Pharmacokinetics

- **Oral bioavailability:** 20%
- **Distribution:** Vd: 1.1 L/kg. Reportedly low protein binding
- **Metabolism:**
  - Hepatic by cytochrome P450 isozymes CYP 2D6 to active metabolite dihydromorphine and CYP 3A4 to nor-dihydrocodeine. A third primary metabolite is dihydrocodeine-6-glucuronide
  - Uridine 5′-diphospho-glucurosyltransferase (UGT) enzymes to glucuronidated dihydrocodeine
- **Onset of action:** 30–45 minutes. Peak plasma concentration 1.5–2 hours after oral administration (immediate-release preparation)

- **Duration of action:** immediate release (IR) ≈ 4–6 hours
- **Clearance:** 300 mL/min
- **Elimiation half-life:** 240 minutes
- **Excretion:** renal excretion

Interactions

- **No specific interactions listed beyond general opioid interactions**

Special circumstances

- Pregnancy: may cause respiratory depression in the neonate. Codeine, its sister drug, has a possible association with respiratory and cardiac defects in first trimester
- Breastfeeding: avoid

Cost

Tablet

- Dihydrocodeine tartrate non-proprietary 30 mg: £0.06/tablet (£7.20–14.40 per month for 30–60 mg four times daily)
- Modified-release: DHC® Continus® 60 mg: £0.09/tablet

Oral solution

- Dihydrocodeine tartrate non-proprietary 2 mg/mL: £7.16/150 mL

Solution for injection

- Dihydrocodeine tartrate non-proprietary 50 mg/1 mL: £9.11/ampoule

Further reading

1. Ammon S, Hofmann U, Griese EU, et al. Pharmacokinetics of dihydrocodeine and its active metabolite after single and multiple oral dosing. Br J Clin Pharmacol 1999;48(3):317–22
2. Joint Formulary Committee. British National Formulary. 2020. London: BMJ Group and Pharmaceutical Press. https://www.bnf.org
3. DePriest AZ, Puet BL, Holt AC, et al. Metabolism and disposition of prescription opioids: a review. Forensic Sci Rev 2015;27(2):115–45
4. Electronic medicines compendium (emc). Dihydrocodeine phosphate tablets 30mg. 2020. https://www.medicines.org.uk/emc/product/10395/smpc
5. Rowell FJ, Seymour RA, Rawlins MD. Pharmacokinetics of intravenous and oral dihydrocodeine and its acid metabolites. Eur J Clin Pharmacol 1983;25(3):419–24
6. Schmidt H, Vormfelde SV, Walchner-Bonjean M, et al. The role of active metabolites in dihydrocodeine effects. Int J Clin Pharmacol Ther 2003;41(3):95–106

7.5 Fentanyl

Class of drugs

- Strong synthetic opioid
- Tertiary amine: synthetic phenylpiperidine derivative

Indications

- Acute pain
- Palliative care
- Sedation/analgesia on intensive care and during procedures

Specific contraindications/caution

(For general opioid contraindications, see 7.1 Overview of opioids, p. 119.)

- Specific: cerebral tumour, diabetes mellitus, impaired consciousness
- Buccal use: mucositis
- Transdermal use: risk of fatal respiratory depression if used on opiate-naïve patients
- IV: respiratory depression persisting post-operatively

Dose

Intravenous

- Induction of anaesthesia and supplementation of analgesia: 1–2 mcg/kg
- Infusion: 3–4.8 mcg/kg/hour (usually on HDU and ICU)
- PCA starting dose of 10–20 mcg every 5 minutes

Epidural

- 50–100 mcg bolus
- 2 mcg/mL if mixed with bupivacaine 0.1% or ropivacaine 0.2% infusion

Intrathecal

- 5–25 mcg bolus

Transdermal patches (12, 25, 50, 100 mcg/hour)

- Duration 72 hours. Equilibrium after 12–24 hours
- Change patches 72-hourly
- Generally avoid in acute and chronic pain

Sublingual/buccal tablet

- 100, 200, 400, 600 and 800 mcg lozenges/tablets (PRN max. four times daily)

Equivalence and conversion

- Transdermal patches (multiply patch dose in micrograms by 3 to obtain the OMEDD in milligrams). For example, a fentanyl patch 25 mcg/hour ≈ OMEDD 75 mg
- IV fentanyl (conversion factor 200) to calculate to an oral morphine equivalent dose. For example, IV fentanyl 100 mcg ≈ oral morphine 20 mg
- IV fentanyl 100 mcg ≈ IV morphine 7 mg

Mode of action

- Highly selective MOP receptor agonist
- Activates pre-synaptic Gi-protein receptor, hyperpolarizing the cell membrane by ↑ K^+ conductance
- Inhibits adenylyl cyclase: ↓ cyclic adenosine monophosphate (cAMP) production; closure of voltage-gated Ca^{2+} channels also occurs

Monitoring of treatment

- Monitor IV use in theatre
- Post-anaesthesia care unit (PACU) or level 2 environment in many hospitals (except PCA)

Pharmacodynamics

- CNS: 50–80 times analgesic potency of morphine. Little hypnosis and sedation. ↓ minimum alveolar concentration of volatile anaesthetic agents, ↑ effect of non-depolarizing muscle relaxants. Miosis secondary to Edinger–Westphal nucleus stimulation. Seizure-like motor activity reported—no demonstrable EEG activity
- Cardiovascular: bradycardia, cardiovascular response to laryngoscopy and intubation obtunded (cardiac output, mean arterial pressure, peripheral vascular resistance and systemic vascular resistance are stable, and pulmonary capillary wedge pressure is unaffected)
- Respiratory: potent respiratory depression (↓ respiratory rate (RR) and tidal volumes (T_V)); diminished ventilatory response to hypoxia and hypercarbia. Potent antitussive. Chest wall rigidity reported. Minimal histamine release and bronchospasm
- Genitourinary: ↑ tone of ureters, bladder detrusor muscle, and vesicular sphincter
- GI: ↓ GI motility, ↓ gastric acid secretion. Sphincter of Oddi spasm and ↑ common bile duct pressure
- Miscellaneous: high doses obtund metabolic stress response to surgery. No effect on ADH and minimal serotonin release

Specific side effects

(For general S/Es, see 7.1 Overview of opioids, p. 119.)

- Easy to develop tolerance and addiction
- Post-operative respiratory depression (secondary peak plasma concentration due to elution from muscle)

Pharmacokinetics

- **Oral bioavailability:** 33%. Transdermal absorption: 47% at 24 hours, 88% at 48 hours, 94% at 72 hours. Drug delivery continues after patch removal
- V_D: 0.88–4.1 L/kg; 81–94% protein-bound. No delayed respiratory depression post-intrathecal administration as rapidly absorbed into spinal cord
- **Metabolism:** hepatic metabolism predominantly by cytochrome P450 isozyme CYP 3A4 by N-dealkylation to norfentanyl/subsequent hydroxylation to hydroxypropionyl derivatives. Inactive metabolites and safe to use in renal impairment
- **Onset of action:** 2–5 minutes (IV and sublingual/buccal)
- **Duration of action:** small dose 30–60 minutes, and high dose (>5 mcg/kg) 4–6 hours
- **Clearance:** 13 mL/kg/min
- **t1/2 elimination:** 141–853 minutes (short duration of action of single dose due to redistribution; infusion prolongs duration of action due to saturation of tissues)
- **Excretion:** renal excretion (10% excreted unaltered in urine). Clearance decreased in renal and hepatic impairment

Interactions

- Incompatible with thiopentone and methohexital

Special circumstances

- **Pregnancy:** as per morphine
- **Breastfeeding:** monitor infant for opioid-induced S/Es
- Not known if removed by haemodialysis

Cost

Sublingual tablet

- 100 mcg tablet: 10-tablet pack: £49.99 (£150 monthly, depending on dose)

Nasal spray

- 50 mcg/metred spray; 10-dose pack: £59.50

Solution for injection

- Fentanyl citrate 50 mcg/mL, 2 mL ampoule: £0.30; 10 mL ampoule: £0.64

Transdermal patches

- 12 mcg/hour, pack of 5: £7 (£14–66 monthly, depending on dose)

Further reading

1. Joint Formulary Committee. British National Formulary. 2020. London: BMJ Group and Pharmaceutical Press. https://www.bnf.org
2. Scarth E, Smith S. Drugs in Anaesthesia and Intensive Care. 5th edition, 2016. Oxford: Oxford University Press

7.6 Methadone

Class of drug, names

- Strong opioid, controlled drug (methadone hydrochloride)
- Tablets: 5 mg
- Injection: 10, 20, and 50 mg/mL
- Oral solution: 1, 10, and 20 mg/mL

Indications

- Methadone (non-proprietary) is primarily used in the treatment of opioid drug addiction
- Treatment of severe pain (commonly in palliative care)
- Terminal cough (in palliative care)

Specific contraindications

(For general opioid contraindications, see 7.1 Overview of opioids, p. 119.)

- Significant obstructive airway disease or respiratory depression
- Severe hepatic impairment
- Ulcerative colitis
- MAOIs inhibitors

Mode of action

- Methadone is both a potent MOP (mu) receptor agonist, with both high affinity and efficacy (R-enantiomer), and a glutamate (NMDA) receptor antagonist (D-enantiomer)
- It is a weak agonist at KOP (kappa) and DOP (delta) receptors

Monitoring

- ECG pre-initiation, and on significant dose increase in patients at risk of long QT syndrome
- Monitoring of hormone levels for all patients on significant doses of long-term opioids, and for methadone patients, particularly prolactin
- Clinical supervision and urine testing on drug treatment programmes (methadone is present in both saliva and sweat)

Methadone-specific side effects

(For general opioid S/Es, see 7.1 Overview of opioids, p. 119.)

- Cardiovascular: bradycardia, QT interval prolongation, and torsades de pointes
- Respiratory: respiratory depression (immediate/delayed) as has long half-life
- Drowsiness is common
- Localized pain, erythema, and swelling, with treatment by SC infusion
- Stigma

Dose

- PO, SC, or IM injection: initially 5–10 mg every 6–8 hours (every 12 hours or once daily if prolonged use)
- PO for opioid withdrawal: 10–30 mg once daily, increased by 5–10 mg daily according to response (maximum weekly dose increase: 30 mg), typical maintenance dose 40–120 mg daily
- PO for terminal cough (linctus): 1–2 mg every 4–6 hours, reduced to 1–2 mg twice daily if prolonged use
- Dose equivalence to oral morphine 1:3–1:20, depending on oral morphine daily dose and the dosing conversion regime used (see Table 7.6.1)
- For opioid rotations with methadone, see 7.13 Opioid rotation and conversion, p. 158

Table 7.6.1 Morphine to methadone conversion ratios

Ayonrinde regime		Mercadante regime		Ripamonti regime	
Oral morphine daily dose	Conversion ratio	Oral morphine daily dose	Conversion ratio	Oral morphine daily dose	Conversion ratio
<100 mg	3:1	30–90 mg	4:1	30–90 mg	4:1
101–300 mg	5:1	90–300 mg	8:1	90–300 mg	6:1
301–600 mg	10:1	>300 mg	12:1	>300 mg	8:1
601–800 mg	12:1				
801–1000 mg	15:1				
>1001 mg	20:1				

Pharmacokinetics

- Methadone is well absorbed but undergoes significant first-pass metabolism, having a variable oral bioavailability of around 50%
- Peak plasma concentration at 4 hours
- Methadone is extensively protein-bound and has relatively high lipid solubility
- Vd: 100–500 L
- The terminal half-life is 12 hours (initially), increasing to 50 hours or more over the first week of use
- The analgesic half-life is often much shorter at 6–8 hours
- Methadone undergoes hepatic metabolism primarily via CYP450 3A4 (and CYP450 2D6 to a lesser extent) to inactive metabolites, but a minority is excreted unchanged in the urine (CYP450 3A4 shows significant intra-individual variability)

Interactions

- CYP450 3A4 and 2D6 inhibitor inducers reduce the plasma concentrations of methadone (examples include carbamazepine, phenytoin, spironolactone, St John's wort, tobacco, alcohol, and rifampicin)
- Methadone appears to initially induce its own metabolism

Special circumstances

- When used in a drug treatment programme during pregnancy, there is a risk of neonatal opioid withdrawal syndrome; this ideally needs to be anticipated and managed in a hospital setting. Methadone should not be used in labour. It is excreted in breast milk
- Methadone is not suitable for children
- Use with caution in the elderly as clearance is reduced
- Clearance is higher in females than in males

Additional information

- Methadone slowly accumulates after initiation, lengthening the half-life and leading to an increased risk of overdose (caution needed when switching from other opioids to methadone)
- Due to its dual effect, methadone might have an advantage in treating chronic neuropathic pain over other opioids (in practice, there has been an increase in mortality associated with its use)
- When used in opioid withdrawal programmes, patients may attempt to trick urine testing by adding methadone directly to their urine (while methadone is excreted directly in the urine, so is its major metabolite 2-Ethylidene-1,5-dimethyl-3,3-diphenylpyrrolidine perchlorate, meaning this is easily spotted)
- Methadone may be associated with a lower rate of tolerance, dependence, and withdrawal. Tolerance may be rapidly lost on discontinuation

Cost

- Methadone 5 mg tablets: £0.05 per 50 tablets (£12–36 per month)
- Methadone 1 mg/mL solution: £1 per 100 mL
- Methadone 10 mg/mL solution: £12 for 150 mL
- Methadone 50 mg/mL for injection, 1 mL ampoule: £1.50 (£45–90 per month)

Further reading

1. Joint Formulary Committee. British National Formulary. 2020. London: BMJ Group and Pharmaceutical Press. https://www.bnf.org
2. Electronic Medicines Compendium (emc). Methadone 5mg hydrochloride tablets. 2020. https://www.medicines.org.uk/emc/product/3568/smpc
3. Ostgathe C, Voltz R, Van Aaken A, et al. Practicability, safety, and efficacy of a 'German model' for opioid conversion to oral levo-methadone. Support Care Cancer 2012;20:2105–10
4. US Food and Drug Administration. Methadone. https://www.accessdata.fda.gov/drugsatfda_docs/label/2018/006134s045lbl.pdf

7.7 Morphine

Class of drugs, names

- Phenanthrene derivative (morphine hydrochloride or morphine sulphate)
- Strong opioid (analgesic, controlled drug)

Indications

Licensed uses

- Acute pain
- Chronic pain
- Pain management in palliative care
- Cough in terminal disease
- Premedication
- PCA
- Myocardial infarction (MI)
- Acute pulmonary oedema
- Dyspnoea at rest in palliative care

Unlicensed uses

- Morphine sulfate solution PO in children aged under 1 year
- Sevredol® tablets in children aged under 3 years
- Suppositories not licensed for rectal use in children

Specific contraindications

(For general opioid contraindications, see 7.1 Overview of opioids, p. 119.)

Hepatic impairment

- Use with caution, can precipitate encephalopathy
- Reduce dose (avoid oral preparations in acute impairment)

Renal impairment

- Avoid use or reduce dose (active metabolite morphine-6-glucuronide accumulates)
- Opioid effects potentiated and prolonged with increased cerebral sensitivity

Dose

Oral

- Initially 10 mg 3- to 4-hourly, titrate to response
- Elderly: 2.5–5 mg 4-hourly

Intravenous, subcutaneous, or intramuscular

- 0.05–0.1 mg/kg 3- to 4-hourly. Doses normally used in opioid-naïve patients: 5–10 mg, titrated to response (dose can be adjusted more frequently during titration). Decreased dose in frail and elderly patients

Intrathecal (100–200 mcg) or epidural (1–2 mg)—preservative-free

- (See 20.8 Intrathecal drug delivery systems, p. 384)

Rectal

- Initially 15–30 mg every 4 hours

Mode of action

- Agonist at mu and kappa receptors
- Increases intracellular Ca^{2+} concentration, increasing K^+ conductance and hyperpolarization of excitable cell membranes
- Decreased membrane excitability decreases pre- and post-synaptic responses

Monitoring of treatment

- Ward-based monitoring in quoted doses (sedation scores, HR, oxygen saturation (SpO_2), RR, BP)
- Closer monitoring if higher doses, e.g. in post-anaesthetic care unit
- Monitor kidney and liver function regularly (in acute post-operative pain, every 2–3 days)

Specific side effects

- For general S/Es, see 7.1 Overview of opioids, p. 119

Pharmacodynamics

- **CVS:** minimal. Orthostatic hypotension, bradycardia
- **RS:** respiratory depression with decreased ventilatory response to hypoxia and hypercarbia. Antitussive. Bronchoconstriction at high doses
- **CNS:** drowsiness, relief of anxiety, euphoria, miosis, seizure activity at high doses
- **GI:** constipation. Decreases gastric, biliary, and pancreatic secretions. Sphincter of Oddi spasm
- **GU:** urinary retention
- **Other:** histamine release, pruritus

Pharmacokinetics

- **Oral bioavailability:** 15–50% (commonly regarded to be 30%). Well absorbed, but extensive first-pass metabolism
- **Distribution:** 20–40% protein-bound in plasma, predominantly to albumin. Vd 3.4–4.7 L/kg (slow equilibration between plasma and CSF; no clear correlation with degree of analgesia and plasma concentration)

- **Metabolism:** hepatic to morphine-3-glucuronide (arousal), morphine-6-glucuronide (analgesia) and normorphine
- **Onset of action:** 30–60 minutes
- **Duration of action:** 3–4 hours
- **Biological half-life:** 2.5–3 hours
- **Clearance:** 12–23 mL/min/kg
- **half-life elimination:** 1.7–4.5 hours
- **Excretion:** predominantly renal as glucuronide conjugates; 10% excreted in faeces as conjugated morphine

Interactions

- Alcohol and antipsychotics: enhance hypotensive and sedative effects when co-administered
- MAOIs: possible CNS excitation or depression with co-administration and up to 2 weeks after cessation
- Moclobemide: possible CNS excitation or depression
- Gabapentin: morphine increases bioavailability
- Esmolol: morphine possibly increases its plasma concentration
- Domperidone and metoclopramide: opioid analgesics antagonize effects on GI activity
- Baclofen and sedative antihistamines: increased sedative effect when co-administered with morphine
- Sodium oxybate: opioids enhance effects; avoid concomitant use

Special circumstances

- Pregnancy: neonatal respiratory depression and withdrawal symptoms, and maternal gastric stasis and aspiration pneumonia reported if used peri-partum
- Breastfeeding: therapeutic doses unlikely to affect infant
- Elderly: possible confusion and oversedation

Additional information

- Can precipitate dependence, tolerance, and addiction, as with other opioids
- Decrease dose gradually to avoid withdrawal and abstinence symptoms, especially if taken for longer periods
- Available in combination with cyclizine (for short-term use in moderate to severe pain)
- Not removed by haemodialysis or peritoneal dialysis

Cost

Immediate-release morphine

- Morphine tablets—Sevredol® 10 mg: £0.10/tablet (for 20–40 mg/day: £6–12 per month)

Modified-release morphine

- Capsules—Zomorph® 10 mg: £0.06/capsule (10 mg twice daily: £3.50 per month)
- MST®—tablets 10 mg: £0.06–0.09/tablet (10 mg twice daily: £4–5 per month)
- MST Continus® suspension (granules) 20 mg: £1.22/sachet (20 mg twice daily: £73 per month)

Oral liquid solutions

- Non-proprietary 10 mg/5 mL: £1.68/100 mL (for 20–40 mg/day: £5–10 per month)
- Oramorph® 10 mg/5 mL: £1.89/100 mL (for 20–40 mg/day: £5.70–11.40 per month)

Solution for injection

- 10 mg/1 mL: £1.10/ampoule
- For IV infusion—50 mg/50 mL: £5.78; 100 mg/50 mL: £6.48

Further reading

1. Joint Formulary Committee. British National Formulary. 2020. London: BMJ Group and Pharmaceutical Press. https://www.bnf.org
2. Scarth E, Smith S. Drugs in Anaesthesia and Intensive Care. 5th edition, 2016. Oxford: Oxford University Press

7.8 Naloxone

Class of drugs, names

- Naloxone hydrochloride substituted oxymorphone derivative
- Opioid receptor antagonist (mu > delta > kappa > sigma)

Indications

- Licensed use: overdose with opioids in medical or non-medical setting
- Reversal of post-operative respiratory depression
- Treatment of clonidine overdose

Caution

- Cardiovascular disease (those receiving cardiotoxic drugs)
- Pregnancy—maternal opioid dependence (precipitation of opioid withdrawal in newborns)
- Patients with opioid dependence—sudden cessation of opioids causes flare-up of pain and opioid withdrawal symptoms
- Titration of dose—titrate dose for each patient to obtain sufficient respiratory response without completely antagonizing the analgesic effects of opioids

Dose in opioid overdose (intravenous)

- >12 years: initially 400 mcg, then 800 mcg up to two doses at 1-minute intervals. Increased to 2 mg for one dose if still no response; 4 mg may be required in severe poisoning. Then review diagnosis
- Child aged 1 month to 11 years: initially 100 mcg/kg; if no response, repeat at 1-minute intervals to maximum of 2 mg, then review diagnosis
- Adequate IV dose is that which maintains satisfactory ventilation for at least 15 minutes
- Continuous infusion (all ages): start rate at 60% of initial resuscitative dose per hour. Titrate to response for all ages

Dose for reversal of post-operative respiratory depression (intravenous)

- >12 years: 100–200 mcg or bolus 1.5–3 mcg/kg. If adequate response, give subsequent doses of 100 mcg every 2 minutes or 100 mcg IM every 1–2 hours

Mode of action

- Competitive antagonist at MOP, DOP, KOP, and sigma opioid receptors
- Negligible affinity to nociceptin opioid peptide (NOP) receptors
- Reversal of MOP receptor effects: sedation, respiratory depression, dysphoria

Monitoring of treatment

- Close monitoring of vital signs (sedation scores, HR, BP, RR, SpO_2) in context of opioid overdose

Side effects

- In presence of opioids: sweating, nausea, restlessness, trembling, vomiting, flushing, and headache
- Rarely arrhythmia, seizures, and pulmonary oedema
- Serious ventricular dysrhythmias in patients with irritable myocardium

Pharmacodynamics

- GI: reverses opioid-induced spasm of sphincter of Oddi
- CNS: slight drowsiness at high doses. Obtunds some forms of stress-induced analgesia. Decreases pain tolerance in those with high pain thresholds
- Cardiovascular: no effect at normal doses. Increased BP with doses >0.3 mg/kg

Pharmacokinetics

- **Oral bioavailability:** 2% oral bioavailability (91% absorbed, but extensive first-pass metabolism)
- **Vd:** 2 L/kg, 46% protein-bound
- **Metabolism:** hepatic metabolism by conjugation to glucuronide
- **Onset of action:** IV, 2 minutes; IM, 5 minutes
- **Duration of action:** approximately 20 minutes
- **Clearance:** 25 mL/min
- **Plasma half-life:** 1.2 hours
- **Excretion:** renal excretion

Special circumstances

- **Pregnancy:** no adverse effects known, but use only if potential benefit outweighs risk (animal studies do not suggest detrimental effects)
- **Neonates/infants:** can be used in the presence of respiratory depression if the mother has been exposed to opioids during the pregnancy

Additional information

- Alleviates pruritus, nausea, and respiratory depression associated with epidural or intrathecal opioids (in small IV boluses of 25–50 mcg)
- Available in combination with buprenorphine (Suboxone®) as an adjunct in the treatment of opioid dependence
- Available in combination with oxycodone (Targinact®) for pain management (associated with less opioid-induced constipation)
- Rarely used for severe idiopathic restless legs syndrome after failure of dopaminergic therapy (no good evidence to support this indication)

- Naloxone (IV 0.5 mg/kg) sometimes used for opioid-induced urinary retention, with minimal worsening of pain severity. This can be found sometimes in children receiving opioids for acute pain management

Cost—injection (non-proprietary)

- 20 mcg/mL, 2 mL ampoule: £5.50
- 400 mcg/mL, 1 mL ampoule: £3.60–4.50
- 1 mg/mL, 2 mL prefilled syringe: £16.80

Further reading

1. Joint Formulary Committee. British National Formulary. 2020. London: BMJ Group and Pharmaceutical Press. https://www.bnf.org
2. Scarth E, Smith S. Drugs in Anaesthesia and Intensive Care. 5th edition, 2016. Oxford: Oxford University Press

7.9 Naltrexone

Class of drugs, names

- Opioid receptor antagonist (competitive)
- Adepend®, Naltrexone®, Nalorex®, Naltrexone hydrochloride

Indications

- Prevention of relapse in previously opioid- or alcohol-dependent patients (to be initiated under specialist supervision, unlicensed for alcohol-dependent patients)
- Naltrexone has also been combined with opioids (morphine, oxycodone), and there is some evidence of reduction in tolerance, possibly enhanced analgesia, and reduced abuse potential
- Methylnaltrexone is a peripherally acting MOP receptor antagonist that is licensed as SC injection in the treatment of opioid-induced constipation
- Naltrexone with bupropion (Mysimba®) is licensed for weight loss in obesity, in conjunction with dietary measures and increased physical activity (especially if patients have cardiac risk factors such as diabetes, hypertension, and dyslipidaemia)

Contraindications

- Avoid in acute hepatitis and severe hepatic and/or renal failure
- In patients who fail a naloxone challenge test (where an injection of naloxone elicits acute effects of opioid withdrawal)
- In patients not opioid-free for 7 days pretreatment
- Uncontrolled hypertension, epilepsy, CNS tumour, bipolar disorder, bulimia, anorexia nervosa
- Patients undergoing acute opioid, alcohol, or BZD withdrawal
- Use of MAOIs with last 14 days

Mode of action

- Naltrexone is a competitive antagonist acting at all three classic opioid receptors (MOP, DOP, KOP), possessing high affinity for the receptors, but no efficacy

Monitoring

- LFTs before and during treatment
- Signs of opioid withdrawal if used in patients on long-term opioids

Side effects

- GI: nausea, vomiting, loss of appetite, thirst, diarrhoea, abdominal pain. The most common reason for discontinuation of naltrexone in trials was nausea
- CNS: headaches, fatigue, irritability, mood swings, sleep disruption
- General effects: muscle pain, sweating, impotence, and delayed ejaculation are also common

Dose

Oral

Opioid/alcohol dependency

- Naltrexone hydrochloride initiated at 25 mg once daily
- Standard dose: 50 mg once daily
- Once established, it can also be used at 100–150 mg once every 2–3 days (maximum weekly dose 350 mg)

Weight management

- Mysimba® 8/90 (naltrexone hydrochloride 8mg/bupropion hydrochloride 90mg)
- Initiate once daily
- Increase by one tablet every week. Maximum four tablets daily

Subcutaneous (opioid-induced constipation)

- Methylnaltrexone 8 mg (38–61 kg) and 12 mg (62–114 kg) used on alternate days normally

Intramuscular (alcohol dependence)

- Vivitrol® 380 mg injection every 4 weeks

Pharmacokinetics

- Oral bioavailability: only 25% (oral dose well absorbed, but extensive first-pass hepatic metabolism)
- Peak plasma levels: within 1 hour
- Vd: 1300 L, 20% protein-bound
- Metabolism:
  - Predominantly reduction (independent of the cytochrome P450 system)
  - Metabolites are clinically inactive. Mainly renally excreted
  - Elimination half-life: 4–12 hours

Interactions

- Should not be used in conjunction with opioid medication
- Caution with any medications that may cause sedation, especially thioridazine

Special circumstances

- Not recommended in children and breastfeeding mothers (due to potential toxicity)
- Pregnancy: naltrexone has been reported to be toxic in animal studies (use only if benefit outweighs risk)

- Elderly: not recommended in patients aged >75 years, and avoid in patients aged >65 years

Additional information

- Reported as useful in cholestatic pruritus
- Naltrexone does not appear to increase or decrease suicide risk in patients
- Hepatotoxic in overdose, though data are limited—but appears non-toxic at a dose of 800 mg/day (very high doses of opioids are needed to re-narcotize a patient on naltrexone, which leads to a large histamine release)
- Naltrexone produces pupillary constriction; the mechanism is unknown
- Tolerance is not an issue with prolonged use

Cost

- Naltrexone 50 mg: £0.80–1.80 per tablet (£25–55 per month)

Further reading

1. Joint Formulary Committee. British National Formulary. 2020. London: BMJ Group and Pharmaceutical Press. https://www.bnf.org
2. Electronic Medicines Compendium (emc). Naltrexone Hydrochloride 50mg filmcoated tablets. 2014. https://www.medicines.org.uk/emc/product/6073/smpc#gref
3. National Institute for Health and Care Excellence (NICE). Naltrexone for the management of opioid dependence. TA115. 2007. https://www.nice.org.uk/guidance/ta115
4. US Food and Drug Administration. Vivitrol (Naltrexone). 2010. https://www.accessdata.fda.gov/drugsatfda_docs/label/2010/021897s015lbl.pdf

7.10 Oxycodone

Class of drugs, names

- Semi-synthetic opioid (oxycodone hydrochloride)
- Abtard®, Carexil®, Longtec®, Oxeltra®, OxyContin®, Oxylan®, Reltebon®, Zomestine® (slow release)
- Capsules: Lynlor®, OxyNorm®, Shortec® (immediate release (IR))
- Oral solution/solution for injection: oxycodone, OxyNorm® (IR)

Indications (licensed)

- Moderate to severe post-operative/palliative care pain

Specific contraindications/caution

(For general opioid contraindications, see 7.1 Overview of opioids, p. 119.)

Hepatic impairment

- Initial dose reduction of 50% in mild impairment (e.g. maximum initial dose 2.5 mg 6-hourly in opioid-naïve patients), adjust according to response
- Avoid in moderate to severe impairment

Renal impairment

- Maximum initial dose 2.5 mg 6-hourly in opioid-naïve patients with mild to moderate impairment
- Avoid when eGFR <10 mL/min/1.73 m^2

Dose

Oral (uptitrate as required)

- Immediate release: initially 5 mg 4- to 6-hourly
- Modified release (MR): initially 10 mg 12-hourly

Intravenous

- Bolus: 1–10 mg 4-hourly PRN by slow IV injection
- Infusion: initially 1–2 mg/hour, titrate to response
- PCA: typically 1 mg/5 minutes

Subcutaneous

- Bolus: initially 5 mg 4-hourly PRN
- Infusion: initially 7.5 mg every 24 hours, titrate to response

Equivalence and conversion

- Oral oxycodone 3 mg ≈ IV oxycodone 1 mg
- Oral morphine equivalence 1.5:1 (oral morphine 15 mg ≈ oral oxycodone 10 mg)

Mode of action

- Agonist at MOP, KOP, and DOP receptors
- ↑ intracellular Ca^{2+} concentration, ↑ K^+ conductance, and hyperpolarization of excitable cell membranes
- Inhibition of adenylyl cyclase: ↓ cAMP production, causing closure of voltage-sensitive Ca^{2+} channels. ↓ membrane excitability, decreasing pre- and post-synaptic responses

Monitoring of treatment

- Close monitoring in context of opioid overdose and tolerance, dependence, and diversion

Specific side effects

- (For opioid S/Es, see 7.1 Overview of opioids, p. 119)

Pharmacodynamics

- Cardiovascular: minimal orthostatic hypotension
- Respiratory: respiratory depression with decreased ventilatory response to hypoxia and hypercarbia. Antitussive. Bronchoconstriction at high doses
- CNS: drowsiness, relief of anxiety, euphoria, miosis, seizure activity at high doses
- GI: constipation
- Genitourinary: urinary retention
- Other: histamine release, pruritus

Pharmacokinetics

- **Oral bioavailability:** 60–87%
- Vd: 2.6 L/kg; 45% protein-bound
- **Metabolism:** hepatic metabolism, CYP450 3A to noroxycodone, CYP450 2D6 to oxymorphone and other conjugated glucuronides
- **Onset of action:** PO IR: P_{max} 1–1.5 hours; PO MR: P_{max} 3 hours
- **Duration of action:** PO IR: 3–6 hours. PR 6–10 hours
- **Clearance:** 800 mL/min
- **Elmination half-life:** IR 3 hours; MR 4.5 hours
- **Excretion:** 19% free drug, 50% conjugated oxycodone, and 14% conjugated oxymorphone excreted in the urine

Interactions

- Alcohol: enhances hypotensive and sedative effects
- Buprenorphine: possible opioid withdrawal
- Telithromycin: inhibits oxycodone metabolism
- Itraconazole, ketoconazole, voriconazole: increases plasma concentration of oxycodone
- Domperidone and metoclopramide: opioid analgesics antagonize the effects on GI activity

Special circumstances

- Pregnancy: penetrates the placenta
- Breastfeeding: avoid (present in milk)
- Elderly: reduce dose

Additional information

- Reduce dose gradually after long-term treatment to avoid withdrawal symptoms
- Not removed by haemodialysis or peritoneal dialysis

Cost

MR tablet (slow release)

- Abtard®, Carexil®, Longtec®, Oxeltra®, OxyContin®, Reltebon® 10 mg: £0.11–0.45/tablet (£6.70–27.00 per month)

Capsule (immediate release)

- Lynlor®, OxyNorm®, Shortec® 10 mg: £0.25–0.41/capsule (at 20–60 mg per day = £13.70–75.00 per month)

Oral solution (immediate release)

- Non-proprietary, OxyNorm® 1 mg/mL: £3.84/100 mL (10 mg = £0.38) (at 20–60 mg per day = £2.30–68.00 per month)

Solution for injection

- Non-proprietary, OxyNorm® 10 mg/1 mL: £1.60/ampoule
- Non-proprietary, OxyNorm® 50 mg/1 mL: £14.02/ampoule

Further reading

1. Joint Formulary Committee. British National Formulary. 2020. London: BMJ Group and Pharmaceutical Press. https://www.bnf.org
2. Scarth E, Smith S. Drugs in Anaesthesia and Intensive Care. 5th edition, 2016. Oxford: Oxford University Press

7.11 Tapentadol

Class of drugs, names

- Strong opioid (controlled drug) (tapentadol hydrochloride)
- Tapentadol hydrochloride (oral solution 20 mg/mL, MR tablets 50–250 mg, IR tablets 50–75 mg)

Indications

- Licensed for moderate to severe pain in acute pain in adults
- Sustained-release formulation for severe chronic pain only

Contraindications (tapentadol-specific)

(For general opioid contraindications, see 7.1 Overview of opioids, p. 119.)

- Known hypersensitivity/allergy to tapentadol
- Paralytic ileus
- Recent use of MAOIs (within 14 days)
- Acute intoxication with another centrally acting drug
- Avoid in severe hepatic impairment and severe renal impairment, epilepsy, seizure susceptibility, and impaired consciousness

Mode of action

- MOP receptor agonist
- Inhibition of noradrenaline uptake
- Therefore, effective at ascending and descending pain pathways

Monitoring

- Pain score, sedation score, and RR
- LFTs recommended for patients with hepatic impairment
- Testing for androgen deficiency (advised only if clinically suspected)
- All patients treated with stronger opioids should be monitored for evidence of misuse

Tapentadol-specific side effects

(For general opioid S/Es, see 7.1 Overview of opioids, p. 119.)

- Less respiratory depression, nausea, vomiting, pruritus, and constipation than with other opioids which are full MOP receptor agonists (e.g. oxycodone)
- Headaches, seizures (rarely)
- Associated with serotonin syndrome (rarely), which may be precipitated if administered with medications that increase serotonin levels such as triptans, TCAs, SSRIs, and SNRIs

Dose

Modified-release

- Starting dose: 50–100 mg every 12 hours (start with 50 mg in opioid-naïve patients)
- After initiation, the dose should be titrated individually to provide adequate analgesia and avoid S/Es (including pain severity, previous treatments, and adjusted according to response)
- Increments of tapentadol 50 mg twice daily every 2–3 days have been shown to be appropriate to achieve adequate analgesia
- Maximum daily dose: 500 mg

Immediate-release

- 50–100 mg every 4–6 hours
- Maximum daily dose: 600 mg (700 mg in first 24 hours)

Other points on dose ranges

- Tapentadol MR can be combined with tapentadol IR for breakthrough pain
- The effective steady-state dose of tapentadol has been shown to be between 300 mg and 350 mg per day
- Other guidelines recommend a daily maximum dose of 250 mg tapentadol (= 80 mg oral morphine equivalent dose)
- When switching from other opioids to tapentadol, a higher initial dose of tapentadol may be required (see Table 7.11.1)
- Abrupt discontinuation of tapentadol may cause withdrawal symptoms (therefore, taper the dose gradually)
- Reduced doses are recommended in patients aged over 65 years and in moderate renal and hepatic impairment

Equivalence to other opioids

- Equianalgesic doses are based on expert opinions (limited data)
- For opioid conversions, the usual equipotent dose reduction of 25–50% is recommended
- The relative potency of tapentadol to oxycodone is estimated to be 1:5 (oral oxycodone MR 10 mg = oral tapentadol 50 mg)
- Morphine equivalence has also been quoted as 3:10 (oral morphine 15 mg = oral tapentadol 50 mg)

Table 7.11.1 Opioid conversion to tapentadol

Current opioid	Current opioid dose			
Hydromorphone, oral (mg/day)	11	12–15	16–19	20–27
Oxycodone, oral (mg/day)	39	50–59	60–79	80–99
Morphine, oral (mg/day)	79	80–119	120–159	160–199
Buprenorphine patches (mcg/hour)	34	35–52.4	52.5–69	70–87.4
Fentanyl patches (mcg/hour)	37	37.5–49.9	50–74	75–86
Starting dose of tapentadol (slow release)	50 mg × 2/day	100 mg × 2/day	150 mg × 2/day	200 mg × 2/day

Modified from Sanchez del Aguila et al., 2015 and with permission from Grunenthal Ltd.

Opioid conversion to tapentadol

The figures provided are an approximate guide to a range of doses of other opioids to one dose of tapentadol MR.

Pharmacokinetics

- **Oral bioavailability:** about 30% due to first-pass metabolism (despite initial high oral absorption)
- **Peak plasma level:** 80 minutes
- Vd: 500–1200 L, 20% protein-bound
- **Metabolism:**
  - 97% metabolized by conjugation with glucuronic acid (high metabolic rate implies extra-hepatic metabolism)
  - A minority part of metabolism is via the cytochrome P450 system
  - The metabolites are clinically inactive, and 99% excreted by the kidney
- **Terminal half-life:** 4 hours

Interactions

- Direct interactions appear minimal as tapentadol metabolism is through a high capacity system that is not easily saturated
- Further, tapentadol is neither highly protein-bound (20%) nor does it appear to interfere with the cytochrome P450 system
- Tapentadol should not be used with other opioids, and caution with other drugs with possible centrally acting depressant effects

Medicines and Healthcare products Regulatory Agency (MHRA)/Commission on Human Medicines (CHM) advice (BNF)

- Prescribe with caution in patients with a history of seizures and epilepsy (can lower seizure threshold, in particular if prescribed with antidepressants, e.g. SSRIs, SNRIs, TCAs, antipsychotics)
- Serotonin syndrome has been reported in combination with serotonergic antidepressants (SSRIs, SNRIs, TCAs)
- Withdrawal of the serotonergic substance usually improves serotonin syndrome rapidly

Special circumstances

- Not licensed for use in children
- However, the oral solution can be used from the age of 2 at a dose of 1.25 mg/kg every 4 hours; do not exceed the calculated dose for a bodyweight on the 97.5th percentile for the given age, with a maximum of 100 mg per dose) (see BNF for Children)
- High serum levels occur in patients with significant hepatic impairment
- Avoid in pregnancy (no information available, risk of respiratory depression and withdrawal in neonates)
- Excreted in breast milk. Avoid with breastfeeding (no information available)

Additional information

- Pharmacokinetics are similar in the elderly and in renal failure, although metabolites may accumulate with significant renal failure

- Tapentadol has reduced abuse potential, compared to opioids, which are full MOP receptor agonists
- Tapentadol has significantly less affinity to opioid receptors than morphine (1/10 to 1/18 weaker than the binding affinity of morphine to mu receptors) but is an equipotent analgesic, suggesting that its actions on noradrenaline reuptake are relevant to the analgesic effect. Its action on opioid receptors account for approximately 30% of its activity, and its action on noradrenaline reuptake accounts for 70% of its activity
- Less activity on opioid receptors and most of its activity on noradrenaline reuptake is a hypothesis to explain a better S/E profile associated with tapentadol. Studies have reported a lower risk of respiratory depression, less tolerance and constipation/nausea/vomiting, and less immunosuppression with tapentadol versus conventional opioids (full MOP agonists)
- Use with caution in patients on centrally acting drugs for Parkinson's disease, and those with dystonia, dementia, or psychiatric conditions (especially elderly patients)
- Advantages of tapentadol versus tramadol: less risk of developing seizures, less confusion or cognitive dysfunction, less risk of serotonergic reactions, safer in mild/moderate renal impairment, less interactions with TCA, SSRIs, and SNRIs, minimal CYP450 metabolism
- Disadvantages of tapentadol versus tramadol: no IV preparation, more expensive; currently, there is less evidence on tapentadol in pain management because it is a newer drug

Cost

- Tapentadol IR oral solution (20 mg/mL): £0.45–0.90 for 50–100 mg (£18 per 100 mL bottle)
- Tapentadol IR tablets 50–75 mg (£0.45–0.67/tablet) (£13.50–81.00 per month)
- Tapentadol MR tablets 50–250 mg (£0.45–2.25/tablet) (£27–133 per month)

Further reading

1. Joint Formulary Committee. British National Formulary. 2020. London: BMJ Group and Pharmaceutical Press. https://www.bnf.org
2. Electronic Medicines Compendium (eMC). Tapentadol drug data sheet. https://www.medicines.org.uk
3. US Food and Drug Administration. Tapentadol. https://www.accessdata.fda.gov/drugsatfda_docs/label/2010/022304s003lbl.pdf
4. Sanchez del Aguila MJ, Schenk M, Kern K-U, et al. Practical considerations for the use of tapentadol prolonged release for the management of severe chronic pain. Clin Ther 2015;37:94–113
5. Grunenthal Medical Department. Switching from other strong opioid analgesics to Palexia SR (tapentadol slow release). 2016. Grunenthal Medical Department, Grunenthal Ltd

7.12 Tramadol

Class of drugs, names

- Moderately strong opioid (tramadol hydrochloride)
- Racemic synthetic aminocyclohexanol opioid

Indications

- Licensed uses: moderate to severe acute/chronic/post-operative pain
- Unlicensed use: intraoperative use—may enhance awareness with light anaesthesia; treatment of post-operative shivering

Tramadol-specific contraindications

(For general opioid contraindications, see 7.1 Overview of opioids, p. 119.)

- Uncontrolled epilepsy
- Avoid in severe hepatic and renal impairment, pregnancy, and breastfeeding
- History of epilepsy, seizure susceptibility, impaired consciousness
- Use with caution in patients with excessive bronchial secretions

Dose

Oral/intramuscular/intravenous

- 50–100 mg 4- to 6-hourly
- To be given slowly when used IV
- Maximum dose 400 mg/day and 600 mg/day in post-operative pain

Hepatic and renal impairment

- ↑ dose interval to 12 hours
- Maximum dose 200 mg/day (not recommended in end-stage renal failure)

Equivalence and conversion

- Morphine equivalence 1:5 (oral morphine 10 mg = oral tramadol 50 mg)

Mode of action

- Non-selective MOP, KOP, and DOP receptor agonist
- Inhibits neuronal noradrenaline reuptake and enhances serotonin (5-HT3) release (activation of descending serotonergic and noradrenergic pathways)

Tramadol-specific side effects

(For general opioid S/Es, see 7.1 Overview opioids, p. 119.)

- Less respiratory depression, dependence, and constipation than other opioids
- Rarely seizures, headaches
- Associated with serotonin syndrome (rarely, may be precipitated if administered with SSRIs or SNRIs)
- Anticholinergic S/Es (dry mouth, confusion, changes in BP), particularly in the elderly or patients on drugs acting on centrally acting NTs such as serotonin and noradrenaline

Pharmacodynamics

- **Cardiovascular:** no significant effects
- **Respiratory:** RR, minute volume, partial pressure of carbon dioxide ($PaCO_2$) largely unchanged in therapeutic doses
- **GI:** no effect on bile duct contractility

Pharmacokinetics

- **Oral bioavailability:** 68–100%
- **Vd:** 2.9–4.37 L/kg; 20% protein-bound; 80% crosses the placenta
- **Metabolism:** hepatic metabolism by cytochrome P450 isozymes CYP2B6, CYP2D6, CYP3A4 (85% is demethylated; O-desmethyltramadol is the only active metabolite)
- **Onset of action:** 15 minutes. Peak plasma concentration 2 hours after PO; 12–15 hours with MR preparation

- **Duration of action:** IR ≈ 6 hours, MR ≈ 12 hours
- **Clearance:** 6.7–10.1 mL/kg/min
- **Elimination half-life:** 4.5–7.5 hours
- **Excretion:** 90% excreted in urine, 10% in faeces

Interactions

- **Precipitates when mixed with diazepam or midazolam**
- Co-administration with:
  - Quinidine: increases tramadol levels 50–60%
  - CYP3A4 inhibitors (ketoconazole, erythromycin) or inducers (St John's wort) alter tramadol levels
  - Digoxin: digoxin toxicity (rare reports)
  - SSRIs/SNRIs: serotonin syndrome
  - MAOIs and α-2 adrenergic blockers increase seizure risk in animal studies
  - Triptans: potential for serotonin syndrome

Special circumstances

- Pregnancy: avoid (embryotoxic in animals)
- Breastfeeding: avoid (although amount likely too small to harm)

Additional information

- Slowly removed by haemodialysis/haemofiltration
- 30% reversed by naloxone
- Available with paracetamol: Tramacet®
- Available with dexketoprofen: Skudexa®

Cost

Soluble/orodispersible tablets

- Zydol®, Zamadol® 50 mg: £0.12–0.13/tablet (£3.60–31.00 per month, depending on dose)

Capsule (immediate-release)

- Zamadol®, Zydol® 50 mg: £0.08/tablet (£2.50–19.00 per month, depending on dose)

Modified-release tablets/capsules

- Tramadol hydrochloride MR non-proprietary, Invodol® SR, Mabron®, Maneo® 100 mg: £0.12–0.75/tablet (£7–90 per month)
- Zamadol® 24-hour 150 mg: £0.38/tablet (£11 per month)
- Maxitram®, Tramquel®, Zamadol® SR 100 mg: £0.20–0.24/tablet (£12–29 per month, depending on dose)

Oral drops

- Tramadol hydrochloride non-proprietary 100 mg/mL: £0.35/mL (£35 per bottle)

Solution for injection

- Tramadol hydrochloride non-proprietary, Zamadol®, Zydol® (100 mg/2 mL): £0.80–1.10 per ampoule

Further reading

1. Joint Formulary Committee. British National Formulary. 2020. London: BMJ Group and Pharmaceutical Press. https://www.bnf.org
2. Smith HS, Pappagallo M, Stahl SM. Essential Pain Pharmacology: The Prescriber's Guide. 1st edition, 2012. Cambridge, UK: Cambridge University Press
3. Scarth E, Smith S. Drugs in Anaesthesia and Intensive Care. 5th edition, 2016. Oxford: Oxford University Press

7.13 Opioid rotation and conversion

Introduction

- Opioid rotation is a technique where the type of an opioid is changed, in an attempt to reduce side effects and maintain or enhance analgesia
- Diminished analgesia can appear when an opioid is being used for longer due to tolerance
- High doses of opioids can also contribute to OIH (increased sensitivity to painful stimuli)
- Instead of increasing opioid doses, rotation to a different opioid can result in dose reduction, with improved analgesia and fewer S/Es
- However, serious adverse events, including death, have been reported with opioid rotations
- Most of the evidence on opioid rotations has been undertaken in cancer pain patients, although there is some evidence in CNCP. The heterogeneity of studies makes clinically useful comparison difficult

Physiological and pharmacological mechanisms

Individual variability to responses to opioids

- Despite a clear understanding of the pharmacology of opioids, we have limited ability to predict an individual patient's response and S/Es
- In cancer pain, 30% of patients fail to benefit from morphine, but many improve with other opioids
- Many opioids (e.g. buprenorphine, fentanyl, oxycodone, codeine, tramadol) are metabolized via the CYP450 system (wide genetic variation, depending on liver function, other concomitant drugs affecting the P450 pathway)

Mechanisms of incomplete cross-tolerance

- Opioids have different levels of affinity and efficacy at MOP receptors, and high affinity of buprenorphine may displace the opioid it is replacing (initially increased risk of withdrawal when converting)
- While most opioids act clinically as pure MOP receptor agonists, pethidine is also a DOP receptor agonist, while oxycodone, codeine, methadone, and pethidine are KOP receptor agonists. Tapentadol, tramadol, and methadone exert some of their actions via non-opioid receptors
- Nearly 20 subtypes of the MOP receptor have been discovered, with different affinities to an opioid (the variability observed between opioids may be caused by MOP subtypes, at least partially)

Indications for an opioid rotation

- Development of intolerable adverse effects to an opioid (some evidence in cancer pain that an opioid rotation can reduce S/Es in up to 50% of patients)
- Poorly controlled pain—some patients respond better to equipotent doses of different opioids
- Patients with CNCP on high doses of opioids (normally oral morphine equivalent daily dose (oMEDD) >100 mg) who are not able to or who do not want to stop or reduce their doses of opioids, especially if the patient has risks of opioid-related adverse (particularly opioid-related respiratory impairment). These patients can be rotated to an opioid with a better safety profile (e.g. from fentanyl patches to buprenorphine)
- Development of renal or hepatic failure (some opioids have a better safety profile, as outlined in 7.1 Overview of opioids, p. 119)
- Opioid misuse and/or dependency—opioid replacement programmes (usually with methadone or buprenorphine) where opioids are provided in a controlled, safe, and monitored way under an addiction medicine service (in addiction medicine, opioid rotations are often not done with equipotent doses)
- The need to change the route of delivery (e.g. cancer patients with dysphagia)

General principles of opioid conversion

- Different onset times, especially between oral and transdermal opioids, as well as short- and long-acting formulations, need to be considered at initiation
- Biopsychosocial factors, current medications, age, BMI, comorbidities, pain aetiology, chronicity, and renal and liver function influence the method used during an opioid rotation and the patient response
- The wide range of 'opioid equivalence' has led to the recommendation that a new opioid is started at 70% of the equipotent opioid dose to minimize the risk of inadvertent overdose (some studies quote a 50% dose equivalent reduction, particularly at high doses, in elderly/frail patients), due to incomplete cross-tolerance
- Patients can access 1/6 to 1/12 of the background dose as breakthrough analgesia (the dose of breakthrough analgesia is normally a lower proportion of the background dose in patients on high doses of background opioids)
- There is a risk that pain may flare up or symptoms of opioid withdrawal may occur during an opioid rotation
- There may be variability of the regimes or doses of opioids used during opioid rotations by clinicians in different settings. The opioid doses used are important, but even more important are a comprehensive patient assessment, individualized titrations according to response, and cautious monitoring of S/Es and efficacy
- An individualized patient approach is needed
- Opioid rotation should be recommended or supervised by an adequately trained and experienced health care practitioner
- Withdrawal symptoms (e.g. sweating, yawning, abdominal cramps, restlessness, anxiety) occur if an opioid is stopped or the dose reduced abruptly
- Patients need to be reviewed after an opioid rotation to assess the efficacy of the rotation, for titration of doses, and to ensure there are no opioid-related adverse effects or S/Es. The timing of the review after an opioid rotation will depend on the clinical situation—some patients may require a review within 24 hours.

Opioid conversion

(See Tables 7.13.1, 7.13.2 and 7.13.3.)

- A large number of opioid conversion charts exist in cancer and non-cancer pain, as well as several guidelines (e.g. in the BNF of the UK)
- Significant variability between charts and often a significant range quoted for an equipotent dose on a number of these charts

Practical points for opioid conversion

1. Assess the patient thoroughly (uncontrolled pain secondary to worsening of an existing condition or due to a new cause)
2. Select the opioid that you want to convert to, and know the limitations of data available (1 + 1 does not always equal to 2 in opioid conversion)
3. Calculate the total dose of opioid that the patient takes (oral/parenteral/transdermal)
4. Calculate the OMEDD using the conversion factors shown in Tables 7.13.1, 7.13.2 and 7.13.3, and reduce the new dose by 20–30% to account for cross-tolerance

Example of rotating from oxycodone 20 mg orally to subcutaneous hydromorphone

1. Oral oxycodone 20 mg × 1.5 = oral morphine 30 mg
2. Oral morphine 30 mg / 5 = oral hydromorphone 6 mg
3. Oral hydromorphone 6 mg / 3 = SC hydromorphone 2 mg
4. Reduce by 20–30% to SC hydromorphone 1.5 mg:

   i. Review the patient and plan regular follow-ups with careful monitoring (daily–weekly–monthly, more frequently for cancer patients; psychological support may be needed)

   ii. In opioid rotation, consider the half-life of the current opioid and the time of onset of action of the new opioid, to avoid breakthrough pain and opioid toxicity (e.g. fentanyl patch to tapentadol: do not use tapentadol until 24 hours after removal of the fentanyl patch)

Table 7.13.1 Equipotent oral opioid doses

Opioid	Equivalent oral doses	Potency in comparison to oral morphine (conversion factor)	Oral:parenteral ratio
Hydromorphone	2 mg	5	3:1
Oxycodone	6.6 mg	1.5	2:1
Morphine	10 mg	1	3:1
Tapentadol	25 mg	0.4	N/A
Tramadol	100 mg	0.1	1.2:1
Dihydrocodeine	100 mg	0.1	N/A
Codeine	100 mg	0.1	2:1

Table 7.13.2 Transdermal opioid patches (conversion from oral morphine)

Oral morphine (mg/day)	12	48	84	Side effects
Buprenorphine patch (mcg/hour)	5	20	35	In 17% (nausea and vomiting in 6.7%)
Oral morphine (mg/day)	**30**	**60**	**120**	**Side effects**
Fentanyl patch (mcg/hour)	12	25	50	In 20% (nausea and vomiting in 10%)

Avoid direct conversion of oral morphine >80 mg to buprenorphine—risk of opioid withdrawal.

Table 7.13.3 Equipotent intravenous opioid doses (e.g. perioperative use)

Opioid	Equivalent IV doses	Potency
Sufentanil	10–20 mcg (0.01–0.02 mg)	500–1000
Remifentanil	50 mcg (0.05 mg)	100–200
Fentanyl	100 mcg (0.1 mg)	100
Alfentanil	1 mg	10
Hydromorphone	2 mg	5
Oxycodone	7 mg	1.5
Morphine	10 mg	1
Pethidine	75 mg	0.15
Tramadol	100 mg	0.1
Codeine	100 mg	0.1

Opioid rotation to methadone (see also 7.6 Methadone, p. 136)

- Methadone = second-line opioid for pain management (NMDA receptor activity is thought to be responsible for lower tolerance)
- Conversion to methadone is not linear due to its pharmacokinetic profile
- There is no consensus on the best regime for an opioid rotation to methadone
- Opioid rotations to methadone are not routinely done for pain management due to its complexities, risks, and pharmacological properties. Depending on the conversion ratio and dosing regimen used, there is a broad range in the doses of methadone
- Methadone is mostly used by pain specialists as an adjuvant
- Input from a specialist in palliative care or addiction medicine or an experienced practitioner is recommended

Steps to do an opioid rotation to methadone

1. Consider factors described above in an opioid rotation and specific factors for methadone (e.g. risks of QTc prolongation/cardiac arrhythmias, drug interactions, ability to monitor patient closely, respiratory disease, and other factors discussed in 7.6 Methadone p. 136))
2. Calculate the current OMEDD and the equivalent dose of methadone. This can be done using the Ayonrinde or Mercadante or Ripamonti conversion ratios (see Table 7.6.1 in 7.6 Methadone, p. 137)
3. Determine the dosing regimen using one of the following protocols:

Morley–Mankin regime (better for inpatients)

- Day 1: stop previous opioid. Commence methadone dose equivalent to 10% of the OMEDD (highest amount 30 mg) PRN 3-hourly
- Day 6: provide average methadone dose used on days 4 and 5 in two divided doses (12-hourly) and methadone PRN at 10–15% of the new methadone background dose

Friedman regime

- Takes into account the patient's age, more conservative at lower doses
- Stop previous opioid and then:
  - Patients <65 years on OMEDD <1000 mg: use **10%** of the OMEDD
  - Patients >65 years on OMEDD <1000 mg or any patient of any age on OMEDD 1000–2000 mg: use **5%** of the OMEDD
  - Patients on OMEDD >2000 mg: use **3%** of the OMEDD

Methadone product information

- Daily dose of oral methadone is determined as a percentage of the OMEDD:
  - OMEDD of <100 mg: methadone dose of 20–30% of the OMEDD
  - OMEDD of 100–300 mg: methadone dose of 10–20% of the OMEDD
  - OMEDD of 300–600 mg: methadone dose of 8–12% of the OMEDD
  - OMEDD of 600–1000 mg: methadone dose of 5–10% of the OMEDD
  - OMEDD of >1000 mg: methadone dose of <5% of the OMEDD

Further reading

1. Agerson AN, Benzon HT. 37. Management of acute and severe pain. In: Barash PG, Cullen BF, Stoelting RK, et al. (eds). Clinical Anesthesia Fundamentals. 2015; pp. 705. Alphen aan den Rijn: Wolters Kluwer
2. Roxane Laboratories. Dolophine hydrochloride. 2006. Columbus, OH: Roxane Laboratories.
3. Gretton S, Droney J. Splice variation of the mu-opioid receptor and its effects on the actions of opioids. Br J Pain 2014;8(4):133–8
4. Practical Pain Management. Opioid calculator. https://opioidcalculator.practicalpainmanagement.com
5. Faculty of Pain Medicine ANZCA. Opioid dose equivalence calculation table. 2021. http://fpm.anzca.edu.au/documents/opioid-dose-equivalence.pdf
6. Faculty of Pain Medicine of The Royal College of Anaesthetists. Dose equivalents and changing opioids. 2020. https://fpm.ac.uk/opioids-aware-structured-approach-opioid-prescribing/dose-equivalents-and-changing-opioids
7. McPherson ML. Demystifying Opioid Conversion Calculations: A Guide for Effective Dosing. 2nd edition, 2018. Bethesda, MD, USA: American Society of Health-System Pharmacists
8. Natusch D. Equianalgesic doses of opioids—their use in clinical practice. Br J Pain 2012;6(1):43–6
9. Faculty of Pain Medicine ANZCA. Opioid Calculator. 2020. Melbourne: ANZCA

CHAPTER 8

Non-steroidal Anti-inflammatory Drugs and Paracetamol

Peter Keogh

CONTENTS

8.1 Overview of non-steroidal anti-inflammatory drugs

Introduction

- NSAIDs refer to both non-selective NSAIDs (nsNSAIDs) and COX-2 inhibitors
- Widely used to treat mild pain as a monotherapy or as a co-analgesic to treat moderate to severe pain

Indications

- Acute pain, subacute pain, chronic pain, cancer-related pain
- Perioperatively, burns, trauma, MSK pain, or conditions with an inflammatory component (e.g. inflammatory phase of CRPS, rheumatoid arthritis (RA), scleroderma, ankylosing spondylitis)
- Co-analgesic as part of a multimodal regimen for moderate to severe pain
- Adjunct for opioid-sparing effects and potential reduction of opioid-related adverse effects
- Some headache disorders
- Antipyretic

Classification

- Salicylic acids: aspirin
- Acetic acid derivatives: indometacin, diclofenac, ketorolac
- Fenamates: mefenamic acid
- Pyrazolones: phenylbutazone
- Propionic acids: ibuprofen, naproxen
- Oxicams: piroxicam, meloxicam

Physiology of cyclo-oxygenase enzymes

- Within the phospholipid bilayer of cell membranes, phospholipase A2 stimulates the production of arachidonic acid precursor. Prostaglandin precursor formation from arachidonic acid is catalysed by COX enzymes which, in turn, produces TXA2, PGI2, and inflammatory

PGs (PGE2, PGF2α, PGD2). Pro-inflammatory leukotrienes are also produced via an alternate lipoxygenase pathway catalysed by 5-lipoxygenase enzyme. There are three COX isoenzymes:

- COX-1 (the constitutive form) is blocked by nsNSAIDs and aspirin. COX-1 is largely responsible for the production of:
  - Cytoprotective PGs—gastric mucosal protection
  - TXA2—promotes platelet aggregation, vasoconstriction
- COX-2 (the inducible form) is blocked by nsNSAIDs, aspirin, and COX-2 inhibitors. COX-2 is largely responsible for the production of:
  - Inflammatory PGs—stimulate production of inflammatory mediators which sensitize peripheral and/or central nociceptors
  - Prostacyclin—Prevents platelet aggregation, vasodilatation, and regulation of renal blood flow
- COX-3—its existence is controversial. May be involved in the mechanism of action of paracetamol

Mechanism of action

- NSAIDs inhibit the COX pathway, reducing the production of PG precursors. The differential between COX-1 and COX-2 inhibition determines the effect and is measured by the drug's selectivity ratio
- Inhibition of the COX-2 pathway results in the following:
  - Anti-inflammatory effect: decreased PG and prostacyclin causes vasodilatation, resulting in decreased tissue oedema
  - Analgesia: decreased sensitization of nociceptive nerve endings by decreased production of PGs and inflammatory mediators such as bradykinins. NSAIDs are effective in headaches by decreasing PG-induced vasodilatation
  - Antipyretic effect: decreased secretion of inflammatory mediators, such as IL1, which elevate body temperature by acting on the hypothalamus

Routes of administration

- Topical, rectal, PO, IM, and IV routes
- Topical NSAIDs may be associated with fewer S/Es

Pharmacokinetics

- Absorption: NSAIDs are weak acids (pKa = 3–5) and rapidly absorbed from the stomach. Slow-release preparations are available
- Distribution: highly protein-bound (>90%), with potential to displace other protein-bound drugs
- Metabolism: hepatic. Oxidation and conjugation to inactive metabolites
- Excretion: mainly in the urine, variable amount in bile

Adverse effects

- More predominant in the elderly, those with comorbidities, and those on NSAIDs which are less COX-2-selective
- All NSAIDs share to different degrees similar mechanistic-based adverse effects
- Nervous system: increased risk of ischaemic stroke—higher risk with COX-2-selective NSAIDs. Rarely headaches, dizziness, drowsiness, insomnia, vertigo, and tinnitus

- CVS: increased risk of MI, independent of baseline cardiovascular risk factors. Higher risk with COX-2-selective NSAIDs. Risks negated with naproxen (up to 1 g daily) and ibuprofen (up to 1.2 g daily). Can also contribute to development of hypertension and pulmonary oedema
- Respiratory system: bronchospasm (increased activity in the lipoxygenase pathway)
- GI system: peptic ulceration, diarrhoea, bleeding—consider enteric-coated formulations, administration with food, and antacid prophylaxis. Slight elevation in hepatic transaminases is common
- Renal system: dysfunction and failure from decreased renal blood flow, decreased GFR, salt and water retention, acute papillary necrosis, and chronic interstitial nephritis
- Coagulation: prolongation of bleeding via inhibition of platelet function (COX-1-mediated)
- Skin hypersensitivity, rash, angio-oedema, urticaria, photosensitivity
- Soft tissue healing: animal studies have shown impaired wound healing by blocking the release of PGs which promote angiogenesis and mediators involved in wound healing. Clinical studies have not identified strong evidence indicating poorer wound healing or anastomotic breakdown
- Bone healing: PGs stimulate osteoblastic and osteoclastic activity. Animal models have shown decreased bone healing with inhibition of PG production. Clinical use of NSAIDs in bone fractures remains controversial

Contraindications

- NSAID-induced hypersensitivity (history of precipitation of asthma, angio-oedema, urticaria, or rhinitis), GI ulceration/bleeding, renal impairment (moderate/severe), major vascular/cardiac surgery, major surgery with a previous history of a thrombotic event (stroke and MI), hypovolaemia, moderate/severe heart failure
- Pregnancy, especially in the third trimester, is associated with an increased risk of closure of the fetal ductus arteriosus *in utero*. Regular use of NSAIDs in early pregnancy is associated with an increased risk of miscarriage
- NSAIDs are not readily excreted in breast milk. Most manufacturers advise caution during breastfeeding and to avoid aspirin use altogether (risk of neonatal Reyes syndrome)

Analgesic efficacy

- A single dose of an NSAID has similar analgesic activity to paracetamol
- NSAIDs have to be used in combination with other agents for moderate to severe pain
- Full analgesic effect should be obtained within a week of initiation of regular NSAID use, but full anti-inflammatory effects may take up to 3 weeks to take effect
- The differences in anti-inflammatory properties between NSAIDs are small, but there is considerable variation in individual response to these drugs
- Sixty per cent of patients respond to any NSAID, and non-responders may respond to another NSAID
- Ibuprofen has fewer adverse effects than other nsNSAIDs, but its anti-inflammatory properties are weaker
- Naproxen combines good analgesic and anti-inflammatory efficacy, with a low (but higher than ibuprofen) incidence of adverse effects
- Diclofenac has similar efficacy to naproxen, but a higher incidence of adverse effects

Acute pain

- NSAIDs form an integral part of multimodal analgesic regimes

- Combined use of NSAIDs and paracetamol is more effective than using NSAIDs or paracetamol alone
- Normally, opioid use is reduced by 30–50% when NSAIDs are also used
- NSAID use reduces the incidence of pneumonia, admission to critical care, and ventilation support in patients with rib fractures

Chronic non-cancer pain

- Limited evidence supports NSAIDs in chronic back pain and osteoarthritis (OA)
- NSAIDs have a role in inflammatory joint conditions such as RA
- NSAIDs probably have no role in neuropathic pain

Cancer-related pain

- Use may be associated with a survival advantage in a range of solid cancers through an as yet unknown mechanism

Additional information

- When prescribing NSAIDs, take into account the patient's individual risk factors and potential benefits
- Prescribe the lowest effective dose for the shortest possible time
- Patients should be counselled on the risk of NSAID use, and reviewed regularly
- Exercise caution in patients who are elderly and have cardiovascular risk factors, diabetes, uncontrolled hypertension, renal dysfunction, major surgery, advanced hepatic impairment, prior history or risk of GI ulceration, and coagulation defects (COX-2 inhibitors may be an acceptable alternative)
- NSAIDs are highly protein-bound and can displace other drugs from plasma proteins. Of note:
  - Increased risk of bleeding when given with SSRIs, selective SNRI, aspirin, warfarin, and other anticoagulants
  - Enhanced risk of lithium toxicity
  - Interactions also with corticosteroids, ACEIs, potassium-sparing diuretics, aminoglycosides, and methotrexate
- Ibuprofen is the most appropriate nsNSAID for use in children
- Naproxen (up to 1 g/day) or ibuprofen (up to 1.2 g/day) are recommended as first-line drugs for adults, based on cardiovascular risk

Further reading

1. Joint Formulary Committee. British National Formulary. 2020. London: BMJ Group and Pharmaceutical Press. https://www.bnf.org
2. Maund E, McDaid C, Rice S, et al. Paracetamol and selective and non-selective non-steroidal anti-inflammatory drugs for the reduction in morphine-related side-effects after major surgery: a systematic review. Br J Anaesth 2011;106(3):292–7
3. Ong C, Lirk P, Tan C, Seymour R. An evidence-based update on nonsteroidal anti-inflammatory drugs. Clin Med Res 2007;5(1):19–34
4. Schug SA, Palmer, GM, Scott, DA, et al. Acute Pain Management: Scientific Evidence. 4th edition, 2015. Melbourne: Australian and New Zealand College of Anaesthetists and Faculty of Pain Medicine

8.2 Cyclo-oxygenase 2 inhibitors

Introduction

- Selective COX-2 inhibitors were developed to decrease the risk of GI adverse effects mediated via COX-1 enzyme inhibition by nsNSAIDs
- The analgesic efficacy of COX-2 inhibitors is similar to that of nsNSAIDs

Classification

- Pyrazole: parecoxib, celecoxib, rofecoxib
- Methylsulphone: etoricoxib
- Phenylacetic acid derivative: lumaricoxib

Mechanism of action

- COX-2 inhibitors reduce the production of PGs which facilitate the inflammatory response to tissue injury
- Less COX-1 inhibition than nsNSAIDs. This has theoretical advantages by maintaining production of protective PGs responsible for positive effects in relation to gastric mucosal protection, platelet function, and renal blood flow
- The interdependence between COX-1 and COX-2 inhibition influences the risks and benefits of different NSAIDs. This is measured by the drug selectivity ratio (e.g. the selectivity ratio for celecoxib is 1:30, etoricoxib 1:344, and parecoxib 1:61)

Characteristics of COX-2 inhibitors versus non-selective NSAIDs

- Modest reduction in serious GI adverse events
- Decreased bleeding (do not significantly impair platelet function)
- Probably less bronchospasm in asthmatics
- Similar analgesic efficacy
- Similar risk of renal impairment
- Similar rates of cardiovascular adverse effects (stroke and MI). Celecoxib and naproxen are associated with the lowest risk
- More expensive

Routes of administration and dosing

- Celecoxib: 200–400 mg PO daily in 2 divided doses 12 hourly (not recommended in children)
- Etoricoxib: 30–90 mg PO once daily
- Parecoxib: IM or IV injection up to 40 mg daily (some sources do not recommend in children)

Pharmacokinetics

- Celecoxib:
  - Absorption: good oral bioavailability
  - Distribution: 97% protein-bound, Vd 5.7 L/kg
  - Metabolism: hepatic by CYP2C9 to inactive metabolites
  - Excretion: renal. Elimination t1/2: 8–12 hours
- Etoricoxib:
  - Absorption: oral bioavailability 95%
  - Distribution: 90% protein-bound, Vd 1.5 L/kg

  - Metabolism: hepatic by CYP3A4 and other cytochrome P450 enzymes to inactive metabolites
  - Excretion: renal. Elimination t1/2: 22 hours
- Parecoxib:
  - Absorption: poor oral bioavailability. Given IM or IV
  - Distribution: 99% protein-bound
  - Metabolism: hepatic conversion of prodrug to valdecoxib, and then by CYP2C9 and CYP3A4 to inactive metabolites
  - Excretion: renal. Elimination t1/2: 8 hours

Additional information

- Rofecoxib was withdrawn from the UK in 2004 over cardiovascular safety concerns. The APPROVe study (2005) showed an increased cardiovascular risk when it was used in patients with a history of colorectal adenomas
- Valdecoxib was withdrawn in the UK in 2005 because of serious skin reactions
- Lumiracoxib was withdrawn in the UK in 2007 because of hepatotoxicity
- VIGOR study (2000): patients with RA treated with rofecoxib had fewer upper GI events than those treated with naproxen
- PRECISION study (2016): celecoxib was non-inferior to ibuprofen or naproxen with regard to cardiovascular adverse effects

Further reading

1. Cashman J, Holdcroft A. Non-steroidal anti-inflammatory agents. In: Holdcroft A, Jaggar S (eds). Core Topics in Pain. 1st edition, 2005; pp. 277–80. Cambridge: Cambridge University Press
2. Husband M, Mehta V. Cyclo-oxygenase-2 inhibitors. Contin Educ Anaesth Crit Care Pain 2013;13(4):131–5
3. Moore RA, Derry S, Aldington D, Wiffen PJ. Single dose oral analgesics for acute postoperative pain in adults—an overview of Cochrane reviews. Cochrane Database Syst Rev 2015;9:CD008659

8.3 Diclofenac

Chemical

- A phenylacetic acid derivative

Presentation

- Tablets: immediate-release, 25 mg and 50 mg; modified-release, 75 mg and 100 mg
- Suppositories: 12.5 mg, 25 mg, 50 mg, and 100 mg
- IV or IM injection: 25 mg/mL and 37.5 mg/mL
- Topical gel: diclofenac sodium 1%
- Others: dermal patch, eye drops, preparations combined with misoprostol

Mechanism of action and important features

- Non-selective COX inhibitor
- Number needed to treat (NNT) (50%) 50 mg = 2.7

Routes of administration and dosing

- Pain in adults:
  - PO: 25–50 mg every 6–8 hours (maximum 150 mg daily)
  - IV or IM injection: 50–75 mg every 4–6 hours (maximum 150 mg daily)
  - Rectally: 75–150 mg daily in divided doses
- Pain in children:
  - PO: >1 year old, 1.5–2.5 mg/kg (maximum 50 mg) three times daily
  - IV or IM injection: >2 years old, 0.3–1 mg/kg 1–3 times daily (maximum 150 mg daily)
  - Rectally: not licensed for <6-year olds, except if >1 year old with juvenile idiopathic arthritis; 8–12 kg, 12.5 mg twice daily, and >12 kg, 1 mg/kg (maximum 50 mg) three times daily

Pharmacokinetics

- Absorption: oral bioavailability 60%
- Distribution: protein-bound 99%, Vd 0.12–0.17 L/kg
- Metabolism: hepatic, predominantly by hydroxylation and methylation, resulting in several phenolic metabolites which are converted to glucuronide conjugates. Two of these metabolites are biologically active, but to a much smaller extent than diclofenac. A small proportion of the metabolism is by glucuronidation of the intact molecule
- Excretion: 60% as metabolites in the urine, 1% unchanged in the urine, and 40% as metabolites in bile. Elimination t1/2: 1.1–1.8 hours

Cost

- 50 mg (28 tablets): £1.63
- 50 mg (ten suppositories): £2.04
- Gel 1.16% (100 g): £4.63
- 75 mg for IV injection (ten ampoules): £9.91–24.00

Further reading

1. Joint Formulary Committee. British National Formulary. 2020. London: BMJ Group and Pharmaceutical Press. https://www.bnf.org
2. Electronic Medicines Compendium. Diclofenac potassium 50 mg tablets. https://www.medicines.org.uk/emc/medicine/24377
3. Peck T, Hill S, Williams M. Pharmacology for Anaesthesia and Intensive Care. 3rd edition, 2008. Cambridge: Cambridge University Press

8.4 Ibuprofen

Chemical

- Phenylpropionic acid derivative

Presentation

- Tablets, capsules, and caplets (immediate-release) 200 mg and 400 mg
- Tablets (modified-release) 800 mg

- Oral suspension 100 mg/5 mL
- Topical gel 5% and 10%
- IV preparation 800 mg/8 mL
- Aqueous cream 10 mg/mL with isopropyl myristate
- Combined with codeine, paracetamol, phenylephrine, and pseudoephedrine

Mechanism of action and important features

- Non-selective COX inhibitor
- Acute pain NNT (50%) 400 mg = 2.5
- Anti-inflammatory properties are weaker than those of other nsNSAIDs
- Increased risk of myocardial thrombotic events minimized up to 1.2 g daily

Routes of administration and dosing

- Adults: 400–800 mg 3–4 times daily (maximum 2.4 g daily or <3.2 g for ≤2 days)
- Children: maximum 30 mg/kg in 3–4 divided doses. In the UK, not licensed in children aged under 3 months or if body weight below 5 kg

Pharmacokinetics

- Absorption: oral bioavailability 87–100%
- Distribution: 99% protein-bound. Vd 0.14 L/kg
- Metabolism: hepatic. Predominantly by hydroxylation and conjugation to inactive metabolites (metabolites A and B)
- Excretion: renal; 10% unchanged in the urine. Elimination t1/2: 1.3–3 hours

Additional information

- Ibuprofen is the most appropriate nsNSAID for use in children
- Dexibuprofen is the active enantiomer of ibuprofen. It has similar properties to ibuprofen and is licensed for the relief of mild to moderate pain and inflammation

Cost

- 48 tablets of 400 mg for as little as £1.20
- Ibuprofen suspension 100 mg/5 mL: £1.59

Further reading

1. Joint Formulary Committee. British National Formulary. 2020. London: BMJ Group and Pharmaceutical Press. https://www.bnf.org
2. Electronic Medicines Compendium. Ibuprofen. https://www.medicines.org.uk/emc/search?q=%22Ibuprofen%22

8.5 Naproxen

Chemical

- Phenylacetic acid derivative

Presentation

- Tablets (immediate-release) 250 mg and 500 mg
- Oral suspension 25 mg/mL
- Preparations combined with esomeprazole and misoprostol

Mechanism of action and important features

- Non-selective COX inhibitor
- NNT (50%) 500 mg = 2.7
- Increased risk of myocardial thrombotic events minimized up to 1 g daily

Routes of administration and dosing

- Pain in adults:
  - PO: 500 mg initially, then 250 mg every 6–8 hours as required (maximum dose after first day 1.25 g daily)
- Pain in children:
  - PO: 5 mg/kg twice daily (maximum 1 g daily)
  - UK—not licensed in children aged under 5 years for juvenile idiopathic arthritis or those under 16 years for musculoskeletal pain or dysmenorrhoea

Pharmacokinetics

- Absorption: oral bioavailability 95%
- Distribution: 99% protein-bound. Vd 0.16 L/kg
- Metabolism: hepatic to 6-0-desmethyl naproxen and other conjugated metabolites
- Excretion: in the urine (97%) and faeces (3%). Elimination t1/2: 12–17 hours

Cost

- 56 tablets of 250 mg: £2.20 (gastroresistant)
- 28 tablets of 250 mg: £2.91 (monthly approximately £6)
- 28 tablets of 500 mg: £2.47 (monthly approximately £5)

Further reading

1. Joint Formulary Committee. British National Formulary. 2020. London: BMJ Group and Pharmaceutical Press. https://www.bnf.org
2. Electronic Medicines Compendium. Boots period pain relief 250 mg gastro-resistant tablets. https://www.medicines.org.uk/emc/medicine/26017

8.6 Paracetamol

Indications

- Analgesia for mild to moderate pain
- Antipyretic

Chemical

- Acetanilide derivative

Presentation

- Tablets, capsules, and caplets (immediate-release) 500 mg
- Oral suspension 120 mg, 250 mg, and 500 mg/5 mL
- Suppositories 60 mg, 120 mg, 125 mg, 200 mg, 250 mg, 500 mg, and 1 g
- IV infusion 10 mg/mL
- Also available in modified-release preparations
- Combined with codeine, tramadol, isometheptene mucate, buclizine, caffeine, and metoclopramide

Mechanism of action

- Poorly understood. Several proposed mechanisms:
    - PG inhibition: inhibition of PG synthesis by weak inhibition of peripheral COX activity, with apparent selectivity for COX-2. It is also believed to work by COX-1 variant inhibition
    - Serotonergic pathway activation: enhanced descending inhibition pathways via 5-HT3 receptor agonism
    - Endocannabinoid enhancement: reuptake inhibition of endocannabinoids via N-arachidonoyl phenol amine, a conjugated metabolite of paracetamol, which is implicated in the activation of TRPV1 receptors, inhibition of nitric oxide

Routes of administration and dosing

- Pain in adults:
    - PO: 0.5–1 g every 4–6 hours (maximum 4 g daily)
    - IV infusion:
        - Adults over 50 kg: 1 g every 4–6 hours (maximum 4 g daily)
        - Adults up to 50 kg: 15 mg/kg every 4–6 hours (maximum 60 mg/kg daily)
    - Rectally: 0.5–1 g every 4–6 hours (maximum 4 g daily)
- Pain in children:
    - PO: 1 month to 18 years 15–20 mg/kg (maximum 1 g) every 4–6 hours, maximum 75 mg/kg daily (maximum 4 g) in divided doses
    - Dose should be based on lean body weight, and not on total body weight, in obese children

Pharmacokinetics

- Absorption: oral bioavailability 70–90%. Rectal bioavailability 68–88%
- Distribution: 0–5% protein-bound. Vd 1 L/kg. Non-ionized at physiological pH, with good lipid solubility and CNS penetration
- Metabolism: hepatic. Predominantly by glucuronidation and sulphation to non-toxic conjugates. Small amount oxidized via cytochrome P450 enzyme system to highly toxic N-acetyl-p-benzoquinone imine (NAPQI). NAPQI is rapidly conjugated with hepatic glutathione to render it harmless
- Excretion: 2–5% unchanged in the urine. Elimination t1/2: 1.9–2.2 hours

Pharmacodynamics

- CNS: analgesia, antipyretic through direct action on the hypothalamus
- Hepatic: hepatotoxic in overdose

Adverse effects and toxicity

- CNS: possible sedation
- CVS: hypotension and flushing with IV infusion
- Respiratory system: bronchospasm
- GI: non-specific GI symptoms
- Hepatic: hepatocellular necrosis in overdose. Following a toxic dose, normal hepatic conjugation pathways become saturated. When hepatic glutathione stores are depleted, NAPQI accumulates. NAPQI forms covalent bonds with sulfhydryl groups in hepatocytes, resulting in centrilobular hepatic necrosis. Treatment is with oral methionine or PO or IV acetylcysteine to provide a source of glutathione
- Renal: acute tubular necrosis in overdose
- Haematological: thrombocytopenia, leucopenia, neutropenia
- Skin: rash

Contraindications

- Hypersensitivity to the active substance or to any of the excipients
- Caution in those allergic to aspirin—5% cross-sensitivity
- Caution in renal ± hepatic impairment and malnourished

Interactions

- Enzyme-inducing drugs may increase the risk of paracetamol toxicity
- Co-administration of paracetamol (4 g/day for at least 4 days) with oral anticoagulants may lead to slight variations in international normalized ratio (INR) values
- Probenecid causes an almost 2-fold reduction in clearance of paracetamol

Additional information

- Pregnancy: not known to be harmful
- Breastfeeding: clinically insignificant amounts excreted in breast milk

Cost

- 500 mg (16 tablets): £0.77 (even as little as £0.13)
- Ten suppositories of 500 mg: £36.50
- Oral suspension 120 mg/5 mL for 100 mL bottle: £2.29

Further reading

1. Joint Formulary Committee. British National Formulary. 2020. London: BMJ Group and Pharmaceutical Press. https://www.bnf.org
2. Sasada M, Smith S. Drugs in Anaesthesia and Intensive Care. 2003. New York, NY: Oxford Medical Publications
3. Sharma C, Mehta V. Paracetamol: mechanisms and updates. Contin Educ Anaesth Crit Care Pain 2014;14(4):153–8

CHAPTER 9

Anticonvulsants

Mohammed Sajad and Alifia Tameem

CONTENTS

9.1 Overview of anticonvulsants

Introduction

- Anticonvulsants reduce the excitability of neurons and hence are important components of multimodal management of neuropathic pain
- Approximately 60% of prescriptions for this group of medications are for non-epilepsy reasons
- They help in reduction of the intensity of pain, as well as improve sleep and decrease anxiety
- Opioid-sparing effect, hence a useful adjunct in perioperative and acute pain

Classification

(See Table 9.1.1.)

Table 9.1.1 First- and second-generation of anticonvulsants

First generation	Second generation
Older, more side effects Examples: carbamazepine, phenytoin, sodium valproate, benzodiazepines	Newer, better side effect profile Examples: gabapentinoids, lamotrigine, topiramate, oxcarbazepine

Mode of action

- Blockade of Na^+ channels, e.g. carbamazepine, oxcarbazepine (OXC), phenytoin, lamotrigine, topiramate
- Blockade of Ca^{2+} channels, e.g. gabapentinoids, lamotrigine, topiramate
- Decreased transmission of glutamate via AMPA receptors, e.g. topiramate
- Modulation and potentiation of GABA via inhibitory GABA receptors, e.g. BZDs, topiramate

Indications

- Treatment of epilepsy
- Treatment of neuropathic pain (neuralgia, MS, post-sympathectomy pain, neuropathic cancer pain, post-traumatic neuralgia, PHN, post-stroke pain, painful diabetic neuropathy, HIV, chemotherapy-induced neuropathic pain)
- Fibromyalgia, anxiety disorders
- Migraine

Analgesic efficacy—pharmacotherapy for neuropathic pain

- Gabapentinoids: high evidence, moderate effect size on pain, as well as on QoL, tolerability/ safety (high for gabapentin and moderate for pregabalin). First line for neuropathic pain—overall NNT: pregabalin 7.7 (6.5–9.4) and gabapentin 6.3 (5.0–8.3)
- Carbamazepine—NNT: 1.7 (1.3–2.2) for trigeminal neuralgia (TN); 2.3 (1.6–3.9) for diabetic neuropathic pain; 3.4 (1.7–105) for post-stroke pain
- Phenytoin—NNT: 2.1 (1.5–3.6) for diabetic neuropathic pain
- Lamotrigine—NNT: 2.1 (1.3–6.1) for TN, 4.0 (2.1–42) for diabetic neuropathic pain
- Topiramate—NNT: 7.4 (4.3–28.5) for diabetic neuropathic pain, with high withdrawal rate

Additional information

- Should be considered in patients who have peripheral or central neuropathic pain and some chronic widespread pain syndromes
- Lowest possible dose to be started and titrated up slowly to balance between effect and S/Es
- Should intolerable S/Es occur, titrate down to the least effective dose which is tolerated by the patient
- Lower doses in the elderly, and in renal and hepatic impairment due to decreased excretion
- Avoid in pregnancy and breastfeeding if possible (for pain)

Further reading

1. Finnerup NB, Attal N, Haroutounian S, et al. Pharmacotherapy for neuropathic pain in adults: a systematic review and meta-analysis. Lancet Neurol 2015;14:162–73
2. Tracey I. Pain 2012 Refresher Courses. 14th World Congress on Pain, 2012. Seattle, WA: IASP Press

9.2 Overview of benzodiazepines

Introduction

- BZDs are a group of drugs used to treat anxiolysis, in turn helping with pain management
- They are used in anaesthesia such as hypnotics and anxiolytics, and help as premedication
- Used as anticonvulsants, especially for management of acute seizures

Classification of benzodiazepines

- Short-acting (up to 6 hours): midazolam, oxazepam
- Intermediate-acting (6–12 hours): lorazepam, temazepam, alprazolam, nitrazepam
- Long-acting (12 hours to 3 days): diazepam, clonazepam (see 13.7 Clonazepam, p. 242)

Mechanism of action

- $GABA_A$ receptor agonist (by allosteric modulation) at specific BZD binding site (α subunit)
- Increase influx and conductance of chloride ion, causing hyperpolarization of the neuronal cell membrane (in the presence of GABA NT)
- Effective CNS depression and muscle relaxation, anxiolytic effects

Indications

- Muscle spasm
- Pain-associated anxiety
- Acute back pain
- Lancinating neuropathic pain
- Case studies showing promise in phantom limb pain (clonazepam)
- Some evidence of BZDs being helpful in tic douloureux, tension headache, and temporomandibular joint disorder
- Insomnia

Contraindications/caution

- Alcohol excess
- Severe depression
- High falls risk
- Concurrent sedative drug use (e.g. opioids)
- Acute angle closure glaucoma
- Obstructive sleep apnoea

Dose

- Minimal effective dose titrated to effect. Avoid sudden increases in dose to prevent oversedation; exact dose varies with agent
- Diazepam: initially PO 2–10 mg daily in divided doses
- Clonazepam: 1–2 mg daily in 3–4 divided doses
- Aim for gradual weaning in long-term users

Side effects

- Excessive sedation, confusion, paradoxical aggression/stimulant effect
- Allergic reaction
- Tolerance, dependence, and withdrawal
- Amongst chronic pain users, BZD use is associated with:
    - Greater pain severity
    - Higher risk of strong opioid use
    - Substance abuse
    - Greater mental health comorbidity
    - Increased emergency health care consultation

Interactions

- **Aim to avoid any concurrent CNS depressant**
- Barbiturates, alcohol, opioids, baclofen
- Antipsychotic agents

Special circumstances

- Pregnancy: weak evidence to suggest association between BZDs and cleft lip and palate, hence best to avoid in pregnancy. Risk of neonatal withdrawal symptoms
- Breastfeeding: considered safe in breastfeeding if <20 mg per 24 hours
- Warn patients about the potential risks when driving and operating machinery
- Will need to contact the Driver and Vehicle Licensing Agency (DVLA) regarding driving
- Can precipitate hepatic encephalopathy in hepatic failure
- Increased cerebral sensitivity in renal patients

Additional information

- Generally well tolerated if used cautiously
- No routine blood concentration monitoring in practice
- Used mainly for non-pain-related reasons (anxiolytics, insomnia, sedation)
- Occasionally, paradoxical disinhibition is experienced
- Based on current evidence, BZDs cannot be recommended for neuropathic pain
- Published case reports of clonazepam successfully used in phantom limb pain
- Flumazenil—reverses BZD effect when given IV in 100 mcg increments. It has a short t1/2 of 1 hour, can precipitate seizures

Diazepam—long-acting benzodiazepine

- Used as muscle relaxant in chronic pain

Pharmacokinetics (diazepam)

- Absorption: rapid gut absorption effective within 15 minutes, 85–100% bioavailability
- Distribution: highly protein-bound (98%), peak plasma concentration in 30–90 minutes
- Metabolism: main active metabolite is desmethyldiazepam; other active metabolites are temazepam and oxazepam. Metabolites undergo glucuronidation and are then excreted in the urine
- Excretion: t1/2 30–60 hours

Cost

- 2 mg (28 tablets): £0.57
- 5 mg (28 tablets): £0.69
- 10 mg (28 tablets): £0.75

Further reading

1. Masada M, Smith S. Drugs in Anaesthesia and Intensive Care. 1st edition, 2003. Oxford: Oxford University Press
2. Jacob S, Nair A. An updated overview on therapeutic drug monitoring of recent antiepileptic drugs. Drugs R D 2016;16(4):303–16
3. Nielsen S, Lintzeris N, Bruno R, et al. Benzodiazepine use among chronic pain patients prescribed opioids: associations with pain, physical and mental health, and health service utilization. Pain Med 2005;16:356–66

9.3 Gabapentin

Class of drugs

- Gabapentin gel 6% (2–10%)
- Acetic acid derivative

Indications

- First-line treatment for painful diabetic neuropathy and PHN
- Fibromyalgia, anxiety, restless legs syndrome, hot flushes, insomnia
- Facial pain, episodic migraine
- Epilepsy (partial seizures)
- Perioperative pain due to its opioid-sparing effects
- Gel for focal neuropathic pain and localized itch

Contraindications/caution

- Diabetes mellitus—worsening glycaemic control
- Manufacturers advise caution in adolescents and patients with low body weight

Dose

- Doses start at 100 mg three times daily up to a maximum of 1200 mg three times daily (3600 mg/day)
- Avoid sudden withdrawal. Aim for dose reduction to stop over 14 days or more
- NNT previously was 4.3–4.7 across all neuropathic conditions, but updated to 9.6

Mode of action

- Although structurally similar to GABA, the mode of action is predominantly by binding to voltage-sensitive Ca^{2+} channels in the CNS and peripheral nervous system, with a 3-fold response:
  - Antagonism of NMDA on glutamate receptors
  - Enhanced action of glutamate decarboxylase, thereby increasing GABA production
  - Enhances release of GABA at synapses
- All responses lead to hyperpolarization of the neuron and inhibit AP propagation

Monitoring

- Monitoring is possible with gabapentin assays. Most patients respond at a therapeutic level of 2–20 mcg/mL
- Monitor for weight gain

Side effects

- Neurological: ataxia, dizziness, drowsiness, fatigue, diplopia, nystagmus, and tremor
- GI: abdominal pain, constipation, dyspepsia, and nausea and vomiting
- Weight gain and peripheral oedema

Pharmacokinetics

- Absorption: slowly from the gut with unpredictable pharmacokinetics, with peak plasma concentration occurring within 3–4 hours; duodenal absorption limited by transporter saturation (LAT1 transporter).

- Bioavailability not linear (note: different characteristic to pregabalin which shows first-order absorption—concentration is linearly dose-dependent)
    - 900 mg/day = 60%
    - 1200 mg/day = 47%
    - 2400 mg/day = 34%
    - 3600 mg/day = 33%
    - 4800 mg/day = 27%
- Distribution: minimal plasma protein binding (<3%)
- Metabolism: negligible
- Excretion: renally as unchanged drug
- Elimination t1/2: 5–7 hours
- Gabapentin is excreted mainly unchanged by renal mechanism; important to reduce doses in renal impairment:
    - Maximum 1.8 g/day if estimated GFR (eGFR) 50–80 mL/min
    - Maximum 900 mg/day if eGFR 30–50 mL/min
    - Maximum 600 mg/day if eGFR 15–30 mL/min
    - Maximum 300 mg/day if eGFR <15 mL/min

Interactions

- Use cautiously with opioids—can potentiate sedation
- Known interactions alter seizure threshold but do not affect pain management
- Bioavailability is reduced with simple antacids

Special circumstances

- Pregnancy: use with caution if benefit outweighs risk
- Breastfeeding: use with caution if benefit outweighs risk
- Children: unlicensed use in those aged <6 years. Dose: 10 mg/kg, maximum 70 mg/kg. If used with opioids, rare risk of severe respiratory depression, as well as increased emotional and behavioural S/Es
- Elderly: increased cognitive S/Es, hence lower doses to be used. Care in renal impairment

Additional information

- Not effective in HIV-induced neuropathy or CRPS

Cost

- 100 mg capsules (100 pack): £2
- 300 mg capsules (100 pack): £3.20
- 600 mg tablets (100 pack): £8.72
- Monthly supply of 100–1200 mg three times daily: £2–17.50
- 50 mg/mL in 150 mL bottle (= 250 mg three times daily for 1 month): £57–67
- Gabapentin gel (prepared by pharmacy): £0.50–2.41 per gram

Further reading

1. Jacob S, Nair A. An updated overview on therapeutic drug monitoring of recent antiepileptic drugs. Drugs R D 2016;16(4):303–16

2. Moore RA, Wiffen PJ, Derry S, et al. Gabapentin for chronic neuropathic pain and fibromyalgia in adults. Cochrane Database Syst Rev 2014;4:CD007938
3. Bockbrader H, Wesche D, Miller R, et al. A comparison of the pharmacokinetics and pharmacodynamics of pregabalin and gabapentin. Clin Pharmacokinet 2010;49(10):661–9

9.4 Pregabalin

Class of drug

- 3-isobutyl derivative of gamma-amino butyric acid (GABA)

Indications

- Chronic and acute neuropathic pain
- PHN
- Generalized anxiety disorder—licensed use

Contraindications/caution

- Pregnancy—folic acid inhibition and neural tube defects

Dose

- Dose started at 150 mg/day in divided doses, increasing slowly to a maximum of 600 mg/day over a few weeks
- Lowest NNT for 50% reduction in pain with 600 mg of pregabalin daily: PHN, 3.9; diabetic neuropathy, 5.6; central neuropathic pain, 5.6; and fibromyalgia, 11

Mode of action

- Mechanism similar to that of gabapentin, with binding of voltage-gated Ca^{2+} channels and release inhibition of excitatory NTs in synapses
- GABA analogue binding to α-2-δ subunit of voltage Ca^{2+} channels
- Reduces Ca^{2+} influx into neurons
- **Inactive at GABA receptors**

Monitoring

- No specific plasma monitoring available
- Monitor for weight gain

Side effects

- CNS: blurred vision, confusion, dizziness, memory impairment, suicidal risk
- Constipation, nausea, peripheral oedema
- Weight gain
- Rarely: low platelets, PR prolongation, creatinine kinase (CK) release

Pharmacokinetics

- Absorption: absorbed more rapidly than gabapentin (3-fold increase). It occurs throughout the small intestine, via multiple transporter mechanisms, and the ascending colon (unlike

gabapentin). Bioavailability >90%. First-order kinetics—concentration is linearly dose-dependent. Peak concentration 1 hour after administration
- Distribution: no protein binding
- Metabolism: negligible (<2%)
- Excretion: primarily eliminated through renal excretion (98%) as unchanged compound in the urine
- t1/2: 5–7 hours
- Effectively cleared through renal haemodialysis in patients with end-stage renal failure
- Pregabalin is excreted mainly unchanged by renal mechanism. Important to reduce the dose in renal impairment:
    - Maximum 300 mg/day if eGFR 30–60 mL/min
    - Maximum 150 mg/day if eGFR 15–30 mL/min
    - Maximum 75 mg/day if eGFR <15 mL/min

Interactions

- Minimal interactions
- Caution with other sedative and anxiolytic drugs

Special circumstances

- Pregnancy: avoid due to major risk of neural tube defects
- Breastfeeding: limited data; avoid for pain management; if used, then monitor infant for sedation. Infants can have withdrawal when breastfeeding stopped
- Children: 2.5–15 mg/kg has been tried. Increased emotional and behavioural S/Es
- Elderly: increased cognitive S/Es, hence lower doses to be used. Care in renal impairment

Additional information

- Withdrawal effect experienced by many patients; care needs to be taken to taper down pregabalin and gabapentin appropriately
- Very few studies available for prophylaxis of chronic pain; however, results from one RCT showed promise in the reduction of incidence of chronic knee pain after total knee arthroplasty with use of pregabalin preoperatively up to 14 days after surgery
- Also improves mood disturbance and sleep in PHN sufferers, while also effective in helping with central pain, sleep, and anxiety in spinal cord injury (SCI) patients
- Easier to titrate, compared to gabapentin
- Pregabalin 50 mg equivalent to gabapentin 300 mg

Cost

- Great variability in cost between manufacturers
- 25 mg (56 capsules) = £2.16 (monthly supply)
- 300 mg (56 tablets) = £4.86 (monthly supply)
- Oral solution: 20 mg/mL in 500 mL bottle: £75 (= 150 mg twice daily for 1 month)

Further reading

1. Gajraj N. Pregabalin: its pharmacology and use in pain management. Acute Pain 2008;10(1):51–2
2. Bockbrader H, Wesche D, Miller R, et al. A comparison of the pharmacokinetics and pharmacodynamics of pregabalin and gabapentin. Clin Pharmacokinet 2010;49(10):661–9

9.5 Carbamazepine

Class of drugs

- Iminostilbene derivative, related to tricyclics

Indications

- Trigeminal neuralgia—first-line treatment (NNT 1.4–1.9)
- Neuropathic pain (NNT 1.6–2.5)
- Epilepsy: generalized tonic–clonic seizures and temporal lobe specifically

Contraindications/caution

- Bone marrow dysfunction, tricyclic hypersensitivity, syndrome of inappropriate antidiuretic hormone (SIADH), porphyria, depression, atrioventricular block, along with MAOIs

Dose

- Recommendations are to start with modified release at low dose (100 mg) every 8–12 hours, with breakthrough dose of shorter-acting 100 mg preparation every 4 hours, maximum 1600 mg/day. Determining dose of longer-acting drug based on S/Es and therapeutic effects
- Expect dosing at around 400–1200 mg/day

Mechanism of action

- Blockade of voltage-gated Na^+ channels in CNS and peripheral nervous system through specific α pore binding
- Dose-dependent blockade reduces neuronal cell excitability, hence preventing firing of APs
- Possible involvement of $GABA_A$ synaptic inhibition
- Some evidence of serotonin reuptake inhibition and enhanced serotonin release
- Inhibits glutamine release

Side effects

- CNS—dizziness, blurred vision, sedation, confusion
- GI—nausea and vomiting, diarrhoea
- Blood dyscrasia—leucopenia, thrombocytopenia, haemolysis
- CVS—depressed atrioventricular conduction
- Skin reactions—urticarial rashes
- SIADH and hyponatraemia
- Rarely—agranulocytosis, Stevens–Johnson syndrome (SJS), psychosis
- Hepatotoxicity, cardiac arrhythmias
- Higher dosing (>1000 mg/day)—can develop cerebellar symptoms (incoordination and ataxia) and cerebellar atrophy

Pharmacokinetics

- Absorption: 100% bioavailability after oral administration
- Distribution: 80–90% protein-bound
- Metabolism: oxidation in the liver to the active metabolite epoxide; can induce its own metabolism with long-term use

- Excretion: initial t1/2 25–65 hours, reduces to 12 hours after maintenance use. Clearance (3.59 L/min) is often consistent and not associated with body weight, age, or size

Interactions

- Liver enzyme inducer—can enhance drug metabolism and hence reduce efficacy of other drugs, particularly oral contraceptive pills
- Higher doses needed in patients taking concurrent phenytoin (approximately 25% higher)
- Carbamazepine's plasma concentration can be reduced by other inducers, e.g. phenytoin, rifampicin, cisplatin, barbiturates, theophylline/aminophylline. Consider increasing the dose if needed
- Reduces anticoagulant property of warfarin (OXC preferable)

Special circumstances

- Pregnancy: higher incidence of neural tube defects; therefore, avoid in pregnancy where possible
- Breastfeeding: can use in breastfeeding if benefits outweigh risks, but consider close monitoring

Additional information

- Less well tolerated, compared to other anticonvulsant drugs (number needed to harm (NNH) 2.6)
- Avoid if known HLA-B1502 (increased risk of SJS)
- Aim for plasma concentrations of 4–12 micromoles/L (measure after 2 weeks of treatment), as risk of unwanted effects significantly increases beyond this range
- Will require monitoring for liver function tests (LFTs), renal function, FBC, Na^+, TFT, and HLA-B1502
- Not cleared by haemodialysis

Cost

- 100 mg (28 tablets): £2.07–4.50 (manufacturer-dependent)
- 400 mg (56 tablets): £5.05
- Monthly cost for a dose of 400–1200 mg/day: approximately £2.50–7.50

Further reading

1. Joint Formulary Committee. British National Formulary. 2020. London: BMJ Group and Pharmaceutical Press. https://www.bnf.org
2. Sasada M, Smith S. Drugs in Anaesthesia and Intensive Care. 1st edition, 2003. Oxford: Oxford University Press
3. Jacob S, Nair A. An updated overview on therapeutic drug monitoring of recent antiepileptic drugs. Drugs R D 2016;16(4):303–16

9.6 Oxcarbazepine

Class of drugs

- Ketoanalogue of carbamazepine

Indications

- Trigeminal neuralgia—NNT comparable to that of carbamazepine
- Use if increasing S/Es with carbamazepine at increasing doses

Contraindications/caution

- Sensitivity to tricyclics or carbamazepine, severe renal impairment, hyponatraemia, depression

Dose

- Dosing 300 mg twice daily, increasing up to 1200 mg twice daily (no more than 600 mg/week increments); maximum: 2400 mg/day
- Carbamazepine:OXC = 1:1.5

Mode of action

- Similar action to that of carbamazepine
- Totally absorbed and partially metabolized to the active hydroxyl metabolite compound monohydroxy derivative (MHD), which also inhibits K^+ channels, as well as Na^+ channels

Monitoring

- Monitor for hyponatraemia, and monitor liver function for acute toxicity

Side effects

- Similar to carbamazepine

Pharmacokinetics

- Absorption: 70% bioavailability
- Distribution: 40% protein-bound
- Metabolism: by the liver to MHD metabolite (pharmacokinetics are complex for OXC)
- Excretion: t1/2 of active MHD is 9 hours (only 2 hours for OXC itself)
- Little effect on CYP450 system

Interactions

- OXC is itself a potent liver enzyme inhibitor, but its concentration can be reduced by other inducers and it may increase the plasma concentration of other drugs

Special circumstances

- Pregnancy: insufficient data available to determine safety
- Breastfeeding: can be used, but monitoring for drowsiness is advised by manufacturers

Additional information

- Better S/E profile than that of carbamazepine
- Avoid with tricyclic compounds and MAOIs
- Reduces effectiveness of contraceptive pill
- May exacerbate narrow angle closure glaucoma
- MHD of OXC is the active metabolite, which is absorbed from the proximal small bowel. May need to consider alternatives in cases of duodenal resection
- 30% cross-allergy with carbamazepine
- Better than carbamazepine when anticoagulated with warfarin

Cost

- 300 mg (50 tablets) = £7.09
- 600 mg (50 tablets) = £38.71
- Monthly supply for 300–1200 mg twice daily: £8.50–93.00
- Oral suspension 60 mg/mL in 250 mL bottle: £49 (monthly supply for 500 mg/day)

Further reading

1. Sasada M, Smith S. Drugs in Anaesthesia and Intensive Care. 1st edition, 2003. Oxford: Oxford University Press
2. Flesch G. Overview of the clinical pharmacokinetics of oxcarbazepine. Clin Drug Investig 2004;24(4):185–203
3. Zhou M, Chen N, He L, et al. Oxcarbazepine for neuropathic pain. Cochrane Database Syst Rev 2013;3:CD007963

9.7 Sodium valproate

Class of drugs

- Valproate and valproic acid are organic carboxylic acid hydrocarbons

Indications

- Epilepsy, neuropathic pain, migraine prophylaxis, bipolar disorder, schizophrenia, dopamine dysregulation syndrome

Contraindications/caution

- Pregnancy
- Pre-existing liver dysfunction
- Metabolic and mitochondrial disorders
- Acute porphyrias
- Systemic lupus erythematosus (SLE)

Dose

- Initial dose 600 mg daily in two divided doses. Increase gradually by 150–300 mg every 3–4 days. Maintenance 1–2 g/day; maximum of 2.5 g/day in divided doses

Mode of action

- Stabilizes inactive Na^+ channels
- Increases brain GABA levels
- Reduces nerve cell excitability

Monitoring

- Therapeutic range 20–100 mg/L

Side effects

- Common S/Es include weakness, nausea, vomiting, sedation, and dizziness

- Less commonly, bleeding, thrombocytopenia, encephalopathy, suicidal ideation, and hypothermia

Pharmacokinetics

- Absorption: 100% bioavailability
- Distribution: highly protein-bound (90%)
- Metabolism: liver glucuronidation (30–50%)
- Excretion: 3% unchanged in the urine
- t1/2: between 8 and 20 hours
- Valproic acid is a potent androgen antagonist and an aromatase inhibitor. Lowers oestrogen concentrations, leading to lower fertility. Can increase gonad androgen biosynthesis via inhibition of histone deacetylases
- Higher rates of menstrual disorder and polycystic ovary syndrome

Interactions

- Multiple interactions mainly via inhibition of CYP2C9, glucuronyl transferase, and epoxide hydrolase
- Displacement of other protein-bound drugs
- Inhibitors of cytochrome P450 (e.g. cimetidine) will increase valproate levels
- Inducers of cytochrome P450 (phenytoin, carbamazepine, barbiturates, and rifampicin) will reduce valproate levels
- Other anticonvulsants—reduced clearance of both drugs
- Warfarin—increased concentration and prolonged bleeding time

Special circumstances

- Pregnancy: not recommended as it causes birth defects, neural tube defects, lower intelligence quotient (IQ), and autism
- Breastfeeding: theoretical risk, but no proven adverse reactions. Can be used with breastfeeding if benefits outweigh risks, but consider close monitoring
- Children: liver dysfunction, especially in children aged under 3 years with metabolic or degenerative disorders
- Elderly: increased sedation in patients with dementia

Additional information

- Evidence for effectiveness in diabetic neuropathy is weak. A Cochrane review in 2011 reported insufficient evidence to use as first-line agent for neuropathic pain
- Lack of data, and RCT results for other neuropathic types of pain are sketchy at best
- For neuropathic pain, its use is limited by dose-dependent S/Es; evidence remains poor for use in chronic neuropathic conditions
- Sodium valproate shows effectiveness in an open trial for treatment of cluster headaches and has the benefit of a single daily dose
- A meta-analysis showed NNT of 5 for 50% reduction in migraine when used as prophylaxis

Cost

- 200 mg (30 tablets): £2.77
- 300 mg (30 tablets): £5.24
- 500 mg (30 tablets): £8.73
- Monthly supply (600–2500 mg/day): approximately £11–44
- Oral solution 200 mg/5 mL in 300 mL bottle: £7.78 (for 600–2500 mg/day monthly supply: £12–50)

Further reading

1. Gill D, Derry S, Wiffen PJ, Moore RA. Valproic acid and sodium valproate for neuropathic pain and fibromyalgia in adults. Cochrane Database Syst Rev 2011;2011(10):CD009183. Published 2011 Oct 5. Doi:10.1002/14651858. CD009183.pub2
2. Linde M, Mulleners WM, Chronicle EP, McCrory DC. Valproate (valproic acid or sodium valproate or a combination of the two) for the prophylaxis of episodic migraine in adults. Cochrane Database Syst Rev 2013 Jun 24;(6):CD010611. Doi: 10.1002/14651858.CD010611. PMID: 23797677

9.8 Phenytoin

Class of drugs

- Hydantoin derivative (glycolylurea)

Indications

- Epilepsy (tonic–clonic and focal) and post-surgery seizure prophylaxis
- Status epilepticus
- Malignant ventricular arrhythmias
- Digoxin toxicity
- Neuropathic pain

Contraindications/caution

- Pregnancy
- Breastfeeding
- Acute porphyrias
- Second-degree or complete heart block
- Sinus bradycardia
- Sinoatrial (SA) node block

Dose

- Starting dose for adults: 3–4 mg/kg daily or 150–300 mg once or twice daily
- Usual maintenance 200–500 mg daily, to be taken preferably with or after food

Mode of action

- Membrane stabilization by binding to Na^+ channels and slowing inward Na^+ and Ca^{2+} flux during depolarization, and delaying outward K^+ flux

- Blockade of further AP generation
- Enhances action of GABA
- May counteract allodynia and hyperalgesia associated with neuropathic pain

Monitoring

- Narrow therapeutic window
- Target 10–20 mg/L of total plasma phenytoin
- Consider free phenytoin levels in reduced protein-binding states

Side effects

- Common—nausea, vomiting, incoordination, appetite loss, acne, hirsutism, gum hypertrophy
- CVS—hypotension, complete heart block, arrhythmias
- CNS—nystagmus, ataxia, tremor, cerebellar atrophy, peripheral neuropathy
- Blood dyscrasias—megaloblastic anaemia, folate deficiency
- Teratogenicity, carcinogenesis
- Skin—SJS, itching, toxic epidermal necrolysis (TEN)
- Drug-induced lupus, immunoglobulin A (IgA) deficiency
- Suicidal thoughts
- Reduced bone density

Pharmacokinetics

- Absorption: bioavailability 85–95% after oral dose
- Distribution: highly protein-bound (90–90%)
- Metabolism: mainly by CYP450 system to 5-(p-hydroxyphenyl)-5-phenylhydantoin (HPPH). It follows mixed-order elimination—first-order kinetics initially, and then rapid saturation of enzymes leads to achievement of zero-order kinetics just above the therapeutic level, hence a narrow therapeutic margin. Rapid accumulation with minor dose increments
- Excretion: 70–80% excreted in the urine and <5% unchanged

Interactions

- Potent inducer of liver enzymes—causes possible widespread interactions
- Metronidazole and isoniazid precipitate phenytoin toxicity
- Reduces effectiveness of warfarin, pethidine, and BZDs
- Highly protein-bound—hence, protein displacement leads to high concentrations of free drugs in some cases
- To be used cautiously with all antiarrhythmics due to risk of bradycardia
- Not cleared by haemodialysis

Special circumstances

- Pregnancy: teratogenic drug—therefore, avoid use
- Breastfeeding: can be used with breastfeeding if benefits outweigh risks, but consider close monitoring
- Children: avoid using for pain
- Elderly: higher risk of S/Es due to difference in kinetics. If prescribed, use smaller doses

Additional information

- Phenytoin is used very infrequently for pain

- A Cochrane review in 2012 to find evidence of its use in chronic pain could not find any good-quality RCT with robust inclusion criteria and a conclusion of 'no evidence of sufficient quality' was made by the authors

Cost

- 100 mg (28 tablets) = £10.07
- 300 mg (28 capsules) = £9.11
- Monthly supply for 200–500 mg daily: £20–30
- Oral solution 6 mg/mL in 500 mL bottle: £4.27
- Solution for injection 250 mg/5 mL vial= £48.79

Further reading

1. McCleane GJ. Intravenous infusion of phenytoin relieves neuropathic pain: a randomized, double-blinded, placebo-controlled, crossover study. Anesth Analg 1999;89:985–8
2. Birse F, Derry S, Moore RA. Phenytoin for neuropathic pain and fibromyalgia in adults. Cochrane Database Syst Rev 2012 May 16;2012(5):CD009485. Doi: 10.1002/14651858.CD009485.pub2. PMID:22592741; PMCID: PMC6481697

9.9 Lamotrigine

Class of drugs

- Phenyltriazine *derivative*

Indications

- Migraines
- Cluster headaches
- Bipolar disorder
- Focal and generalized seizures

Contraindications/caution

- Known sensitivity
- Use cautiously in patients with anaemia and generalized blood dyscrasia

Dose

- Start at 25 mg once daily, alternate days for 14 days, then daily for 14 days, increased to 50 mg once daily for a further 14 days. Increase up to 100 mg every 7–14 days, in steps
- Maintenance 100–200 mg daily in 1–2 divided doses, increased if necessary, up to 500 mg daily
- If restarting after 5 days' interval, the dose should be titrated again
- NNT = 4

Mode of action

- Triazine derivative inhibiting voltage-gated Na^+ channels, causing hyperpolarization of neuronal cell membrane and preventing the release of certain excitatory amino acids—of note, glutamate
- Also inhibits 5-HT receptors and L-, N-, and P-type Ca^{2+} channels

Monitoring

- No special plasma monitoring available

Side effects

- There have been reports of idiosyncratic skin reactions like SJS and TEN. Other non-specific rashes have been reported. An allergic reaction risk is related to the initial concentration of lamotrigine in plasma; hence, low-dose initiation and slow uptitration are recommended
- Well tolerated overall, with S/Es similar to those of gabapentin such as somnolence and dizziness
- CNS—blurred vision, aggression, agitation, ataxia, diplopia, dizziness, drowsiness, headache, insomnia, nausea, nystagmus, tremor
- MSK—arthralgia, back pain
- GI—diarrhoea, dry mouth, nausea, vomiting
- Skin—rash

Pharmacokinetics

- Absorption: 98% bioavailability after oral dose, first-order kinetics
- Distribution: 55% protein-bound
- Metabolism: via glucuronic acid conjugation in the liver to inactive metabolites
- Excretion: elimination t1/2 29 hours

Interactions

- Liver enzyme inducers can shorten the t1/2 of lamotrigine, so dose increases may be required
- Oestrogen-containing drugs reduce serum levels of lamotrigine, so women on such medications may require a higher dose
- Interaction with valproate enhances the action of both drugs and potentiates drug S/Es. Rare cases of neuroleptic malignant syndrome have also been reported

Special circumstances

- Pregnancy: not recommended during first trimester as increased risk of cleft lip and palate
- Breastfeeding: expressed in breast milk; manufacturers recommend to avoid if breastfeeding
- Children: rash is the most common S/E

Additional information

- A Cochrane review in 2013 revealed no convincing evidence for the use of lamotrigine in chronic pain; in fact, trials showed a higher rate of unwanted S/Es, when compared to placebo

Cost

- 25 mg (56 tablets): £1.70
- 100 mg (56 tablets): £3.12
- 200 mg (56 tablets): £3.92
- Monthly supply for 200–500 mg/day: £2–6

Further reading

1. Lynch M, Watson C. The pharmacotherapy of chronic pain: a review. Pain Res Manag 2006;11(1):11–38
2. Wiffen PJ, Derry S, Moore RA. Lamotrigine for acute and chronic pain. Cochrane Database of Systematic reviews 2011, Issue 2. Art. No.: CD006044. DOI: 10.1002/14651858.CD006044.pub3

9.10 Topiramate

Class of drugs

- Sulfamate-substituted monosaccharide compound, unlike any other anticonvulsants in use

Indications

- Epilepsy, weight loss, migraine prophylaxis, bipolar disorder, borderline personality disorder, alcoholism
- Cluster headaches
- Migraines

Contraindications/cautions

- Acute porphyria
- Kidney stones—topiramate changes urine pH, hence an increased risk of causing renal stones
- Acroparaesthesia due to inhibition of carbonic anhydrase

Dose

- Start at 25 mg once daily for 1 week at night and then can be increased by 25–50 mg every week. Usual dose of 50–100 mg/day in two divided doses
- Maximum 200 mg daily

Mode of action

- Modulates voltage-gated Na^+ channels and voltage-gated Ca^{2+} channels
- Inhibits carbonic anhydrase
- Enhances action of GABA
- Blocks neurotransmission and prevents the release of excitatory amino acids—of note, glutamate

Monitoring

- Serum/plasma level can be monitored for epilepsy or overdose
- Levels usually <10 mg/L

Side effects

- Common S/Es include weight loss, nausea, fatigue, and cognitive dysfunction
- Difficulty with word finding is specific to topiramate and seen in one-third of patients
- Use limited by dose-dependent S/Es

Pharmacokinetics

- Absorption: rapid absorption from the gut, 80% bioavailability
- Distribution: 13–17% protein-bound

- Metabolism: hydroxylation, hydrolysis, and glucuronidation
- Excretion: 70% excreted unchanged in the urine
- t1/2: 19–25 hours

Interactions

- Topiramate can alter the concentration of other anticonvulsant drugs. Use cautiously in epileptic patients using phenytoin, valproate, carbamazepine, lithium, barbiturates, and metformin
- Hyperammonaemia and CNS toxicity reported when combined with valproic acid

Special circumstances

- Pregnancy: avoid as proven link with cleft palate when taken in first trimester
- Breastfeeding: avoid, as per manufacturer, as small amounts in breast milk
- Children: unlicensed use for migraine prophylaxis; can cause vertigo, fever, and vomiting
- Elderly: increased cognitive impairment and risk of falling

Additional information

- An RCT in 2006 showed positive changes in pain sensitivity, subjective disability, health-related QoL, and weight loss when used for chronic lower back pain
- Used in neuropathic pain, but limited by dose-dependent S/Es, while evidence remains poor for use in chronic neuropathic conditions
- Used successfully in cases of trigeminal neuralgia in MS patients, although evidence for its use in non-MS subjects is less dramatic
- Used in migraine prophylaxis as can cause cerebral vasodilatation
- Has undergone trials for other conditions, including PTSD, infantile spasms, periventricular leucomalacia, and hypoxic–ischaemic injury
- Promotes weight loss in overweight people

Cost

- 25 mg (60 tablets): £9.50
- 50 mg (60 tablets): £9.50
- Monthly supply for 50–100 mg: £9.50
- Oral suspension 10 mg/mL in 150 mL bottle: £129 (monthly: £129–200)

Further reading

1. Chong M, Libretto S. The rationale and use of topiramate for treating neuropathic pain. Clin J Pain 2003;19(1):59–68
2. Linde M, Mulleners WM, Chronicle EP, McCrory DC. Topiramate for the prophylaxis of episodic migraine in adults. Cochrane Database Syst Rev 2013 Jun 24;2013(6):CD10610. Doi: 10.1002/14654858.CD010610. PMID:23797676; PMCID: PMC7388931
3. Zvartau-Hind M, Din M, Gilani A, et al. Topiramate relieves refractory trigeminal neuralgia in MS patients. Neurology 2000;55(10):1587–8

CHAPTER 10

Antidepressants

Hadi Bedran, Enrique Collantes, Peter Keogh, and Matthew Wong

CONTENTS

10.1 Overview of antidepressants

Introduction

- Prevalence of chronic pain and mood disorders is common and varies, depending on the clinical setting studied (around 50% in chronic pain clinics)
- Simultaneous treatment of chronic pain and mood disorders is needed to achieve good outcomes
- Antidepressants can be used as part of a multidisciplinary approach addressing the physical, psychological (psychiatric or psychological), and social (work, litigation, social support network) contributors to pain, disability, and distress
- Consider the use of non-pharmacological strategies to improve mood and pain. These can include training in relaxation, mindfulness, and other forms of psychotherapy such as acceptance and commitment therapy (ACT), cognitive behavioural therapy (CBT), dialectical behaviour therapy (DBT), supportive therapies, family/couples/marital therapies, and psychodynamic therapies

Classification

- MAOIs: phenelzine, isocarboxazid
- TCAs: amitriptyline, nortriptyline, imipramine
- SSRIs: citalopram, sertraline, fluoxetine
- SNRIs: duloxetine, venlafaxine, desvenlafaxine, milnacipran
- Tetracyclic/unicyclic antidepressants: mirtazapine
- Serotonin antagonist and reuptake inhibitors: trazadone
- Melatonergic and serotonin reuptake inhibitors: valdoxan

Mode of action

- Improve mood and pain, and vice versa. The exact mode of action is unknown, but some mechanisms of action may be through:

  - Restoring the imbalance or deficiency of key NTs (serotonin, noradrenaline, dopamine, glutamate, GABA) widely distributed throughout the brain
  - Potentiating descending inhibitory pathways at the spinal level (e.g. acting on opioid receptors in the DH) and other areas of the CNS such as PAG

Indications

- Treatment of anxiety and depressive disorders
- Symptomatic treatment of common presentations such as anxiety, insomnia, and irritability
- Direct treatment of neuropathic pain:
  - General consensus is that TCAs are the most effective antidepressants but have the most adverse effects
  - Most of the evidence is from diabetic neuropathy and PHN
  - Antidepressants can be used in acute neuropathic pain, based on experience from chronic neuropathic pain

Analgesic efficacy—pharmacotherapy for neuropathic pain

- First line (TCA or SNRI or gabapentinoids):
  - TCA (amitriptyline 25–150 mg): moderate evidence, moderate effect size (NNT 3.6), low to moderate tolerability/safety (NNH 13.4)
  - SNRI (duloxetine 60–120 mg): high evidence, moderate effect size (NNT 6.4), moderate tolerability/safety (NNH 11.8)
  - Gabapentinoids (pregabalin 150–600 mg or gabapentin 1200–3600 mg): high evidence, moderate effect size, tolerability/safety (high for gabapentin and moderate for pregabalin)
- Second line: tramadol or capsaicin patch 8% or topical lidocaine
- Third line: strong opioids or botulinum toxin type A (BTX-A)

Administration and dose

- Given by the oral route
- To be considered in patients with neuropathic pain, particularly if associated with symptoms of insomnia (TCA) and low mood and/or anxiety (TCA/SNRI)
- Initiation at low dose (taking into account risk factors for toxicity) and titrated according to effect. Titrations of different antidepressants is affected by the pharmacokinetics and inter-individual variations in drug handling
- The lowest effective dose should be maintained
- Should intolerable S/Es occur, the patient should be stepped back down to the highest dose tolerated
- Caution and use lower doses in the elderly and in renal and hepatic impairment due to decreased excretion
- When started, possible increased risk of suicide-related events in those with a depressive/psychiatric condition. An adequate risk assessment for suicide needs to be done before commencing antidepressants, and appropriate ongoing support is required
- Beware that when antidepressants are weaned, potentially there can be a deterioration in the mental state and increased suicidal ideation
- Beware the withdrawal phenomenon when discontinuing particularly SSRIs and SNRIs. Titrate the dose down slowly (at least a minimum of every 2 weeks) if the dose has been high or for a prolonged duration. Monitor closely for withdrawal symptoms such as nausea, vomiting, dizziness, agitation, anxiety, headache, and other symptoms

- Discuss with patients and other clinicians discontinuing antidepressants if these are no longer needed as they cause S/Es. When and how to do this is different patient by patient

Additional information

- Generally, avoid using antidepressants for pain management in pregnancy, breastfeeding, and children. If the benefits outweigh the risks, use the safest and most effective antidepressant
- There is conflicting evidence of whether combining antidepressants with other analgesics for pain management is useful

Further reading

1. Hooten M. Chronic pain and depression. In: Wilson P, Jensen T, Watson P, Haythornthwaite JA (eds). Clinical Pain Management: Chronic Pain. 2008; pp. 241–53. London: Hodder
2. Finnerup NB, Attal N, Haroutounian S, et al. Pharmacotherapy for neuropathic pain in adults: a systematic review and meta-analysis. Lancet Neurol 2015;14:162–73

10.2 Tricyclic antidepressants

Indications

- Depression
- Neuropathic pain:
  - Effective in diabetic neuropathy, PHN, HIV sensory neuropathy, central post-stroke pain, post-mastectomy pain, trigeminal neuralgia
  - Efficacy NNT 2–3 and NNH 13.4
  - Sedative effects can be useful in patients with sleep disturbances
- Prophylaxis of migraine

Contraindications

- Acute porphyrias; arrhythmias; manic phase of bipolar disorder; heart block; recent MI, severe liver disease (relative), simultaneous use of other medications such as tramadol, warfarin, SSRIs, MAOIs

Dose

- Starting dose 10–25 mg nocte, gradually increased if necessary
- Neuropathic pain: 10–50 mg daily
- Depression or migraine prophylaxis: maximum daily dose 150 mg

Mode of action

- Reuptake inhibition of serotonin and noradrenaline (via the metabolite nortriptyline)
- Receptor blockade: muscarinic cholinergic, α-1 adrenergic, histamine H1, NMDA
- Ion channel blockade: Na^+, Ca^{2+}

Monitoring

- Patients should be monitored closely for changes in behaviour, clinical worsening of the mental state, and suicidal tendencies; this should be done during the initial 1–2 months of therapy and dosage adjustments

Side effects

- Common: dry mouth, constipation, fatigue, drowsiness, dizziness, postural hypotension, blurred vision, urinary hesitancy, confusion (elderly), risk of falls
- Rare: dysarthria, sexual dysfunction, extrapyramidal symptoms, tremor, oedema, cardiac conduction defects
- Very rare: neuroleptic malignant syndrome, precipitation of angle closure glaucoma
- Frequency unknown: arrhythmias, paraesthesiae, rash, taste disturbance, nausea, vivid dreams

Relevant pharmacokinetics

- Absorption/distribution: oral bioavailability 45%, peak serum level 4 hours, 95% protein-bound, large Vd
- Metabolism: significant variability in patients due to genetic variability. Amitriptyline undergoes N-demethylation into its primary active metabolite nortriptyline by hepatic CYP2C19. This secondary amine is hydroxylated by CYP2D6 and conjugated to glucuronide and sulphates
- Excretion: mostly as inactive conjugates in the urine, minimal amounts in faeces. Elimination t1/2: 13–36 hours

Relevant pharmacodynamics

- CVS: postural hypotension, sinus tachycardia, dysrhythmia, increase in AV conduction time, prolonged PR and QT intervals
- CNS: sedation, fatigue, respiratory depression in toxic doses

Interactions

- SSRI: increased adverse effects
- Adrenaline/noradrenaline/phenylephrine: increased effects
- Alcohol: increased CNS depression
- Antiarrhythmic drugs: increased risk of ventricular arrhythmias
- Antipsychotics: increased sedation, additive anticholinergic effects
- Barbiturates: decreased activity
- Clonidine: antihypertensive effects reduced or abolished
- Lithium: risk of neurotoxicity
- MAOIs: mutual enhancement, hypertension, hyperpyrexia, convulsions, and coma
- Tramadol: increased risk of seizures and serotonergic syndrome

Special circumstances

- Renal impairment: use with caution, but normally dose reductions are not needed
- Hepatic impairment: dose reduction in severe liver impairment
- Pregnancy: use with caution; consider if benefits outweigh risks
- Lactation: the amount secreted into breast milk is too small to be harmful
- Elderly: susceptible to many of the S/Es; low doses, with close monitoring
- Driving: drowsiness may affect the performance of skilled tasks

Additional information

- Nortriptyline (5–50 mg) can sometimes be more effective, with fewer S/Es, than amitriptyline
- TCAs can attenuate the cardiovascular effects of adrenaline during general anaesthesia
- Overdosage: associated with a relatively high rate of fatality
- Withdrawal symptoms: the risk is increased if the antidepressant is stopped suddenly after regular administration for 8 weeks or more. The dose should preferably be reduced gradually over about 4 weeks

Cost

- Amitriptyline 10 mg (28 tablets): £0.89
- Amitriptyline 25 mg (28 tablets): £0.76
- Amitriptyline 50 mg (28 tablets): £2.02
- Nortriptyline 10 mg (28 tablets): £1.85
- Nortriptyline 25 mg (28 tablets): £2.27
- Nortriptyline 50 mg (30 tablets): £21.13
- Prices for oral solutions are significantly higher than for tablet form (10 mg/mL for 250 mL bottle: £246; 1-month supply for 10–50 mg/day: £10–50)

Further reading

1. Joint Formulary Committee. British National Formulary. 2020. London: BMJ Group and Pharmaceutical Press. https://www.bnf.org
2. Finnerup NB, Attal N, Haroutounian S, et al. Pharmacotherapy for neuropathic pain in adults: a systematic review and meta-analysis. Lancet Neurol 2015;14:162–73
3. Sindrup SH, Otto M, Finnerup NB, et al. Antidepressants in the treatment of neuropathic pain. Basic Clin Pharmacol Toxicol 2005;96:399–409

10.3 Serotonin and noradrenaline reuptake inhibitors

Indications

- Neuropathic pain
- Major depressive disorder
- Anxiety disorder

Mechanism of action

- The exact analgesic mechanisms of action of SNRIs is unknown but may be through blockade of reuptake of serotonin and/or noradrenaline
- Venlafaxine has a dose-related effect:
  - Low dose: serotonin blocked
  - Medium dose: serotonin and noradrenaline blocked
  - High dose: serotonin, noradrenaline, and dopamine blocked

Analgesic efficacy

- SNRIs and TCAs are more effective than SSRIs for the management of neuropathic pain
- Duloxetine: NNT 5.8, NNH (minor) 11.8, and NNH (major) 17
- Venlafaxine: NNT 6.4, NNH (minor) 9.6, and NNH (major) 16.2
- Evidence indicates that duloxetine (60–120 mg daily) provides:
  - Analgesia for diabetic neuropathy and other presentations of neuropathic pain
  - Analgesia and improved QoL in fibromyalgia, but no effect on sleep or fatigue
- In diabetic polyneuropathy, venlafaxine and duloxetine are superior to TCAs with regard to both analgesia and S/Es

Routes of administration and dosing

- Duloxetine: commence at 30 mg, increased to 60 mg daily, maximum 120 mg daily

- Venlafaxine: 75 mg daily in two divided doses, maximum 375 mg daily. Dose-related effect (analgesic at higher doses)
- Renal impairment (creatinine clearance <30 mL/min): duloxetine and venlafaxine dose reduction
- Liver impairment: duloxetine should not be used; venlafaxine dose reduction

Pharmacokinetics

- Duloxetine:
  - Absorption: bioavailability 50%
  - Distribution: 96% protein-bound
  - Metabolism: hepatic via cytochrome P450 (especially CYP1A2 and CYP2D); large inter-subject variability in response
  - Excretion: elimination t1/2: 8–17 hours, mainly in the urine
- Venlafaxine:
  - Absorption: bioavailability 92%
  - Distribution: 60% protein-bound, Vd 5 L/kg
  - Metabolism: hepatic via cytochrome P450 to weakly active metabolites
  - Excretion: renal

Adverse effects

- Cardiovascular: prolongation of QT interval, torsades de pointes
- GI: duloxetine can commonly cause nausea and vomiting
- Haematological: increased bleeding risk from blocking serotonin reuptake into platelets
- Metabolic: hyponatraemia
- Nervous system:
  - Worsening of depressive symptoms/increase suicide-related event risk, mostly when initiated
  - Paradoxical anxiety, insomnia, delirium, akathisia, seizures, headache, dizziness
  - Serotonin syndrome—avoid serotonergic medicines, including triptans and tramadol
- Skin/MSK: rash, myalgia, arthralgia

Contraindications

- Patients on MAOIs—risk of serotonin-type syndrome
- Prolonged QT syndrome or if taking other drugs that prolong the QT interval
- Caution in diabetics—may alter glucose control
- Caution in epileptics—may lower seizure threshold
- Caution in patients with bleeding abnormalities or co-administered anticoagulants
- May precipitate closed angle glaucoma in susceptible patients

Additional information

- Pregnancy:
  - Duloxetine: caution recommended
  - Venlafaxine: not recommended
- Breastfeeding:
  - Duloxetine, venlafaxine: not recommended
- Children:
  - Duloxetine, venlafaxine: avoid under 18 years of age

- Desvenlafaxine (metabolite of venlafaxine) is sometimes better tolerated. Dose 50–200 mg daily
- Milnacipran is a more recent selective SNRI licensed for fibromyalgia and neuropathic pain (not in the UK). It has been found to provide pain relief to a minority of people

Cost

- Duloxetine 30 mg capsules (28 pack): £22.40
- Duloxetine 60 mg capsules (28 pack): £27.72
- Venlafaxine 37.5 mg tablet (56 pack): £7.95
- Venlafaxine 75 mg tablet (56 pack): £15.95

Further reading

1. Joint Formulary Committee. British National Formulary. 2020. London: BMJ Group and Pharmaceutical Press. https://www.bnf.org
2. Finnerup NB, Attal N, Haroutounian S, et al. Pharmacotherapy for neuropathic pain in adults: a systematic review and meta-analysis. Lancet Neurol 2015;14:162–73
3. Gilron I. Treatment of neuropathic pain: antiepileptic and antidepressant drugs. Pain. In: Raja SN, Sommer CL (eds). Refresher Courses, 15th World Congress on Pain. 2014; pp. 225–37. Buenos Aires: IASP Publisher
4. Ryder S, Stannard C. Treatment of chronic pain: antidepressant, antiepileptic and antiarrhythmic drugs. Contin Educ Anaesth Crit Care Pain 2005;5(1):18–21

10.4 Selective serotonin reuptake inhibitors

Indications

- Major depressive disorder
- Anxiety disorder
- Neuropathic pain (poor evidence)

Efficacy

- SNRIs and TCAs are better analgesics than SSRIs in the management of neuropathic pain
- SSRIs are safer in overdose than TCAs
- Effective at targeting anxiety, depression, and arousal

Mechanism of action

- The exact analgesic mechanism is unknown but may be through blockade of reuptake of serotonin with no, or minimal, effect on noradrenaline
- Citalopram is the most selective SSRI, with minimal effect on noradrenaline, dopamine, and GABA uptake

Routes of administration and dosing

- Citalopram: 20–40 mg PO daily
- Sertraline: 50–200 mg PO daily
- Fluoxetine: 20–60 mg PO daily

Pharmacokinetics

- Citalopram:
  - Absorption: bioavailability 80%
  - Distribution: 80% protein-bound, Vd 12.3 L/kg
  - Metabolism: hepatic via cytochrome P450 (especially CYP2C19, but also CYP3A4) to active metabolites with (weaker) SSRI activity. Displays linear kinetics, with steady state achieved in 1–2 weeks
  - Excretion: elimination t1/2 1.5 days, 85% via the liver and 15% via the kidneys
- Sertraline:
  - Absorption: good oral bioavailability
  - Distribution: 98% protein-bound
  - Metabolism: hepatic via cytochrome P450 (mainly CYP3A4, CYP2C19, and CYP2B6)
  - Excretion: elimination t1/2 26 hours, 50% via the liver and 50% via the kidneys
- Fluoxetine:
  - Absorption: good oral bioavailability
  - Distribution: 95% protein-bound, Vd 20–40 L/kg
  - Metabolism: hepatic via cytochrome P450 to active norfluoxetine
  - Excretion: elimination t1/2 4–6 days for fluoxetine and 4–16 days for norfluoxetine (hence persistence of the drug for 5–6 weeks after discontinuation)

Adverse effects

- Nervous system: worsening of depressive symptoms/increased suicide-related event risk, mostly when initiated. Paradoxical anxiety, insomnia, delirium, akathisia, seizures, headache, dizziness. Serotonin syndrome—avoid serotonergic medicines, including triptans and tramadol. Citalopram appears to have the least adverse effects on the nervous system of the SSRIs
- Cardiovascular: prolongation of QT interval, torsades de pointes. Interaction with linezolid (citalopram), causing severe hypertension
- Metabolic: hyponatraemia
- Haematological: increased bleeding risk from blocking serotonin reuptake into platelets
- Skin/MSK: rash, myalgia, arthralgia

Contraindications

- Patients on MAOIs—risk of serotonin-type syndrome
- Prolonged QT syndrome or if taking other drugs that prolong the QT interval
- Caution in diabetics—may alter glucose control
- Caution in epileptics—may lower seizure threshold
- Caution in patients with bleeding abnormalities or co-administered anticoagulants
- May precipitate closed angle glaucoma in susceptible patients

Special considerations

- Pregnancy
  - Citalopram considered safe by manufacturer
  - Sertraline and fluoxetine: not recommended
- Breastfeeding
  - Citalopram and fluoxetine: caution recommended
  - Sertraline: not recommended

- Children
  - Citalopram: avoid in those under 18 years of age
  - Sertraline only for treatment of obsessive–compulsive disorder (OCD)
  - Fluoxetine licensed in children over 8 years of age

Additional information

- Agomelatine is a melatonin receptor agonist and a selective serotonin receptor antagonist which is sleep-enhancing, and can be used with other antidepressants (off-label). LFT monitoring is required (28 tablets cost £30)

Cost

- Citalopram 10 mg tablets (28 pack): £0.90
- Citalopram 40 mg tablets (28 pack): £1.46
- Sertraline 50 mg tablets (28 pack): £4.50
- Sertraline 100 mg tablets (28 pack): £7.99
- Fluoxetine 20 mg capsules (30 pack): £1.15
- Fluoxetine 40 mg capsules (30 pack): £1.80

Further reading

1. Gilron I. Treatment of neuropathic pain: antiepileptic and antidepressant drugs. Pain. In: Raja SN, Sommer CL (eds). Refresher Courses, 15th World Congress on Pain. 2014; pp. 225–37. Buenos Aires, IASP Publisher
2. Ryder S, Stannard C. Treatment of chronic pain: antidepressant, antiepileptic and antiarrhythmic drugs. Contin Educ Anaesth Crit Care Pain 2005;5(1):18–21

10.5 Mirtazapine

Indications

- Moderate/major depression—particularly if the patient also has anorexia, weight loss, and insomnia

Contraindications

- Hypersensitivity to mirtazapine
- Concomitant use or within 2 weeks from cessation of MAOIs

Dose

- Starting dose 15–30 mg/day; range is 15–45 mg/day
- In elderly patients, the starting dose can be lower (7.5 mg)
- Caution is required in moderate/severe liver and renal impairment as clearance is reduced
- Lower doses used for depression and insomnia. At higher doses, there are less sedative effects

Mode of action

- Antagonist at pre-synaptic α-2 adrenergic inhibitory receptors on both serotonin and noradrenaline pre-synaptic axons, resulting in an increased release of noradrenaline

- Potent antagonist of 5-HT2 and 5-HT3 receptors. There is increased 5-HT1 activity due to selective enhancement of 5-HT1 receptors
- Potent antagonist of histamine (H1) receptors, contributing to its sedative effects
- Moderate peripheral α-1 adrenergic antagonist which can lead to orthostatic hypotension
- Moderate antagonist at muscarinic receptors which may explain low anticholinergic S/Es
- Its mechanism of action is not related to noradrenaline or serotonin reuptake blockade
- At lower doses, it improves sleep as it has a higher affinity for histamine receptors. At higher doses, there is less sedating effect because there is less antihistamine effect and more noradrenergic transmission

Monitoring

- Patients should be advised to report any fever, sore throat, stomatitis, or other signs of infection during treatment. Blood count should be performed and the drug stopped immediately if blood dyscrasia is suspected
- Close monitoring is required when simultaneously used with serotonergic active substances

Side effects

- Common: sedation, dry mouth, weight gain, increased appetite, dizziness, fatigue
- Less common: abnormal dreams, tremor, nausea, arthralgia
- Rare: myoclonus, elevation of transaminase levels, bone marrow suppression, hyponatraemia, toxic epidermal necrolysis, Stevens-Johnson syndrome

Relevant pharmacokinetics/pharmacodynamics

- Absorption: oral bioavailability 50%, reaching peak plasma levels after 2 hours of oral intake
- Metabolism: demethylation and oxidation in the liver by cytochrome P450 enzymes. The demethyl metabolite is pharmacologically active
- Elimination: via the urine (75%) and faeces (15%). Mean t1/2 is 20–40 hours. Steady state is reached after 304 days
- Mirtazapine can cause minor/moderate cognitive impairment (e.g. impaired ability to drive, use machines, etc.)

Interactions

- Warfarin: INR can be increased
- MAOIs/serotonergic active substances: risk of serotonin-associated effects
- BZDs/antihistamines/opioids/antipsychotics: sedating properties may be enhanced
- Alcohol: mirtazapine may worsen the CNS-depressant effect of alcohol
- CYP3A4 inducers (e.g. carbamazepine, phenytoin): can increase mirtazapine clearance by about 2-fold
- CYP3A4 inhibitors (e.g. HIV protease inhibitors, azole antifungals): mirtazapine dose may have to be decreased due to reduced clearance
- Paroxetine, amitriptyline, risperidone, or lithium: interaction studies did not indicate any relevant pharmacokinetic interactions

Special circumstances

- Pregnancy: limited data do not indicate an increased risk of congenital malformations
- Breastfeeding: excreted in breast milk only in very small amounts
- Elderly: reduced clearance
- Sometimes used as an antiemetic mostly in palliative care—evidence is controversial

- Can be a good agent in underweight, depressed patients as can increase appetite and weight

Additional information

- Some elderly patients can develop insomnia when mirtazapine is used at higher doses, such as 45 mg, due to increased noradrenaline concentrations. Some patients on higher doses take mirtazapine in the morning, aiming for less interference with sleep

Cost

- Mirtazapine 15 mg tablets (28 pack): £1.22
- Mirtazapine 30 mg tablets (28 pack): £1.09
- Mirtazapine 45 mg tablets (28 pack): £1.32
- Oral solution formulations are significantly more expensive

Further reading

1. REMERON® (mirtazapine) Tablets. 2007. https://www.accessdata.fda.gov/drugsatfda_docs/label/2007/020415s019,021208s010lbl.pdf
2. British National Formulary. Mirtazapine. https://bnf.nice.org.uk/drug/mirtazapine.html
3. Riediger C, Schuster T, Barlinn K, et al. Adverse effects of antidepressants for chronic pain: a systematic review and meta-analysis. Front Neurol 2017;8:307. https://www.frontiersin.org/articles/10.3389/fneur.2017.00307/full
4. Electronic Medicines Compendium. Mirtazapine 15mg tablets. https://www.medicines.org.uk/emc/product/531/smpc
5. Kim S-W, Shin I-S, Kim J-M, et al. Factors potentiating the risk of mirtazapine-associated restless legs syndrome. Hum Psychopharmacol 2008;23(7):615–20. https://onlinelibrary.wiley.com/doi/abs/10.1002/hup.965

CHAPTER 11

Neurolytic Agents

Hadi Bedran

CONTENTS

11.1 Ethyl alcohol

Indications

- Alcohol is one of the main agents used for chemical neurolysis
- Predominantly indicated in patients with a short life expectancy for management of cancer pain intractable to other modalities

Contraindications

- Absolute: known allergy to ethyl alcohol
- Relative: patients taking medications which inhibit alcohol dehydrogenase

Dose

Concentration used

- Complete nerve destruction with concentrations of 100% or 95%
- Partial nerve destruction with concentration of 50%
- Analgesia has been achieved with concentration of 33%
- Absolute alcohol is ideal for some peripheral nerve neurolytic blocks

Volumes used

- Neuraxial blocks: normally 0.3–0.7 mL of alcohol per dermatome
- Peripheral blocks need larger volumes, as alcohol rapidly spreads after it is injected from its site of action. In lumbar sympathetic/coeliac plexus, 10–20 mL of alcohol may be used bilaterally

Mode of action

- Non-selective destruction of nerve tissue by precipitation of cell membrane proteins, extraction of lipid compounds, demyelination, and subsequent Wallerian degeneration
- When alcohol is injected near the sympathetic chain, it destroys the ganglion cells and thus blocks all post-ganglionic fibres to all effector organs

Monitoring

- Cardiac arrhythmias, hypotension, and skin and non-target tissue necrosis can occur
- Patients on medications that inhibit alcohol dehydrogenase can develop disulfiram-like reactions: flushing, vomiting, sweating, marked hypotension, and dizziness

Adverse effects

- Alcoholic neuropathy (common), hypoaesthesia, neuritis, deafferentation pain, motor deficit when mixed nerves are ablated, unintentional damage to non-targeted tissue and thrombosis if given IV
- In neuro-axial blocks or blocks close to the spinal cord can get the adverse effects already described and the following: bowel or urinary incontinence, neuralgias (e.g. genitofemoral neuralgia with lumbar sympathectomy), arterial vasospasm (spasm of the artery of Adamkiewicz can cause paraplegia)

Relevant pharmacokinetics/pharmacodynamics

- Alcohol spreads rapidly from the injection site. When injected in the CSF, only 10% of the initial dose remains at the site of injection after 10 minutes and about 4% remains after 30 minutes
- Between 90% and 98% of ethyl alcohol that enters the body is completely oxidized in the liver, principally by alcohol dehydrogenase
- Denervation and pain relief accrue over a few days after injection, usually after 1 week

Interactions

- Safe to be mixed with LAs, usually 1:1 ratio

Additional information

- Alcohol is hypobaric in nature relative to the CSF. The position of the patient must be with the painful site in the uppermost and lateral decubitus position. After injection, the patient can be rolled anteriorly approximately 45° to place the dorsal (sensory) root uppermost
- Alcoholic neuritis occurs frequently following thoracic paravertebral sympathetic block. This may be due to the close proximity of the sympathetic ganglia to the intercostal nerves. As a prophylactic measure, it is recommended to inject LA during insertion of the needle, at the site of injection before the alcohol is injected and on withdrawing the needle
- Perineural injection of alcohol is followed immediately by severe burning pain along the nerve's distribution, which lasts about a minute, before giving way to a warm, numb sensation. Pain on injection may be diminished by prior injection of LA and using sedation during the procedure

Further reading

1. Hicks F, Simpson KH. Nerve Blocks in Palliative Care. 2004. Oxford: Oxford University Press
2. Jain S, Gupta R. Neurolytic agents in clinical practice. 2nd edition, 2001. Philadelphia, PA: WB Saunders
3. Zhou L, Craig J, Parekh N. Current concepts of neurolysis and clinical applications. J Analgesics 2014;2:16–22

11.2 Phenol

Class of drug

- Neurolytic drug made of carbolic acid, phenic acid, phenylic acid, phenyl hydroxide, hydroxybenzene, and oxybenzene
- Can be prepared by the hospital pharmacy by dissolving 1 g of phenol in 15 mL of water (6.67%)

Indications

- Phenol is one of the main agents used for chemical neurolysis. Predominantly indicated in palliative patients with a short life expectancy for management of intractable neuropathic pain refractory to other management modalities caused by:
  - Cancer pain
  - Persistent non-cancer pain
  - Sympathetic-mediated pain intractable to other modalities
- Used with caution for sclerotherapy of haemorrhoids (by injection)

Contraindications

- Oily phenol injection: neonates or children
- Allergy to any of the constituents of phenol

Dose

- Sclerotherapy for haemorrhoids: 2–3 mL of phenol 5% in oil; maximum 10 mL
- Neural/intrathecal: concentrations of 4–10% are typically used with sterile water or glycerol. In neuraxial blocks hyperbaric solutions (e.g. with glycerol) are preferred

Mode of action

- Concentrations of <5% cause protein denaturation
- Concentrations of >5% cause protein coagulation, non-specific segmental demyelination, and Wallerian degeneration
- Phenol has LA properties at lower concentrations

Monitoring

- Signs of cardiac and CNS instability after every single use in neurolysis

Side effects

- Topical preparations: blanching, corrosion, pain, local ulceration, sterile abscess formation
- Perineural/intrathecal injections: neuritis, deafferentation pain, unintentional damage to non-targeted tissue, motor deficit, hypoaesthesia

Relevant pharmacokinetics/pharmacodynamics

- Hyperbaric relative to the CSF
- Absorption: rapidly absorbed through the skin and into the lungs. After intrathecal injection, its concentration decreases rapidly to 30% of the original concentration in 60 seconds and to 0.1% within 15 minutes
- Metabolism: conjugation to glucuronides and oxidation by liver enzymes
- Clearance: the kidneys are the primary route of elimination

- Therapeutic effects: the process of neural degeneration takes about 14 days, and regeneration is completed in about 14 weeks

Adverse effects

- Toxic systemic doses of phenol (>8.5 g) are associated with convulsions, followed by CNS depression, and finally cardiovascular collapse
- Chronic poisoning results in skin eruptions, GI symptoms, and renal toxicity
- Clinical doses of between 1 and 10 mL of 1–10% solutions (up to 1000 mg) unlikely to cause serious toxicity
- Unintentional damage to non-targeted tissue, neuralgias, deafferentation pain and thrombosis if given IV
- In neuro-axial blocks or blocks close to the spinal cord can also develop bowel or urinary incontinence and arterial vasospasm (spasm of the artery of Adamkiewicz can cause paraplegia)

Interactions

- None known

Additional information

- Parental exposure to phenol and its related compounds is associated with spontaneous abortion
- Phenol causes minimal discomfort when injected, whereas ethyl alcohol produces discomfort when administered
- Less intense and shorter duration of block, when compared to alcohol

Further reading

1. Drugbank. Owned by the Governors of the University of Alberta. https://www.drugbank.ca/drugs/DB03255
2. Mandl F. Aqueous solution of phenol as a substitute for alcohol in sympathetic block. J Int Coll Surg 1950;13:566
3. Nathan PW, Sears TA. Effects of phenol on nervous conduction. J Physiol 1960;150:565
4. Wood KM. The use of phenol as a neurolytic agent: a review. Pain 1978;5:205

CHAPTER 12

Corticosteroids

Sadiq Bhayani, Bethany Fitzmaurice, and Alifia Tameem

CONTENTS

12.1 Overview of corticosteroids

Introduction

- The adrenal cortex releases two classes of corticosteroids into circulation: GCs and mineralocorticoids
- In this chapter, we focus on GCs and their synthetic analogues
- Estimated human cortisol production = 5–10 mg/m^2/day, equivalent to 20–30 mg/day of hydrocortisone and 5–7 mg/day of prednisolone
- Anticipate HPA axis suppression with >30 mg/day of hydrocortisone/7.5 mg/day of prednisolone/0.75 mg of dexamethasone for >3 weeks, i.e. 'supraphysiological' doses
- The British Pain Society/Faculty of Pain Medicine Consensus statement:
  - Corticosteroid use for neuraxial interventions—ongoing debate due to reports of catastrophic neurological complications
  - Sufficient evidence to support continued use of corticosteroids in epidural injections for acute symptom relief, especially in the presence of acute radicular pain with disc herniation
  - Limited evidence that particulate corticosteroid preparations have better efficacy than non-particulate preparations
  - Particulate steroids must not be used for transforaminal cervical epidural injections
  - Caution with interlaminar cervical epidurals and thoracic/lumbar/caudal routes
  - Patients at increased risk if previous spinal surgery
  - Small risk of neurotoxicity with inadvertent intrathecal injection due to preservatives (polyethylene glycol (PEG) in Depo-Medrone®). Many clinicians now prefer to use triamcinolone or dexamethasone
  - Consent—use of epidural corticosteroids is outside the product licence and should be incorporated into the consent process

Pain-related indications

- Not licensed in pain interventions for any route other than intra-articular

Acute pain

- Acute herpes zoster, PHN prevention (remains speculative)
- SLE (oral or local injection, e.g. enthesitis, tendonitis)
- Polymyalgia rheumatica and giant cell arteritis—low-dose corticosteroids are the mainstay of treatment
- Sickle cell crisis—a short course of high-dose methylprednisolone may decrease crisis duration
- Post-operative pain—dexamethasone 0.1–0.2 mg/kg, opioid-sparing effect
- Acute painful inflammatory conditions, including CRPS, carpal tunnel syndrome, adhesive capsulitis, and painful cervical or lumbar radiculopathy

Chronic pain

- Epidural for radicular pain, intra-articular, muscular (trigger point injection (TPI)), specific nerves
- Cluster headaches—transitional prophylactic treatment
- PHN—intrathecal methylprednisolone: pain relief demonstrated
- CRPS—PO prednisolone 10 mg three times daily demonstrated efficacy in acute CRPS (<13 weeks)
- RA—to control pain or to bridge therapy of slower-acting agents
- Temporomandibular dysfunction—topical or local injection

Cancer pain

- Cerebral oedema headache (lower intracranial pressure (ICP))
- Hepatic capsular stretch pain from liver metastases (reduce capsular inflammation)
- Neuropathic pain and compressive symptoms (reduce perineural oedema); can reverse early nerve compression
- Steroid enemas in treatment of tenesmus
- Chemotherapy-induced arthropathy
- Myeloma and associated pain: dexamethasone classed as chemotherapeutic agent

(See Table 12.1.1.)

Table 12.1.1 Classification of corticosteroids

Naturally occurring or synthetic	Particulate (poorly soluble) or non-particulate (soluble)	Preservative or preservative-free
Naturally occurring: Hydrocortisone (cortisol) Cortisone Corticosterone *Synthetic:* Prednisone Prednisolone Methylprednisolone Betamethasone Dexamethasone Triamcinolone	According to water solubility and aggregation characteristics '*Particulate*' = aggregates larger than red blood cells (6–8 micrometres) All synthetic corticosteroids are particulate, except dexamethasone (0.5 micrometres) and betamethasone	Multistate outbreak (2012) of fungal meningitis in patients receiving contaminated preservative-free methylprednisolone acetate (MPA) Majority include preservatives for sterility and enhanced shelf-life

Mode of action

Therapeutic effects

- *Gene regulation:*
  - Corticosteroids are gene-active hormones, targeting DNA molecules and inducing or repressing the synthesis of specific messenger ribonucleic acid (mRNA) within a few minutes, although the physiological response may take hours to days to develop
  - Synthetic GCs have a higher affinity for the receptor, are less rapidly inactivated, and have little or no mineralocorticoid activity
- *Anti-inflammatory action:*
  - Potent inhibition of cytokines, various inflammatory mediators, production and recruitment of inflammatory cells, and NO synthase
  - Inhibit plasma exudation at inflammatory sites and prevent intracellular water sequestration, thus preventing cell swelling and destruction
- *Mechanisms in pain relief:*
  - Enhance pain-relieving effects of LA by anti-inflammatory and direct analgesic effects (inhibitory effects on C-fibre conduction)
  - Modulate pain pathways—decrease both peripheral and central neuronal hyperexcitability
  - Long-term pain reduction may be secondary to changes in gene expression
  - Injection into the epidural space allows a higher local concentration than systemic administration
  - Co-administration of LA interrupts sustained abnormal neural activity that perpetuates pain
  - Anti-swelling and anti-inflammatory effects on nerve root and surrounding tissue, aiming to create sufficient space and mobility of the nerve root to reduce or abolish pain

Metabolic effects

- Carbohydrates—stimulate hepatic gluconeogenesis, increase hepatic glycogen content, and inhibit insulin-mediated peripheral blood glucose uptake
- Proteins—decrease anabolism, stimulate catabolism, and deplete the protein matrix of the vertebral column (trabecular bone), with minimal effect on long bones (compact bone)
- Lipids—permissive effect on lipolytic hormones and fat redistribution

Immunosuppressive effects

- Modulate immune response, with leucocytosis but reduced antibody production, impair phagocytosis, reduce the number and function of circulating T-lymphocytes, and reduce (or decrease) the production inflammatory mediators

Vascular reactivity

- Allow efficient response to circulating catecholamines, positive inotropy

Routes of administration and dosing

- Little agreement about dose or type, with/without LA, volume, or frequency of injections
- Dose and duration do not predict the extent of adrenal suppression as ACTH
- If no benefit obtained after two injections, additional injections rarely efficacious
- Repeated injections usually limited to three per year

Table 12.1.2 Corticosteroid potencies and dosing

Drug	Equivalent glucocorticoid dosing (mg)	Relative glucocorticoid activity	Relative mineralocorticoid activity	Duration of action (hours)	Plasma half-life (minutes)
Short-acting					
Cortisone	25	0.8	0.8	8–12	60
Hydrocortisone (cortisol)	20	1.0	1.0	8–12	90
Intermediate-acting					
Prednisone	5	4	0.6	24–36	60
Prednisolone	5	4	0.6	24–36	200
Methylprednisolone	4	5	0.5	24–36	180
Triamcinolone	4	5	0	24–36	300
Long-acting					
Dexamethasone	0.75	20–30	0	36–54	200
Betamethasone	0.6	20–30	0	36–54	200

(See Table 12.1.2.)

- Note: $t_{1/2}$ does not represent the duration of action—this is best represented by the duration of ACTH suppression
- Short-acting: advantageous when rapid clinical effect desired, e.g. allergic reactions (highest mineralocorticoid potency)
- Long-acting: prolonged anti-inflammatory effects (weakest mineralocorticoid potency)

Side effects and toxicity

- Fluid retention, hyperglycaemia, elevated BP, mood changes, menstrual irregularities, gastritis, Cushing's syndrome, increased appetite, weight gain, infections, delayed wound healing, and acneiform eruptions. Short courses (<2–3 weeks) are safe, and S/Es rare
- Local S/Es:
    - Repeated intra-articular injections—severe joint destruction, bone necrosis, Charcot-like deformities
    - Injection/leakage in skin—dermal and subdermal atrophy
    - Intrathecal methylprednisolone—sterile meningitis and arachnoiditis (related to polyethylene preservative)
    - Swelling, tenderness, warmth, infection, post-injection pain flare-up—can last up to 2 days. Soft tissue atrophy, depigmentation, periarticular calcifications, and tendon rupture
- Systemic S/Es:
    - Minimal changes in fasting blood glucose or lipid levels after a single epidural injection of dexamethasone usually
    - Depot preparations used for epidural injections may produce ACTH suppression and Cushing's syndrome lasting up to a few weeks, even following a single epidural injection of 60 mg of methylprednisolone or triamcinolone
    - Single lumbar epidural injection of triamcinolone 80 mg can cause profound HPA axis suppression for 3 weeks and marked reduction in insulin sensitivity
    - Intra-articular steroid injections—patients can have detectable levels in circulation

- More serious S/Es with long-term supraphysiological doses:
  - Immunosuppressive:

    Chickenpox and measles are of particular concern
  - Allergy
  - Endocrine: secondary adrenocortical insufficiency and atrophy (3 months minimum after treatment cessation), hypopituitarism, Cushing's syndrome, withdrawal syndrome (headache, pyrexia, myalgia), often called 'steroid pseudorheumatism'
  - Increased blood glucose, predisposition to diabetes, worsened pre-existing diabetes, increased appetite and weight gain
  - Psychiatric: affective and psychotic disorders, insomnia, confusion
  - Neurological: amnesia, dizziness, headaches, vertigo
  - Ocular: cataracts, glaucoma, exophthalmos, retinal detachment
  - Cardiac: dyslipidaemia, hypertension
  - Vascular/haematological: increased thrombosis risk, leucocytosis
  - GI: peptic ulcer, GI perforation, oesophagitis, oesophageal candidiasis, nausea and vomiting, dyspepsia, abdominal distension, peritonitis, pancreatitis
  - MSK: osteoporosis, growth retardation, muscular weakness and atrophy, osteonecrosis, vertebral compression fractures, aseptic necrosis of femoral and humeral heads, arthralgia, myalgia, tendon rupture
  - Renal and urinary: caution in renal insufficiency
  - Dermatological: impaired wound healing, thin and fragile skin and atrophy, hirsutism, petechiae, erythema, hyperhidrosis, hyper- or hypopigmentation, rash, pruritus, acne, suppression of skin tests
  - Reproductive: irregular menstruation

Pharmacokinetics

- Absorption: small and lipid-soluble, readily absorbed from GI tract, enter target cells by simple diffusion
- Distribution: transported in plasma by corticosteroid-binding globulin (CBG) and albumin—do not bind to synthetic steroids readily. CBG has low capacity and may become saturated when therapeutic doses of steroids are used. Albumin binds both natural and synthetic steroids. CBG and albumin-bound steroids are biologically inactive
- Metabolism: by CYP3A enzyme system, reduction of the double bond between C4 and C5; occurs mainly in hepatocytes. Cortisone and prednisone are inactive until converted *in vivo* to hydrocortisone and prednisolone, respectively. Cortisol (hydrocortisone) is an active agent, whereas the inactive drug cortisone must be converted by the liver to cortisol for biological activity
- Excretion: renal

Analgesic efficacy

- No difference in pain and function scores between particulate and non-particulate steroids
- Epidural corticosteroids: NNT 7 for 75% pain relief at 60 days, 13 for 50% pain relief at 1 year
- Transforaminal: steroid onto ventral aspect of nerve root sleeve and dorsal aspect of disc herniation is theoretically more effective
- Efficacy less with radicular pain that has lasted >3 months and previous back surgery
- The less soluble an agent (acetate suspensions), the longer it remains in the joint or epidural space and theoretically the more prolonged effect
- Several recommendations:

- Interlaminar and caudal epidural steroid injection (ESI): lower risk due to known vascular anatomy
- Cervical transforaminal ESI (TFESI): vertebral artery in the foramen at every level—use non-particulate corticosteroid only
- Thoracic TFESI: risk of presence of an artery is higher than lumbar spine, but lower than cervical spine—ribs obscuring ability to detect vascular flow on fluoroscopy hence recommend non-particulate corticosteroid
- Lumbar TFESI: risk of arterial presence is lowest. Dexamethasone preferred as first line. Higher-risk particulates should be reserved for patients non-responsive to non-particulate formulations
- Non-particulate steroids should be used as first line for TFESI in all cervical injections and lumbar injections above L3

Contraindications and cautions

- Hypersensitivity to the drug or excipient
- Should not inject into unstable joints, presence of active infection in or near joints
- Should not inject into Achilles tendon
- Co-treatment with CYP3A inhibitors—increase risk of systemic S/Es
- Live virus vaccines contraindicated in patients receiving immunosuppressive doses of corticosteroids
- Inactivated viral or bacterial vaccines—expected serum antibody response may not be obtained

Interactions

- CYP3A4 inhibitors—increased plasma concentrations of corticosteroid
- CYP3A4 inducers—may need to increase dose
- Corticosteroids can reduce effects of anticholinesterases in myasthenia gravis
- Enhanced hypokalaemic effects with diuretics, carbenoxolone, B2 agonists, and theophylline
- Caution with cardiac glycosides—hypokalaemia may result in toxicity
- Antagonism of competitive neuromuscular blocking drugs
- Renal clearance of salicylates is increased by corticosteroids

Special considerations

- Pregnancy:
  - Variable between individual corticosteroids. Prednisone and prednisolone are inactivated by the placenta
  - Increased incidence of low birthweights and cataracts in infants
  - Not known to be teratogenic in humans
  - Animal studies show increased incidence of cleft palate, and brain development affected
  - May theoretically lead to neonatal hypoadrenalism, but rarely clinically important
  - FDA (Food and Drug Administration) Pregnancy Categories for Drugs: prednisolone is schedule D for first trimester, and schedule C for second and third trimesters (schedule C = human risk cannot be ruled out; schedule D = evidence of risk to human fetus)
- Breastfeeding:
  - Corticosteroids pass into breast milk, and infants may have a degree of adrenal suppression
- Paediatrics:
  - Dose-related growth retardation which may be irreversible

    - May accelerate epiphyseal closure
- Patients should carry a 'Steroid Treatment' card detailing: prescriber, drug, dosage, and treatment duration
- Effects may be enhanced in hypothyroidism and cirrhosis, and reduced in hyperthyroidism
- Corticosteroids inhibit growth-promoting effect of human growth hormone

Additional information

- Withdrawal syndrome may occur without evidence of adrenal insufficiency
- Particulate corticosteroids particle size order: methylprednisolone > triamcinolone > betamethasone
- Recommended corticosteroid for epidural injection: betamethasone > triamcinolone
- Proposed mechanisms of injury with corticosteroids:
    - Inadvertent arterial injection arrow pointing rightwards infarction
    - Animal studies: direct injection into artery—no neurological injury with dexamethasone
    - Chemical vascular injury
    - Direct neurotoxic effects of additives and preservatives—benzyl alcohol, PEG, polysorbate 80, ethylenediaminetetraacetate (EDTA)
    - Vasospasm due to needle trauma or dye

Further reading

1. British Pain Society/Faculty of Pain Medicine (RCA) Consensus Statement on the use of Corticosteroids for Neuraxial Procedures in the UK. 2018. https://www.britishpainsociety.org/static/uploads/resources/files/BPS_FPM_Steroid_Statement_FINAL.pdf
2. Knezevic AA, Jovanovic F, Voronov D, et al. Do corticosteroids still have a place in the treatment of chronic pain. Front Pharmacol 2018;9:1229. https://doi.org/10.3389/fphar.2018.01229
3. Peck TE, Hill SA, Williams M (eds). Pharmacology for Anaesthesia and Intensive Care. 2003. London: Greenwich Medical Media
4. Stannard C, Booth S (eds). Churchill's Pocketbooks of Pain. 2nd edition, 2004. London: Elsevier Churchill Livingstone
5. Electronic Medicines Compendium. https://www.medicines.org.uk/emc

12.2 Triamcinolone acetonide

Name (brands)

- Kenalog® intra-articular/IM injection

Presentation

- 40 mg/mL of sterile aqueous suspension, 1 mL glass vial
- Excipient with known effect: 15 mg/mL of benzyl alcohol
- Other excipients: polysorbate 80, sodium carboxymethyl cellulose, sodium chloride
- Particulate

Pain-related indications

- Intra-articular:
    - RA, OA with inflammatory component, bursitis, epicondylitis, tenosynovitis

- IM (where sustained systemic treatment required):
  - Collagen disorders, dermatological diseases, rheumatic, GI, or respiratory disorders, neoplastic diseases
- Safety and efficacy of administration by other routes are yet to be established

Contraindications/caution

- IV, intrathecal, and intraocular routes are contraindicated
- Incidence of blindness after nasal turbinate and intralesional injections in the face/head

Routes of administration and dosing

- Intra-articular:
  - Small joints 5–10 mg; large joints up to 40 mg; multiple joint involvement up to 80 mg
  - For sheaths of short tendons, Adcortyl® injection (triamcinolone acetonide 10 mg/mL) is recommended
- IM:
  - Deep into gluteal muscle to avoid SC fat atrophy. Avoid deltoids
  - Adults and children >12 years: suggested initial dose 40 mg

Mode of action

- High-potency GC, with low mineralocorticoid activity

Pharmacokinetics

- Absorption:
  - May be absorbed into systemic circulation from synovial spaces
  - Deep IM depot injection: almost 100% bioavailability, absorbed slowly. Provides an extended duration of therapeutic effect and fewer S/Es, compared with oral therapy
  - Following a single 80 mg dose, adrenal suppression occurs within 24–48 hours, gradually returning to normal within 3 weeks, correlating with the extended duration of therapeutic action
- Metabolism:
  - Hepatic, CYP3A4 substrate, 6-β-hydroxylation

Interactions

- Reports of clinically significant drug interactions in patients receiving triamcinolone acetonide and ritonavir

Special circumstances

- Elderly: common S/Es are more serious, particularly osteoporosis, diabetes, hypertension, hypokalaemia, thin skin, and immunodeficiency
- Children 6–12 years: suggested initial dose of 40 mg, not recommended in those aged <6 years
- Must not be given to premature babies or neonates due to benzyl alcohol; can cause toxic and anaphylactoid reactions in infants and children aged up to 3 years
- Pregnancy: crosses the placenta
- Breastfeeding: no data available

Additional information

- Note: does not contain PEG, hence decreased risk of neurotoxicity

Cost

- 40 mg/mL (five vials): £7.45

Further reading

1. Benzon H, Rathmell J, Wu CL, et al. Raj's Practical Management of Pain. 4th edition, 2008. Philadelphia, PA: Elsevier
2. Electronic Medicines Compendium. https://www.medicines.org.uk/emc

12.3 Methylprednisolone acetate

Name (brands)

- Depo-Medrone® or Depo-Medrol®
- Also available: Depo-Medrone® with lidocaine (methylprednisolone 4%, lidocaine hydrochloride 1%)
- Solu-Medrone® or Solu-Medrol®

Presentation

- White aqueous sterile suspension for injection
- Each vial contains 1, 2, or 3 mL of Depo-Medrone® 40 mg/mL
- Excipients—PEG, sodium chloride, myristyl-γ-picolinium chloride, water for injection
- Particulate

Pain-related indications

- IM administration (for prolonged systemic effect in rheumatological disorders)
- Intra-articular administration
- Periarticular, into bursae, into tendon sheaths (not into the substance of tendons)
- Intralesional, e.g. keloid scars

Contraindications/caution

- Avoid injection into the deltoid—high incidence of SC atrophy
- Avoid intralesional administration too superficially—SC atrophy and depigmentation

Routes of administration and dosing

- IM;
  - Single 80 mg injection expected to last average of 2 weeks
- Rheumatic disorders and collagen diseases 40–120 mg (1–3 mL) per week
- Intra-articular (RA, OA):
  - 4–80 mg; where appropriate, the dose may be repeated at intervals of 7–35 days
  - Large joint 20–80 mg; medium joint 10–40 mg; small joint 4–10 mg
  - Spinal joints, unstable joints, and joints devoid of superficial synovial space are not suitable

- Into the bursa, periarticular, into the tendon sheath:
  - 4–30 mg; repeat injections may be necessary

Mode of action

- High GC effects, low mineralocorticoid effects

Side effects

- Systemic absorption of methylprednisolone occurs following intra-articular injection
- Adrenal cortical atrophy occurs if received higher than physiological doses (approximately 6 mg of methylprednisolone) for >3 weeks
- Rapid IV administration of methylprednisolone is associated with cardiovascular collapse
- Overdose:
  - Reports of acute toxicity and/or death are rare. No specific antidote; treatment is supportive. Methylprednisolone is dialysable

Pharmacokinetics

- Absorption:
  - When injected, provides slow release of the active steroid to the target site
- Distribution:
  - Widely distributed into tissues, crosses the BBB, secreted in breast milk. Plasma protein binding: approximately 77%
- Metabolism:
  - Hepatic, inactive metabolites (mainly 20α- and 20β-hydroxymethylprednisolone)
- Excretion:
  - No dose adjustments required in renal impairment

Special circumstances

- Paediatrics: infants and children are at particular risk from raised ICP
- Elderly: no information to suggest a dose change is warranted
- Fertility: impairs fertility in animal studies
- Pregnancy: methylprednisolone crosses the placenta
- Breastfeeding: excreted in small amounts in breast milk. Up to 40 mg daily is safe. May be theoretical risk of hypoadrenalism in doses higher than this, but benefits of breastfeeding outweigh this risk
- Neonates—avoid as contains benzyl alcohol

Additional information

- Enhanced effect in patients with hypothyroidism
- Intrathecal methylprednisolone—promising treatment for PHN
- Post-mortem studies of PHN patients noted SC inflammation, and PHN patients may have high levels of IL8 in the CSF. This treatment may theoretically decrease pro-inflammatory mediators (which may contribute to central sensitization), neuraxial inflammation, and PHN pain as a result.
- Studies have shown a significant decrease in PHN pain (both burning and lancinating). CSF concentrations of IL8 were also significantly decreased

Cost

- 1 vial 40 mg/mL = £3.44
- 1 vial 80 mg/2 mL = £6.18
- 1 vial 120 mg/3 mL = £8.96
- Methylprednisolone acetate 40 mg and lidocaine hydrochloride 10 mg in 1 mL vial = £3.94, 2 mL vial = £7.06

Further reading

1. Vadivelu N, Urman RD, Roberta H. Essentials of Pain Management. 2015. London: Springer
2. Electronic Medicines Compendium. https://www.medicines.org.uk/emc

12.4 Dexamethasone

Presentation

- Clear glass ampoule, 1 mL or 2 mL, clear colourless solution
- Dexamethasone (Hospira®), 3.3 mg/mL:
    - 1 mL solution for injection contains 4 mg of dexamethasone phosphate equivalent to 3.32 mg of dexamethasone base
    - Excipients—sodium citrate, disodium edetate, sodium sulphite anhydrous, sodium hydroxide, and hydrochloric acid
- Dexamethasone preservative-free (Aspen®) 3.8 mg/mL:
    - 1 mL solution for injection contains 5 mg of dexamethasone sodium phosphate equivalent to 3.8 mg of dexamethasone base
    - Excipients—glycerol, disodium edetate, sodium hydroxide, or phosphoric acid, stored in the fridge
- Non-particulate and devoid of benzyl alcohol and PEG

Pain-related indications

- Adjuvant analgesic and symptomatic treatment of cord compression in palliative care settings
- Cancer pain: reduces tumour oedema, and thereby pressure on surrounding structures. Analgesic effect is greatest in a confined space:
    - Headache associated with raised ICP from cerebral tumours
    - Nerve compression pain, often in conjunction with other analgesics/adjuvants
    - Malignant bone pain
- Particularly useful for neuropathic, visceral, and bone pain syndromes in patients with advanced malignant disease
    - Standard dose is 16–24 mg/day, can be given once daily due to its long t1/2, but divided doses usually used to mitigate high-dose toxic effects such as psychosis and severe blood glucose abnormalities in diabetic patients
    - Doses as high as 100 mg may be given in severe pain crises, similar to doses used in acute neurological emergencies
    - IV boluses should be given over several minutes to avoid untoward reactions such as burning sensations

Routes of administration and dosing

- All dosing recommendations are given in units of dexamethasone base

- Dose range usually 4–16 mg/24 hours
  - Suitable for intra-articular or soft tissue injection
- Recurrent or inoperable brain tumours: usually 1.7 mg twice to three times daily
- Large joint 1.7–3.3 mg; small joints 0.66–0.8 mg; bursae 1.7–2.5 mg; tendon sheaths 0.33–0.8 mg; soft tissue infiltration 1.7–5 mg
- Frequency = ranges from 3 days to 3 weeks

Mode of action

- Predominant GC activity and minimal mineralocorticoid activity, making it the least toxic choice
- Second highest GC potency after betamethasone

Side effects

- Enhanced GC activity of dexamethasone leads to more hyperglycaemia, compared with other steroids
- Sleep disturbance and restlessness may start within hours of a large dose

Pharmacokinetics

- Absorption
  - Well absorbed by mouth and inhalation; following injection, dexamethasone is rapidly hydrolysed to dexamethasone, with peak plasma levels within 5 minutes
- Distribution:
  - Plasma protein binding approximately 77% (less than most other corticosteroids)
  - Penetrates into tissue fluid and CSF
- Metabolism:
  - High uptake by the liver, kidneys, and adrenal glands, with slow hepatic metabolism
  - Plasma t1/2 3.5–4.5 hours, but effects outlive plasma concentrations; thus, biological t1/2 is of greater relevance (36–54 hours)
- Excretion:
  - Up to 65% of a dose excreted in the urine in 24 hours, mainly as unconjugated steroids

Special circumstances

- Neonates: only preservative-free solutions should be administered
- Paediatrics: dosage should be limited to a single dose on alternate days
- Pregnancy: readily crosses the placenta, with minimal inactivation
- Breastfeeding: no data available for dexamethasone
- Palliative care: can be diluted with sodium chloride and given by continuous subcutaneous infusion (CSCI)

Additional information

- Burning or tingling after IV administration, particularly in perineal area
- Number and activity of spermatozoa may be affected in men
- Theoretical disadvantages: easy washout from epidural space, reports of convulsions after intrathecal injection in animals
- Has been shown to prolong anaesthesia and analgesia, alongside LA, in nerve blockade

Cost

- 500 mcg (28 tablets): £6.40
- 2 mg (50 tablets): £6.84
- 4 mg (50 tablets): £83
- Dexamethasone (base) 3.3 mg/mL (ten ampoules) = £15.00–22.63
- Dexamethasone (base) 6.6 mg/2 mL (ten ampoules) = £22.00–24.00

Further reading

1. Electronic Medicines Compendium. https://www.medicines.org.uk/emc
2. Drugs.com. Dexamethasone. https://www.drugs.com/ingredient/dexamethasone.html

12.5 Hydrocortisone

Presentation

- Hydrocortisone acetate 25 mg/mL suspension for injection
- IV/IM—white powder as sodium succinate, for reconstitution with water for injection
- Glass ampoule, suspension for injection
- Excipients: benzyl alcohol, sodium chloride, sodium carboxymethyl cellulose, polysorbate 80)

Pain-related indications

- Intra-articular or periarticular: for RA and OA, when few joints are involved
- Non-articular: for symptomatic treatment of inflammatory conditions such as inflamed tendon sheaths and bursae

Contraindications/caution

- Injection into spinal or other non-diarthrodial joints

Routes of administration and dosing

- Intra-articular: 5–50 mg, depending on size of patient and joint
- May be repeated at intervals of 21 days
- No more than three joints should be treated on any one day
- Adults: 5–50 mg, depending on joint size
- Children: 5–30 mg daily in divided doses

Mode of action

- Both GC and mineralocorticoid activity
- Cortisone has minimal activity and must be converted to hydrocortisone in the liver first

Side effects

- Overdose: no specific antidote available. Symptoms: nausea and vomiting, sodium and water retention, hyperglycaemia, GI bleeding
- Treatment is symptomatic

Pharmacokinetics

- Absorption:
  - Slow systemic absorption following intra-articular or soft tissue injection. Onset after IV/IM injection is 2–4 hours; lasts 8 hours
- Distribution:
  - Plasma protein binding >90%
- Metabolism:
  - Metabolized in the liver and most body tissues to hydrogenated and degraded forms such as tetrahydrocortisone and tetrahydrocortisol
- Excretion:
  - In the urine, mainly as conjugated glucuronides, and a very small proportion is excreted unchanged

Special circumstances

- Pregnancy: cortisone readily crosses the placenta
- Breastfeeding: no specific data available for cortisone. Doses of up to 200 mg daily unlikely to cause systemic effects in infants

Additional information

- Hydrocortisone is dialysable
- In overdose, can administer IV cimetidine or ranitidine to prevent GI bleeding

Cost

- 10 mg and 20 mg (30 tablets): £7.04–7.52
- 100 mg/mL solution for injection (five ampoules): £10.60
- Hydrocortisone cream 0.5% and 1% (15 g): £1.07–1.22 (2.5% = £4.99)

Further reading

1. Smith T, Pinnock C, Lin T. Fundamentals of Anaesthesia. 4th edition, 2016. Cambridge: Cambridge University Press
2. Electronic Medicines Compendium. https://www.medicines.org.uk/emc

12.6 Betamethasone

Name (brands)

- Celestone® or Betnesol® 4 mg/mL solution for injection (betamethasone acetate) = soluble ester with rapid action, particulate
- Soluspan® (betamethasone)—only slightly soluble, affords sustained activity, considered non-particulate, given its soluble nature, not commercially available
- Celestone® Soluspan®—commercially available; contains both betamethasone acetate and phosphate and shows extensive aggregation of particles; reported cases of paralysis in the literature

Presentation of Betnesol®

- 1 mL ampoule contains a clear colourless or pale yellow, sterile aqueous solution
- Each ampoule contains 5.3 mg of betamethasone sodium phosphate is equivalent to 4 mg of betamethasone
- Excipients with known effect: sodium metabisulphite 0.1% w/v, 0.678 mg sodium per mL

Pain-related indications

- Soft tissue lesions, e.g. tennis elbow, tenosynovitis, bursitis

Contraindications/caution

- Not recommended intrathecally

Routes of administration and dosing

- Can be given slow IV, deep IM, subconjunctivally, or as local soft tissue injection, depending on indication
- Local injection dose = 4–20 mg in adults, smaller doses in children. This dose can be repeated on 2–3 occasions, depending on response (up to four times in 24 hours)

Mode of action

- Has the highest GC potency, and although it is a depot-type injectate, it has the least particulate material

Pharmacokinetics

- Following IM injection—betamethasone appears to be readily absorbed, with peak plasma concentration detected at 12.92 hours

Interactions

- Concomitant use of betamethasone with quetiapine may result in increased metabolism of quetiapine, so a higher dose may be needed

Special circumstances

- Pregnancy: betamethasone readily crosses the placenta. May result in transient suppression of fetal heart rate (FHR)
- Myocardial hypertrophy and gastro-oesophageal reflux have been reported in association with *in utero* exposure to betamethasone

Additional information

- Betamethasone acetate thought to act as prodrug or reservoir, conferring extended-release characteristics

Cost

- 4 mg/1 mL solution for injection (five ampoules): £30.26
- 0.1% cream (30 g): £1.14

Further reading

1. Electronic Medicines Compendium. https://www.medicines.org.uk/emc
2. Salem II, Najib NM. Pharmacokinetics of betamethasone after single-dose intramuscular administration of betamethasone phosphate and betamethasone acetate to healthy

subjects. Clin Ther 2012;34(1):214–20. https://www.clinicaltherapeutics.com/article/S0149-2918(11)00774-0/pdf

12.7 Steroid passport

- For an example of a steroid passport used at the University Hospitals of Leicester, see Figs. 12.7.1 and 12.7.2
- Patients/doctors can document the steroid-based interventions which patients receive from various specialties

Steroid injections

- Steroids that are injected into muscles or joints may cause some pain and swelling at the site of the injection, but this should pass within a few days
- Steroid injections can also cause muscle or tendon weakness on repeated injections
- Because of the risk of side effects, steroid injections are often only given at intervals of at least 4 months and a maximum of three injections in a year is usually recommended

Please kindly keep this passport safe and ask your doctor to fill in this passport every time you have a steroid injection. It is very important to carry this passport every time you have an injection.

No	Date of injection	Type of steroid	Dosage in mgs
1			
2			
3			
4			
5			
6			
7			
8			
9			
10			

Post procedure care following chronic pain intervention

- Use ice (cold) packs on the treated area today
- Use warmth on the treated area from tomorrow
- Take your regular pain medications as usual
- Don't worry if your pain gets worse for the first few days immediately after your injection. This is known as flare up pain
- If the injection has helped you may be offered a repeat injection if appropriate. If you get no benefit from the injection you may go to your GP to be referred back to the pain clinic for further assessment and discuss further management options
- Injection treatment is one of the multiple options for pain management and they are not cure for your pain
- Use any time you have reduced pain to work on any physiotherapy exercises you may have been doing

Figure 12.7.1 Example of a steroid passport used at the University Hospitals of Leicester

Steroid injections / steroid passport
Pain Management Service
Information for Patients
University Hospitals of Leicester NHS
NHS Trust
Caring at its best

Figure 12.7.2 Steroid passport as a booklet

About steroid injections

Steroid injections

Steroids that are injected into muscles or joints may cause some pain and swelling at the site of the injection but this should pass within a few days. Steroid injections can also cause muscle or tendon weakness on repeated injections. Because of the risk of side effects, steroid injections are often only given at intervals of at least four months and a maximum of three injections in a year is usually recommended.

Corticosteroids side effects

Corticosteroids are powerful medications that can sometimes have a wide range of side effects. They will only be used if the potential benefits are thought to outweigh this risk.

The risk of experiencing side effects largely depends on:

The type of steroid you're taking – steroid tablets (oral corticosteroids) are more likely to cause side effects than inhalers or injections.

The dose – the higher the dose, the greater the risk of developing side effects.

The length of treatment – for example, you're more likely to develop side effects if you take steroid tablets for more than three weeks.

Your age – young children and the elderly are more likely to experience side effects benefits are thought to outweigh this risk.

2

About steroid injections

Why are steroid injections for pain limited to only a few a year?

Steroid injections can also cause side effects including; skin thinning, loss of colour in the skin, facial flushing, insomnia, moodiness and high blood sugar. The risk of side effects increases with the number of steroid injections you receive.

Steroid injections contain drugs that mimic the effects of the hormones cortisone and hydrocortisone which can disrupt your body's natural hormone balance. Delaying repeat injections allows your body to return to its normal balance so it's important to carefully weigh the potential risks and benefits of long-term steroid injections.

Systemic side effects of steroids

- Increased appetite which can potentially lead to weight gain if you find it difficult to control what you eat.
- Acne.
- Rapid mood swings and mood changes – such as becoming aggressive, irritable and short-tempered with people.
- Thin skin that bruises easily.
- Muscle weakness.
- Delayed wound healing.
- A combination of fatty deposits that develop in the face, stretch marks across the body and acne – known as Cushing's syndrome.
- Weakening of bones (osteoporosis).
- Diabetes (or may worsen existing diabetes).
- High blood pressure.
- Glaucoma and cataracts (eye conditions).

3

About steroid injections

- Stomach ulcers – you may be prescribed an additional medication called a proton pump inhibitor (PPI) to reduce this risk.
- Mental health problems such as depression, suicidal thoughts, anxiety, confusion and hallucinations. See your GP if you experience any of these problems.
- Increased risk of infections, particularly chickenpox, shingles and measles – avoid close contact with anyone who has an infection and seek medical advice immediately if you think you may have been exposed.

4

Steroid Passport

Please kindly keep this passport safe and ask your doctor to fill in this passport every time you have a steroid injection. It is very important to carry this passport every time you have an injection.

No	Date of injection	Type of steroid	Dose in mgs
1			
2			
3			
4			
5			
6			
7			
8			
9			
10			

5

Figure 12.7.2 Continued

Post procedure care following chronic pain intervention

- Use ice (cold) packs on the treated area today.
- Use warmth on the treated area from tomorrow.
- Take your regular pain medications as usual.
- Don't worry if your pain gets worse for the first few days immediately after your injection. This is known as flare up pain.
- Keep a pain diary. Score your pain every day and keep diary for 1 month.
  0 = No pain
  10 = Worst pain
- The pain nurse will call you in 6-8 weeks time to ask how your pain has been. If the injection have helped you may be offered a repeat injection if appropriate. If you get no benefit from the injection you may be booked back to see the doctor in the pain clinic for further assessment and discuss further management options.
- Injection treatment is one of the multiple options for pain management and they are not cure for your pain.
- Use any time you have reduced pain to work on any physiotherapy exercises you may have been doing.

Pre- procedure pain score- /10

6

Day	Pain Score (1-10)
1	
2	
3	
4	
5	
6	
7	
8	
9	
10	
11	
12	
13	
14	
15	
16	
17	
18	
19	
20	
21	
22	
23	
24	
25	
26	
27	
28	
29	
30	

7

Figure 12.7.2 Continued

Corticosteroid side effects

- Corticosteroids are powerful medications that can sometimes have a wide range of side effects
- They will only be used if the potential benefits are thought to outweigh this risk

The risk of experiencing side effects largely depends on

- The type of steroid you are taking—steroid tablets (oral corticosteroids) are more likely to cause side effects than inhalers or injections
- The dose—the higher the dose, the greater the risk of developing side effects
- The length of treatment—for example, you are more likely to develop side effects if you take steroid tablets for more than three weeks
- Your age—young children and the elderly are more likely to experience side effects; benefits are thought to outweigh this risk

Why are steroid injections for pain limited to only a few a year?

- Steroid injections can also cause side effects, including skin thinning, loss of colour, facial flushing, insomnia, moodiness, and high blood sugar
- The risk of side effects increases with the number of steroid injections you receive
- Steroid injections contain drugs that mimic the effect of the hormones cortisone and hydrocortisone, which can disturb your body's natural hormone balance
- Delaying repeat injections allows your body to return to its normal balance, so it is important to carefully weigh the potential risks and benefits of long-term steroid injections

Systemic side effects of steroids

- Increased appetite which can potentially lead to weight gain if you find it difficult to control what you eat
- Acne
- Rapid mood swings and mood changes—such as becoming aggressive, irritable, and short-tempered with people
- Thin skin that bruises easily
- Muscle weakness
- Delayed wound healing
- A combination of fatty deposits that develop in the face, stretch marks across the body, and acne—known as Cushing's syndrome
- Weakening of bones (osteoporosis)
- Diabetes (or may worsen existing diabetes)
- High blood pressure
- Glaucoma and cataracts (eye conditions)
- Stomach ulcers—you may be prescribed an additional medication called a proton pump inhibitor (PPI) to reduce this risk
- Mental health problems such as depression, suicidal thoughts, anxiety, confusion, and hallucinations. See your GP if you experience any of these problems
- Increased risk of infections, particularly chickenpox, shingles, and measles—avoid close contact with anyone who has an infection, and seek medical advice immediately if you think you may have been exposed

Post-procedure care following chronic pain intervention

- Use ice (cold) packs on the treated area today
- Use warmth on the treated area from tomorrow
- Take your regular pain medications as usual
- Don't worry if your pain gets worse for the first few days immediately after your injection. This is known as flare-up pain
- If the injection has helped, you may be offered a repeat injection if appropriate. If you get no benefit from the injection, you may go to your GP to be referred back to the pain clinic for further assessment and discuss further management options
- Injection treatment is one of the multiple options for pain management and they are not a cure for your pain
- Use any time you have reduced pain to work on any physiotherapy exercises you may have been doing

CHAPTER 13

Miscellaneous

Hadi Bedran, Udaya Chakka, Bethany Fitzmaurice, Praveen Ganty, James Jack, Peter Keogh, Arumugam Pitchiah, Kavita Poply, Manamohan Rangaiah, Jan Rudiger, Maria Stasiowska, Alifia Tameem, and Matthew Wong

CONTENTS

13.1 Baclofen

Indications

- Painful spasticity from MS, spinal lesions, cerebral events, or other pathologies causing pain from muscle spasms
- Limited role as monotherapy for primary treatment of pain

Contraindications

- Precaution in diabetics, stroke, peptic ulceration, renal/respiratory/hepatic failure
- Avoid in patients with mental health disorders, seizures, and heart failure (negative inotropic effect)
- Intrathecal delivery in patients with contraindications to invasive neuromodulation

Dose

- Oral administration:
  - Usually high doses are required for analgesia
  - Normally started at 5 mg 2–3 times daily
  - Usual daily dose: 5–10 mg three times daily
  - Maximum daily dose: 120 mg
  - Children: 0.3 mg/kg/day
  - Reduced doses in renal impairment
- Intrathecal administration (see 20.8 Intrathecal drug delivery systems, p. 384):
  - Only used in selective cases of severe neuropathic/nociceptive chronic painful spasticity refractory to oral antispastic drugs and conservative treatments

- Trial of intrathecal baclofen should be done before implanting an external or internal intrathecal pump system. Some institutions perform 2-3 diagnostic blocks 24 hours apart of a single shot baclofen intrathecal administration 25mcg, 50mcg and 75-100mcg in a monitored health care setting. Test dose is performed to assess effectiveness, adverse effects and determine the starting dose of baclofen if a pump is inserted
- Tolerance/tachyphylaxis occurs in a fifth of patients
- Doses of above 1 mg daily are normally not recommended

Mode of action

- Depression of monosynaptic and polysynaptic reflex transmission by stimulating $GABA_B$ receptors. Secondary effect may be inhibition of glutamate and aspartate

Monitoring

- Careful adjustment is often necessary to meet the requirements of each individual patient
- Elevated aspartate aminotransferase, alkaline phosphatase, and glucose have been recorded. These should be monitored in patients with liver disease or diabetes mellitus

Side effects

- Very common: sedation, somnolence, nausea
- Common: dry mouth, respiratory depression, light-headedness, confusion, dizziness, headache, insomnia, depression, euphoric mood, myalgia, ataxia, tremor, nystagmus, hallucination, nightmare, visual impairment, GI disorder, rash
- Rare: abdominal pain, abnormal LFTs, dysarthria, erectile dysfunction, paraesthesiae, taste disturbances, urinary retention

Relevant pharmacokinetics

- Absorption: rapidly and completely absorbed after oral administration. Peak plasma concentrations 0.5–1.5 hours after oral administration
- Distribution: active substance concentrations are approximately 8.5 times lower in the CSF than in the plasma
- Metabolism: minimal. Deamination yields a pharmacologically inactive metabolite
- Excretion: plasma elimination t1/2 is 3–4 hours. Excreted largely unchanged in the urine
- Renal impairment: dosage adjustment is required
- Hepatic impairment: no change in dose required

Relevant pharmacodynamics

- CNS depressant properties and anti-nociceptive effects
- Increased gastric acid secretion

Interactions

- Antidepressants: pronounced muscular hypotonia
- Antihypertensives: marked hypotension
- CNS depressants: increased sedation and risk of respiratory depression
- Lithium: aggravated hyperkinetic symptoms
- Levodopa/dopa decarboxylase inhibitors: confusion, hallucinations, agitation, worsening symptoms of parkinsonism
- Opioids: enhanced CNS and respiratory depressant effects of opioids

Special circumstances

- Pregnancy: crosses the placental barrier and should be avoided
- Breastfeeding: quantities of active substance passing into breast milk are unlikely to cause undesirable effects in infants
- Children: can be used for pain from muscular spasticity of cerebral origin or secondary to spinal cord diseases of infectious, degenerative, traumatic, neoplastic, or unknown origin
- Driving: patients experiencing adverse reactions such as dizziness, somnolence, and visual impairment should be advised to refrain from driving or operating machinery

Additional information

- Patient selection: it is likely to be of most benefit in patients whose spasticity constitutes a severe handicap to their activities
- Abrupt withdrawal can cause:
  - Confusion, delirium, hallucination, psychosis, dyskinesia, tachycardia, hyperthermia
  - Serotonin syndrome
  - Temporary aggravation of spasticity
  - Can be life-threatening in patients on high doses (mainly patients on intrathecal baclofen pumps)
- Overdose can present with somnolence, respiratory depression, seizures, hypotonia, autonomic instability, and bradycardia
- Excipients: baclofen tablets contain lactose
- Alternative medications with antispasmodic properties that can be considered include botulinum toxin, dantrolene, NSAIDs, BZDs, topiramate, gabapentin/pregabalin, and tizanidine

Cost

- 10 mg (84 tablets): £1.64
- Oral solution 5 mg/5 mL for 300 mL bottle: £4.72

Further reading

1. British National Formulary. Baclofen. https://bnf.nice.org.uk/drug/baclofen.html
2. NHS Commissioning Board Clinical Reference Group for Neurosciences. Clinical commissioning policy: intrathecal baclofen (ITB). 2013. https://www.england.nhs.uk/wp-content/uploads/2013/04/d04-p-c.pdf
3. Electronic Medicines Compendium. Baclofen tablets 10mg. https://www.medicines.org.uk/emc/product/2594/smpc

13.2 Bisphosphonates

Introduction, class of drugs

- Bisphosphonates are commonly prescribed for the prevention and treatment of a range of skeletal conditions where there exists an imbalance between bone formation and bone resorption
- Bisphosphonates are chemically stable derivatives of inorganic pyrophosphate, a naturally occurring compound in which two phosphate groups are linked by esterification
- Generally, they are available in generic names.

Table 13.2.1 Classification of bisphosphonates

Bisphosphonates	Examples	Relative potencies for osteoclast inhibition
First generation	Etidronate	1
	Tiludronic acid	10
Second generation	Pamidronate	100
	Alendronic acid	500
	Ibandronic acid	1000
Third generation	Risedronate	2000
	Zoledronic acid	10 000

- Pamidronate is an amino-bisphosphonate, available in 3 mg/mL, 9 mg/mL, and 15 mg/mL concentrations.

(See Table 13.2.1.)

They can also be divided into non-nitrogen-containing (earlier generation) and nitrogen-containing (newer generation which are more potent).

Indications

- Primary agents in the management of conditions associated with osteoclast-mediated bone loss due to osteoporosis, Paget's disease of bone, bony metastasis, multiple myeloma, and hypercalcaemia of pregnancy
- Also used in the treatment of heritable skeletal disorders in children and postmenopausal and GC- and transplant-induced osteoporosis
- In chronic pain, pamidronate is used for the management of early CRPS

Contraindications

- Previous hypersensitive reactions to other bisphosphonates and mannitol
- Cautioned in patients with elderly with cardiac disease, previous thyroid surgery, patients at risk of hypocalcaemia—may precipitate symptomatic hypocalcemia including tetany and renal impairment

Routes of administration and dosing

- Bisphosphonates can be administered by either oral or parenteral route
- Parenteral route can be considered for use in patients with contraindications to oral bisphosphonates (e.g. oesophageal disease, inability to sit up right after an oral dose, expected poor adherence to oral route, failure to respond with oral agents). However, recent development of pharmacologically equivalent oral preparations, allowing either once-weekly or once-monthly administration, has improved patient compliance

Osteoporosis

1. Alendronic acid 10 mg daily or 70 mg once weekly
2. Risedronate 5 mg once daily; alternately 35 mg once weekly

Early CRPS

- Patients with suspected/established CRPS (especially in the first 6 months of presentation) may benefit from a single dose of pamidronate 60 mg by IV administration

Mechanism of action

- The main mechanism is inhibition of bone resorption
- Bisphosphonates have a very high affinity for mineralized bone, like their natural analogue pyrophosphate. Bisphosphonates strongly adsorb to hydroxyapatite (calcium phosphate) crystals in bone, which may reduce bony dissolution
- They also inhibit osteoclast activity
- Bisphosphonates also function to limit both osteoblast and osteoclast apoptosis

Monitoring

- Assessment of renal function plays an important role. Regular checking of serum electrolytes, Ca^{2+}, and phosphates are needed, as electrolyte imbalance can cause convulsions in vulnerable patients
- Dental examination is advisable prior to initiation of treatment in vulnerable patients

Adverse effects

- Hypertension, injection site reaction, alopecia, loss of appetite, anaemia, arthralgia, constipation, diarrhoea, influenza-like illness, malaise, anaphylactic reaction, and bronchospasm

Specific risks

- Arthralgia
- Osteonecrosis of the jaw: can occur predominantly in cancer patients receiving chemotherapy or corticosteroids and with certain pre-existing dental conditions (periodontal disease, poorly fitting dentures, or local trauma). Dental examination is recommended prior to treatment
- Atypical femur fracture: often bilateral fractures with minimal or no trauma were reported. This risk increases in patients taking GCs
- Potential increased risk of atrial fibrillation (more studies are warranted)

Pharmacodynamics and kinetics

- Bisphosphonates are poorly absorbed through the GI tract
- The oral bioavailability of alendronate, risedronate, and ibandronate ranges from 0.6% to 1%
- The oral dosing of bisphosphonates requires consumption on an empty stomach, with advice for no food intake for nearly 60 minutes
- The skeleton takes up 50% of the absorbed drug, with the remainder excreted unchanged by the renal route
- Pamidronate is not metabolized in the human body; its elimination $t1/2$ is 28 hours ± 7 hours, and the renal route is the main route of excretion. Avoid if the GFR is <30 mL/min/1.73 m^2. No dose adjustment is necessary in mild to moderate hepatic impairment

Special circumstances

- Avoid in pregnancy (may cause fetal effects) and in breastfeeding

Cost

- Pamidronate disodium 60 mg/20 mL solution: £110

Further reading

1. Cremers S, Drake MT, Ebetino FH, et al. Pharmacology of bisphosphonates. Br J Clin Pharmacol 2019;85:1052–62
2. Giusti A, Bianchi G. Treatment of complex regional pain syndrome type 1 with bisphosphonates. RMD Open 2015;1:e000056.
3. Joint Formulary Committee. British National Formulary. London: 2020. BMJ Group and Pharmaceutical Press. https://www.bnf.org

13.3 Botulinum toxin

Class of drug and brand names

- Botulinum toxin type A (BTX-A): Azzalure® (Galderma), Bocouture® (Merz), Botox® (Allergan), Dysport® (Ipsen), Xeomin® (Merz)
- Botulinum toxin type B (BTX-B): Neurobloc® (Eisai)

Indications

- Licensed for use in overactive bladder, urinary incontinence from detrusor overactivity, prophylaxis of chronic migraine, spasticity in cervical dystonia, axillary hyperhidrosis, blepharospasm associated with dystonia, and strabismus (children)
- Unlicensed for use in prophylaxis of episodic migraine, upper or lower limb spasticity in children, trigeminal neuralgia, neuropathic pain, and myofascial pain

Contraindications

- Hypersensitivity to botulinum toxin or components in the formulation
- Infection
- Urinary tract infection or retention when used for intradetrusor injections

Caution

- Risk of respiratory failure and/or swallowing difficulties from muscular paralysis in patients
- Bronchitis and upper respiratory tract infections with Botox® injections for upper limb spasticity
- Compromised respiratory/bulbar function with parotid/neck muscle injections
- Neuromuscular disorders

Dose

- Maximal cumulative dose should not exceed 400 units in a 3-month interval
- Individual doses injected vary per muscle group and indication for injection

Mode of action

- Blocks the release of ACh from cholinergic neurons at the NMJ, autonomic ganglia, post-ganglionic parasympathetic nerve terminals, and sympathetic nerve endings that release ACh
- Inhibits the release of GABA, noradrenaline, and glutamate in the brain and spinal cord
- Central and peripheral actions on sensory nerves:
  - Inhibits CGRP and SP production at the DRG
  - Inhibits the release of pro-inflammatory and nociceptive NTs in the peripheral nervous system and dorsal horn

    - Attenuates neuroinflammation and central sensitization

Relevant pharmacokinetics/pharmacodynamics

- Local effects from IM Botulinum injections—produce transient flaccid paralysis
- Onset of action is 24–72 hours
- Peak effect at 5–7 days
- Duration of action for 8–12 weeks

Side effects

- Common adverse reactions (≥5%) from injections in the following conditions:
    - Overactive bladder/detrusor instability: urinary tract infection, dysuria, urinary retention
    - Chronic migraine: neck pain, headache
    - Spasticity: pain in extremity
    - Cervical dystonia: dysphagia, upper respiratory tract infection, neck pain, headache, increased cough, flu syndrome, back pain, rhinitis
    - Axillary hyperhidrosis: injection site pain and haemorrhage, non-axillary sweating, pharyngitis, flu syndrome

Interactions

- Potentiated effect of Botulinum when used with aminoglycosides, neuromuscular blockers/muscle relaxants, Mg^{2+}

Special circumstances

- Pregnancy: may cause fetal harm
- Breastfeeding: avoid; low risk of systemic absorption
- Children: safety and efficacy only established in patients <16 years old for treating cervical dystonia, and in those <12 years old for treating blepharospasm and strabismus

Cost

- Xeomin® and Bocouture®, 50-unit vial: £72
- Allergan® 300-unit vial: £276

Further reading

1. Joint Formulary Committee. Botulinum toxin type A. British National Formulary (online). London: BMJ Group and Pharmaceutical Press
2. Oh HM, Chung ME. Botulinum toxin for neuropathic pain: a review of the literature. Toxins (Basel) 2015;7(8):3127–54

13.4 Calcitonin

Introduction

- Calcitonin is a polypeptide hormone secreted by the parafollicular cells of the thyroid gland, with a primary role in Ca^{2+} homeostasis
- Evidence of calcitonin for pain management is controversial and mostly from small studies

Indications

- Disorders of bone metabolism: osteoporosis, Paget's disease, hypercalcaemia of malignancy, and prevention of acute bone loss due to sudden immobilization (e.g. after a fracture)
- Phantom limb pain: effective in acute phantom limb pain (<7 days post-amputation), but not in the chronic setting
- Acute pain from osteoporotic vertebral fractures and bony metastases
- Refractory neuropathic pain

Contraindications

- Hypocalcaemia
- Caution in heart failure as can reduce cardiac output

Dosage

- Preparations: salmon calcitonin (IV, IM, SC, and intranasal preparations) and intranasal preparations of calcitonin
- Hypercalcaemia and prevention of acute bone loss due to sudden immobilization: 100 units in single or divided doses (less than daily dose of 400 units) SC or IV
- Phantom limb pain: 200 units SC or IV in 100 mL of normal saline for 3 days
- Children 5–10 units/kg IV in normal saline administered over 6 hours
- Treatment limited to the shortest possible time to minimize the risk of malignancy. Poor-quality evidence suggests an association between calcitonin and cancer development

Mode of action

- Mechanism of action in pain relief is unclear. Some hypotheses include:
  - Inhibition of osteoclastic bone resorption, altering both the number and/or the resorptive activity of osteoclasts
  - Binding to calcitonin receptors on serotonergic neurons in the thalamus, PAG matter, and raphe nucleus, targeting the descending inhibitory pain pathways
  - Normalization of Na^+ channel expression on damaged peripheral nerves
  - Reduced production of cytokines and inflammatory PGs peripherally
  - Potential binding to opioid receptors (kappa or delta) and release of endogenous β-endorphins

Pharmacokinetics

- Bioavailability: 65–70%, normally given IV, SC, or IM
- Terminal t1/2: approximately 60 minutes following IM or SC administration
- Apparent Vd: 0.15–0.3 L/kg
- Metabolism: mostly to inactive metabolites in the kidney, blood, and peripheral tissues

Interactions

- Reduces the concentration of lithium

Special circumstances

- Believed to be safe in pregnancy: does not cross the placental barrier. However, assess on an individual case basis and consider risk versus benefit for both mother and fetus. Contact your local department of medicines information for advice

- Not established if safe during lactation and in children. Human data lacking, but excretion into milk not expected as calcitonin has a high molecular weight. Calcitonin has been shown to inhibit lactation in animals

Adverse effects

- Can lead to hypocalcaemic tetany if the patient was hypocalcaemic before administration
- Common: nausea, vomiting, facial flushing, diarrhoea, thrombophlebitis, headaches, drowsiness. Antiemetics are commonly given pre-emptively to prevent nausea and vomiting
- Cancer: the Committee for Medicinal Products for Human Use found that a higher proportion of patients treated with calcitonin for long periods of time develop cancer of various types, compared with patients taking placebo. The increase in cancer rates ranged from 0.7% (oral formulation) to 2.4% (nasal formulation). The studies have poor-quality cancer assessment methodology and calcitonin continues to have a licence for its clinical use

Cost

- Injectable solution: five ampoules (50 units/mL): £167
- Injectable solution: five ampoules (100 units/mL): £220
- Injectable solution: five ampoules (400 units/mL): £352

Further reading

1. Martinez-Zapata MJ, Roqué i Figuls M, Català E, et al. Calcitonin for metastatic bone pain. Cochrane Database Syst Rev 2006;3:CD003223
2. Schug SA, Palmer GM, Scott DA, et al. Acute Pain Management: Scientific Evidence. 4th edition, 2015. Melbourne: Australian and New Zealand College of Anaesthetists and Faculty of Pain Medicine

13.5 Cannabis

Introduction

- Natural cannabis products are illegal in most countries worldwide
- The prevalence of cannabis use in patients attending chronic pain clinics is approximately 12–15%
- Compounds are derived from *Cannabis sativa*, *Cannabis ruderalis*, and *Cannabis indica* species
- Natural preparations contain over 100 metabolically active compounds, including:
  - THC
  - CBD
  - Cannabinol (CBN)
  - Cannabigerol (CBG)
  - Tetrahydrocannabivarin (THCV)
  - Non-cannabinoid compounds

Indications

- The evidence to support the efficacy, tolerability, and safety profile of cannabinoids in the treatment of acute and chronic pain is currently limited

- Nonetheless, cannabinoids may be considered in highly selected patients after failure of multiple pharmacological and non-pharmacological therapies for the following conditions:
  - CNCP: neuropathic pain or spasticity-related pain in MS
  - Chemotherapy-induced nausea and vomiting (CINV)
  - Palliative care: appetite stimulation, weight gain, antiemesis, analgesia
  - Paediatric epilepsy
  - Other conditions in which it has been used: Parkinson's disease, anxiety disorder, fibromyalgia, PTSD, sleep disorders, Tourette's syndrome

Analgesic efficacy

- A meta-analysis (including 104 studies, 47 RCTs, and 9958 participants) on the effectiveness of cannabinoids in CNCP of mixed aetiology showed:
  - NNT for 30% pain reduction: 24 (95% CI 15–61)
  - NNH: 6 (95% CI 5–8)
  - No significant impacts on physical or emotional functioning; low-quality evidence of improved sleep and patient global impression of change
- Currently no strong support for use in CNCP, due to lack of robust evidence

Cannabis-based medications and licensed indications

- Natural cannabis products:
  - Nabiximols (Sativex®): THC:CBD ratio 1:1—MS and intractable cancer pain
  - Whole plant extract (Cannador®): plant-based, THC:CBD ratio 2:1—no licensed indications
- Synthetic preparations:
  - Nabilone (Cesamet®, Canemes®): synthetic THC—CINV
  - Rimonabant (Acomplia®): CB1 receptor inverse agonist and mu opioid receptor antagonist—licensed for obesity and smoking cessation. Withdrawn in Europe in 2008 due to mental health adverse effects
  - Dronabinol (Marinol®): synthetic THC—CINV
  - Synthetic CBD (Subsys®): synthetic CBD—intractable cancer pain

Mechanism of action

- Endocannabinoid system agonism implicated for analgesia in inflammatory and neuropathic pain states
- Anandamide and *2-arachidonoylglycerol* are the two major endocannabinoids derived from membrane phospholipids
- Cannabinoids bind to cannabinoid GPCRs, causing membrane hyperpolarization and inhibition of NT release. Main features of the endocannabinoid system include:
  - Cannabinoid receptor type 1:
    - Mainly CNS (PAG, RVM, thalamus), but also peripheral neuronal tissues at pre-synaptic sympathetic nerves
    - Involved in modulation of the NTs ACh, dopamine, GABA, D-aspartate, cholecystokinin, glutamate, serotonin, and noradrenaline
    - Involved in pain perception, movement, brain reward/addiction, mood, and cognition systems
  - Cannabinoid receptor type 2:
    - Mainly in the peripheral immune system (macrophages, lymphocytes, natural killer cells, mast cells), but also in glial cells of the CNS
    - Inhibition of release of pro-inflammatory cytokines and movement of immune cells

- Cannabinoid system also modulates:
  - Ascending nociceptive and descending anti-nociceptive pathways in the spinal cord and higher relay centres
  - Afferent sensitization in the peripheral nervous system

Routes of administration and dosing

- PO, sublingual, inhaled, topical
- Titration period followed by maintenance therapy
- Nabiximols (Sativex®): oro-mucosal spray containing THC 2.7 mg and CBD 2.5 mg per 100 microlitres spray (maximum 16 doses daily)
- Whole plant extract (Cannador®): THC 2.5 g and CBD 1.2 mg per oral capsule
- Dronabinol (Marinol®): 2.5/5/10 mg oral capsule. Maximum dose 20 mg daily
- Nabilone (Cesamet®): 0.25/0.5/1 mg oral capsule. Maximum dose 6 mg daily

Pharmacokinetics

- Absorption:
  - Depends on route and highly variable between patients
  - Inhaled (smoking, vaporizers): rapid onset of action, bioavailability of around 18%, levels falling within 2 hours, inaccurate dosing
  - Oral: poor absorption, low bioavailability, difficult to titrate
  - Sublingual: Sativex® (spay) achieves peak plasma levels in 45–120 minutes
- Distribution: highly lipophilic, high protein binding, accumulates in fatty tissues
- Metabolism: THC and CBD are metabolized by CYP450 enzymes
- Excretion: faeces (majority) and renal. Long elimination t1/2 of 24–36 hours due to high lipid solubility

Pharmacodynamics

- Nervous system: psychoactive properties (THC as primary psychoactive component), sedation, anxiolysis, analgesia
- GI: appetite stimulant, antiemetic
- Immunological: inflammatory cytokine inhibitor

Contraindications

- Unstable ischaemic heart disease (IHD) or arrhythmias
- Severe renal or hepatic disease
- Active mental health disorder, especially psychosis, family history of psychosis, history or risk of aberrant drug behaviour
- Co-administered sedatives, including alcohol

Adverse effects

- Low acute toxicity in commercially prepared drugs. The higher the frequency, dose, and duration of use, the more likely adverse effects
- Nervous system: dizziness, sedation, dry mouth, dysphoria, impaired cognition and memory
- Use in younger age (<25 years old) associated with:
  - Reduction in frontal and parietal brain lobe volumes
  - Poorer educational achievements, lower IQ
  - Precipitation of the onset of mental health disorders, poorer treatment compliance, and increased hospitalization rates and risk of self-harm

- Cardiovascular: hypo- and hypertension, tachy- and bradycardia
- Respiratory: if smoked, associated effects of additional compounds of tobacco
- Endocrine: lowers testosterone levels and quality/number of sperm
- Mental health: hallucinations, psychosis, depression, anxiety, mania, self-harm, strong relationship between schizophrenia and cannabis use
- Drug and alcohol: cannabis dependence syndrome (10%)

Interactions

- Inhibition of cytochrome P450 isoenzymes, including CYP2D6 and CYP3A4

Further reading

1. Mücke M, Phillips T, Radbruch L, et al. Cannabis-based medicines for chronic neuropathic pain in adults. Cochrane Database Syst Rev 2018;3:CD012182
2. Raja S, Sommer C. Pain 2014 Refresher Courses. Treatment of neuropathic pain: opioids, cannabinoids, and topical agents. 15th World Congress on Pain, 2014. Seattle, WA: IASP Press
3. Stockings E, Campbell G, Hall W, et al. Cannabis and cannabinoids for the treatment of people with chronic noncancer pain conditions. Pain 2018;159(10):1932–54

13.6 Capsaicin

Class of drugs

- Extract from chilli peppers belonging to the *Solanaceae* family

Formulations and brand names (pricing)

- Zacin® 0.025% topical cream—250 mcg/g (45 g: £17.71)
- Axsain® 0.075% topical cream—750 mcg/g (45 g: £14.58)
- Qutenza® 8% patch—179 mg per patch (£210.00 per patch)

Pharmacodynamics—mechanism of action

Action of capsaicin on Transient Receptor Potential Vanilloid (TRPV)

- Receptor on C-fibres
- TRPV1 is a ligand-gated non-selective cation channel of the TRP family that could be activated by a variety of noxious stimuli
- Chronic exposure to capsaicin first stimulates, then desensitizes this channel to noxious stimuli, including capsaicin (tolerance develops with chronic use)

Local depletion of substance P

- As Substance P is depleted, there is inadequate chemical stimulus available to activate C-fibres

Pharmacokinetics

- Minimal systemic absorption from skin
- Can be excreted in breast milk if the 8% patch is used
- Can stimulate bradykinin release

Indications

- OA, PHN, painful diabetic neuropathy
- Qutenza® (8% patch) is licensed by the FDA only for PHN (the only other topical product licensed for PHN is 5% lidocaine plaster)
- Unlicensed use: back pain, painful diabetic neuropathy, some forms of refractory pruritus

Contraindications/cautions

- Broken skin, active ulceration (for both the patient and the individual applying the medication!)
- Avoid: contact with eyes, hot shower or bath just before or after application, inhalation of capsaicin vapour
- Not to be used under tight bandages
- Caution as capsaicin can increase cough, especially in patients on ACEIs (due to its agonist action on TRPV present in the respiratory tract)
- **Note: only wear nitrile gloves for application since latex does *not* provide protection from capsaicin!**
- Caution in patients with hypertension as capsaicin could accentuate hypertension, and rarely accentuate AV nodal block

Application of Qutenza® patches

- Qutenza® (8% patch) could be applied every 12 weeks—a single patch is applied for up to 30–60 minutes
- Prepare the affected area by mapping the painful area, then apply LA topically or use oral analgesic (e.g. tramadol 50–100 mg) to reduce the intense burning sensation
- Up to a maximum of four patches is recommended per application

Side effects

- Most common is severe skin burning (if not premedicated with adequate topical LA)—treated by short-acting opioids, and by application of ice to the affected area
- Nausea is rare, transient increase of blood pressure

Special circumstances

- Safe in patients with hepatic or renal impairment
- Not licensed for use in patients younger than 18 years
- Caution in breastfeeding women since capsaicin has been isolated from milk (in rats)

Additional information

- Use nitrile gloves for application of capsaicin
- Evaluate the patient for uncontrolled hypertension or chronic cough before considering capsaicin treatment (relative contraindication)
- Avoid contact with mucous membranes—wash hands thoroughly
- Disposal of unused patches and used products in biohazard dispensers as per local policy (could be an irritant to those who come into contact if disposed of in regular clinical waste)

Further reading

1. Joint Formulary Committee. British National Formulary. 2020. London: BMJ Group and Pharmaceutical Press. https://www.bnf.org
2. Smith HS, Pappagallo M, Stahl SM (eds). Essential Pain Pharmacology: The Prescriber's Guide. 1st edition, 2012. Cambridge: Cambridge University Press
3. Brunton LL, Hilal-Dandan R, Knollmann BC. Goodman & Gilman's The Pharmacological Basis of Therapeutics. 13th edition, 2017. New York, NY: McGraw-Hill

13.7 Clonazepam

Class of drugs

- Benzodiazepine (BZD)

Indications

- Epilepsy
- Myoclonus
- Panic disorder
- Movement disorder (akathisia)
- Insomnia
- Muscle spasticity
- Not recommended for treating neuropathic pain

Contraindications

- Respiratory depression and acute pulmonary insufficiency
- Marked neuromuscular respiratory weakness, including unstable myasthenia gravis
- Alcohol or recreational drug abuse

Dose

- Initial dose 1 mg daily for 3–4 days and increased according to response over 2–4 weeks, to a usual maintenance dose of 4–8 mg in 3–4 divided doses
- Children:
  - <1 year: initially 250 mcg, which can be increased to 0.5–1 mg daily
  - 1–5 years: initially 250 mcg, which can be increased to 1–3 mg daily
  - 5–12 years: initially 500 mcg, which can be increased to 3–6 mg
- Caution in hepatic and renal impairment
- Patients can develop coma due to increased cerebral sensitivity. Where necessary, BZDs with shorter t1/2 should be used
- Avoid long-term use due to its S/Es and contraindications

Mode of action

- Structurally a 1,4-BZD. Its primary mode of action is to facilitate GABAergic transmission in the brain by a direct effect on GABA receptors, by inhibiting firing of raphe cells which are located in the midbrain and pons

Side effects

- Common: respiratory depression, drowsiness, dizziness, cognitive impairment, headaches, sleep disturbances, slurred speech, dry mouth, constipation, and blurred vision. Can worsen depression
- Occasional: dysphoria and blood disorders
- Very rare: psychosis and suicidal ideations; although the mechanism underlying these risks is not known, available data do not exclude the possibility of increased risk either (therefore, the patient's mental state should be monitored)

Pharmacokinetics

- Absorption: oral bioavailability of 90%, with peak concentrations reached within 1–4 hours of oral administration
- Distribution: 85% protein-bound
- Metabolism: highly metabolized before undergoing acetylation, hydroxylation, and glucuronidation
- Excretion: <2% in the urine

Interactions

- Reduced plasma concentration when given with carbamazepine and phenytoin
- Increased risk of neurotoxicity when given with lithium
- Increased risk of S/Es when given with sodium valproate
- Increased sedative effects when given with TCAs, antipsychotics, opioids, or other sedatives

Special circumstances

- Special precaution in the elderly with the dose initiated at 500 mcg and titrated very cautiously to higher doses
- The safety profile in pregnancy is less clear. Some inconclusive data associate its intake during pregnancy with cardiac and facial malformations. If BZDs are necessary, chlordiazepoxide and diazepam may be safer options

Additional information

- Drowsiness caused by clonazepam may affect performance of skilled tasks (e.g. driving, use of machinery)
- Current limitations of point-of-care immunoassays suggest testing by mass spectrometry to ensure better accuracy
- Avoid long-term use to mitigate the risk of development of dependence and S/Es listed above

Cost

- Clonazepam 500 mcg (100 tablets): £31.67
- Clonazepam 2 mg (100 tablets): £34.33
- Monthly cost for 0.5–1 mg/day: £9.50–19

Further reading

1. Joint Formulary Committee. British National Formulary. 2020. London: BMJ Group and Pharmaceutical Press. https://www.bnf.org
2. Corrigan R, Derry S, Wiffen PJ, Moore RA. Clonazepam for neuropathic pain and fibromyalgia in adults. Cochrane Database Syst Rev 2012;5:CD009486.

13.8 Clonidine

Class of drugs

- Centrally acting α-2 adrenergic agonist which reduces sympathetic outflow

Indications

- Management of alcohol, opioid, and nicotine withdrawal symptoms
- Hot flushes and excessive sweating in menopause
- Migraine prophylaxis
- Prevention and management of anxiety and delirium (e.g. after surgery, critical ill patients etc.)
- Acute pain:
    - Not a first line agent in acute pain management due to associated S/Es and other agents are more effective for acute pain management
    - Effective adjunct to opioid-tolerant patients and in complex acute pain predominantly due to its anxiolytic effects
    - Neuraxial blockade (intrathecal, epidural): as an adjunct to LAs, clonidine improves the duration of analgesia, reduces systemic use of opioids, and prolongs the time needed until first-rescue analgesia
    - Peripheral regional blockade and perineural infusions: improves duration of action of analgesia and anaesthesia
    - Weak evidence to support the use of clonidine for intra-articular use (knee arthroscopy) and surgical site infiltration following mastectomy
- Chronic pain:
    - *Neuropathic pain:*
        - Diabetic neuropathy: topical clonidine may provide some benefit
        - At level of neuropathic pain in SCI: intrathecal clonidine and morphine have proven to be useful
        - Intractable cancer neuropathic pain: neuroaxial clonidine can be useful
    - CRPS: epidural or topical clonidine may provide pain relief in refractory cases
    - Pain from muscular spasticity: can reduce pain from muscle spasms
    - Chronic post-surgical pain—weak evidence demonstrates that epidural clonidine and steroid may improve pain relief and sleep in post-thoracotomy pain

Caution

- Avoid in patients with hypotension, bradycardia, sedation, or cognitive dysfunction, and those at risk of falls
- Severe renal impairment: reduce dosage

Dose

- PO 50–600 mcg in divided doses
- IV 50–300 mcg in divided doses
- Neuraxial 15–30 mcg

Mode of action

- Activates α-2 (pre-synaptic) receptors in the brain, DH of the spinal cord, DRG, and sensory neurons. It reduces noradrenaline release and sympathetic outflow at both central and peripheral adrenergic terminals, causing sedation, anxiolysis, reduction in anaesthetic requirement, and gastric motility

- Anti-nociceptive action:
  - DH of the spinal cord: reduces the release of noradrenaline and enhances the action of descending inhibitory pathways
  - Peripheral sensory neuron terminals: blocks adrenergic receptors (α-1, α-2) expressed on sensory neurons or on post-ganglionic sympathetic terminals following a nerve injury
  - Imidazoline receptor agonist: activation causes analgesia. These receptors are located in the brain, spinal cord, and peripheral nerve endings
  - Clonidine has the intrinsic ability to block C- and A-delta fibres
  - Causes local vasoconstriction and may prolong the duration of LAs

Side effects

- Common: hypotension, bradycardia, sedation, dry mouth, and rebound hypertension
- If used over a prolonged period, it may cause withdrawal symptoms if stopped abruptly

Pharmacokinetics

- Oral bioavailability: 75–95%
- Onset of action: 30–60 minutes; peak plasma levels: 1–3 hours
- Elimination t1/2: 6–26 hours
- Excretion: 60–65% excreted unchanged in the urine

Interactions

- Antiepileptics, alcohol, sedatives, and anxiolytics: potentiates sedative and depressant effects
- Digoxin: may worsen arrhythmias

Special circumstances

- Avoid in pregnancy and lactation: crosses the placental barrier, secreted in breast milk
- Avoid long-term use in children

Cost

- Oral 25 mcg, 112 tablets: £4
- Oral 100 mcg, 100 tablets: £8
- Oral 10 mcg/mL 100 mL bottle: £68

Further reading

1. Campbell CM, Kipnes MS, Stouch BC, et al. Randomized control trial of topical clonidine for treatment of painful diabetic neuropathy. Pain 2012;153:1815–23
2. Kumar A, Maitra S, Khanna P, et al. Clonidine for management of chronic pain: a brief review of the current evidences. Saudi J Anaesth 2014;8(1):92–6

13.9 Contrast agents

Introduction

- Contrast agents have been used in pain management practice to ensure correct positioning of the needle tip, to confirm the intended target, to identify intravascular uptake, and to distinguish between different anatomical structures
- This facilitates the deposition of diagnostic/therapeutic agents near the targeted area

Classification

(See Table 13.9.1.)

- Broadly, radiocontrast agents can be divided into either positive (these agents absorb X-ray to produce darker shadows of tissues in question) or negative (transparent to X-ray)
- *Positive* contrast agents are commonly used, as they are radio-opaque. They can also be divided into iodinated and non-iodinated agents (gadolinium-based)
- Iodinated agents are commonly used and they are divided into ionic and non-ionic agents, based on water solubility and charge of the iodinated molecule. They can be monomers or dimers (based on molecular structure) and can also be classified based on osmolality

- Omnipaque™ 240 contains 240 mg/mL of organic iodine
- Omnipaque™ 300 contains 300 mg/mL of organic iodine
- Niopam® 200 contains 200 mg/mL of organic iodine

Indications

- Intravascular: digital subtraction angiography (DSA), CT angiography
- Intrathecal: myelography
- Others: discogram, epiduroscopy, arthrography, nerve root/ganglion/plexus identification
- Enteral: GI problems

Contraindications

- Known allergy to contrast agents or allergy to iodine

Dose

- Varies depending on the procedure (from a few mL to a few hundred mL)
- Use the lowest dose possible. For simple pain interventions, usually 1–3 mL of contrast is sufficient

Mechanism of action

- Iodine is responsible for causing radio-opacity in iodinated contrast agents and it outlines the structures better when there exists a density difference between the structures

Table 13.9.1 Types of radiocontrast agents

Iodinated	Ionic (charged particles)	Non-ionic
Monomer	Osmolality—high Viscosity—low Examples: diatrizoate (Uorgrafin®), iothalamate (Conray®)	Osmolality—low to intermediate Viscosity—intermediate Iohexol (Omnipaque™) Iopamidol (Niopam®) Both licensed for intrathecal use as non-ionic Commonly used in pain interventions
Dimer	Osmolality—intermediate Viscosity—intermediate Example: ioxaglate (Hexabrix®)	Osmolality—low Viscosity—highest Example: iotrolan (Isovist®)

Relevant pharmacokinetics/pharmacodynamics

- Contrast agents share a tri-iodinated benzene ring structure
- The t1/2 of redistribution of the intravascular compartment is between 2 and 5 minutes and equivalent to that of the extracellular fluid. Contrast agents are carried free in plasma
- Serum protein binding is <5%
- There is no evidence of biotransformation of these agents and elimination is almost entirely through the kidneys

Adverse reactions

- Idiosyncratic anaphylactoid—self-limiting minor adverse events, such as pain and rash, to life-threatening reactions
- Dose-dependent reactions—cardiac S/Es, seizures, nephropathy. Uncommon with simple pain interventions if non-vascular injections and small doses used
- Higher risk of adverse effects with high osmolar and ionic agents

Risk factors for adverse reactions

- History of previous reaction, allergy, asthma, dehydration, pre-existing renal disease, sickle cell anaemia, polycythaemia, myeloma, and use of NSAIDs

Interactions

- Contrast agents themselves do not directly interact with other agents. However, caution must be exercised with Omnipaque™ in patients with a history of epilepsy, renal disease, chronic alcoholism, and MS
- Niopam can affect iodine uptake by thyroid tissue more than Omnipaque™ can, and should be used cautiously in hyperthyroid patients

Special circumstances

- There are no studies on use of Omnipaque™ in pregnant women. It is advisable to supplement breastfeeding with bottle feeding following Omnipaque™ use for 24 hours, as contrast agents are excreted unchanged in breast milk

Additional information

- Drugs which lower the seizure threshold, especially phenothiazine-based antihistamines and antiemetics, are not recommended to be used along with Omnipaque™
- Contrast agents are nearly twice more viscous at 20°C than at body temperature
- Warming the contrast agents can offer better flow rates in angiography as viscosity decreases

Further reading

1. Beckett KR, Moriarity AK, Langer JM. Safe use of contrast media: What the radiologist needs to know. RadioGraphics 2015 35:6:1738–1750
2. Rathmell, James P. Radiographic contrast agents. In: Rathmell JP (ed). Atlas of Image-Guided Intervention in Regional Anesthesia and Pain Medicine. 2006; pp. 16–22. Philadelphia, PA: Lippincott Williams and Wilkins

13.10 Hyaluronidase

Class of drugs

- Enzyme used to render tissues more readily permeable to injected fluids

Indications—licensed uses

- Enhances permeation of SC or IM injections
- Enhances permeation of LAs
- Enhances permeation of ophthalmic LAs
- Hypodermoclysis (introduction of fluids by SC infusion)
- Extravasation: infiltrate as soon as possible into the affected area
- Haematoma: infiltrate into the affected area

Contraindications

- Avoid sites where infection/malignancy present
- Corneal application, IV administration
- In anaesthesia in premature labour
- To enhance absorption and dispersion of dopamine and/or adrenoceptor agonists
- To reduce swelling of bites/stings

Caution

- Elderly: control speed and total volume; of administration avoid overhydration, especially in renal impairment

Dose

- SC/IM/local infiltration: 1500 units to be dissolved directly into the solution to be injected (check compatibility)
- Some use up to 3000 units per injection (for epidural adhesiolysis)
- To the eye: 15 units/mL mixed with LA solution for ophthalmic block
- Hypodermoclysis/extravasation/haematoma: dissolve 1500 units in 1 mL of water/0.9% saline

Mode of action

- Reversibly depolymerizes hyaluronic acid, a polysaccharide present in connective tissue, increasing tissue permeability
- Hyaluronidase as adjuvant to epidural steroid increases its efficacy and duration of action by reducing fibrosis and oedema in tissues and lysing the adhesions, thus facilitating the spread of the injected substance

Monitoring of treatment

- No additional monitoring required beyond that in place for procedure

Side effects

- Common: oedema
- Rare: bleeding, bruising, infection, local irritation
- Frequency not known: anaphylaxis, severe allergy

Interactions

- With aspirin or dexamethasone (larger amounts of hyaluronidase may be required)

Special circumstances

- Pregnancy: caution
- Breastfeeding: caution

Additional information

- Store refrigerated at 2–8°C

Cost

- Hyaluronidase 1500-unit powder for injection: £13.65/ampoule

Further reading

1. Joint Formulary Committee. British National Formulary. 2020. London: BMJ Group and Pharmaceutical Press. https://www.bnf.org
2. Yentis S, Hirsch N, Smith G. Anaesthesia and Intensive Care A–Z. 6th edition, 2018. Edinburgh: Elsevier
3. Menzel EJ, Farr C. Hyaluronidase and its substrate hyaluronan: biochemistry, biological activities and therapeutic uses. Cancer Lett 1998;131:3–11

13.11 Ketamine

Class of drugs

- Ketamine is a water-soluble aryl-cyclo-alkylamine and is structurally related to cyclidines

Indications

- Anaesthetic induction agent, especially suitable for patients who are cardiovascularly unstable
- Sole anaesthetic agent for short procedures such as burns dressing
- Potent perioperative analgesic at sub-anaesthetic doses
- Opioid-sparing effect
- As third-line agent in resistant pain conditions, particularly with a neuropathic component (CRPS type 1, PHN, orofacial pain, and phantom limb pain)
- Third-line drug in opioid- and adjunct-resistant cancer pain
- New evidence emerging on its role as an antidepressant

Contraindications

- Malignant hypertension, certain heart conditions, raised ICP, eclampsia, psychiatric conditions

Routes of administration

- IV, IM, PO, nasal, rectal, and intrathecal routes

Dose

- *Anaesthetic:* 1.5–2 mg/kg IV; 10 mg/kg IM with onset time 2–8 minutes
- *Acute pain:* 0.1–0.5 mg/kg IV bolus dose and 0.05–0.2 mg/kg/hour continued as IV infusion
- *Chronic pain:* 10–40 mg four times daily PO, titrate according to individual. Ketamine infusion can be done for neuropathic pain as a day case procedure at 0.15–0.3 mg/kg over 30 minutes
- *Cancer:* racemic ketamine 1 mg/kg/day or S (+) ketamine (0.5–2 mg/kg/24 hours) infusion up to 600 mg/day as an IV infusion, 67.2 mg/day via intrathecal route
- *Palliative:* PO doses of 50–100 mg four times daily have been used

Mechanism of action

- Primarily acts as non-competitive antagonist at NMDA receptor Ca^{2+} channel pore which can counteract wind-up or central sensitization
- Agonist at α and β adrenergic receptors
- Antagonistic effect at CNS muscarinic receptors

Monitoring

- Repeated ketamine administration may require careful liver enzyme monitoring

Adverse effects

- CNS: drowsiness, nausea and vomiting, visual/auditory hallucinations, paranoid effects, anxiety, and euphoria
- CVS: direct negative inotropic effect (high-dose infusion) and indirect stimulatory effect (low-dose infusion). Ketamine causes tachycardia, increases systemic and pulmonary hypertension, and increases cardiac output and myocardial oxygen consumption
- Hepatic: reversible hepatic enzyme elevation
- Renal: both upper and lower renal tract symptoms may occur. Ketamine-induced uropathy includes complex changes in the bladder and upper urinary tract changes. Regular and prolonged use of high doses may lead to cystitis (limit dose to <160 mg/day)
- GI tract: causes upper GI symptoms, including nausea, GI bleeding, and anaemia

Relevant pharmacodynamics/pharmacokinetics

- Ketamine molecule is freely water-soluble, with a molecular weight of 238 g/mol. Its pKa is 7.5
- It is formulated as a slightly acidic aqueous solution (pH 3.5–5.5)
- Ketalar® is a racemic mixture of equal proportions of two enantiomers
- The active S (+) enantiomer is stronger than both racemic (twice) and R (−) enantiomer (four times)
- Due to high lipid solubility, it has extensive distribution. Vd ranges from 1.5 to 3.2 L/kg. It has low protein binding between 10% and 30%
- High lipid solubility and low plasma binding facilitate rapid transfer across the BBB
- Extensive first-pass metabolism, hence poor oral bioavailability of 15%—the predominant route of metabolism is via the liver involving N-demethylation and producing norketamine. Norketamine has nearly one-third the anaesthetic potency, as well as analgesic properties
- Conjugated metabolites are excreted mainly via the renal route

Interactions

- Ketamine and norketamine are metabolized by the CYP450 family
- Opioids, alcohol, sedatives, anxiolytics potentiate the depressant effects

Special circumstances

- Ketamine in sub-anaesthetic doses may adversely affect pregnancy outcomes (based on animal studies)

Additional information

- Oral ketamine has limited shelf life. Controlled drug; although inexpensive, ketamine prescription is resource-intensive and needs regular monitoring and repeat prescriptions
- Potential for drug abuse, so avoid in vulnerable patients

Cost

- Ketamine for injection—200 mg/20 mL one vial: £5 (£50 for ten vials)
- Ketamine for injection—500 mg/10 mL one vial: £8.80 (£70 for ten vials)

Further reading

1. Zanos P, Moaddel R, Morris PJ, et al. Ketamine and ketamine metabolite pharmacology: insights into therapeutic mechanisms. Pharmacol Rev 2018;70(3):621–62
2. Expert Committee on Drug Dependence. Ketamine—update review report. 2014. Geneva: World Health Organization

13.12 Methocarbamol

Introduction

- Central muscle relaxant indicated for treating skeletal muscle spasms
- Alternative to baclofen/diazepam in pain medicine

Mechanism of action

- Unclear, but may cause inhibition of carbonic anhydrase and CNS depression. It may decrease nerve transmission at the spinal and supraspinal levels and also prolong the refractory period of muscle cells

Dose

- Initial dosage: 1500 mg four times daily, initially for 2–3 days, Maintenance: PO 750 mg 4-hourly, and then 1500 mg three times daily or 1000 mg four times daily. Maximum: 4 g/day
- Each tablet contains 750 mg and the injectable solution has 100 mg/mL
- Methods of administration: PO/IV/IM

Uses

Skeletal muscle spasm associated with acute musculoskeletal pain

- Parenteral: 1 g IV/IM; additional doses three times daily; not to exceed 3 g/day

- Enteral dose: 1500 mg PO four times daily for 48–72 hours; no more than 8 g/day and reduce to 4–4.5 g/day in divided doses

Tetanus

- Adjunct therapy: initially 1–2 g IV injection (at 300 mg/min), up to a total dose of 3 g; may repeat 1–2 g IV 6-hourly until PO tolerated; total 24 g PO
- IM administration: not to exceed 500 mg (5 mL undiluted)

Pharmacokinetics

- Rapidly absorbed PO, with high therapeutic index
- Onset 30 minutes; peak serum levels 1–2 hours; peak plasma concentration: 16–30 mcg/mL
- Protein binding: 46–50%
- Metabolism: conjugation, dealkylation, and hydroxylation
- Metabolites: glucuronide and sulphate conjugates of 3-(2-hydroxyphenoxy)-1,2-propanediol-1-carbamate and 3-(4-hydroxy-2-methoxyphenoxy)-1,2-propanediol-1-carbamate
- Elimination t1/2: 0.9–1.8 hours

Duration of treatment

- Depends on symptoms but should not exceed 30 days

Side effects

- Common: dizziness, headache, light-headedness, mild sedation
- Nausea and vomiting, dyspepsia, metallic taste, jaundice
- Rare: fever, angio-oedema, hypersensitive reactions, conjunctivitis, nasal congestion, flushing, bradycardia, syncope
- *Very rare:* blurred vision, drowsiness, tremor, convulsion, restlessness, anxiety, confusion, anorexia, leucopenia, anaphylaxis

Contraindications

- Hypersensitivity, coma or pre-coma states, brain injury or epilepsy
- Myasthenia gravis

Interactions

- May potentiate CNS depressant effects with opioids, BZDs, antihistamines, antipsychotics (clozapine), and antidepressants (mirtazapine)

Caution

- In renal impairment, **avoid parenteral** form due to the presence of PEG
- May change the colour of urine to brown, black, or green
- Drivers and machine operators to be warned as CNS depressant
- Drug overdose—seizures, coma, and fatality with supportive treatment
- Abuse potential is less

Special circumstances

- Pregnancy—Category C (use only if benefits outweigh risks)
- Lactation: unknown if it is excreted in breast milk

- Elderly—halve the dose
- Hepatic impairment—t1/2 elimination is prolonged; hence, increase the dosing interval
- Children—safety and efficacy not been established

Additional information

- In the emergency department, patients with acute, non-traumatic, non-radicular low back pain, combining naproxen with methocarbamol did not improve functional outcomes, compared with naproxen + placebo

Cost

- 750 mg 100 tablets: £12.65 (monthly cost for 1.5–4 g/day: approximately £7–25)

Further reading

1. Joint Formulary Committee. British National Formulary. 2020. London: BMJ Group and Pharmaceutical Press. https://www.bnf.org
2. Electronic Medicines Compendium. Methocarbamol. https://www.medicines.org.uk/emc/search?q=methocarbamol
3. Medscape. https://reference.medscape.com
4. Witenko C, Moorman-Li R, Motycka C, et al. Considerations for the appropriate use of skeletal muscle relaxants for the management of acute low back pain. P T 2014;39(6):427–435

13.13 Methoxyflurane

Introduction

- Introduced in early 1960s, as a low-dose self-administered analgesic, but was withdrawn in 2005 due to safety reasons
- Re-emerged in 2015 as Penthrox®
- Used in Australia for >40 years for trauma-related pain and procedural pain in children and adults

Name

- Penthrox® 99.9% (999 mg per 1 g)

Class of drugs

- Fluorinated hydrocarbon group of volatile anaesthetic agents

Presentation

- Each bottle contains 3 mL of volatile liquid
- Clear, almost colourless, characteristic fruity odour

Indications

- Emergency relief of moderate to severe pain in conscious adults with trauma and related pain
- Outpatient medical and surgical procedures, including colonoscopy, changes in burns dressings, and prostate biopsies (Australasia)

Contraindications/caution

- Hypersensitivity
- Malignant hyperthermia
- Clinically significant cardiovascular instability, respiratory depression, and altered consciousness
- Renal impairment:
  - Causes significant nephrotoxicity at high doses (serum levels >40 micromoles/L)
- Liver impairment:
  - Previous halogenated hydrocarbon anaesthesia, especially if within 3 months, may increase potential for hepatic injury
- Not appropriate for breakthrough pain in chronic pain conditions or in trauma pain in closely repeated episodes
- Occupational exposure: use with activated carbon (AC) chamber which adsorbs exhaled methoxyflurane

Routes of administration and dosing

- Self-administered under supervision
- Handheld Penthrox® inhaler, custom-built
- One 3 mL bottle is a single dose; second bottle only where needed
- Recommended dosing schedule: no more than 6 mL in a single day; administration on consecutive days not recommended; total weekly dose should not exceed 15 mL

Mode of action

- Mechanism of analgesic action not fully elucidated
- Onset is rapid; 6–10 inhalations and then inhale intermittently to maintain analgesia (self-titrate)
- Duration of action: continuous inhalation of 3 mL bottle—analgesia for up to 25–30 minutes

Side effects (limited by nature of self-administration)

- Hypotension and bradycardia. Not significant at analgesic doses
- Sedation, dizziness, euphoria, reduced concentration, headache, restlessness, mood changes
- Cough, hypoxia, dry mouth, nausea, vomiting
- Hepatic and renal failure

Pharmacokinetics

- Absorption:
  - Enters the lungs as vapour; rapidly transported into blood—therefore, rapid onset of analgesic action
- Distribution:
  - Highly lipophilic, diffuses into adipose tissue → reservoir, slowly released over days
- Metabolism:
  - Hepatic—dichlorination and O-demethylation, mediated by CYP450, metabolized to free fluoride and oxalic acid which are responsible for renal damage
- Elimination:
  - Approximately 60% excreted in the urine as organic fluorine, fluoride, and oxalic acid
  - Remainder exhaled unaltered or as CO_2

Interactions

- No reported drug interactions when used at analgesic doses (3–6 mL)
- Hepatic enzyme inducers—potential toxicity
- Avoid with concurrent use of nephrotoxic drugs
- Avoid using sevoflurane following methoxyflurane analgesia; sevoflurane increases serum fluoride levels
- Additive depressant effects with CNS depressants

Special circumstances

- Children: not for use in those aged <18 years
- Renal and hepatic impairment: caution
- Pregnancy: animal studies—no observed harmful effects
- Obstetric analgesia—single report of neonatal respiratory depression associated with a high fetal level of methoxyflurane
- Breastfeeding: insufficient data on excretion in human milk
- Ability to drive/operate machinery: minor influence

Additional information

- No clear evidence of carcinogenic or mutagenic properties
- Does not affect sperm cells in mice
- Crosses the placenta in animal studies, but no evidence of embryotoxic or teratogenic properties
- Delayed fetal development was observed with repeated dosing

Cost

- Vapour 3 mL bottle: £17.89

Further reading

1. Porter K, Dayan AD, Middleton PM. The role of inhaled methoxyflurane in acute pain management. Open Access Emerg Med 2018;10:149–64
2. Jephcott C, Grummet J, Nguyen N, et al. A review of the safety and efficacy of inhaled methoxyflurane as an analgesic for outpatient procedures. Br J Anaesth 2018;120(5):1040–8
3. Electronic Medicines Compendium. https://www.medicines.org.uk/emc

13.14 Nitrous oxide

N_2O is an inhalation anaesthetic agent which was first extracted in 1772 by Joseph Priestley and was further developed for analgesia by H. Davy (1799)

Chemical properties

- At room temperature, it is colourless and non-flammable but supports combustion
- Sweet taste and odour, soluble in water
- Stored in French blue cylinders as a liquid
- Preparation: ammonium nitrate (NH_4NO_3) $\rightarrow$ 2 H_2O + N_2O

- Weak general anaesthetic properties, used mainly as a carrier gas with volatile inhalational agents
- Minimum alveolar concentration (MAC)—105
- Low blood/gas partition coefficient of 0.46—rapid onset of action
- The filling ratio is 0.75, and critical temperature 36.5°C

Pharmacokinetics

- Kinetics—administered by inhalation and absorbed by diffusion through the lungs; eliminated via respiration (<0.004% metabolized)
- Elimination t1/2: 5 minutes

Uses

- Analgesic and CNS depressant
- General anaesthesia as a N_2O and oxygen mixture—70%:30%, respectively
- Entonox®: 50:50 (N_2O:oxygen) in dental surgery, in obstetrics for labour analgesia, and for procedural pain, e.g. change of burns dressing
- In the UK, the maximum permissible level is 100 ppm

Mechanism of action

- Exact mechanism is unclear but may act on GABA and glycine receptors and ligand-gated ion channels which are mainly inhibitory

Effects

- Mild depressant effects on the myocardium, increased sympathetic activity
- Mild decrease in respiratory T_V and increased RR
- Increases cerebral blood flow
- Demonstrates concentration effect and second gas effect

Side effects

- Nausea, vomiting
- Prolonged use (>6 hours) interferes with methionine synthesis and decreases thymidine and DNA synthesis
- May cause megaloblastic anaemia and peripheral neuropathy due to vitamin B12 deficiency

Interactions

- Potentiates hypotension with amitriptyline and antihypertensives (β-blockers, diuretics, ACEIs)
- CNS depression with sedatives, alcohol, and CNS depressants (BZDs, gabapentinoids)

Potential for abuse

- N_2O is not a controlled drug (second most popular recreational drug amongst young people)
- Environmental effects: contributes to greenhouse gas effects, global warming, and ozone layer depletion

Contraindications

- Expands air spaces (contraindicated in patients with pneumothorax, ocular surgery using intraocular gas, intestinal obstruction, etc.)

Special circumstances

- Pregnancy—may affect fertility and fetal development after exposure to high concentrations for prolonged periods
- May depress neonatal respiration

Applications of N_2O/research of N_2O in pain medicine

- The analgesic effects of N_2O may be linked to interactions between endogenous opioids and the descending noradrenergic system
- NMDA antagonism of N_2O may offer a significant benefit in the reduction of chronic post-surgical pain and OIH
- N_2O is as efficient as, and safer than, various other analgesic methods used during colonoscopy procedures, but further trials are necessary
- The ENIGMA-II trial showed that N_2O does not increase the risk of death or cardiovascular complications (note: ENIGMA-I trial: N_2O was associated with an increased long-term risk of MI, but not of death or stroke)

Further reading

1. Leslie K, Myles PS, Chan MT, et al. Nitrous oxide and long-term morbidity and mortality in the ENIGMA trial. Anesth Analg 2011;112(2):387–93
2. Chan MT, Wan AC, Gin T, et al. Chronic postsurgical pain after nitrous oxide anesthesia. Pain 2011;152(11):2514–20

13.15 Orphenadrine

Name, class of drugs

- Orphenadrine oral solution (50 mg/5 mL)
- Anti-Parkinson medication (anti-muscarinic)

Indications

- Parkinsonism
- Drug-induced extrapyramidal symptoms
- Unlicensed for nociceptive MSK pain symptoms
- May also reduce tremor and rigidity

Contraindications

- Acute porphyrias
- GI obstruction
- Myasthenia gravis
- Caution in cardiovascular disease, the elderly, hypertension, angle closure glaucoma, prostatic hypertrophy, psychotic disorders, and pyrexia

Dose

- Orphenadrine 50 mg three times daily (in combination with paracetamol 1 g three times daily)
- Orphenadrine may be increased in steps of 50 mg every 2–3 days according to response

- Usual daily dose: 150–300 mg
- Maximum daily dose: 400 mg
- Reduced dose in renal and liver failure

Mode of action

- Post-ganglionic anticholinergic, antihistaminergic, and LA properties
- CNS depressant with skeletal muscle relaxant effects (precise mechanism of action not known)
- Does not directly relax skeletal muscle
- Therapeutic action may be related to analgesic properties
- May reduce skeletal muscle spasm (possibly through an atropine-like central action on cerebral motor centres or on the medulla)

Side effects

- Constipation, dry mouth, nausea, vomiting, tachycardia, dizziness, sedation, confusion, euphoria, hallucinations, impaired memory, anxiety, restlessness, insomnia, urinary retention, blurred vision, and rash
- Angle closure glaucoma occurs very rarely
- Potential to impair mental alertness or physical coordination—use caution when driving or operating machinery until effects on the individual are known

Pharmacokinetics

Bioavailability

- Readily absorbed following oral intake

Distribution

- In animals, detected in all organs (not known in humans)
- Unknown if in breast milk

Metabolism

- Almost completely metabolized to at least eight metabolites
- Not fully determined

Elimination

- Eliminated principally in the urine as metabolites
- As unchanged drug (in small amounts)

Half-life

- Approximately 14 hours

Interactions

- Many drugs have anti-muscarinic effects; concomitant use of two or more such drugs can increase S/Es such as dry mouth, urinary retention, and constipation; concomitant use can also lead to confusion in the elderly
- Interactions are possible with TCAs, antihistamines, clozapine, codeine, domperidone, haloperidol, levodopa, MAOIs, memantine, metoclopramide, nefopam, nitrates, parasympathicomimetics, and phenothiazines
- Increased sedative effects with alcohol

Special circumstances

- In the elderly: reduce dose (at lower end of range recommended)
- Caution in pregnancy and breastfeeding (may cross the placenta)
- Caution in renal and hepatic impairment
- May affect driving ability
- Safety and efficacy not established in those under 12 years of age

Additional information

- Orphenadrine is anti-muscarinic and can theoretically exacerbate epilepsy and trigger seizures. The patient needs to be warned that their antiepileptics may necessitate an increase in dose if that is the case
- Avoid abrupt withdrawal

Cost

- 150 mL bottle (50 mg/5 mL): £42.45 (£1.42 per 50 mg)
- Per month: £127–255, depending on the dose

Further reading

1. Joint Formulary Committee. British National Formulary. 2020. London: BMJ Group and Pharmaceutical Press. https://www.bnf.org
2. ASHP. Drugs.com. 2020. https://www.drugs.com/monograph/orphenadrine-citrate.html

13.16 Vitamin D

Introduction

- Vitamin D is a fat-soluble vitamin, produced endogenously and obtained through food (either naturally or with fortification) and through supplements
- It controls the amount of calcium and phosphate in our body, which are needed for healthy bones, muscles, and the immune system
- Vitamin D deficiency is a worldwide epidemic and approximately 1 billion people are vitamin D-deficient
- In the UK, 1 in 5 people have low vitamin D
- All estimated average requirements (EARs) or recommended daily allowances (RDAs) assume that there is minimal or no sun exposure
- Serum concentration of Vitamin D (see table 13.16.1)

Table 13.16.1 Serum concentration of vitamin D

Vitamin D	**Plasma level (nmol/L)**
Deficiency	<50
Insufficient	51–74
Normal (varies)	**75–250**
Potentially harmful	>250

Class of drugs

- Vitamin D is a secosteroid, synthesized in the skin with energy from ultraviolet B light
- It is hydroxylated into 25(OH)D (pro-form) and then into 1,25$(OH)_2$D (active form)

Causes of deficiency

- Low sun exposure
- Inadequate dietary intake
- Use of creams with ultraviolet (UV) filter (protection >8)
- Hyperpigmented skin
- Malabsorption
- Increased catabolism (use of anticonvulsants, ATT, antiretrovirals)
- Deficient 25-hydroxylation/1α hydroxylation

What happens with vitamin D deficiency

- Rickets in infants and osteomalacia in adults
- Impairs proximal muscle function and predisposes to falls in those who are vulnerable
- Long-standing deficiency is a risk factor for osteoporosis
- Insufficiency increases the rate of cardio-metabolic disorders, leading to an increased risk of IHD and stroke

Dose

- Supplementtaion of vitamin D can be either to prevent or to treat deficiency
- Vitamin D is available as D3 (colecalciferol) and D2 (calciferol)
- Both D3 and D2 are equally active in humans

Loading dose

- Colecalciferol D3: aim for cumulative dose of 300000 units (usually 50000 units/week)
- Calciferol D2: between 40000 units and 100000 units per day (based on pathology)

Maintenance

- For prevention—usually 400 units daily; for treatment of deficiency—800 units daily

Mechanism of action

- Vitamin D is a potent inducer of antimicrobial peptide on immune cells.
- It reduces the release of pro-inflammatory cytokines, suppresses T cell response, and inhibits the synthesis of Prostaglandin E2
- Antiproliferative effects on several types of cancer cells

Monitoring

- Ca^{2+} concentration should be checked in patients receiving vitamin D at least once weekly initially

Contraindications

- Hypercalcaemia, metastatic calcification

Adverse effects

- Abdominal pain, headache, hypercalcaemia, hypercalciuria, nausea, constipation, decreased appetite

- **Overdose** causes anorexia, nausea, vomiting, weight loss, polyuria, and increased plasma and urinary concentrations of Ca^{2+} and phosphates

Pharmacodynamics and kinetics

- Vitamin D is a fat-soluble vitamin, and its absorption depends on the gut's ability to absorb dietary fat, particularly from the duodenum
- Once in circulation, it binds to vitamin D-binding protein for transport and is stored in adipose tissue
- After hydroxylation, it exerts its physiological action by binding to intracellular vitamin D receptor and promotes intestinal Ca^{2+} and phosphate absorption, renal tubular Ca^{2+} reabsorption, and Ca^{2+} mobilization from bones
- Vitamin D is excreted mainly through bile

Special circumstances

- Therapeutic doses in pregnancy unlikely harmful
- In breastfeeding, high doses can cause hypercalcaemia in infants
- Monitor Ca2+ levels in renal impairment

Additional information

- Insufficient vitamin D levels increases pain in fibromyalgia and other chronic MSK pain conditions
- Low vitamin D levels are linked to increased statin- related myalgias
- In patients with cancer pain, low levels of vitamin D can be associated with high opioid requirement
- Low 25(OH)D levels are present in patients suffering from chronic pain, but a Cochrane review in 2015 established that supplementing chronic pain patients with vitamin D was safe, but not consistently efficacious over placebo, hence does not support vitamin D treatment as an independent treatment for chronic pain conditions (e.g. fibromyalgia, non- specific MSK pain)
- Although obesity and overweight are associated with low circulating 25(OH)D levels, there is inconclusive evidence regarding its effect on bone health

Further reading

1. British National Formulary. Colecalciferol. https://bnf.nice.org.uk/drug/colecalciferol.html
2. Charoenngam N, Shirvani A, Holick MF. Vitamin D for skeletal and non-skeletal health: what we should know. J Clin Orthop Trauma 2019;10(6):1082–93
3. Helde-Frankling M, Björkhem-Bergman L. Vitamin D in pain management. Int J Mol Sci 2017;18(10):2170

Clinical Pharmacology

Sabina Bachtold, Shyam Balasubramanian, Rahul Guru, Katharine Howells, James Jack, Sandeep Kapur, Jan Rudiger, and Alifia Tameem

CONTENTS

14.1 Analgesic ladders

- In 1986, the World Health Organization (WHO) published a document entitled *Cancer Pain Relief*, which set out the principles of use of analgesics in cancer pain management, based on the use of a 'three-step analgesic ladder' (see Fig. 14.1.1). An updated version was published in 1996
- The guidelines arose from evidence of poor management of cancer pain in both developing and developed countries
- One of the reasons for this situation was the reluctance of health professionals to use 'strong' opioids because of misplaced fears of addiction and tolerance amongst patients, and of illegal use amongst the wider community
- This legitimized and increased the prescribing of 'strong' opioids amongst patients with moderate to severe cancer pain, but also extended its use for non-cancer pain
- The WHO analgesic ladder has a role in management of patients with acute pain, but a limited role in CNCP
- This three-step approach of administering the right drug in the right dose at the right time is inexpensive and 70–90% effective for cancer, but this has led to opioid overprescribing and an opioid epidemic in non-cancer pain
- In the case of cancer pain in children, the WHO recommends a two-step ladder
- Adapted analgesic ladder for acute, chronic non-cancer, and cancer pain (see Fig. 14.1.2)

Principles

- 'By the mouth' (wherever possible)—a different route of administration should be considered if the oral route is not suitable
- 'By the clock'—patients should be given regular analgesia such that the next dose is delivered before the previous one wears off plus rescue doses at 50–100% of the regular dose
- 'By the ladder'—if pain occurs, there should be prompt oral administration of drugs in the following order: non-opioids (aspirin and paracetamol); then, as necessary, mild opioids

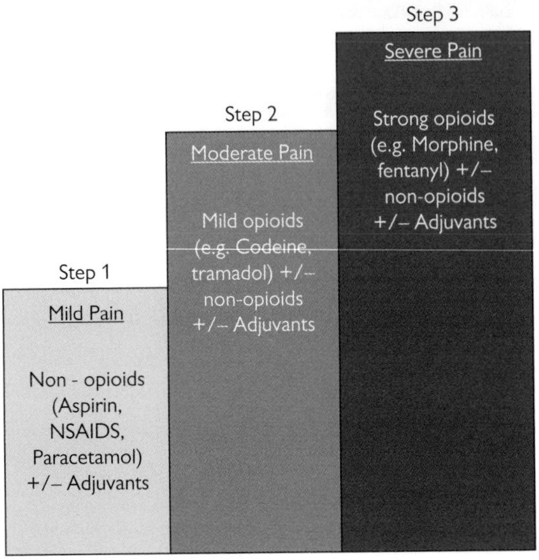

Figure 14.1.1 The WHO analgesic ladder—a three-step approach for cancer and acute pain

Reproduced with permission from Tameem, A. (2016). Analgesic ladders. In Plunkett, E., Johnson, E., Pierson, A., (Eds). *Returning to Work in Anaesthesia: Back on the circuit.* Cambridge, United Kingdom: Cambridge University Press

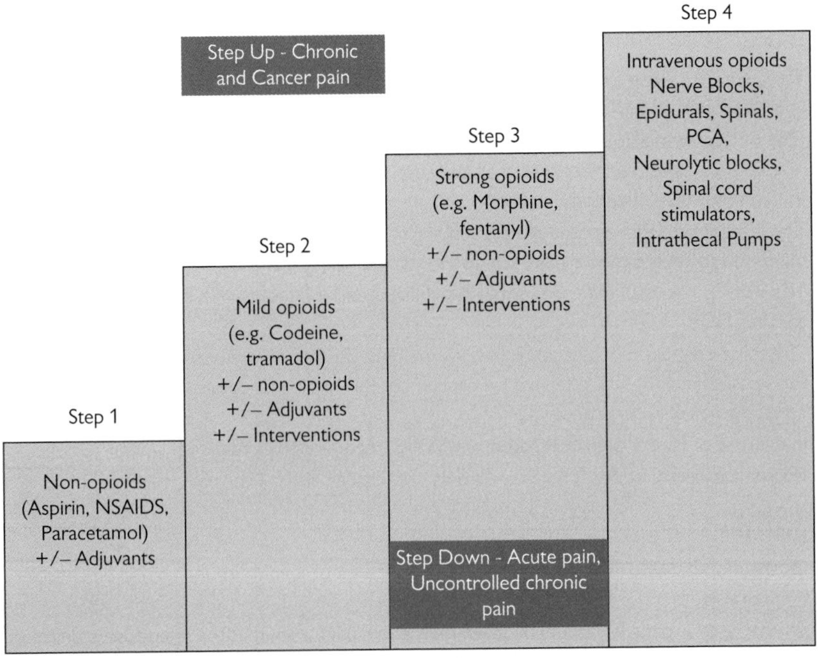

Figure 14.1.2 Adapted analgesic ladder for acute, chronic non-cancer, and cancer pain

Reproduced with permission from Tameem, A. (2016). Analgesic ladders. In Plunkett, E., Johnson, E., Pierson, A., (Eds). *Returning to Work in Anaesthesia: Back on the circuit.* Cambridge, United Kingdom: Cambridge University Press

(codeine); then strong opioids, such as morphine, until the patient is free of pain. The patient should be treated with drugs on the step that corresponds to their pain. For example, if they score pain as severe, they should be treated with drugs from step 3 (strong opioids)

- 'By the individual'—there are no standard doses for opioids; the right dose is the one that relieves the individual's pain. Other analgesics have a standard maximum dose, whereas opioids are titrated to achieve adequate analgesia with minimal S/Es
- 'Attention to detail'—individualized care involving the patient, family, and carers is vital to provide adequate analgesia

Medications

- Simple analgesics: paracetamol, NSAIDs, e.g. ibuprofen, naproxen, diclofenac, COX-2 inhibitors
- Weak opioids: codeine, dihydrocodeine
- Strong opioids: tramadol, morphine, oxycodone, fentanyl, methadone
- Adjuvants: used to enhance pain relief or treat specific types of pain, to treat adverse effects of analgesics, and to treat concomitant psychological disturbances, including insomnia, anxiety, and depression:
  - Antidepressants: TCAs, SSRIs, and selective noradrenaline reuptake inhibitors
  - Anticonvulsants: gabapentinoids, carbamazepine, oxcarbazepine, sodium valproate, lamotrigine, phenytoin
  - NMDA receptor antagonists: ketamine
  - α-2 agonists: clonidine, dexmedetomidine
  - Anxiolytics: BZDs (diazepam), hydroxyzine
  - Others: steroids, baclofen, cannabinoids, lidocaine 5% patch, topical capsaicin, LAs (IV lidocaine, mexiletine)
  - Antiemetics (chlorpromazine, prochlorperazine) and laxatives

The WHO analgesic ladder, despite its limitations in non-cancer pain, does provide a good framework to manage pain

Further reading

1. World Health Organization. Cancer pain relief. 1st edition, 1986; 2nd edition, 1996. Geneva: World Health Organization
2. Reid C, Davies A. The World Health Organization three-step analgesic ladder comes of age. Palliat Med 2004;18(3):175–6

14.2 Pre-emptive and preventative analgesia in acute pain

Pre-emptive analgesia

Definition

- Administration of preoperative treatment is more effective than the identical treatment administered after surgical incision or during surgery. The key point is the timing of administration of the analgesic treatment before the onset of the noxious stimuli or skin incision during surgery
- *Note: an analgesic treatment given pre-emptively can also be preventative*

History

- Crile in 1913 suggested that pain after surgery might be amplified by noxious stimuli following surgical incision. The use of a multimodal analgesia, including regional LA blocks, was thought to potentially reduce this
- Wall in 1988 described 'pre-emptive pre-operative analgesia'
- Woolf in 1983 and 1991 described evidence of a central component of post-injury pain hypersensitivity in experimental studies and went on to suggest that changes in timing of analgesia could affect post-operative pain control
- Kissin in 1994 and Katz in 2002 found that individual clinical studies have reported conflicting outcomes when comparing 'pre-incisional' with 'post-incisional' interventions. In part, this may relate to variability in definitions, deficiencies in clinical trial design, and differences in the outcomes available to laboratory and clinical investigators

Efficacy

- There are many techniques described, with conflicting reports on their efficacy. The evidence is strongest for epidural neural blockade; for example, one study has shown that following thoracotomy, pre-emptive thoracic epidural analgesia reduces the severity of acute pain on coughing for up to 48 hours

Mechanism of action

- Reduced central sensitization associated with a nociceptive stimulus. By administering the analgesic agent prior to an acute nociceptive stimulus, subsequent DH changes associated with central sensitization and hypersensitivity are reduced, compared with administration of the analgesic before the surgical insult has occurred and the pain is established
- The development of chronic pain may be reduced through this alteration in sensory processing

Preventative analgesia

Definition

- Preventative analgesia is **persistence** of an analgesic effect beyond the expected duration of action of the agents or interventions
- Administration of a preventative analgesic agent leads to a reduction in post-operative pain and/or analgesic consumption, when compared to another treatment, placebo treatment, or no treatment. This therapeutic effect is observed at a point in time beyond the expected duration of action of the intervention (e.g. 5.5 $t1/2$ of the drug)
- The agent or technique is used preoperatively, intraoperatively, or post-operatively

History

- Kissin in 1994 suggested the term 'preventative' analgesia to be more clinically relevant than 'pre-emptive' analgesia
- Dahl in 2004 described the importance of continuing the analgesic agent into the post-operative recovery period to allow ongoing reduction in central sensitization
- Katz in 2011 described the focus of preventative analgesia or interventions not being on the timing of their administration, but on their overall ability to impact on reducing the nociceptive barrage associated with noxious preoperative, intraoperative, and post-operative stimuli

Efficacy

- There is evidence to support that ketamine is an effective preventative analgesic

- LAs (either systemic or perineural) are preventative analgesics, reducing acute pain in the perioperative period. Intraoperative neuraxial block and systemic LAs may be effective in major abdominal procedures
- The evidence for whether NSAIDs and gabapentinoids are preventative analgesics is less convincing

Mechanism of action

- Persistent analgesic effect is achieved by minimizing sensitization induced by noxious perioperative stimuli, leading to reduction of central sensitization and 'wind-up'. This action occurs in different ways, depending on the drug or technique involved, and may reduce the risk of developing chronic pain
- Peripheral sensitization is reduced by a decrease in the local inflammatory response caused by tissue damage. For example, NSAIDs reduce the production of PGs that lead to transduction and increased conduction of nociceptive impulses to nociceptive selective and wide dynamic range neurons in the DH, resulting in altered responsiveness of these neurons
- A reduction in the barrage of pain signals from nociceptors to neurons in the DH leads to less hyperresponsiveness and hence decreased central sensitization

Further reading

1. Mishra AK, Afzal M, Mookerjee SS et al. Pre-emptive analgesia: recent trends and evidences. Indian J Pain 2013;27(3):114–20
2. Katz J, Clarke H, Seltzer Z. Preventive analgesia: quo vadimus? Anesth Analg 2011;113:1242–53
3. Kissin I. Pre-emptive analgesia: terminology and clinical relevance. Anesth Analg 1994;79(4):809–10
4. McQuay HJ. Pre-emptive analgesia: a systematic review of clinical studies. Ann Med 1995;27:249–56
5. Schug SA, Palmer GM, Scott DA, et al. Acute pain management: scientific evidence. 4th edition, 2015. Melbourne: Australian and New Zealand College of Anaesthetists and Faculty of Pain Medicine
6. Wall PD. The prevention of postoperative pain. Pain 1988;33:289–90
7. Woolf CJ. Central mechanisms in acute pain. In: Bond MR, Charlton JE, Woolf CJ (eds). Proceedings of the World Congress on Pain. 6th edition, 1991; pp: 25–34. Amsterdam: Elsevier

14.3 Management of patients with a substance use disorder

Introduction

- Management of patients with acute and/or chronic pain on prescription drugs can be challenging
- Opioid prescription drug abuse is the most common. There has been large-scale prescription of opioids for all types of pain since the early 1990s, owing to publications asserting that the risk of addiction and abuse is low in patients receiving opioids for chronic pain
- The prevalence of prescription opioid abuse ranges from 1% to 40% in patients with CNCP due to difficulties in diagnosing abuse in this patient population
- While patients did benefit from increased access to opioids, there has been an alarming increase in opioid misuse, abuse, and opioid-related mortality and morbidity
- Other prescription drugs that are abused include BZDs, gabapentinoids, barbiturates, and cannabis

Definitions

- For important definitions on substance abuse and addictive behaviours, see 4.5 Tolerance, dependence, addiction, and pseudoaddiction, p. 87

Withdrawal

- Opioid withdrawal occurs when the opioid dose is stopped or rapidly tapered, or when an opioid antagonist is given
- There may be psychological effects, which include craving and agitation, and physical symptoms such as diarrhoea, palpitations, or tachycardia

Diversion

- Diversion is the transfer of prescribed opioids for unlawful use
- Prescription opioids may be passed on or sold to persons other than the patient, for therapeutic or recreational use
- Doctors have a legal and ethical responsibility to uphold the law and to protect society from drug misuse
- Opioids must be responsibly prescribed, and health care professionals must be vigilant for, and guard against, misuse, while also ensuring that patients have the required medication available

Assessment of patients

- Should be done in a **multidisciplinary pain clinic** by applying the biopsychosocial model, using pharmacotherapy, physical therapies, cognitive behavioural/psychological therapies, and exercise
- A single practitioner/pain clinic/GP surgery and a single pharmacy should be responsible for opioid prescriptions and dispensing, respectively
- A thorough history (especially of substance abuse and medication list with doses) and physical examination are of utmost importance
- Signs of medication abuse:
    - Include signs of intoxication or withdrawal, requesting for early reissuing of opioids, approaching a second physician and/or pharmacy, stealing or buying opioids from other patients or on the Internet, exaggerated pain behaviour, inefficacy of alternative treatments, needle marks, being assertive, aggressive, or emotionally labile, a vague or crisp history of symptoms, and refusing tests such as urine toxicology
- Predictors of prescription drug abuse include:
    - Social factors: family history of substance misuse, substance misusers in social network, current victim of abuse, occupational risk
    - Psychological factors: abuse, trauma, anxiety disorders, PDs, current or previous substance abuse
- Psychological screening:
    - Psychological disorders are common in patients with substance abuse. A psychologist should assess and manage these issues. Tools such as the HADS should be used
    - Use tools to assist in identifying at-risk patients: tools include CAGE-AID (adapted to include drugs), Prescription Drug Use Questionnaire (PDUQ), Screening Instrument for Substance Abuse Potential (SISAP), the Screener and Opioid Assessment for Patients with Pain (SOAPP), and the Opioid Risk Tool (ORT)
- **Pill counts**: evaluate the use of prescribed opioids, which can also be part of an adherence monitoring programme to reduce opioid abuse. Attempt should be made to differentiate between addiction and pseudoaddiction

- Assess the **four As** (analgesia, activities of daily living, adverse effects, and aberrant drug-related behaviours)
- Investigations:
  - Urine toxicology, γ-glutamyl transpeptidase, hepatitis B and C antigen titres, and HIV tests should be considered
  - Urine toxicology: immunoassay urine screens are often used as the first line of analysis and detect the presence of prescription and illicit drugs. Gas chromatography/mass spectrometry urine screens quantify the extent of illicit and prescription drug use

Patient stratification

- Low risk (can be managed in primary care): patients have no history of substance abuse or positive predictors. They admit to taking extra doses and can be managed by education and close follow-ups
- Medium risk (need specialist support): patients may have a history of substance abuse and some positive predictors. Specialist advice or referral is needed for these patients
- High risk (need specialist management): patients have a history of active substance abuse and/or an untreated psychiatric disorder. These patients need an urgent referral to addiction specialist services

Management

- High and complex patient needs: these patients have greater needs than opioid-naïve patients, making multidisciplinary team input necessary. They may also need referral to addiction services and social services
- Explanation of management plan: clear **goals** of treatment should be established and frequent assessment of progress towards these goals should be done. Patients should be explained about the **adverse effects of opioids**, the amount of opioid analgesia they can expect, that opioids are not the answer to all the pain, and that non-opioid drugs and non-pharmacological interventions will be beneficial for them. All discussions must be **clearly documented** and communicated to other members of the health care team
- Choice and route of opioid: the **same opioid** should be used, as this will make dose calculation easier and will avoid S/Es of a new agent. The oral route is preferred as this allows easier dose titration. **Long-acting preparations are of lower abuse potential**
- Short-acting preparations and lipid-soluble opioids result in a rapid increase in opioid blood and CNS concentrations, which can give a 'high' feeling
- Lipid-soluble opioids (fentanyl and pethidine) and short-acting preparations of other opioids (morphine, oxycodone, hydromorphone) are to be avoided
- Transdermal preparations can be useful in such patients as they do not cause a rapid rise in plasma concentrations
- The entire amount of opioid should preferably be given as long-acting preparations
- In select cases, breakthrough analgesia may be provided with short-acting opioids, but these patients need to be carefully monitored
- These patients are tolerant of the usual doses of opioids, so they need higher doses, along with the maintenance dose of their usual opioid
- Contracts/opioid therapy agreement: these are agreements that clarify the roles, responsibilities, and limitations between the prescriber and the patient. It is advisable to use contracts when prescribing long-term opioids. If the conditions of the contract are not met, opioid therapy may be withdrawn. A **trilateral agreement** between the pain physician, the GP, and the patient is made if the GP will be prescribing the opioids

- **Close monitoring** (including monthly urine toxicology and compliance checking) and cognitive behavioural counselling: these have shown to improve opioid prescription compliance in high-risk patients
- Patients with psychopathology and psychiatric disorders need input from a psychologist and/or psychiatrist, and adequate **social support** through social services is important. This includes financial support, housing, and help if in an abusive relationship
- Non-opioid pharmacotherapy: NSAIDs, paracetamol, antidepressants (TCAs, selective noradrenaline reuptake inhibitors), and gabapentinoids (gabapentin and pregabalin) can be added as part of a multimodal analgesic regimen
- Pain interventions: where indicated, interventions such as facet joint blocks, ESIs, and TPIs, amongst others, should be offered

Acute pain management in patients abusing prescription opioids

- These patients are opioid-tolerant and consequently require higher doses than opioid-naïve patients
- There is no specific dose at which patients are considered opioid-tolerant; however, the FDA has issued guidelines for defining opioid-tolerant patients
- Opioid-tolerant patient: one taking 60 mg of oral morphine per day or an equianalgesic dose of another opioid for 1 week or longer

Difficulties faced in the assessment of pain in opioid-dependent patients

- Standard methods of assessment of pain and response to therapy are less accurate in these patients, and distrust between these patients and physicians can act as a barrier in the assessment and provision of optimal pain treatment
- Patients fear that their analgesic medication will be withheld, leading to anxiety, fear of withdrawal, and drug-seeking behaviour
- Fear of respiratory S/Es at unusually high doses that these patients require leads to health care providers underprescribing opioids
- It may be difficult to obtain an accurate history of the dose of opioids being taken
- Patients often report higher pain scores, may fabricate pain behaviour, and have increased opioid requirements
- Patients may be abusing other drugs and may divert prescribed opioids

Assessment of pain in opioid-dependent patients

- Discuss clearly the pain management plan and build an environment of trust with the patient
- A good rapport will help in accurately ascertaining which drugs the patient is taking and understanding expectations
- The dose of opioids and other drugs should be obtained as accurately as possible. This will help in calculating the total dose of drug to be given per day
- Early involvement of the **inpatient pain team (IPT)** is required. In patients going for surgery, preoperative engagement with the IPT should be considered
- It is important to get information about the patient's drug history from the primary care physician and addiction team (if known to them)
- These patients have a high prevalence of psychiatric comorbidities, such as anxiety and depression, which need to be addressed

- Along with the usual pain assessment tools, such as VAS and NRS, other measures, such as ability to breathe deeply, cough, ambulate, and engage with physiotherapy, signs of withdrawal, opioid S/Es, and mood, should be assessed
- Urine screening could be considered to help formulate a better management plan
- Assessment of psychiatric comorbidities, medical comorbidities, and social factors
- Do not attempt counselling about substance abuse and/or detoxification in the acute pain stage

Prescribing opioids and other analgesics during an episode of acute pain

- Continue baseline opioid: determine the baseline opioid requirement per day. This amount should be given to prevent withdrawal
  - Route: the patient's normal route (oral or transdermal) should be continued, if possible. In general, the oral route is preferred. Long-acting opioids should be given if the oral route is used
  - If the patient is unable to take opioids orally, a continuous infusion, PCA, or intermittent boluses can be given. PCA will usually need to be at a higher dose than usual, including increased bolus dose and addition of a background infusion
- Choice of opioid: try to use the same opioid the patient was taking, as this will make it easier to calculate the total drug required and prevent S/Es from a new agent
- Additional or breakthrough analgesia: along with the background dose of opioid, additional opioids can be provided by PCA or intermittent boluses of opioids. NSAIDs, paracetamol, ketamine, GCs (dexamethasone), magnesium, gabapentinoids (gabapentin and pregabalin), and α-2 agonists (clonidine and dexmedetomidine) can be added as part of the multimodal analgesic regimen. Regional analgesia and central neuraxial analgesia should be used where appropriate
- Role of adjuvants: drugs such as ketamine (low dose), GCs, magnesium, gabapentinoids, and α-2 agonists improve analgesia and can also be used to manage OIH and opioid tolerance
- Patients on opioid substitution therapy (OST): certain patients may be on OST such as methadone or buprenorphine. This needs to be continued and other opioids and analgesics are added to provide optimal analgesia
- Discharge analgesia: these patients need to be discharged on opioid medication and should be referred to the pain clinic and/or addiction clinic for continued management and support

Further reading

1. Smith HS, McCleane G. Opioids issues. In: Smith HS (ed). Current Therapy in Pain. 2009; pp. 408–421. Philadelphia, PA: Saunders
2. Simpson GK, Jackson M. Perioperative management of opioid-tolerant patient. BJA Educ 2016;17:124–8
3. Tordoff SG, Ganty P. Chronic pain and prescription opioid misuse. Contin Educ Anaesth Crit Care Pain 2010;10(5):158–61
4. Jamison RN, Serraillier J, Michna E. Assessment and treatment of abuse risk in opioid prescribing for chronic pain. Pain Res Treat 2011;2011:941808
5. Quinlan J, Cox F. Acute pain management in patients with drug dependence syndrome. Pain Rep 2017;2(4):e611
6. Cheatle M, Comer D, Wunsch M, et al. Treating pain in addicted patients: recommendations from an expert panel. Popul Health Manag 2014;17(2):79–89

14.4 Serotonin syndrome

Introduction

- Impaired mental state, increased muscle activity, and autonomic instability secondary to excessive serotonin (5-HT) activity in the brainstem and spinal cord
- Seen in SSRI overdose, particularly in combination with other antidepressant drugs such as SNRIs, MAOIs, and TCAs
- Also associated with use of tramadol, tapentadol, pethidine, fentanyl, metoclopramide, ondansetron, amphetamines, and cocaine—particularly if these are taken with SSRIs and SNRIs

Diagnosis

- Diagnosis is made clinically (based on presentation and drug history)
- Differential diagnosis: neuroleptic malignant syndrome, malignant hyperthermia, anticholinergic toxicity, heat stroke, meningitis

Clinical presentation

- Incidence: rare (approximately 15% of SSRI overdoses develop serotonin syndrome)

Clinical triad of abnormalities

- *Cognitive effects:* confusion, headache, agitation, hypomania, hallucinations, coma
- *Autonomic effects:* shivering, sweating, hyperthermia (can be >40°C), vasoconstriction, tachycardia, nausea, diarrhoea
- *Somatic effects:* myoclonus, hyperreflexia, clonus, tremor

Complications

- Disseminated intravascular coagulation, cardiac failure, renal failure, rhabdomyolysis

Treatment

- Cessation of precipitant drugs
- Activated charcoal has a role if given within 1 hour of ingestion
- 5-HT antagonists: cyproheptadine first line, methysergide. Consider olanzapine for severe cases
- Supportive care, including control of autonomic instability:
  - BZDs to control myoclonus and reduce hyperthermia
  - Active cooling if hyperthermia severe
  - Muscle relaxation with intubation and ventilation for severe cases—avoid suxamethonium due to increased K^+ levels
  - Maintain high urine output to limit renal dysfunction

Prognosis

- Usually resolves within 24 hours; death has been reported rarely. Muscle pain and weakness can persist for months

Additional information

- Serotonin syndrome presents with hyperkinesia and clonus
- In contrast to bradykinesia and extrapyramidal 'lead pipe' rigidity that is seen in neuroleptic malignant syndrome

Further reading

1. Boyer EW, Shannon M. The serotonin syndrome. N Engl J Med 2005;352(11):1112–20
2. Chechani V. Serotonin syndrome presenting as hypotonic coma and apnea: potentially fatal complications of selective serotonin receptor inhibitor therapy. Crit Care Med 2002;30(2):473–6
3. Dunkley EJ, Isbister GK, Sibbritt D, et al. The Hunter serotonin toxicity criteria: simple and accurate diagnostic decision rules for serotonin toxicity. QJM 2003;96(9):635–42
4. Isbister G, Bowe S, Dawson A, Whyte I. Relative toxicity of selective serotonin reuptake inhibitors (SSRIs) in overdose. J Toxicol Clin Toxicol 2004;42(3):277–85
5. Volpi-Abadie J, Kaye AM, Kaye AD. Serotonin syndrome. Ochsner J 2013;13(4):533–40

14.5 Placebo and nocebo

Placebo

- A *placebo* is defined by Shapiro and Morris as 'any therapy or component of therapy used for its nonspecific, psychological or psychophysiological effect or that is used for its presumed specific effect, but is without specific activity for the condition being treated'
- The *placebo effect* describes 'the positive response some patients/participants experience after receiving a placebo. When present, this response has a perceptible and measurable beneficial effect that may be subjective (e.g. pain reduction) or objective (e.g. improved blood pressure). These effects are believed to be related to intrinsic factors (e.g. personal expectations or learnt responses) and/or extrinsic (e.g. provider, environment, technology, and contextual) factors'
- Placebo effects have an important role in three areas: (1) as controls in experimental studies to determine specific effects and enable blinding; (2) in placebo research; and (3) as a tool in clinical practice

Nocebo

- Nocebo derives from the word *nocere*, meaning '*I shall harm*'
- The *nocebo effect* is 'the negative response some patients/participants experience after receiving a placebo. These effects range from minor discomforts (e.g. headache, nausea) to life-threatening complications'
- The underlying mechanisms are both psychological (conditioning, negative expectations) and neurobiological (via cholecystokinin, dopamine, and endogenous opioids)
- Nocebo effects can influence clinical outcomes and treatment adherence. Gaining a deeper understanding of the nocebo effect may help in identifying factors that lead to maladaptive responses. For instance, clinicians communicate via both verbal and non-verbal techniques, some of which may unintentionally impart negative suggestions that may trigger a nocebo response. Therefore, carefully balanced clinician–patient communication (positive framing, contextualized informed consent) and exploring patients' treatment beliefs may mitigate the nocebo effects

History

- In medieval times, mourners were hired to attend funerals, but because their emotions were considered insincere, they were called '*placebos*', from the Latin for '*I will please*'
- Henry Beecher (an eminent American anaesthesiologist and medical ethicist), in 1955, published a paper entitled '*The powerful placebo*', in which he wrote: '*placebos have a high*

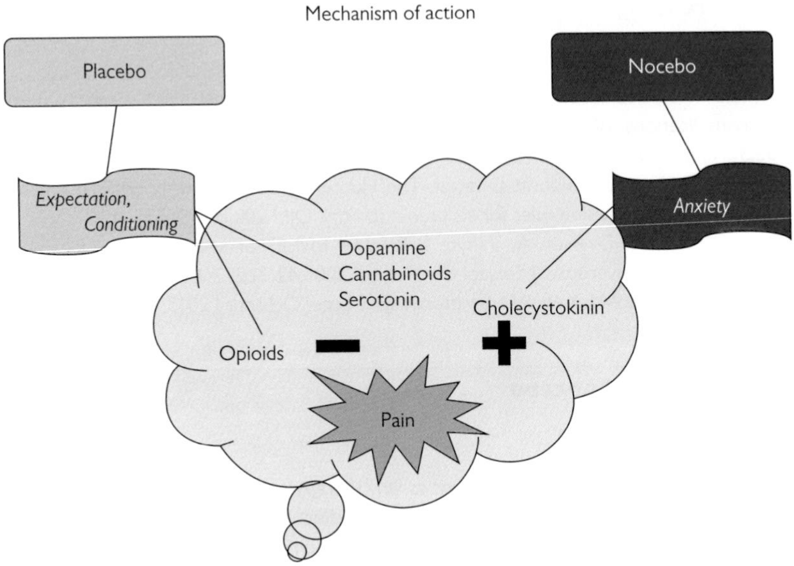

Figure 14.5.1 Mechanisms of placebo analgesia

degree of therapeutic effectiveness in treating subjective responses.' This paper, in which he noted that placebos are effective 30% of the time, had a profound effect on clinical research

Mechanisms of placebo analgesia

(See Fig. 14.5.1.)

Psychological mechanisms

- Psychological traits such as empathy, dispositional optimism, hypnotic suggestibility, neuroticism, altruism, and the locus of ego-reliance have been linked to the efficacy of placebo analgesia

Brain mechanisms

- Placebo analgesic effects have been shown to produce activity changes and enhanced functional coupling in the dorsolateral prefrontal cortex (DLPFC), the rostral anterior cingulate cortex (rACC), and the subcortical regions, including the hypothalamus, amygdala, and PAG
- The DLPFC initiates the placebo analgesic response. The rACC is connected to the PAG and correlates with modulation of placebo analgesia
- fMRI shows that the activity at the level of the spinal cord is modulated by placebo analgesia
- Placebo analgesia may be due to the endogenous release of neuropeptides such as opioids, cholecystokinins, dopamine, serotonin, and cannabinoids, an effect which may be reversed by naloxone

Genetics and the placebo response

- The study of genomic effects on the placebo response has been termed the 'placebome'
- Genetic polymorphism in the expressing of the dopaminergic and serotonergic mechanisms which are responsible for placebo analgesia may mean that placebo responses vary by genotype
- In general, the placebo arm is considered to be an adequate control for outcomes in the active treatment arm of RCTs. However, if the placebo response does indeed vary by genotype, we might expect challenges with confounding, potential gene–drug–placebo effect modification, and disease-specific effects

Recent advances

- Open-label placebo (OLP) breaks from the received wisdom that clinical administration of a placebo requires deception (or double-blind conditions) to be effective—several studies have directly tested the effect of an OLP prescription, and all indicated that patients reported benefits after taking pills presented honestly as placebos
- It has been postulated that 'engendering hope when participants feel hopeless about their condition can be therapeutic'
- Another possible explanation is the Hawthorne (or observer) effect: a person who is aware of being studied/observed often feels better, even if nothing has actually changed—this is also why patients say they feel better when their attending doctor or nurse is attentive and has good bedside manners

Conclusion

- As our understanding of the placebo evolves, it is worth bearing in mind the advice by the American Institute of Medicine: '*placebo (can) conceivably be a form of treatment of pain, especially in light of the shortcoming of other modalities or benefits they bring in their right*'

Further reading

1. Medoff ZM, Colloca L. Placebo analgesia: understanding the mechanisms. Pain Manag 2015;5(2):89–96
2. Carvalho C, Caetano JM, Cunha L, et al. Open-label placebo treatment in chronic low back pain: a randomized controlled trial. Pain 2016;157:2766–72
3. Kapur S, Dunham R, Balasubramanian S. Pain and Placebo. J Pain Relief 2021;10(4):370

Copyright

PAIN INTERVENTIONS

Overview of Interventions

Adnan Al-Kaisy, Simon Braude, Enrique Collantes, Sumit Gulati, Ashok Puttapa, Jan Rudiger, Haggai Sharon, and Alifia Tameem

CONTENTS

15.1 Overview of pain interventions

Introduction

- A pain block is an invasive intervention intended to reduce a patient's pain levels and improve their mobility, activity levels, sleep, and QoL
- Interventional pain management should be part of a multidisciplinary management plan

Factors affecting patient selection and specific intervention offered

- Clinical history:
  - The nature, distribution, and frequency of pain
  - Previous surgery or interventions for pain management
  - The impact of pain on the patient's daily routine, working life, and QoL
  - Assessment of the patient's physical, psychological, and environmental factors
- Pain-orientated clinical examination:
  - MSK ± neurological examination
  - Areas of tenderness
  - Positive/negative features of neuropathic pain
- Investigations (these may vary as per procedures):
  - Blood tests (haematology, biochemistry, coagulation, glycaemic profile)
  - X-rays, CT scans, MRI,US, bone scans
  - Nerve conduction studies (NCS)
- Exclude serious pathology (e.g. infection, fracture, cauda equina syndrome, tumour)
- Identify the underlying cause of the pain
- Advanced interventional procedures should be done in a multidisciplinary pain management unit and after more conservative therapies have been tried
- Resources, adequately trained staff, evidence, and cost of the procedure should be taken into consideration

Patient factors affecting suitability for procedure

- Pain symptoms, signs and investigations correlate with the planned procedure
- Patients and clinicians must have realistic expectations of the outcome of the procedure
- Patients understand that they need to engage actively and take responsibility for their pain management strategy
- Consideration of factors that may be associated with poorer outcomes in interventional pain medicine (e.g. catastrophization, uncontrolled mental health disorders, low self-efficacy, unrealistic expectations, active substance use disorder, use of passive pain management strategies, secondary gain, fear avoidance behaviours, inappropriate use of opioids or other medications, ongoing compensation)
- Absolute and relative contraindications:
  - Medically unwell—poorly controlled cardiovascular, respiratory, renal, and other medical conditions
  - Coagulopathy and/or intake of antiplatelet or anticoagulant drugs
  - Active infections and avoid if high risk of developing infections (e.g. diabetes, immunosuppression)
  - Pregnancy (especially procedures involving ionizing radiation)

Consent

- Mutual decision process between the patient and the clinician(s)—this should be a staged process (e.g. discussion in clinic, use of Internet resources or leaflets, final consent signed or countersigned on the day of the procedure)
- Communication must be clear, and the patient must be able to understand its nature, possible risks, and complications (e.g. failure, discomfort, bruising, haematoma, infection, flare-up of pain symptoms, allergic reaction, temporary/permanent neurological symptoms, damage to surrounding structures and other complications specific for the procedure being performed)
- Discussion of realistic outcomes (e.g. possible failure of the procedure to relieve pain, reduction of pain severity, improvement in function, reduction of use of analgesia, reduction of S/Es from medications)
- Explaining the evidence of the intervention
- Discussion of potential alternative treatments and impact of not having the specific intervention
- Maximizing the patient's ability to make decisions themselves and respecting those decisions
- Answering the patient's questions and respecting their autonomy
- The clinician is responsible for ensuring the patient has capacity to consent for a procedure
- The team involved must be competent to perform the procedure
- Patients can have access to a second opinion if required

Performance of the procedure

- Use of a checklist is recommended during procedures (see Fig. 15.1.1)

Pre-procedure instructions to the patient

- Adjustment of medications (e.g. anticoagulants, hypoglycaemics, etc.)
- Fasting instructions may or may not be needed
- Information about the planned procedure(s) (e.g. local or pain faculty leaflets, Internet resources)
- Further management after the procedure (e.g. physiotherapy, psychology, occupational therapy (OT), biomedical treatments/resources in primary ± secondary care)
- Ensuring adequate support is available for attending the procedure appointment and discharge afterwards (e.g. hospital transport, relative, partner, or friend picking the patient up and staying with them overnight)

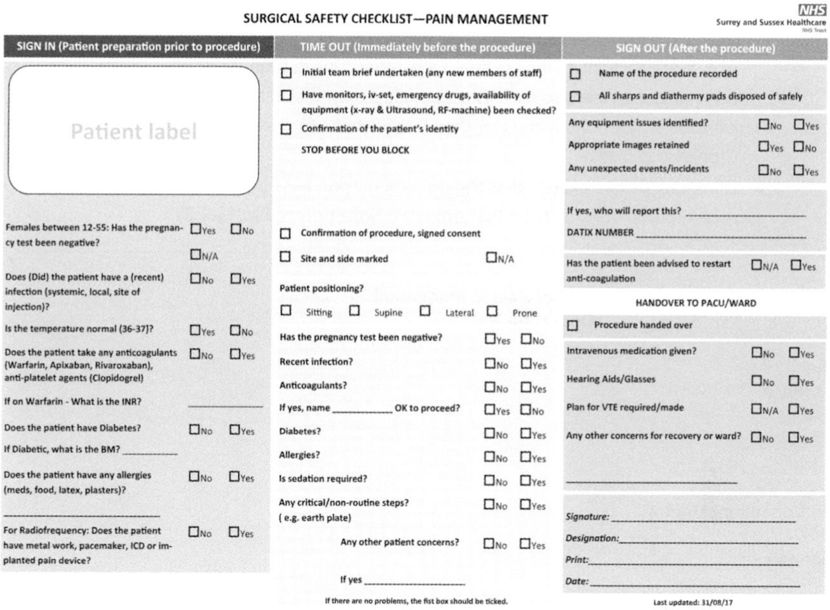
SURGICAL SAFETY CHECKLIST—PAIN MANAGEMENT

NHS Surrey and Sussex Healthcare NHS Trust

SIGN IN (Patient preparation prior to procedure)

Patient label

Females between 12-55: Has the pregnancy test been negative? ☐Yes ☐No ☐N/A

Does (Did) the patient have a (recent) infection (systemic, local, site of injection)? ☐No ☐Yes

Is the temperature normal (36-37)? ☐Yes ☐No

Does the patient take any anticoagulants (Warfarin, Apixaban, Rivaroxaban), anti-platelet agents (Clopidogrel) ☐No ☐Yes

If on Warfarin - What is the INR? ______

Does the patient have Diabetes? ☐No ☐Yes

If Diabetic, what is the BM? ______

Does the patient have any allergies (meds, food, latex, plasters)? ☐No ☐Yes

______

For Radiofrequency: Does the patient have metal work, pacemaker, ICD or implanted pain device? ☐No ☐Yes

TIME OUT (Immediately before the procedure)

☐ Initial team brief undertaken (any new members of staff)

☐ Have monitors, iv-set, emergency drugs, availability of equipment (x-ray & Ultrasound, RF-machine) been checked?

☐ Confirmation of the patient's identity

STOP BEFORE YOU BLOCK

☐ Confirmation of procedure, signed consent

☐ Site and side marked ☐N/A

Patient positioning?

☐ Sitting ☐ Supine ☐ Lateral ☐ Prone

Has the pregnancy test been negative? ☐Yes ☐No

Recent infection? ☐No ☐Yes

Anticoagulants? ☐No ☐Yes

If yes, name ______ OK to proceed? ☐Yes ☐No

Diabetes? ☐No ☐Yes

Allergies? ☐No ☐Yes

Is sedation required? ☐No ☐Yes

Any critical/non-routine steps? (e.g. earth plate) ☐No ☐Yes

Any other patient concerns? ☐No ☐Yes

If yes ______

If there are no problems, the fist box should be ticked.

SIGN OUT (After the procedure)

☐ Name of the procedure recorded

☐ All sharps and diathermy pads disposed of safely

Any equipment issues identified? ☐No ☐Yes

Appropriate images retained ☐Yes ☐No

Any unexpected events/incidents ☐No ☐Yes

If yes, who will report this? ______

DATIX NUMBER ______

Has the patient been advised to restart anti-coagulation ☐N/A ☐Yes

HANDOVER TO PACU/WARD

☐ Procedure handed over

Intravenous medication given? ☐No ☐Yes

Hearing Aids/Glasses ☐No ☐Yes

Plan for VTE required/made ☐N/A ☐Yes

Any other concerns for recovery or ward? ☐No ☐Yes

______

Signature: ______

Designation: ______

Print: ______

Date: ______

Last updated: 31/08/17

Figure 15.1.1 Sample checklist for interventional pain management procedures
Reproduced courtesy of Surrey and Sussex NHS Trust

Performance of procedure

- Available resources and adherence to local/national guidelines to perform the treatment as per national safety standards
- Infection prevention and control
- Appropriate patient monitoring (ECG, BP, pulse oximetry, glycaemic levels, capnography). If patient requires general anaesthesia to have the care of an Anaesthetic Team with the appropriate resources and monitoring as per national safety standards
- Availability of required resources (cannulation equipment, IV fluids, vasoactive drugs, Intralipid®), and staff must be competent in advanced resuscitation
- Light sedation may be offered, where appropriate, for pain procedures if adequate facilities and support are available. The most commonly used agents are midazolam 1–2 mg, propofol 10–20 mg boluses, fentanyl 25–100 mcg, and alfentanil 0.25–1 mg.
- Generic equipment required:
  - Needles: 25G and 23G 38 mm hypodermic needles for skin and SC skin infiltration and specific needles for the procedure (e.g. spinal needles, Tuohy needles, Racz introducer needle and Racz catheter, regional block needles)
  - IV cannula as required
  - Imaging required for the procedure (fluoroscopy, CT, USS, MRI, or other). Contrast may be needed to determine the correct position of the needle with fluoroscopy and CT
  - LA:
    - Short-acting LA (e.g. lidocaine 1%) for skin/SC tissues
    - Injectate—low concentration to avoid motor block, but depends on procedure
    - Bupivacaine/levobupivacaine 0.1–0.5%, ropivacaine 0.2–1%, lidocaine 1% or other

- Adjuvants can be used in an attempt to prolong the duration of some blocks, such as steroids, but the benefit of steroids is not entirely clear at the time of the publication (e.g. methylprednisolone acetate 'Depo-Medrone®', triamcinolone 'Kenalog®', or non-particulate steroids such as dexamethasone). Other adjuvants that can be used are adrenaline bicarbonate and clonidine (for further information, see Chapters 6, 12, 13.8 Clonidine, p. 244)
- Clinicians should ensure that the documentation of procedures is consistent with recommendations of their National Pain Society (see Fig. 15.1.2)

Department of Pain Management
Operation Notes

Date:
First Name:
Surname:
Date of Birth:
Hospital:

Pain Consultant/Doctor:

Diagnosis:

Anaesthetist:

Procedure:		**Side**: Left/Right/Bilateral **Level** if applicable:
Venflon gauge:	22G / 20G / 18G / 16G	Venflon site:
Sedation:	yes/no	Midazolam_____mg; Fentanyl_____mcg; Propofol_____mg; Other _______________
Guidance:	Fluoroscopy / Ultrasound / None	
Position:	Supine / Prone / Lateral / Sitting	
Asepsis:	Cap / Mask / Gown / Gloves 0.5% Chlorhexidine / 2% Chlorhexidine / Betadine Air-dried: yes/no	
Local infiltration:	______mL of______% lidocaine	
Needle:	_____G Spinal/Insulated RF/Hypodermic/Tuohy/Block needle/NR Fit	
Contrast:	Omnipaque 240 / 300; yes / no; _________mL Niopam _________mL	
Local anaesthetic:	______mL of______%Bupivacaine / Lidocaine / Other_____	
Steroid:	______mg of Triamcinolone / Depo-Medrone / Dexamethasone	
Diluent:		

Postop care and Comments:
Spray / Dressing
Monitoring:
Home when safe and mobile
Discharge / Follow-up

Figure 15.1.2 Sample of procedure documentation

Post-procedure instructions

- Monitoring for S/Es of the intervention in a recovery area—ensure patients have normal lower limb function and are able to pass urine prior to discharge; a member of staff should support them when mobilizing after the procedure (e.g. standing up, walking to the toilet)
- Patients must have clear instructions and contact details, should they develop S/Es after discharge (in acute cases, the emergency department of the nearest acute hospital should be attended)
- Patients should be followed up and assessed post-procedure (e.g. by telephone or clinic appointment) (see Fig. 15.1.3). Reduction in pain severity or distribution and impact on QoL should be assessed, ideally with an outcome questionnaire (e.g. NRS and timeline, Oswestry Disability Index, HADS, BPI, PCS, PSEQ, Global Impression of outcome)

Dr ....
Dept of Pain Management

Patient Details

Protocol for evaluation of effect of the test block for a diagnostic investigation

Type of injection: ________________________________

Date: ________________________________

Pain Evaluation

Please indicate how much of your 'normal' pain you have left at every time interval as per the chart (0% means no pain and 100% means your pain is unchanged)

Please mark with an 'X' on the chart

	0% (no pain)	100% (worst pain)
Before the block 100%	◄	►
1 hour after block	◄	►
2 hours after block	◄	►
4 hours after block	◄	►
6 hours after block	◄	►
8 hours after block	◄	►
12 hours after block	◄	►
1 week after block	◄	►
2 weeks after block	◄	►

When did the pain return to your 'usual' level? Date: ________________

Figure 15.1.3 Sample of post-procedure self-evaluation questionnaire

Further reading

1. British Pain Society and Faculty of Pain Medicine of the Royal College of Anaesthetists. Standards of Good Practice for Spinal Interventional Procedures in Pain Medicine. 2020. https://www.britishpainsociety.org/static/uploads/resources/files/BPS_and_FPM_Spinal_Intervention_Guidelines_PDF_Final_May_2020_2_new_ISBN.pdf
2. General Medical Council. Consent: patients and doctors making decisions together. 2020. https://www.gmc-uk.org/-/media/documents/gmc-guidance-for-doctors---decision-making-and-consent-english_pdf-84191055.pdf
3. Academy of Medical Royal Colleges, Standards and Guidance. Safe sedation practice for healthcare procedures. 2016. https://www.aomrc.org.uk/wp-content/uploads/2016/05/Safe_Sedation_Practice_1213.pdf
4. Pain Spa. https://www.painspa.co.uk
5. Anaesthesia Advice. https://www.anaesthesia-advice.com
6. World Health Organization. https://www.who.int/teams/integrated-health-services/patient-safety/research/safe-surgery

15.2 Safety in interventional pain procedures

Introduction

- One of the best-known aphorisms in medical practice is 'Primum Non Nocere'—First Do No Harm—reflecting the basic fact that complications from medical care may sometimes overshadow the diseases they were meant to alleviate in the first place
- This is especially true in the practice of interventional pain medicine where complications in treating what is otherwise a non-life-threatening condition can have catastrophic implications for the patient, as well as for the treating physician
- In a closed claims study, Fitzgibbon and colleagues found 97% of closed claims in pain management malpractice suits were related to invasive procedures
- There are many potential adverse effects of these interventions, with the most feared complications being direct spinal cord or nerve injury (mostly in the setting of deep sedation), injury to critical blood supply (especially, but not limited to, spinal radicular arteries, anterior spinal artery and vertebral arteries, epidural haematomas resulting in spinal compression), infections, especially neuraxial infections, and pneumothorax
- Being mindful of the risks involved in interventional pain medicine and adopting a routine that incorporates the considerations outlined below into your daily practice will undoubtedly serve to protect both you and the patient from professional and personal tragedies

General considerations

- There are many factors that play a role in increasing the likelihood of complications from pain interventions
- These can be broadly divided into physician- (and other staff member), equipment- (errors, technical faults), and patient-related factors

Physician-related

- These include insufficient knowledge or experience of the physician, communication problems between staff members, and unawareness of institutional and expert panels' safety rules and regulations and recommendations

- More mundane factors, such as workload, tiredness, and lapses in concentration, may also play a major role in reducing procedural safety

Equipment-related

- There is a wide variety of technical aspects to interventional pain medicine, from the choice of specific needles for specific procedures (e.g. sharp versus blunt needles, straight versus curved needles) to more complex radiofrequency (RF) devices, spinal cord stimulators, and intrathecal pumps
- All have their own safety profiles, maintenance requirements, and recommended pre-procedural and intra-procedural safety checks
- Good knowledge of these and extreme care regarding their implementation are required from any professional conducting pain procedures

Patient-related

- Poor patient selection may be a crucial factor in local complication rates
- Elderly patients, complex medical comorbidities, polypharmacy, bleeding diatheses and pharmacological anticoagulation, immunosuppression, extreme obesity, diabetes, abnormal anatomy, complex physical disabilities, cognitive impairment, and previous complications or adverse reactions all significantly increase the risk of serious adverse effects from any interventional approach

Practical considerations

- By adhering to simple and rather common sense rules and adopting a safety-oriented working routine, it is possible to minimize the risk of severe complications and adverse events

Physician-related

- Keep updated and maintain your skills (this cannot be overstated)
- Never perform procedures with which you are not familiar and comfortable without expert supervision
- It is imperative that you possess some sort of formal training in the procedures you are performing (e.g. completion of a recognized fellowship programme, Fellow of Interventional Pain Practice (FIPP), Certified Interventional Pain Sonologist (CIPS) certification)
- Be informed of the latest recommendations/guidelines and act according to acceptable best practice, evidence, and safety guidelines of recognized professional organizations and expert opinions (e.g. do not use particulate steroid injections for transforaminal cervical injections, use blunt needles for certain procedures, etc.)
- Do not perform procedures when you are sleep-deprived, shortly after international travel across >3 time zones, or if you are unwell or unfit
- Never perform an interventional procedure based on a single plane view—you should always verify the needle position in two planes
- It is advisable to inject contrast and observe the run-off. If in doubt, take more images in different planes. You may also consider a test dose of lidocaine
- If you are still unsure, either adjust and reassess or abort
- When considering a complicated, unusual, or controversial procedure, always consult a colleague beforehand and document this in the patient's records
- Be extremely careful with every procedure in the upper body, especially head and neck procedures
- Sedation **significantly increases** the risk of serious complications and is to be avoided, if possible. Routine use of sedation for common procedures should be discouraged

- This is especially true for high-risk procedures, as mentioned earlier, and targeted interventions of the peripheral nerves
- **Remember**, a patient who talks is a patient who breathes and would also let you know if you inadvertently touch neural tissue
- Monitor patients for a sufficient period after the procedure (extend the monitoring period after a difficult procedure, an unusual patient reaction, or a prior history of complications, after giving large quantities of LAs, after head and neck procedures, or in at-risk patients)

Equipment-related

- Meticulously follow the maintenance and daily care instructions of your equipment. Store equipment only in conditions recommended by the manufacturer
- Never use equipment with which you are not familiar without supervision
- In devices with safety settings, make sure these are active
- Never use medications without first double-checking the expiry dates and doses administered
- Always have in hand adequate equipment to cope with a medical emergency. This is especially true for every procedure under sedation, every patient who is at risk, and every procedure in the head, neck, or thorax

Patient-related

- Patient selection and tailored preparation are vital. Familiarize yourself with the risk factors for interventional procedures as outlined earlier and in the literature
- Take a careful history, especially focusing on allergies, medical conditions, medications (especially anticoagulants and immunomodulators), food supplements, and previous procedures and complications. Make sure you make necessary adjustments of medications if required (e.g. steroid supplementation if steroid-dependent, changing insulin doses as required, stopping antiplatelet/anticoagulation if indicated, reducing high doses of opioids)
- If necessary, clear the procedure in advance with relevant consulting physicians
- Always consider whether you need to make specific adjustments for the patient's habitus (obesity or cachexia), abnormal anatomy (such as local tumour infiltration and anatomical variants), or specific limitations (e.g. inability to lie in a certain position for long periods)
- Patient education—make sure the patient understands the procedure, the alternatives, possible expected physiological implications (e.g. hyperglycaemia if steroids are given, diarrhoea in coeliac plexus block), and possible adverse events and their incidence
- If there is a need for translation, arrange for a translator and do not rely on poor language understanding or gesticulations
- After the procedure, make sure the patient understands post-operative care instructions (glucose blood monitoring, mobility, etc.). Take extra care to ensure the patient understands when he/she should seek medical advice
- Make sure to mark the body area you will be targeting and always double-check with the patient immediately prior to the procedure

Further reading

1. Benzon HT, Huntoon MA, Rathmell JP. Improving the safety of epidural steroid injections. JAMA 2015;313(17):1713–14
2. Fitzgibbon DR, Posner KL, Domino KB, et al. Chronic pain management: American Society of Anaesthesiologists Closed Claims Project. Anaesthesiology 2004;100:98–105

3. Wang LH, McKenzie-Brown AM, Hord A. The Handbook of C-Arm Fluoroscopy-Guided Spinal Injections. 1st edition, 2006. Boca Raton: CRC Press
4. Manchikanti L, Abdi S, Atluri S, et al. An update of comprehensive evidence-based guidelines for interventional techniques in chronic spinal pain. Part II: guidance and recommendations. Pain Physician 2013;16(2 Suppl):S49–283
5. Thampi SP, Rekhala V, Vontobel T, Nukula V. Patient safety in interventional pain procedures. Phys Med Rehabil Clin N Am 2012;23(2):423–32
6. Windsor RE, Storm S, Sugar R. Prevention and management of complications resulting from common spinal injections. Pain Physician 2003;6(4):473–83

15.3 Fluoroscopy, computed tomography, and ultrasound-guided procedures

Introduction

- Procedures for pain relief can be done using fluoroscopy (X-ray), CT, and US guidance for improved patient safety and outcomes

Fluoroscopy

Basic principles

- Use of X-ray radiation to visualize osseous structures
- Use of an emitter from which X-rays emerge and an image intensifier which transmits images to a processing module
- The X-ray generator is portable and C-arm-shaped, which allows for biplanar imaging of structures
- Key parameters include:
  - Voltage determining the strength of X-ray penetrability (e.g. 90 kV provides better penetration than 70 kV, but higher exposure to ionizing radiation)
  - Current determining the quantity of radiation, and hence image density
  - Magnification determining the size of the radiation cone

Advantages of fluoroscopy-guided interventions

- Familiarity with clinicians
- Good visualization of bony structures
- Ability to visualize the injectate by visualizing radio-opaque contrast to reduce iatrogenic complications and to deliver the treatment to the correct anatomical target

Disadvantages of fluoroscopy-guided interventions

- Lack of visualization of soft tissues such as blood vessels, nerves, visceral membranes, and other structures
- Two-dimensional views—therefore, several views from different angles are needed
- Exposure to ionizing radiation for both patients and staff
- Bulky and difficult-to-move equipment

Ultrasound

Basic principles

- Based on sound waves transmitted from, and received by, the US transducer
- Transducers contain a piezoelectric crystal and when a current is applied across the crystal, it will expand and contract as the polarity of the voltage changes

- The speed of sound in tissue varies and sound waves are reflected at different tissue interfaces
- Sound absorption is directly proportional to the frequency of the US beam, and therefore, high-frequency probes give good resolution but lack penetration
- The operator may use an in-plane or out-of-plane approach
- A hyperechoic (brighter) image is seen at a tissue interface with different acoustic impedance, e.g. soft tissue to bone
- A hypoechoic (darker) image is seen across tissues with similar acoustic impedance, e.g. muscle and fat

Advantages of ultrasound-guided interventions

- Visualization of nerves, arteries, and veins
- Real-time visualization
- No ionizing radiation
- Portability
- Good resolution of MSK tissue, and therefore can be used for TPIs
- Visualization of peripheral nerves has led to increasing use in regional anaesthesia and improved operator skills
- Can see diffusion of injectate without use of radio-opaque contrast
- Uses less personnel and resources
- Evidence of superiority for regional procedures, compared to landmark technique (precision and safety)
- Safety and accuracy of USS guided procedures can be increased by the use of a nerve stimulator attached to the needle

Disadvantages of ultrasound-guided interventions

- Cannot visualize past bone
- Difficulty with obese patients or increased tissue depth
- Operator-dependent

Computed tomography

Basic principles

- Three-dimensional imaging technique with rotating radiation beam
- Produces several cross-sectional images

Advantages of CT-guided interventions

- Excellent spatial resolution and soft tissue contrast
- Low chance of vessel, nerve, or visceral injury
- Useful in patients with complex or difficult anatomy
- Reducing the body area scanned and intermittent scanning can reduce radiation
- Shows precise location of needle tip and surrounding structures

Disadvantages of CT-guided interventions

- Lack of space, facilities, or expertise
- Higher doses of radiation for patient and staff

- Cumulative radiation may be an issue if repeat injections are needed instead of a single diagnostic block
- Oblique angle of injection or increased depth to skin surface may increase the difficulty of the procedure due to needle placement difficulty
- Expense, skill, patient claustrophobia, availability of staff and equipment may be a hindrance

Further reading

1. Brandner B, Nagaratnam M. Interventional techniques for chronic pain. In: Dickman A, Simpson KH. Chronic Pain (Oxford Pain Management Library). 2008; Chapter 8: 1–28. Oxford: Oxford University Press.
2. Carty S, Nicholls B. Ultrasound-guided regional anaesthesia. Contin Educ Anaesth Crit Care Pain 2007;7(1):20–4
3. Malajikian K, Finelli D. Basics of computed tomography. In: Narouze SN (ed). Multimodality Imaging Guidance in Interventional Pain Management. 2016; pp. 38–74. Oxford: Oxford University Press. http://oxfordmedicine.com/view/10.1093/med/9780199908004.001.0001/med-9780199908004-chapter-3
4. Nader A, John G, Kendall M. Basics of Ultrasound. In: Narouze SN (ed). Multimodality Imaging Guidance in Interventional Pain Management. 2016; pp. 25–37. Oxford: Oxford University Press. http://oxfordmedicine.com/view/10.1093/med/9780199908004.001.0001/med-9780199908004-chapter-2
5. Patel V. Basics of fluoroscopy. In: Narouze SN (ed). Multimodality Imaging Guidance in Interventional Pain Management. 2016; pp. 3–24. Oxford: Oxford University Press. http://oxfordmedicine.com/view/10.1093/med/9780199908004.001.0001/med-9780199908004-chapter-1
6. Simpson G, Nicholls B. Use of ultrasound in chronic pain medicine. Part 1: neuraxial and sympathetic blocks. Contin Educ Anaesth Crit Care Pain 2013;13(5):145–51

15.4 Chemical neurolysis

Introduction

- The purpose of chemical neurolysis is to cause an irreversible disruption to neural transmission. This should induce changes of Wallerian degeneration and produce long-lasting impact on the neural fibres
- The irreversible nature of the changes produced means that any S/Es caused by chemical neurolysis need to be carefully considered
- Chemical neurolysis may occur in the context of different patient factors and anatomical locations, and a variety of agents/concentrations can be used
- The advantage of some chemical neurolytic procedures is that a one-off procedure can provide a long duration of pain relief
- Neurolysis can also be performed with surgery, RF, or cryotherapy

Patient factors

- The patient will need to give informed consent prior to having a procedure involving neurolysis
- The patient should have tried conservative strategies such as medications or temporary nerve blockade

- Patient comorbidities, such as cardiac disease, clotting disorders, and others, may affect the safety, potential S/Es, and patient tolerability
- The procedure should be performed in an appropriately monitored environment and where potential complications can be managed
- Chemical neurolysis is mostly used in a palliative care setting in patients with limited life expectancy

Location

- Chemical neurolysis may be performed in the CNS or peripheral nervous system
- Intrathecal neurolysis may be used in complex cancer pain management:
  - Phenol or alcohol can be used, depending on the spread of the disease, given the hyperbaricity of phenol and the hypobaricity of alcohol
  - S/Es may include deafferentation, neuropathic pain, motor or sensory loss, arachnoiditis, and bowel and bladder dysfunction
- Commonly performed peripheral blocks using chemical neurolysis include:
  - Coeliac plexus block to treat upper abdominal visceral pain, with success reported in pancreatic cancer management. Alcohol may be preferred to phenol due to its greater ability to diffuse into target tissues and lesser affinity for vascular tissues. Some clinicians prefer to use phenol as it is not painful when injected
  - Superior hypogastric plexus blocks are used in managing gynaecological cancer pain

Agents used

- Phenol—6–10% concentration
- Alcohol—33–100% concentration
- Glycerol—reports of relieving pain for trigeminal neuralgia
- Ammonium salts—preferential effect on C-fibres, with minimal effect on A-fibres, but overall efficacy is questionable

Patient position

- Patient position during the procedure will affect the spread of the agent
- It is recommended the patient stays in a certain position for around 45 minutes after the procedure, to allow the agent to affect the specific target structures

Post-procedure care

- The patient should be monitored for S/Es, depending on the procedure, and given instructions on discharge
- Patients should be reviewed post-procedure
- Should the patient experience a significant degree of pain relief, medications such as opioids can be carefully downtitrated. After some neurolytic procedures, opioids can be decreased immediately by 30–50%

Further reading

1. Scott-Warren J, Bhaskar A. Cancer pain management: part II: interventional techniques. Contin Educ Anaesth Crit Care Pain 2015;15(2):68–72
2. Sharma M, Simpson K, Bennett M, Gupta S. Practical Management of Complex Cancer Pain (Oxford Specialist Handbooks in Pain Medicine). 2014. Oxford: Oxford University Press

15.5 Radiation and Ionising radiation (medical exposure) regulations

Introduction

- Radiation is a serious risk factor, making it important to know the basic guidelines of radiology to ensure the safety of the operators, staff and patients
- The first fluoroscopy device was developed by Thomas Edison and other scientists, and introduced in 1900

Physics

- Radiation is the dispersion of energy through electromagnetic waves or particles
- Radiation ionizes the atom by breaking off the electrons from their orbits—ionizing radiation consists of charged particles
- Electromagnetic energy is a type of energy radiating at light speed in the form of sine wave
- An X-ray is a typical electromagnetic radiation
- X-rays have shorter wavelengths and higher frequencies, and have higher energy levels

Fluoroscopy

- Fluoroscopy is a live imaging technique using X-rays
- The components are: a radiography tube which provides the source of energy to produce X-rays; an attached filter which modifies the X-ray energy spectrum; a collimator that restricts the focus area; an anti-scatter grid reducing the number of photons scattering on the image receptor; an image receptor; and an image intensifier

Units used for radiation exposure and dose

- Exposure units in Roentgen (R) and in SI units Coulomb/kg
- Radiation absorbed dose (RAD) and in SI unit Gray (Gy)
- 100 RAD = 1 Gy
- Radiation Equivalent in Man (REM) and in SI unit Sievert (Sv)
- Sievert—quantified biological effect of ionizing radiations
- 100 REM = 1 Sv
- For X-rays, 1 Sv = 1 Gy
- X-ray chest ≈ 0.02 mSv
- CT abdomen/pelvis ≈ 11 mSv (550 X-ray chest)
- Annual Maximum Permissible Radiation Doses (see Table 15.5.1)
- Minimum target organ radiation doses to produce organ pathologic effects (see Table 15.5.2)

Table 15.5.1 Annual maximum permissible radiation doses

	mSv	REM
Thyroid	0.5	50
Extremities	0.5	50
Eye lens	0.15	15
Gonads	0.5	50
Whole body	0.05	5
Pregnancy (to fetus)	0.0005	0.5

Table 15.5.2 Minimum target organ radiation doses to produce organ pathologic effects

	RAD	Gy
Eye lens (cataract)	200	2
Skin burns (acute)	300	3
Sterility	400	4
Skin (erythema)	500	5
Permanent alopecia	700	7
Whole body (haemopoietic failure) (4–6 weeks)	200–700	2–7

Factors affecting X-ray quality

- Penetration capability depends on X-ray energy, filtration, distance, and structure of the X-ray tube anode
- X-ray energy can be increased by increasing the power supply (voltage)

Scattered radiation

- Scattered rays from the primary substance; occurs as a result of collision of electrons
- Secondary radiation occurs when scattered X-ray radiation passes through an object. The patient becomes the primary source of scattered radiation during exposure time

Fluoroscopy usage types

- Continuous fluoroscopy, which is the most dangerous in terms of radiation safety
- High-speed fluoroscopy, used where normal fluoroscopy is inadequate
- Pulsed fluoroscopy, with image speed and frames per second rate; the most preferable format

Effects of radiation

1. Direct (definitive/deterministic) effect: evident with the result of dying cells. It can occur with high linear energy transfers (LETs) and the ratio of dying cells increases with increased radiation doses. Associated with cataract, infertility, hair loss, and skin issues
2. Indirect (cytoplastic/stochastic) effect: the severity of the effects is unrelated to the dose of radiation exposure. It can occur with low LETs via production of free radicals, and doses used for radiation are additive. Cytoplastic effects of radiation may cause mutagenic effects such as cancer and leukaemia. Radiation causes neuroplasticity, which initiates DNA damage. Cancer risk is higher at extremes of age and in females
3. Acute effect: can occur within hours to days after high doses of radiation exposure, even for a brief period, causing cell death
4. Haemopoietic cells are the most affected by radiation exposure as they have a replication rate, followed by cells of the reproductive system, then the GI system, and lastly by nerves and muscles

Radiation safety

There are three basic rules to be considered for radiation protection: time, distance, and use of protective material.

- Hold the X-ray tube low: the X-ray tube should be kept under the table or patient, so that the scattered beam is pointed downwards

Table 15.5.3 DAP and screening time

	DAP (Gy/cm^2)	Screening time (s)
Lumbar medial branch blocks	2.5	60
Sacroiliac joint injection	1.63	43

- To keep away from the source of radiation: one should stand 3m away from the table to reduce the beam level
- Consider the scattering profile: using thyroid-protective lead and special lead-sided protective glasses may protect from scattered beam
- Wear protective lead
- Track the beam dose and time. The dose–area product (DAP) and screening time should be kept to a minimum. There are no standards, but a rough guide, for example, could be as mentioned in Table 15.5.3

- Save the last image
- Use the pulse mode, rather than continuous screening
- Limit the beam size (collimation)
- The source should be close to the object to reduce scatter; avoid magnification
- The device should undergo regular technical checks

Personal radiation measurement devices

- Dosimeters are devices carried by personnel who work with radiation to determine radiation exposure—best worn on the chest pocket under the apron

IRMER (Ionising Radiation (Medical Exposure) Regulations 2017)

- The main aim is to achieve exposure 'as low as reasonably practical' (ALARP)
- Practitioner—takes responsibility/justification for individual exposure
- Operator—is responsible for the delivery of radiation and its practical aspects
- Referrer—is responsible for providing adequate medical information to the practitioner to help them decide whether the necessary radiation exposure will be beneficial or not

Summary

- Fluoroscopy is a highly essential technique for interventional pain procedures; however, it can bring many risks and dangers with it
- One must be very careful when using fluoroscopy, used for the shortest possible time and ALARP
- All pain physicians should have radiation safety training and all exposure should always be justified

Further reading

1. Lichtherte S, le Polain de Waroux B. Diagnostic reference levels for X-ray investigations in pain management units in Belgium. Radiat Prot Dosimetry 2012;150(4):520–2

2. Hanu Cernat D, Duarte R, Raphael JH, et al. Type of interventional pain procedure, body weight and presence of spinal pathology are determinants of the level of radiation exposure for fluoroscopically guided pain procedures. Pain Practice 2012;12(6):434–9
3. Taylor J, Chandramohan M, Simpson K. Radiation for the anaesthetist. Contin Educ Anaesth Crit Care Pain 2013;13(2):59–62

15.6 Radiofrequency denervation

Introduction

- Kirschner introduced percutaneous current lesions in 1931 for the treatment of patients with trigeminal neuralgia
- Its use became further established in 1950s and 1960s

Physics

- The RF voltage from the generator is set up between the (active) electrode and the (dispersive) ground plate, which is placed on a non-hairy part of the body
- RF current flows through the tissue, resulting in an electric field through the circuit completed within the body
- This creates an electric force on the ions in tissue electrolytes, causing them to oscillate at a high rate
- Frictional dissipation of the ionic current within the fluid medium causes tissue heating, producing a lesion

Mechanism of action

- The heat generated in the nerve cells at the electrode tip causes coagulation, which is believed to interrupt pain conduction
- Large lesion size is known to improve efficacy. This depends on the diameter of the electrode and the length of the uninsulated electrode tip

Technique

- The RF needle is placed under fluoroscopic guidance, with the tip lying parallel and adjacent to the nerve tissue in order to create the largest lesion
- Cooled RF and Trident needles have an end-on needle position

Indications

- Percutaneous cervical cordotomy:
  - In unilateral, incident, and/or neurogenic pain in advanced cancer patients
  - Lateral approach through the C1–C2 intervertebral space: a 22G RF needle with a 2 mm active tip is placed in the spinothalamic tract in the spinal cord, followed by sensory (cold or warm sensation) and motor stimulation and RF ablation
  - An RF lesion is made, resulting in a tip temperature of 90°C for 10 seconds
- Trigeminal neuralgia:
  - In drug-resistant cases and where microvascular decompression is not indicated or not possible
  - A 22G RF needle with a 2 mm active tip is placed in the foramen ovale through the cheek musculature

- A sensory stimulation threshold below 0.2 V is achieved and an RF lesion of 60–65°C for 60 seconds is made. Long-term success rates vary from 80% to 90%
- Anaesthesia dolorosa has made balloon decompression a preferred option

- Cluster headache:
  - Sphenopalatine ganglion RF ablation is performed by laterally placing the needle through the triangle formed by the zygoma and the muscular and articular processes of the mandible
  - Paraesthesiae should not be felt at <1.0 V and an RF lesion is achieved at 80°C for 60 seconds
  - In episodic cluster headache, complete pain relief has been achieved in 60% of patients, and in chronic cluster headache in 30% of patients
- Lumbo-sacral pain:
  - Following a positive medial branch block for facet joint pain, an 18G RF needle with a 10 mm curved tip is placed in a caudal to cranial and a lateral to medial position, with an angle from the midline of 60° at the junction of the transverse process and the superior articular process
  - After advancing the RF needle to the posterior foraminal line, motor stimulation is used (<1 V) to confirm multifidus stimulation and no radicular stimulation
  - An RF lesion is obtained at 80°C for 60 seconds, and the needle rotated to repeat the lesion
  - Extensive literature has led the Spine Intervention Society (SIS) and the National Institute for Health and Care Excellence (NICE) to recommend RF denervation for pain relief of 12 months or longer. The NNT is between 1.1 and 1.5
  - For SIJ denervation, a palisade technique of multiple needles or a single needle (Simplicity™ RF cannula) is used to create a lesion at the lateral border of the S1, S2, and S3 foramen for the lateral branches of the corresponding dorsal rami, along with an L5 dorsal ramus lesion
- Cervical facetogenic pain and cervicogenic headache:
  - Following a positive medial branch block, a 22G or 18G RF needle with a 5 mm or 10 mm active tip is placed under fluoroscopic guidance parallel to and on the articular pillar (across the C2–3 facet joint for the third occipital nerve)
  - Several RCTs and well-designed studies have demonstrated pain relief of up to 422 days in over 70% of patients
- Abdominal pain:
  - A splanchnic RF lesion is created at T12 or L1 after a positive diagnostic LA injection
  - A 20G, 15 cm, RF needle with a 10 mm active tip is placed overlying the side of the vertebral body at the junction of the lower and middle third of the vertebra, after the spinous processes are projected over the facetal joint column on the opposite side
  - The needle tip is advanced to the anterior border of the vertebral body
  - Following sensory stimulation of up to 2 V, an RF lesion is created at 80°C for 60 seconds
- Lower limb pain with autonomic dysfunction:
  - Lumbar sympathetic ganglion RF is performed at L3 and L4 levels in a fashion similar to splanchnic RF

Further reading

1. Kapural L, Mekhail N. Radiofrequency ablation for chronic pain control. Curr Pain Headache Rep 2001;5:517–25. https://doi.org/10.1007/s11916-001-0069-z

2. Crul BJ, Van Zundert JHM, Van Kleef M. Radiofrequency lesioning and treatment of chronic pain. In: Breivik H, Campbell WI, Nicholas MK (eds). Clinical pain management - Practice and procedures. 2nd edition, 2008; pp. 389–403. London: Hodder Arnold
3. International Spine Intervention Society. Lumbar medial branch blocks. In: Bogduk N (ed.). Practice guidelines for spinal diagnostic and treatment procedures. 2nd edition, 2013; pp. 457–488. San Francisco, CA: International Spine Intervention Society
4. Cohen SP, Bhaskar A, Bhatia A et al. Consensus practice guidelines on interventions for lumbar facet joint pain from a multispecialty, international working group.

   Regional Anesthesia & Pain Medicine. Published Online: 03 April 2020. doi: 10.1136/rapm-2019-101243

15.7 Pulsed radiofrequency

Introduction

- First PRF procedure performed on a lumbar DRG in February 1996

Physics

- PRF applies short pulses of RF signals from an RF generator to the tissue through an insulated needle with an exposed active tip of 5 mm or 10 mm
- A commonly used sequence is a pulse frequency of 2 Hz and a pulse width of 20 ms per 500 ms, permitting 480 ms of silent phase
- The RF oscillation frequency is about 420 kHz, which is the same as for conventional RF
- In PRF, because the pulse duration is only a small percentage of the time between pulses, the average tissue temperature rise for the same RF voltage is much less and the production of heat during these pulses depends on the power deposition
- Higher voltages can be applied to the electrode in PRF than are commonly used in RF without raising the average tissue temperature into the denaturation range of above 45°C
- However, as the electric fields wane rapidly with increasing distance from the tip, there is very little destruction to the tissue

Mechanism of action

- Neuromodulatory effect by alteration in synaptic transmission
- The low frequency of pulses and high voltages induce long-term depression of synaptic transmission at the spinal cord, and antagonizes the long-term potentiation that leads to chronic pain states
- Ion channel disruption and resting and threshold potential alterations are other possible effects

Technique

- A needle is placed under image guidance, with the exposed tip adjacent to the neural tissue

Indications

- Radicular pain:
  - PRF was compared to conventional RF at 42°C for patients with lumbo-sacral radicular pain. The global perceived effect was significantly better in the PRF group
  - In a prospective cohort study of 65 patients, the reduction in NRS and Oswestry Disability Index was statistically significant, compared to the baseline

    - Cervical DRG was studied in one RCT and PRF was shown to be more effective than placebo at 3 months' follow-up
    - In two observational studies, it had >50% pain reduction in >60% of patients. This effect appeared to be sustained at 1-year follow-up
    - PRF adjacent to the cervical DRG is recommended due to the high risk of transforaminal steroids in the cervical region
    - It could be considered for the treatment of lumbo-sacral radicular pain
- Trigeminal neuralgia:
    - PRF of the Gasserian ganglion could be an alternative, with fewer S/Es; unlike conventional ablative treatments that can cause anaesthesia dolorosa or hypoaesthesia
    - The duration of effect may be somewhat shorter than that of conventional RF; however, repeat intervention seems to have comparable results as the initial one
- Occipital neuralgia:
    - In an RCT of 81 patients, pain reduction was significantly greater in the PRF group, compared with the steroid group; this persisted through the 6 months' follow-up. S/Es were minor and transient in both groups, which makes PRF a useful option
- Shoulder pain:
    - In three RCTs and four observational studies, treatment lasted for 6 months. The effect of PRF on the suprascapular nerve was better than that of sham intervention and comparable to TENS
- Knee pain:
    - Intra-articular, DRG, and peripheral nerve (femoral, saphenous, common peroneal, tibial) and plexuses (peripatellar, subsartorial, and popliteal) have been studied and the results are mixed
    - PRF of sensory nerves should be preferred for the treatment of neuropathic pain, while avoiding neuroma formation and deafferentation pain induced by ablative techniques

Further reading

1. Vanneste T, Van Lantschoot A, Van Boxem K, et al. Pulsed radiofrequency in chronic pain. Curr Opin Anaesthesiol 2017;30(5):577–82
2. Chua NHL, Vissers KC, Sluijter ME. Pulsed radiofrequency treatment in interventional pain management: mechanisms and potential indications—a review. Acta Neurochir (Wien) 2011;153(4):763–71. https://doi-org.proxy.library.rcsi.ie/10.1007/s00701-010-0881-5

CHAPTER 16

Head and Neck

Ann-Katrin Fritz and Jan Rudiger

CONTENTS

16.1 Cranial nerves

Importance of good anatomical knowledge

- Basic functions of cranial nerves (CNs)
- Examination techniques of CNs
- To assess and treat pain conditions involving CNs

Olfactory nerve (I)—sensory

- Function: smell
- Test with coffee and cinnamon

Optic nerve (II)—sensory

- Function: vision (via retina and optic disc)
- Test: visual acuity, colour, fields; light and accommodation reflex; fundoscopy

Oculomotor nerve (III)—motor, parasympathetic

- Function: movement of eyeball (inferior, medial, and superior via inferior, medial, and superior rectus muscles, inferior oblique muscle), eyelid movement (levator palpebrae superioris muscle)
- Parasympathetic preganglionic fibres: accommodation and pupillary light reflexes (via pupillary sphincter and ciliary muscles from the Edinger–Westphal nucleus)
- Test: gaze, accommodation, rule out double vision

Trochlear nerve (IV)—motor

- Function: motor movement via the superior oblique muscle (to depress and internally rotate the eyeball)
- Test: eye movement (vertical diplopia, worse when looking down and inwards), head tilt (away from affected side)

- Clinical relevance: microvascular damage (diabetes, hypertension), congenital, thrombophlebitis of sinus cavernosus, raised ICP

Trigeminal nerve (V)—largest cranial nerve with three divisions, mixed

- Ophthalmic nerve (V1)—sensory:
  - Function: sensation to superior face and anterior scalp
  - Test: touch to forehead on each side with cotton wool
  - Additional test: corneal reflex (afferent component)
- Maxillary nerve (V2)—sensory:
  - Function: sensation to midface, including maxillary sinus, upper teeth, and gum
  - Test: touch to cheeks with cotton wool
- Mandibular nerve (V3)—sensory + motor:
  - Function: sensation to lower face, including lower teeth and gums
  - Test: touch to cheeks with cotton wool
  - Additional test: temporalis and masseter muscle function (bulk, ability to open the mouth against resistance and jaw jerk)
- Clinical relevance:
  - Trigeminal neuralgia (usually unilateral) or MS (can be bilateral)

Abducens nerve (VI)—motor

- Function: motor supply of lateral rectus muscle
- Test: eye abduction

Facial nerve (VII)—mixed

- Function: facial expression, taste, salivation, lacrimation, corneal reflex
- Sensory (taste): anterior two-thirds of the tongue (via chorda tympani)
- Motor supply to orbicularis oculi, ear muscles, buccinator muscle, lips, chin, and platysma
- Parasympathetic fibres to salivary and lacrimal glands and mucosal glands
- Test: try to open the eyes against active lid closure, showing the teeth, creasing up the forehead, puff out the cheeks against resistance, corneal reflex (efferent part)
- Clinical relevance: Bell's palsy

Vestibulocochlear nerve = auditory nerve (VIII)—sensory

- Function: hearing and balance
- Test: sound (snapping fingers next to the ear; Weber's and Rinne's tests)
- Clinical relevance: neurofibromatosis type 2

Glossopharyngeal nerve (XI)—mixed

- Function: sensation, taste, motor, carotid body and sinus, parotid gland
- Sensory: pharynx, tonsils, soft palate, and posterior third of the tongue
- Taste: posterior third of the tongue
- Motor: stylopharyngeus muscle
- Parasympathetic: parotid gland
- Test: gag reflex
- Clinical relevance: glossopharyngeal neuralgia

Vagus nerve (X)—mixed

- Function: sensory, taste, autonomic
- Sensory: external ear, larynx, pharynx, taste between the epiglottis and the tongue
- Motor: vocal cords via recurrent laryngeal nerve (left side crosses the aortic arch), most muscles of the larynx and pharynx, and smooth muscles of GI tract
- Parasympathetic supply to thoracic and abdominal visceral organs (cardiac, pulmonary, gastric, hepatic, and coeliac plexus)
- Test: swallowing, speech, and symmetry of the uvula
- Clinical relevance: vagal nerve stimulation for treatment of cluster headaches

Accessory nerve (XI)—motor

- Function: motor supply to sternocleidomastoid and trapezius muscle
- Test: shrugging the shoulders and turn the head against resistance
- Clinical relevance: torticollis (neurovascular compression), winging of the shoulder blade, and secondary shoulder pain

Hypoglossal nerve (XII)—motor

- Function: motor supply to intrinsic and extrinsic tongue muscles (except palatoglossal muscle)
- Test: tongue muscle wasting, fasciculation, and symmetry

Further reading

1. Medistudents. Cranial nerve examination. 2018. https://www.medistudents.com/osce-skills/cranial-nerve-examination
2. Sanders C. Summary of the cranial nerves. 2019. https://teachmeanatomy.info/head/cranial-nerves/summary/

16.2 Anatomy of the trigeminal nerve and trigeminal ganglion block

Anatomy of the trigeminal nerve (fifth cranial nerve)

- Largest cranial nerve with large sensory and small motor roots
- Majority of sensory supply to the face, orbit, nose, and mouth
- Three divisions (V1 and V2—purely sensory; V3—sensory and motor)
- Each division has parasympathetic fibres to glands
- Trigeminal ganglion = Gasserian ganglion

V1—ophthalmic branch

- Through the superior orbital fissure
- Branches: frontal, lacrimal, nasociliary
- Sensory: forehead and scalp, upper eyelid, conjunctiva + cornea, frontal and ethmoid sinuses, dorsum of the nose (small branches to the dura)
- Parasympathetic: lacrimal gland

V2—maxillary branch

- Through the foramen rotundum (posterior to the pterygopalatine fossa)
- 14 terminal branches
- Sensory: lower eyelid and conjunctiva, cheeks, maxillary sinus, nasal cavity and lateral nose, upper lip, upper teeth + gingiva, superior palate
- Parasympathetic: lacrimal gland, nasal glands

V3—mandibular branch

- Through the foramen ovale
- Four terminal branches: buccal, inferior alveolar, auriculotemporal, lingual
- Sensory: mucosa and floor of oral cavity, external ear, lower lip, chin, lower teeth and gingiva, sensation to anterior two-thirds of the tongue (taste via chorda tympani of the facial nerve)
- Parasympathetic: parotid, submandibular, sublingual glands
- Motor supply: muscles of mastication (masseter, temporal, medial, and lateral pterygoid muscles) and tensor veli palatini, tensor tympani, mylohyoid, and anterior belly of digastric muscles

All three branches

- All three divisions form the trigeminal ganglion (Gasserian ganglion), which lies on the floor of the middle cranial fossa of the skull
- The trigeminal nuclear complex is located in the midbrain, pons, medulla, and upper cervical cord as far as C4
- Three sensory trigeminal nuclei (spinal nucleus—pain conduction), one motor nucleus (lies in the pons)
- *1st ON:* noxious stimuli to the face → main trigeminal nuclei and spinal nucleus (clenching of jaw, chattering of teeth)
- *2nd ON:* spinal nuclei—crosses the midline → thalamus (trigeminal thalamic tract) (vulnerable to pressure at the edge of the dura mater, e.g. meningioma, trauma)
- *3rd ON:* thalamic nuclei → somatosensory cortex, insula, cingulate cortex

Trigeminal ganglion block

Indications

- Trigeminal neuralgia (tic douloureux)—therapy-refractory
- Atypical trigeminal neuralgia
- Intractable chronic cluster headaches
- Herpes zoster
- Chronic idiopathic facial pain
- Cancer-related pain palliation

Contraindications

- Patient refusal
- Increased ICP
- Local or systemic infection
- Coagulopathy, thrombocytopenia, or inability to stop anticoagulation drugs
- Distorted or complicated anatomy
- Immunocompromised patients (e.g. facial malignancies) → high risk of infection
- Untreated severe psychopathology

Patient preparation and positioning

- Anaesthetic assessment as conscious sedation is required
- Review of potential anticoagulation drug use or possible risk of thrombocytopenia or coagulopathy
- Patient positioned supine, with head on radiolucent head ring, with IV access and full Association of Anaesthetists of Great Britain and Ireland (AAGBI) monitoring
- Conscious sedation by anaesthetic colleague with supplemental oxygen
- Prophylactic antibiotic administration may be indicated to reduce risk of meningitis

Technique (PRF/RF lesioning)

- Skin preparation, with ipsilateral eye closed and careful draping
- Posteroanterior (PA) view with square nasal septum
- 25–30° caudal tilt for submental view
- Oblique ipsilaterally by 20–30° to get the foramen ovale into view just medial to the ramus of the mandible (lemon-shaped)
- Mark skin entry point about 2 cm lateral to the angle of the mouth
- Anaesthetize the skin with a 25G needle and lidocaine
- Gradually advance a 10 cm 22G RF needle with a 5 mm straight tip towards the foramen ovale, with intermittent fluoroscopy
- Once the needle is engaged in soft tissue, change to lateral view for depth indication
- Further advance the needle to aim for the angle produced by the clivus and petrous portion of the temporal bone
- Recheck the oblique view to confirm the needle advancing towards the medial or middle third of the foramen ovale
- Advance the needle through the foramen ovale on lateral view, making sure the needle tip stays below the clivus
- Remove the stylet and aspirate
- CSF leak may occur if the dural layer surrounding the ganglion is pierced with a sharp needle and the tip positioned in the trigeminal cistern; this will need repositioning only if injection of medication is planned
- Reposition the needle if blood occurs—abort the procedure if blood is aspirated despite repositioning of the needle twice

Thermal rhizotomy

- Sensory test at 100 Hz 0.1–0.5 V (elicits paraesthesiae in affected area)
- Motor test at 2 Hz up to 2 V—mandibular contractions (motor branch)
- 1 mL of LA ± 2 mg of dexamethasone—wait for 1 minute
- Lesioning at 60°C with sedation for 60 seconds
- Recheck sensory response and also corneal reflex (V1) in awake patient
- Repeat in 5°C increments to a maximum of 80°C

Complications

- Bleeding
- Retrobulbar haematoma
- Meningitis

- Local infection
- High spinal (if LA injected)
- Anaesthesia dolorosa up to 4%
- Corneal anaesthesia, hypoaesthesia, keratitis, and ulceration
- Masseter weakness after lesioning of V3

Additional information

- Sensory loss of the treated division is to be expected as a S/E in up to 98% (needs to be explained to the patient and documented prior to chemical or thermal lesioning)
- Injection of LA despite a CSF leak could lead to a high spinal block
- If masseter contraction is seen on motor testing, the needle may be advanced a bit further (check lateral view) prior to RF lesioning
- Avoid entering other foramina: inferior orbital fissure (superiorly), foramen lacerum with carotid artery (postero-medially), and jugular foramen and carotid canal (postero-inferiorly)

Further reading

1. Gauci CA. Manual of RF Techniques. 3rd edition, 2011. Ridderkerk, NL: CoMedical
2. Pazhaniappan N. The trigeminal nerve (CN V). 2020. https://teachmeanatomy.info/head/cranial-nerves/trigeminal-nerve/
3. Kanpolat Y, Savas A, Bekar A, Berk C. Percutaneous controlled radiofrequency trigeminal rhizotomy for the treatment of idiopathic trigeminal neuralgia: 25-year experience with 1,600 patients. Neurosurgery 2001;48(3):524–32

16.3 Sphenopalatine ganglion block

Anatomy of the sphenopalatine ganglion (SPG) = pterygopalatine ganglion

- Large extracranial ganglion (5 mm in size) located in the pterygopalatine fossa (1 cm-wide and 2 cm-high pyramidal structure)
- Complex neural centre, parasympathetic ganglion
- Efferent portion of the trigeminal autonomic reflex

Sensory supply

- Two sphenopalatine branches of the maxillary nerve supply the SPG; most fibres pass directly into the palatine nerves, while a few enter the ganglion

Sympathetic supply

- Post-ganglionic fibres come from the superior cervical ganglion via the carotid plexus and deep petrosal nerves and the greater petrosal nerves to the SPG

Parasympathetic supply

- Preganglionic innervation comes from the superior salivary nucleus of the facial nerve in the pons through the greater petrosal nerve
- In the SPG, the preganglionic fibres synapse with the post-ganglionic fibres

- Post-ganglionic fibres (vasodilator and secretory fibres) travel with the deep branches of the maxillary trigeminal nerve to the mucosa of the nose, soft palate, tonsils, uvula, roof of the mouth, upper lip and gums, and upper part of the pharynx
- Post-ganglionic fibres via the maxillary trigeminal nerve to the nasal, palatine, and pharyngeal glands
- Further post-ganglionic fibres via the zygomatic nerve and lacrimal nerve (ophthalmic nerve) to the lacrimal gland

Branches of the SPG

1. Orbital branches (ethmoid and sphenoidal sinuses, mucosal glands)
2. Posterior superior and inferior nasal branches (nasal cavity and glands, upper part of the septum)
3. Nasopalatine nerve (frontal part of the palate, palatine glands, and mucosa of the upper incisors and canines)
4. Greater and lesser palatine nerves (nasal cavity; gums, mucosa, and glands of the hard and soft palate)
5. Pharyngeal nerve (pharyngeal mucosa and glands)

Indications for SPG block

- Potential benefits must outweigh risks due to the invasive nature of the procedure
- Intractable, medically resistant pain to conventional treatment (e.g. medication, Botox® injections, greater occipital nerve (GON) block) for:
  - Cluster headache, chronic persistent migraine, trigeminal autonomic cephalgias
  - Intractable orofacial pain syndromes and atypical facial pain
  - Herpes zoster in the ophthalmic division of the trigeminal nerve

Contraindications

- Patient's refusal or inability to obtain consent
- Localized or systemic infection
- Coagulopathy or thrombocytopenia
- LA allergy
- Distorted or complicated anatomy (e.g. after surgery, infection)
- Immunocompromised patients (facial malignancies) due to high risk of infection
- No clear causation between anatomy and symptoms

Patient preparation and positioning

- Consent, including detailed explanation of all potential complications
- Review medication, and rule out anticoagulation and potential allergies to skin prep and injectate
- Examine the area of injection for potential infection
- IV access, full monitoring, trained assistant, and resuscitation equipment
- Positioning: supine with head ring, head in the C-arm

Technique (infra-zygomatic anterior or coronoid approach) under fluoroscopy

- Described is the infra-zygomatic approach; alternatives are the transnasal approach (used in ear, nose, and throat (ENT) surgery with topical 4% cocaine) and transoral approach (often used by dentists)

- Fluoroscopy: start in the lateral view to identify the maxilla, lateral pterygoid plate, and coronoid notch—ensure the pterygoid plates are overlapped
- Skin entry point is just inferior to the zygomatic arch either through the coronoid notch (transcoronoid approach) or anterior to the mandible (anterior approach)
- Mark the skin entry point; anaesthetize with a 25G hypobaric needle and 1% lidocaine, and position a 90 mm 22G spinal needle in tunnel vision
- Immediate lateral view to check the depth as the needle is being advanced towards the lateral nasal wall
- Aspirate and inject 0.1–0.2 mL of contrast agent under live screening to outline the pterygoid fossa and exclude intravascular placement
- Inject 1–2 mL of 0.25–0.5% levobupivacaine with non-particulate steroid
- Monitor the patient carefully post-operatively for 40–60 minutes for bleeding and neurological deficit

Complications

- Epistaxis due to piercing of the lateral nasal wall
- Intravascular injection, bleeding, and haematoma (cheek most common) → injury to maxillary artery or branches
- Infection (especially if nasal or oral mucosa pierced)
- Reflex bradycardia during RF lesioning (parasympathetic fibres in the SPG)
- Facial numbness and paralysis
- Double vision (spread of LA to the abducens nerve via the inferior orbital fissure)
- Dry eye (especially with neuroablation; often temporary)
- Fever
- Flare-up of symptoms
- Shift of headache side

Additional information

- RF ablation can be performed in cancer pain, intractable headache, and facial pain syndromes
- Neuroablation techniques are only feasible with the infra-zygomatic approach
- Aspiration of air means the needle tip is too advanced into the nasal cavity
- Limit injectate to 1–2 mL to avoid spread of LA into the abducens nerve

Further reading

1. Dauber W, Feneis H. Anatomisches Bildwörterbuch der internationalen Nomenklatur. 9th edition, 1998. Stuttgart: Thieme Georg Verlag
2. Wikipedia. Pterygopalatine ganglion. 2021. https://en.wikipedia.org/wiki/Pterygopalatine_ganglion
3. Mojica J, Mo B, Ng A. Sphenopalatine ganglion block in the management of chronic headaches. Curr Pain Headache Rep 2017;21(6):27
4. Robbins NS, Robertson CE, Kaplan E, et al. The sphenopalatine ganglion: anatomy, pathophysiology, and therapeutic targeting in headache. Headache 2016;56(2):240–58

16.4 Greater occipital nerve, minor occipital nerve, and third occipital nerve

Anatomy—introduction

- Cervico-trigeminal nucleus—pain of occipital neuralgia/cervicogenic headaches is referred to structures innervated by the trigeminal nerve, including the eyes, temples, and forehead, due to the C1–3 origin of the occipital nerves that share a relay station in the brainstem with the trigeminal cell bodies
- Occasionally, there can be a connection between the greater and lesser occipital nerve

Greater occipital nerve

- Receives fibres from the dorsal primary rami of the second cervical nerve roots
- Exits the C2 foramen laterally to cross over the inferior oblique muscle at the level of the atlanto-occipital joint
- Pierces the semispinalis muscle and the lateral edge of the conjoined tendon on its ascent to the superior nuchal ridge at which point the occipital artery runs just lateral to it
- Sensory innervation to the medial portion of the posterior scalp
- Location is variable with 5–28 mm from the midline, and the GON is medial to the occipital artery

Lesser or minor occipital nerve (LON)

- Receives fibres from the posterior rami of the second and third cervical nerves
- Travels along the border of the sternocleidomastoid muscle as part of the superficial cervical plexus
- Sensory innervation of the lateral portion of the posterior scalp, including the postero-superior surface of the pinna of the ear
- Can have an anomalous origin from the trunk of the suprascapular nerve

Third occipital nerve (TON)

- Medial sensory branch of the posterior division of C3, which supplies the midline of the occipital region (medial to the GON) and innervates the C2/3 facet joint
- Supplies proprioceptive fibres to the semispinalis muscle
- Susceptible to acceleration–deceleration trauma together with the C2/3 joint

Indications

- Occipital neuralgia (entrapment or injury to occipital nerves):
    - Shooting or stabbing pain in cranial portion of the neck with or without a referral pattern to the occiput, temples, forehead, and retrobulbar area (allodynia, paraesthesiae, and numbness)
    - Impairment of vision and ocular pain (67%), tinnitus (33%), dizziness (50%), nausea (50%), and congested nose (17%) can be present (connection with CN VIII, IX, and X, and cervical sympathetic plexus)
    - Examination: tender to pressure over course of the nerves, positive Tinel's sign, diagnosis confirmed by diagnostic nerve block
- History of whiplash injury or similar trauma
- Medication-refractory migraine-type headache
- Cluster headache

Contraindications

- Patient refusal
- Localized or systemic infection
- Coagulopathy or thrombocytopenia
- Distorted or complicated anatomy such as Arnold–Chiari syndrome, cervical instability, or acute fracture

Patient preparation and positioning

- Full monitoring ± IV access (risk of bradycardia)
- Seated position, neck flexed, with head supported on the hands
- Prone if fluoroscopy-guided, with pillow under the chest to allow head flexion
- Skin prepared with appropriate agent

Injection technique (GON)

Landmark technique

- Palpate the occipital nuchal ridge in the midline and inject perpendicularly with a 23G needle after careful aspiration at a point that is 2 cm lateral and 2 cm inferior to that point

Fluoroscopy-guided

- No longer commonly used due to advances in US; however, may be preferable in whiplash patients with cervicogenic headache
- LON block at C2/3 level
- PRF considered if LA infiltration does not provide sufficient analgesia
- Injection of botulinum toxin is controversial unless part of PREEMPT (Phase 3 REsearch Evaluating Migraine Prophylaxis Therapy) which may relieve muscle tension

Ultrasound-guided

- Linear probe
- Identify the bifid C2 spinous process with a horizontal probe position, then move laterally with the medial border of the probe still over the C2 spinous process and the lateral border of the probe towards the C1 transverse process
- The GON crosses the inferior oblique muscle (on top of it) and lies underneath the semispinalis capitis muscle

Complications

- Haematoma
- Infection
- Temporary dizziness, gait disturbance, discomfort at injection site, headache
- Mild ataxia and unsteadiness due to loss of tonic neck reflexes
- Alopecia and skin atrophy
- Intravascular injection, bradycardia
- Total spinal or brain injury if skull defect present and needle passes through (cave: trauma patients)

Additional information

- Subcutaneous occipital nerve stimulation has shown good results in refractory occipital neuralgia
- Warn the patient about potential numbness around the occiput and upper neck plus dizziness

- Apply pressure over the injection site for a few minutes to reduce the risk of haematoma
- Observe the patient for at least 10 minutes before discharge
- Hypoaesthesia is not required for headache relief
- Patients should not drive a car until any signs of ataxia and unsteadiness have resolved
- Patients with a history of posterior fossa surgery or blunt trauma to the occiput may have a skull defect which may lead to injection intracranially, resulting in brain injury or a total spinal block
- Lasting benefit for occipital neuralgia or cervicogenic headache requiring a series of injections
- Better outcome may be achieved in combination with pharmacotherapy and physical therapy
- Persistent pain that only responds briefly to a GON block may benefit from Botox A, PRF of the GON, RF lesioning of the GON, or prolotherapy

Further reading

1. Greher M, Moriggl B, Curatolo M, et al. Sonographic visualization and ultrasound-guided blockade of the greater occipital nerve: a comparison of two selective techniques confirmed by anatomical dissection. Br J Anaesth 2010;104(5):637–42
2. Shields KG, Levy MJ, Goadsby PJ. Alopecia and cutaneous atrophy after greater occipital nerve infiltration with corticosteroid. Neurology 2004;63(11):2193–4
3. Simpson G, Krol A, Silver D, Nicholls B. 5.1 Greater occipital nerve block. In: Simpson G, Krol A, Silver D, Nicholls B (eds). Ultrasound-guided Interventions in Chronic Pain Management. 2019; pp. 126–9. UK: European Society of Regional Anaesthsia & Pain Therapy (ESRA)
4. Vanelderen P, Lataster A, Levy R, et al. Occipital neuralgia. In: Van Zundert J, Patijn J, Hartrick CT, et al. (eds). Evidence-based Interventional Pain Medicine. 2012; pp. 49–54. Chichester: Wiley-Blackwell

16.5 Cervical facet joint/medial branch blocks and radiofrequency denervation

Cervical facet joint pain

- Neck pain is common
- Prevalence of facet joint-related neck pain reported as 25–65% (possibly over 50% of patients attending the pain clinic for neck pain, more common than lumbar facet joint pain)
- Pain referral pattern from cervical facet joints: C2/3—into the occipital aspect of the head as cervicogenic headache; C3/4 and C4/5—between the base of the skull and the first thoracic vertebra over the postero-lateral aspect of the neck to the medial aspect of the shoulder girdle; C4/5 and C5/6—referred to the shoulder girdle and upper part of the scapula; C6/7—over the scapula (see Fig. 16.5.1)
- Cervical facet joint syndrome: axial neck pain, tenderness on palpation of the posterior paravertebral cervical areas, pain and limitation of extension and rotation, absence of neurological symptoms in the arms

History

- Exclude red flag symptoms (e.g. malignancy, myelopathy, instability/trauma, vertebral artery insufficiency, immunocompromise)
- Pain mostly unilateral and not past the shoulder
- Rotation and retroflexion are usually painful and limited

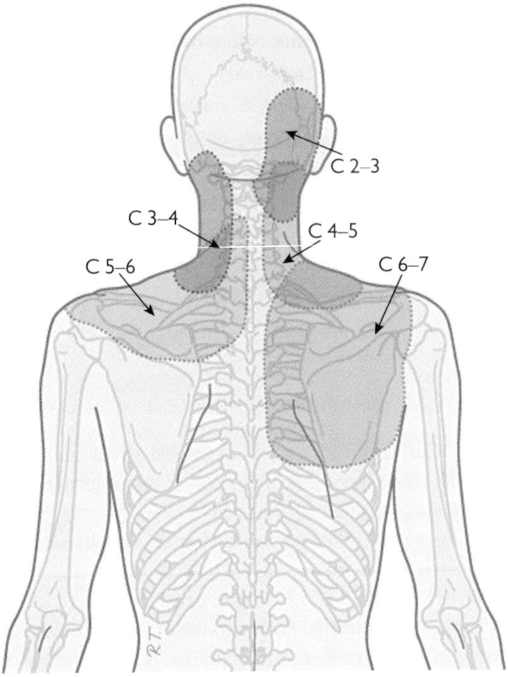

Figure 16.5.1 Radiation pattern of cervical pain

Examination

- Rotation in neutral position—entire cervical column
- Rotation in forward flexion—higher cervical segments
- Rotation in retroflexion (head extension)—lower cervical segments
- Palpation—local tenderness over facet joints (pressure of at least 4kg)
- If neck pain is accompanied by shoulder pain, exclude shoulder pathology

Investigations

- X-ray, CT, MRI (tumour, infection, fracture, degeneration, facet sclerosis, osteophytes)
- Diagnostic cervical facet joint injections or medial branch block (MBB) regarded as successful if >50% pain relief when affected levels are injected (to proceed with RF denervation)

Anatomy of cervical facet joints

- Comprises the joints from C2/3 to C7/T1 at an angle of 45° with the longitudinal axis through the cervical spine
- Cervical facet joints have <1 mL volume
- Higher density of mechanoreceptors, compared to lumbar facet joints
- Pairs on each side formed by the inferior articular process of the superior vertebral segment and the superior articular process of the inferior vertebral segment
- Allows extension, flexion, and rotation
- Innervation by the medial branches of the dorsal rami above and below the joint

- C2/3 joint also supplied by the third optical nerve, which, like the C3 medial branch, originates from the C3 dorsal ramus
- The medial branches are bound by fascia and cross around the waist of the articular processes of the respective numbered vertebra
- At C7, the medial branches are located higher than at C3–C6, due to the transverse process, and 70% are located across the C6/7 facet joint

Indications

- Arthritic or traumatic chronic neck pain, cervicogenic headache, suboccipital headache, axial neck pain, and/or upper thoracic pain
- Neck pain and/or headache with neck movements: flexion, extension, and rotation
- Pain intensity >5/10 and functional disability (neck disability index)
- Failure to respond to conservative management, including physiotherapy, postural optimization, and pharmacotherapy

Contraindications

- Infection
- Inability to consent
- Anticoagulation, antiplatelet therapy, or coagulopathy
- Pregnancy
- Needle phobia
- Severely distorted anatomy

Patient preparation and positioning

- Informed consent (full explanation of potential complications)
- Examination for confirmation of extent of disease, recent average pain score (baseline), and exclusion of infection
- Review for potential bleeding risk (cervical area more vascular than lumbar area)
- IV access and full monitoring
- Exclusion of allergies to drugs, skin prep
- Positioning depends on patient ability and preference of practitioner (supine and lateral for diagnostic blocks; lateral or prone may be preferred for denervations with a posterior approach)

Technique

Medial branch blocks

- Two cervical medial branches must be blocked for each facet joint (above and below the joint)
- Posterior or lateral approach to reach crossing = centre points of the waist of the articular pillar, with the exception of the third optical nerve
- Lateral approach (most suited for C3–6): with patient in supine position and the head on radiolucent head ring; identify articular pillars on lateral view
- Aim for the spine on screen horizontally, with the head on the left, shoulders on the right, and cervical spinous processes heading downwards
- Avoid any double shadows and adjust C-arm accordingly in all planes
- Superficial SC infiltration of LA with a 25G needle and insert a 50 mm spinal needle from postero-laterally towards the centre of the rectangle of the articular pillar and bony contact

- Confirm position on anteroposterior (AP) view—the needle tip should sit in the groove
- Inject 0.25 mL of LA, with or without non-particulate steroid, at each level after careful aspiration
- Assess efficacy of block within 10–20 minutes of block, and document
- Mean duration in a study: 14–16 weeks (3.5 injections per year)

Radiofrequency denervation

- After successful, but short-lasting medial branch blocks
- Posterior approach preferred for better lesion size, but particularly for lower C6/7 denervation—patient in lateral or prone position
- Start with AP view to aim for groove or waist of articular pillars
- Insert a 5 cm 22G needle with a 3–5 mm active straight tip slightly more caudally (one level below) for a slightly tangential approach to the medial branch
- Position as per MBB (centre of the rectangle) and check needle position is posterior to the neural foramen on lateral view
- Aim for impedance of 300–500 Ohm (higher = periostium; lower = intravascular)
- Perform sensory testing at 50 Hz and motor testing at 2 Hz in awake patient
- Aim for sensory response at <0.5 V and negative motor response (triple the sensory threshold) prior to injection of 0.25 mL of LA and lesion at 80°C for 1 minute
- Inject 0.5 mL of LA with non-particulate steroid (e.g. dexamethasone) after the lesion to reduce post-procedural discomfort unless contraindicated

Complications

- Infection
- Bleeding
- Neural trauma—especially nerve root damage
- Dural puncture
- Spinal cord damage
- Weakness or numbness in the arms (usually temporary)
- Dizziness, flushing, sweating, nausea, hypotension, vasovagal reaction, syncope
- Headaches
- Flare-up of pain, especially with denervation

Additional information

- Atlanto-occipital and atlanto-axial joints are anterior joints and not considered facet joints
- Ideally perform two diagnostic test blocks with low volume (0.25 mL) prior to denervation
- Some clinicians recommend two diagnostic blocks (to decrease the number of false positives, but increased false negatives), and others just one diagnostic block (decreased burden for patient with repeated injections, very few negative responses)
- Higher volumes of LA may hamper adjacent sensory test in denervation or give false positive results in diagnostic MBBs
- Do not denervate bilaterally at the same sitting due to the risk of drop head syndrome
- Do not denervate if the needle tip is positioned too close to the neuroforamen and without negative motor test (i.e. no widespread neck, shoulder, or upper limb movement on motor stimulation)
- The needle must never lie anterior to an imaginary line passing through the posterior margin of the intervertebral foramen

Further reading

1. Gauci CA. Manual of RF Techniques. 3rd edition, 2011. Ridderkerk: CoMedical
2. Kweon TD, Kim JY, Lee HY, et al. Anatomical analysis of medial branches of dorsal rami of cervical nerves for radiofrequency thermocoagulation. Reg Anesth Pain Med 2014;39(6):465–71
3. Simpson G, Krol A, Silver D, Nicholls B. 4.2 Cervical medial branch blocks. In: Simpson G, Krol A, Silver D, Nicholls B (eds). Ultrasound-guided Interventions in Chronic Pain Management. 2019; pp. 60–67. UK: European Society of Regional Anaesthesia & Pain Therapy (ESRA)
4. Simpson G, Krol A, Silver D, Nicholls B. 4.3 Cervical facet joint injections. In: Simpson G, Krol A, Silver D, Nicholls B (eds). Ultrasound-guided Interventions in Chronic Pain Management. 2019; pp. 68–70. UK: European Society of Regional Anaesthesia & Pain Therapy (ESRA)
5. Van Eerd M, Patijn J, Lataster A, et al. Cervical facet pain. Pain Pract 2010;10(2):113–23
6. Van Eerd M, Patijn J, Lataster A, et al. 5. Cervical facet pain. In: Van Zundert J, Patijn J, Hartrick CT, et al. (eds). Evidence-based Interventional Pain Medicine. 2012; pp. 31–39. Chichester Wiley-Blackwell

CHAPTER 17

Thorax and Abdomen

Shyam Balasubramanian, Laura Beard, Mohamed Dorgham, Rahul Guru, Doug Stangoe, and Alifia Tameem

CONTENTS

17.1 Thoracic facet joint/medial branch blocks and radiofrequency denervation

Anatomy

- Facet joints are synovial joints with a true joint capsule and are one of the weight-bearing structures in the vertebral column
- Each facet joint is formed by the articulation of the superior articular process of the vertebra below and the inferior articular process of the vertebra above
- The thoracic facet joints are steeply angulated to the axial plane (60–70°) and at 20–30° from the frontal to the sagittal plane
- The superior and inferior articular processes of the thoracic spine cannot be identified separately
- Innervation: the dorsal ramus at each level gives off a medial branch, which supplies the facet joint at the same level and the facet joint below. Therefore, each facet joint receives innervation from the dorsal ramus at the same level and from the level above
- The medial branch crosses the superolateral corner of the transverse process (TP) and then passes medially and inferiorly
- At the mid-thoracic level (T5–T8), an inflection occurs superior to the superolateral corner of the TP
- See Figure 17.1.1

Indications

- Diagnostic block with LA to predict whether RF lesioning will provide long-lasting pain relief in conditions causing thoracic spinal pain (dull or sharp, aching, and usually radiates anteriorly across the chest)
- These conditions include: arthritis, inflammation, trauma, acceleration–deceleration injuries, and osteoporotic or osteolytic vertebral fractures

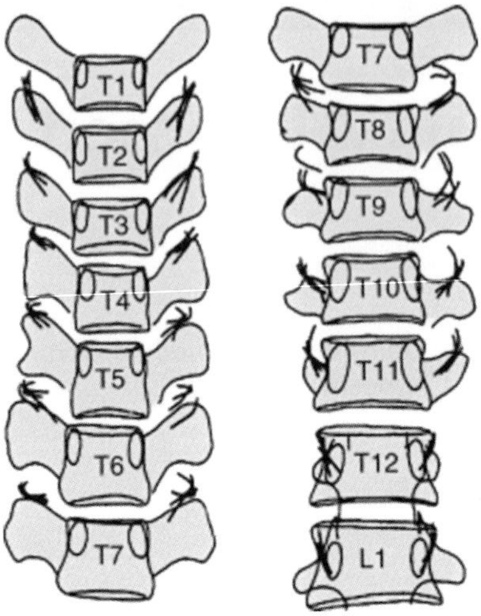

Figure 17.1.1 Courses of the thoracic medial branches across the transverse processes of the vertebrae

Reproduced with permission from Waldman, S. (2014). *Atlas of Interventional Pain Management*, Fourth Edition. Amsterdam, Netherlands: Saunders, an imprint of Elsevier

Contraindications

- Similar to other interventions

Patient preparation and positioning

- Standard protocol followed
- The patient is positioned prone, with pillows under the chest. This allows for flexion of the thoracic spine
- The C-arm is aligned to obtain an AP view of the thoracolumbar region and the target level is identified by counting the corresponding rib either from the thoracolumbar region (T12) upwards or from T1 downwards

Medial branch block

- Once the thoracic medial branch level to be block is located, the endplate of the vertebral body is squared on fluoroscopy
- Oblique rotation of the C-arm helps visualize the junction of the vertebra and TP
- A 22G, 70/90 mm spinal needle is inserted to be positioned either on the middle third of the TP or advanced to the superolateral margin of the TP to lie over the bone at that level
- A total of 0.5–1 mL of lidocaine 1% or bupivacaine 0.25% is injected

Radiofrequency treatment of the medial branch

- An RF needle (10 cm long, with a 10 mm active tip) is used instead of a spinal needle
- Placement is similar to that for MBB, attempting to place the RF needle parallel to the middle third or at the superolateral margin of the TP (see Fig. 17.1.2)
- For the technique, similar principles apply as with all RFs (see 15.6 Radiofrequency denervation, p. 294)

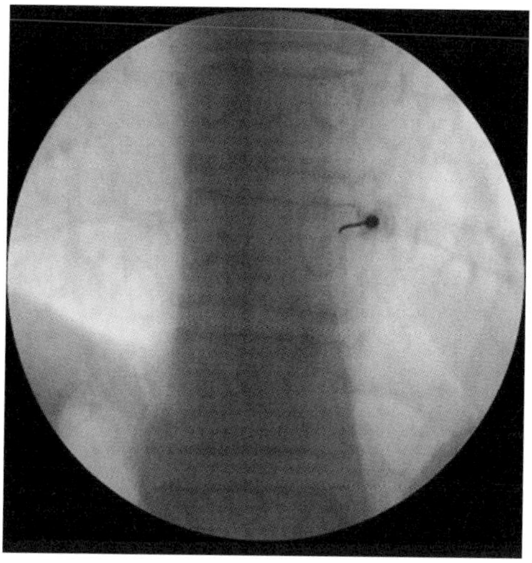

Figure 17.1.2 Radiofrequency needle in the superolateral position for thoracic medial branch block

Reproduced with permission from Waldman, S. (2014). *Atlas of Interventional Pain Management*, Fourth Edition. Amsterdam, Netherlands: Saunders, an imprint of Elsevier

Facet joint injection

- Recognition of the facet joint is facilitated by a caudal tilt of the C-arm
- The needle (22G, 70/90 mm spinal needle) insertion point may be over the pedicle, 1–2 segments caudally due to the steep angulation of the thoracic facets, advanced into the joint space
- Contrast should be mixed with the LA and a small amount (0.4–0.6 mL of the mix) can be injected, avoiding larger volumes
- This is not a recommended procedure due to very narrow joint space

Complications

- For both MBBs and RF denervation:
  - Failure of procedure to reduce pain
  - Infection
  - Pneumothorax
- For RF denervation:
  - Injury to spinal nerve roots—characterized by paraesthesiae, sensory and/or motor loss in the distribution of the spinal nerve root
  - Worsening of pain for 2–4 weeks
  - Dysaesthesia and allodynia of the overlying skin (for a few weeks) as a result of partial denervation of the lateral branch

Additional information

- The course of the medial branch to the facet joints in the thoracic region is quite variable; therefore, some authors advise multiple targets for RF lesion extending from the superolateral margin of the TP to the lamina

- The TPs are larger in the upper thoracic region. They get smaller in the lower thoracic region (T10–T12) and can be difficult to visualize. Therefore, the pedicle can be used as a landmark for needle insertion
- The T12 medial branch lies at the junction of the superior articular process and the TP (similar to the lumbar medial branches)
- The C-arm should be aligned in such a way that the corresponding rib lies cephalad to the TP. This will reduce the chances of pneumothorax as the needle is likely to hit the rib, rather than the pleura, if advanced too deep
- RF denervation is indicated when 50% or greater improvement in pain and function (lasting for the duration of action of the LA) after MBB is obtained

Evidence

- Block for symptomatic relief of facet-related pain—'level 2B'
- RF ablation after positive diagnostic block (extrapolated from cervical and lumbar data)—'level 1B'

Further reading

1. Gauci CA. Thoracic facet joint denervation. In: Gaucci C (ed). Manual of RF Techniques. 2004; pp. 67–78. Ridderkerk: CoMedical
2. Rathmell JP. Facet injection: intra-articular injection, medial branch block, and radiofrequency treatment. In: Rathmell JP (ed). Atlas of Image-guided Intervention in Regional Anesthesia and Pain Medicine. 2006; pp. 80–117. Philadelphia, PA: Lippincott Williams and Wilkins
3. Desai MJ. Thoracic radiofrequency ablation. Techniques in Regional Anesthesia and Pain Management. 2015 (19);126–130
4. Waldman SD. Thoracic facet block: radiofrequency lesioning of the medial branch of the primary posterior rami. In: Waldman SD (ed). Atlas of Interventional Pain Management. 2021; pp. 372–375. Philadelphia, PA: Saunders

17.2 Intercostal nerve block

Anatomy of intercostal nerves

- Anterior rami of the thoracic spinal nerves T1–T12
- Enters the corresponding intercostal space lateral to the intervertebral foramen
- Proximal to the angle of the rib, it travels forward in the subcostal groove between the innermost and internal intercostal muscles and inferior to intercostal vessels
- Gives branches to the skin, parietal pleura, intercostal muscles (three layers of external, internal, and innermost), and serratus muscles
- T7–T12 also innervate the anterior abdominal wall, parietal peritoneum, and anterior abdominal muscles, including the external oblique (EO), internal oblique (IO), transverse abdominis (TA), and rectus abdominis (RA) muscles

Indications

- Analgesia for thoracotomy, intercostal drains
- Rib fractures
- PHN

- Breast and upper abdominal surgery

Contraindications

- Similar to other interventions

Patient preparation and positioning

- Patient positioning: sitting, lateral, or prone position. Best position is achieved when the spine is arched and the arms extended forward in the sitting position (hugging a pillow) or hanging over the side of the bed in the prone position, as it helps to retract the scapula laterally
- For abdominal surgery, T5–T12
- For breast surgery, T2–T6
- For thoracic incisions, 1–2 levels above and below the planned level
- 3–5 mL of LA at each level

Landmark technique

- The inferior border of the rib to be blocked is marked at the angle of the rib
- A 22G block needle is inserted cephalad until it makes contact with the rib
- The needle is 'walked off' the inferior border of the rib and advanced by 1–3 mm anteriorly
- A subtle 'pop' is felt when through the fascia of the internal intercostal muscle
- Correct placement will result in ipsilateral numbness of the corresponding intercostal levels

Ultrasound-guided technique

- A linear, high-frequency probe in the sagittal plane
- 10–15 cm lateral to the spinous process (see Fig. 17.2.1)
- A 21–22G, 50 mm needle used, depth of around 0.5–1.5 cm
- The adjacent ribs are visualized as round shadows, and the pleura as a hyperechoic line
- The innermost intercostal muscle lies just above the pleura

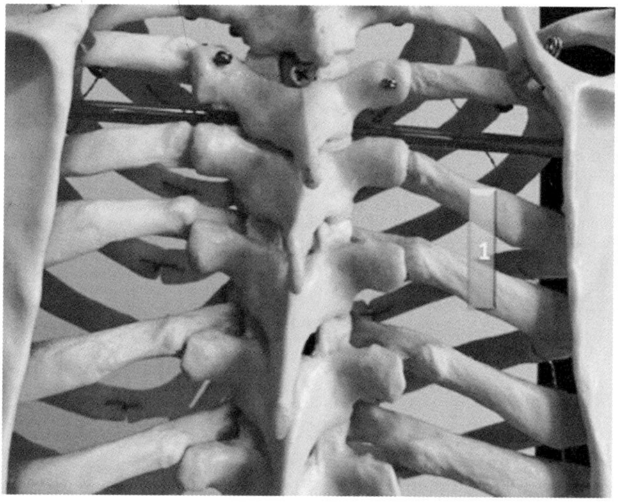

Figure 17.2.1 Placement of the linear ultrasound probe

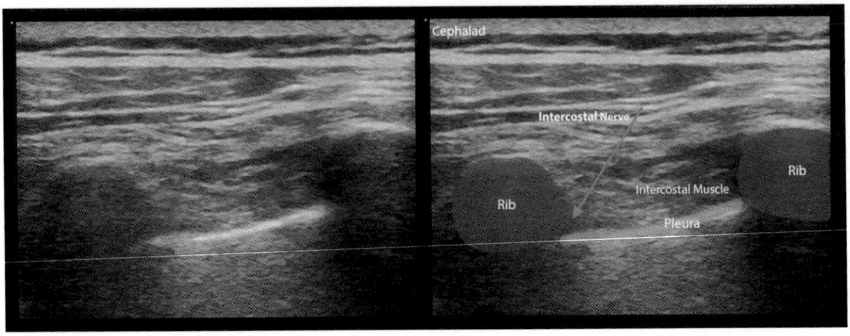

Figure 17.2.2 Sagittal position of the probe—sonoanatomy, in-plane approach (unlabelled and labelled)

- The neurovascular bundle lies in a triangular space below the superior rib, between the internal and innermost muscles, which is the target site for injection (see Fig. 17.2.2)
- In-plane or out-of-plane approach; correct placement identified by displacing the pleura anteriorly
- Lower risk of intravascular injection and pneumothorax, and allows injection more posteriorly which also increases the chance of lateral branch block

Special points

- A persistent 'comet tail' sign of the lung and pleural movement synchronized with breathing after injection excludes pneumothorax
- For cancer and chronic pain, neurolytic/conventional or PRF ablation may provide longer-term benefit

Further reading

1. Albrecht E, Bloc S, Cadas H, et al. The Book of Ultrasound-guided Regional Anaesthesia. 2nd edition, 2018 (Kindle edition). Lausanne: SACAR
2. Hutchins J, Sanchez J, Andrade R, et al. Ultrasound guided paravertebral catheter versus intercostal blocks for postoperative pain control in video assisted thoracoscopic surgery: a prospective randomized trial. J Cardiothorac Vasc Anesth 2017;31(2):458463

17.3 Thoracic paravertebral block

Anatomy

- The thoracic paravertebral space is a wedge-shaped space on either side of the vertebral column
- Contents:
  - Spinal nerves and its branches
  - Sympathetic trunk
  - Adipose tissue

- Anatomical relations:
  - Anterolateral—parietal pleura, endothoracic fascia
  - Posteriorly—superior costotransverse ligament (SCL)
  - Medially—vertebral bodies and intervertebral discs, communicates with the epidural space via the intervertebral foramen
  - Laterally—communicates with the posterior intercostal space
  - Inferiorly—extends till the origin of the psoas muscle at L1
  - Superiorly—communicates with the cervical paravertebral space

Indications

- Perioperative analgesia for thoracic, chest wall, and breast surgery
- Acute pain management for rib fractures

Contraindications

- Similar to other interventions
- Coagulopathy

Patient preparation and positioning

- Aseptic precautions
- A 22G needle for single shot block, 18G or 16G for continuous block with catheter insertion
- 15–20mL of LA will spread 2–3 levels
- Patient position—sitting, lateral decubitus with the block side up, or prone

Technique

Anatomical landmark

- Needle insertion point is 2.5 cm lateral to the uppermost point of the spinous process. Advance the needle perpendicular to the skin until the needle tip hits the TP. Withdraw and redirect the needle cephalad or caudal carefully 1.5–2.0 cm past the depth where the TP is located
- A change in resistance or a pop is felt as the needle traverses the SCL

Ultrasound-guided techniques

- High-frequency linear US transducer probe (2–5 cm)

Transverse technique

- The transducer is positioned in the transverse plane at the selected level, lateral to the spinous process between the two ribs (see Fig. 17.3.1)
- The thoracic paravertebral space appears as a wedge-shaped hypoechoic area bounded between two hyperechoic lines—the pleura anteriorly which moves with respiration, and the internal intercostal membrane (IIm) or the SCL posteriorly (see Fig. 17.3.2)
- The aim is to get the needle tip through the IIm/SCL and superficial to the pleura

Out-of-plane technique

- Insert the needle until it hits the TP, walk off to pierce the SCL

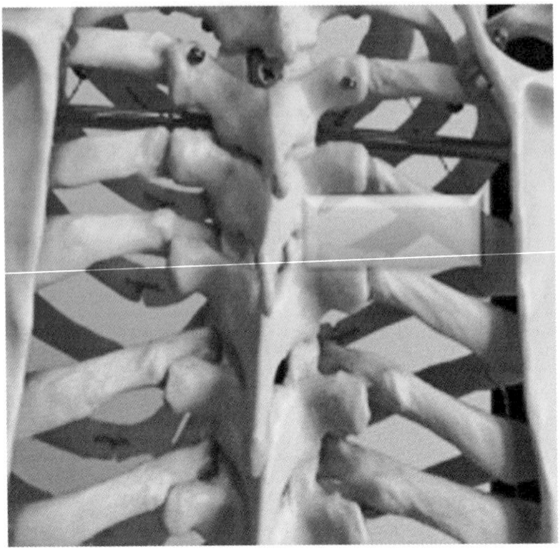

Figure 17.3.1 Transverse placement of the probe

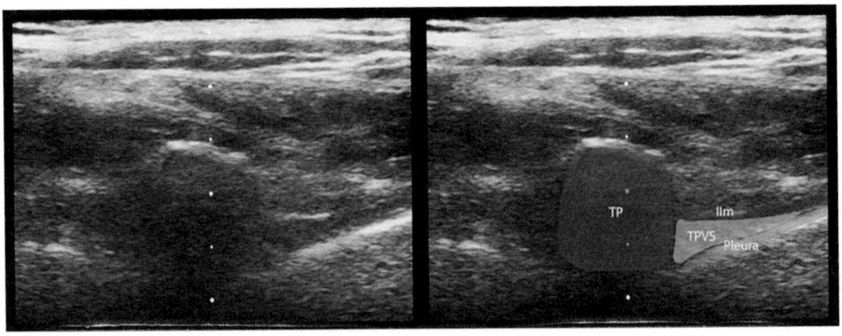

Figure 17.3.2 Transverse position of the probe—sonoanatomy (unlabelled versus labelled). Ilm, internal intercostal membrane (or SCL); TP, transverse process; TPVS, thoracic paravertebral space

In-plane technique

- Insertion is lateral to medial, with the bevel cephalad to avoid pleural, neural, or vascular injury

Longitudinal/parasagittal technique

- The transducer is placed longitudinally 5–10 cm lateral to the spinous process where the ribs appear as rounded shadows and the parietal pleura as a hyperechoic line underneath
- The transducer is then moved medially to less rounded and deeper shadows of the TPs (see Fig. 17.3.3)
- Tilt the transducer in the sagittal axis to a slightly oblique angle, with the upper part of the transducer medial
- The thoracic paravertebral space is the hypoechoic space bounded by the hyperechoic SCL and the pleura (see Fig. 17.3.4)

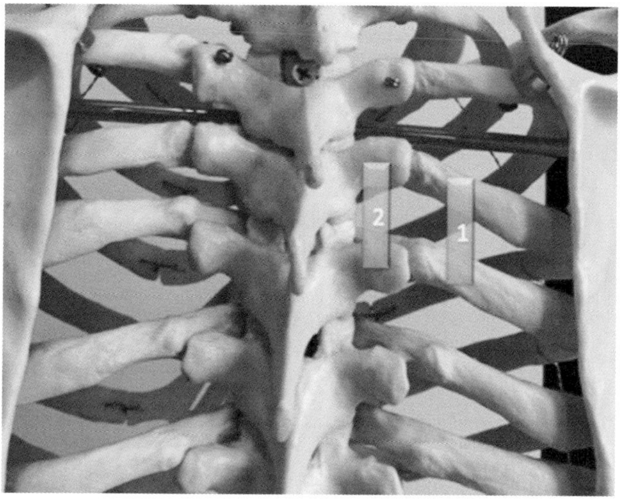

Figure 17.3.3 Longitudinal position of the probe

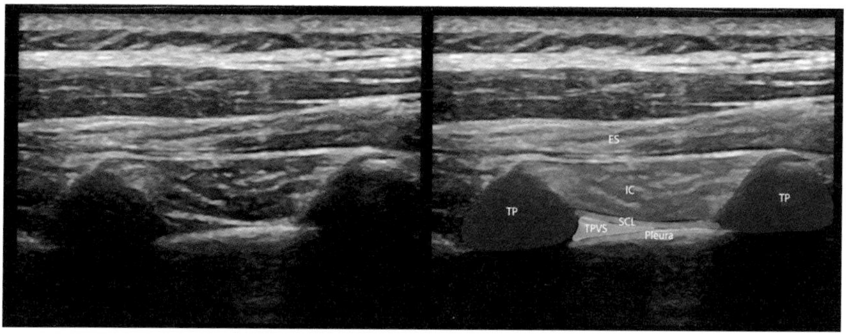

Figure 17.3.4 Longitudinal/parasagittal sonoanatomy (unlabelled versus labelled). IC, intercostal muscles; ES, erector spinae muscle; SCL, superior costotransverse ligament, TP, transverse process; TPVS, thoracic paravertebral space

- Out-of-plane technique: insert the needle until it hits the TP and walk off below the IIm/SCL
- In-plane technique: insert the needle cephalad or caudal and ensure the tip lies below the hyperechoic SCL. The acute angle of needle insertion can render the needle tip visualization more difficult

Complications

- Pleural puncture is reported to be 5% with US in a cadaveric study, higher than with the anatomical landmark technique (1.1%)
- Epidural/intrathecal spread
- Bleeding
- Infection
- Failure

Additional information

- Prone position useful in chronic pain patients as fluoroscopy can be used in conjunction
- The thoracic paravertebral space may be deeper in the upper thoracic regions
- Loss of resistance is subtle
- Real-time USS of LA injection should ideally result in anterior displacement of the pleura, considered as objective evidence of correct block placement
- A lateral-to-medial approach and high-pressure injection increase the risk of epidural spread
- An in-plane, parasagittal approach and an out-of-plane transverse approach are recommended for catheter placement

Further reading

1. Cowie B, McGlade D, Ivanusic J, et al. Ultrasound-guided thoracic paravertebral blockade: a cadaveric study. Anesth Analg 2010;110:1735–9
2. Luyet C, Herrmann G, Ross S, et al. Ultrasound guided placement of catheters in human cadavers. Br J Anaesth 2011;106:246–54
3. O'Riain SC, Donnell BO, Cuffe T, et al. Thoracic paravertebral block using real-time ultrasound guidance. Anesth Analg 2010;110:248–51

17.4 Analgesia for rib fractures

Definition

- Rib fractures are caused by blunt or penetrating forces to the chest
- Flail segments occur when three or more contiguous ribs are fractured in two or more places

Incidence

- 10% of all patients admitted with traumatic injuries
- Common after road traffic collisions and falls from height
- Mortality is approximately 12%, higher in the elderly and those who develop pneumonia
- Elderly patients sustain higher levels of injury from lower mechanisms
- Associated with other injuries in 90% of patients

Pathophysiology

- Respiratory complications are common, either due to the initial primary injury or from secondary insults
- Inadequate analgesia increases the risk of developing secondary complications
- Risk factors that increase mortality and morbidity (see Table 17.4.1)

Table 17.4.1 Risk factors that increase mortality and morbidity

Patient factors	Trauma-related factors
• Increasing age • Pneumonia • Pre-existing comorbidities	• Flail chest • Bilateral fractures • Multiple rib fractures >3 • Pulmonary contusions • Presence of other injuries (polytrauma)

Primary respiratory complications (from the initial injury)

- Contusions, haemothorax, pneumothorax, lung laceration

Secondary respiratory complications

(See Fig. 17.4.1.)

- Pneumonia (up to 31% of patients)
- Acute respiratory distress syndrome (ARDS)
- Need for ventilatory support:
  - Non-invasive—high-flow nasal oxygen, continuous positive airway pressure (CPAP), bilevel positive airway pressure (BiPAP)
  - Invasive—endotracheal intubation and mechanical ventilation ± tracheostomy

Risk scoring systems

- Help risk-stratify and expedite the pain management of high-risk groups
- Two commonly used scoring systems include the Rib Fracture Score (RFS), discussed below, and the radiologically assessed Rib Score

Rib Fracture Score

$$\text{RFS} = (\text{breaks} \times \text{sides}) + \text{age factor}$$

- Breaks = total number of fractures to the ribs (not the number of fractured ribs)
- Sides = score 1 if unilateral, score 2 if bilateral
- Age factor = score 0: <50 years; score 1: 51–60 years; score 2: 61–70 years; score 3: 71–80 years; score 4: ≥80 years
- A score of ≥15 suggests severe and urgent treatment should be initiated, preferably with regional analgesia

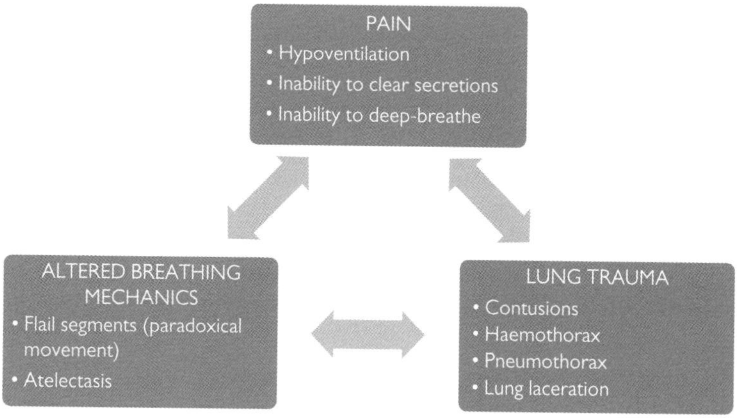

Figure 17.4.1 Secondary respiratory complications are influenced by pain, altered breathing mechanics, and lung trauma

Diagnosis (history, examination/investigations, differential diagnosis)

History

- Event history, other injuries, risk of pathological rib fractures, post-CPR rib fractures
- Respiratory symptoms: chest pain—worse on moving, breathing, and coughing; if delayed presentation, are features of pneumonia present?
- Past medical history: respiratory disease (e.g. chronic obstructive pulmonary disease (COPD), smoking, exercise tolerance)

Examination

- Full Advanced Trauma Life Support (ATLS) assessment with primary and secondary survey
- Focused respiratory examination should assess for:
  - Chest movement (flail segments/paradoxical chest movement)
  - Tracheal deviation (tension pneumothorax)
  - Chest auscultation (reduced breath sounds = pneumothorax/haemothorax; crepitations = contusion/consolidation)
  - Chest percussion (hyperresonance = pneumothorax; hyporesonance = haemothorax/pleural effusion)
  - Signs of respiratory distress: use of accessory muscles, rapid respiratory rate, low oxygen saturation (SpO_2) <94% (air)

Investigations

- Arterial blood gas: low PaO_2 and/or high A–a gradient, raised $PaCO_2$
- Chest X-ray (CXR): pneumothorax, effusion, consolidation, oedema/contusion; rib fractures may be missed
- CT: gives detailed information on number, level, location, and displacement of the rib/ribs, and identifies lung pathology

Treatment

- Early and effective analgesia with multimodal approaches reduces the risk of respiratory complications and subsequent morbidity/mortality (see Table 17.4.2)
- Enables compliance with physiotherapy
- Surgical rib fixation for those with significant chest injuries/flail segments is increasing

Table 17.4.2 Multimodal analgesia

Pharmacological	Interventional*	Operative
Paracetamol Non-steroidal agents (NSAIDs) Neuropathic agents (gabapentin/pregabalin) Codeine Tramadol Morphine (intermittent PO/IV bolus, PCA, continuous infusion in high dependency unit (HDU)/intensive care unit (ICU)) Ketamine infusion	Thoracic epidural Paravertebral catheter Intercostal nerve blocks Erector spinae plane catheter Serratus anterior plane catheter	Surgical rib fixation

* Catheter insertion, rather than a single shot injected, is suggested.

Assessment of pain

- Static (at rest) and dynamic (on movement/coughing) pain scores
- Incentive spirometry as an objective assessment of analgesic adequacy

Challenges of analgesic management

- Regional analgesia is favoured, but <20% of patients actually receive thoracic epidural analgesia or paravertebral analgesia due to patient, injury, and service provision factors

Patient factors

- Multiple comorbidities that prevent insertion, anticoagulant medications

Injury factors

- Spinal trauma and head injuries, significant hypotension

Service provision

- Advanced level of skills required, out of hours, increased level of observation/monitoring required post-thoracic epidural/paravertebral insertion
- Limitations of thoracic epidurals and paravertebral analgesia have led to a rapid rise in popularity of the novel **thoracic wall fascial plane blocks**—serratus anterior and erector spinae planes discussed below
- Intercostal block (see 17.2 Intercostal nerve block, p. 318) and paravertebral block (see 17.3 Thoracic paravertebral block, p. 320) are discussed
- With fascial plane blocks, larger volumes of LAs, typically 20-30 mL are needed, hence caution with LA toxicity, especially when bilateral blocks/catheters are used

Serratus anterior plane

(See Fig. 17.4.2)

Indications

- Most effective in anterior–lateral fractures
- Also effective in breast surgery, thoracotomy, and chest drain insertion

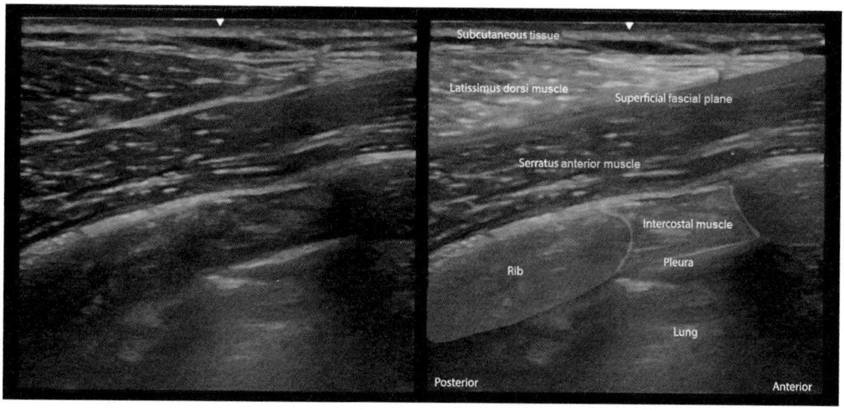

Figure 17.4.2 Serratus anterior plane sonoanatomy (unlabelled versus labelled)

Mechanism of action

- Anaesthesia of the lateral cutaneous nerve, with variable involvement of the long thoracic, intercostal, and thoracodorsal nerves
- Covers anterior–lateral hemithorax T2–T9

Insertion

- Supine or lateral positioning with US-guided in-plane needling
- Transverse orientation of the probe
- Anterior–posterior needle trajectory at the level of the fourth rib in mid-axillary line
- Identify the superficial serratus plane between the serratus anterior and the latissimus dorsi muscles; hydro-dissect the fascial plane to enable catheter insertion
- Deep injection can be performed between the rib/intercostal muscle and the serratus anterior muscle. This is a more advanced technique due to the close proximity of the intercostal vessels and pleura

Advantages

- Reliable analgesia, supine position, easy to learn, no autonomic block, and block/catheters can be inserted bilaterally

Caution

- Avoid the thoracodorsal vessels that run in the superficial plane
- Close proximity to the pleura

Erector spinae plane

(See Fig. 17.4.3)

Indications

- May be most effective for posterior rib fractures
- Bilateral injections/catheter insertions can be performed

Mechanism of action

- Anaesthesia of the posterior (dorsal) rami of the spinal nerves
- Possible anterior spread to the paravertebral space
- Analgesia of the hemithorax

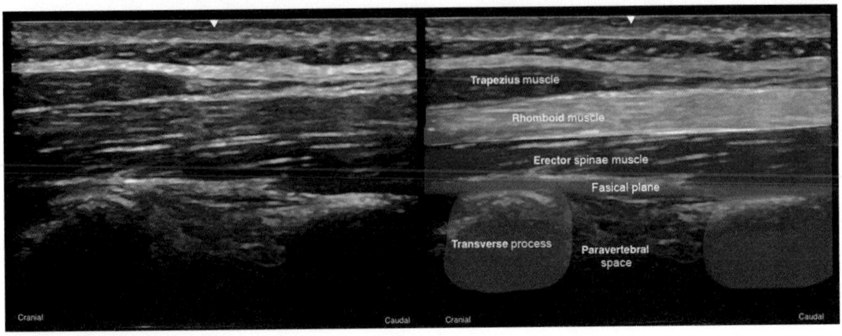

Figure 17.4.3 Erector spinae plane sonoanatomy (unlabelled versus labelled)

Insertion

- Lateral or sitting position, with US-guided in-plane needling
- Paramedian sagittal orientation of the probe and cranial–caudal needle trajectory
- Hydro-dissect the fascial plane between the Transverse Process and the erector spinae muscle

Caution

- Close proximity to the spinal nerves and pleura

PAIN MANAGEMENT ALGORITHM

RIB FRACTURE SCORE = (Breaks × Sides) + Age + Smoking factors

Breaks: Number of Fractures

Sides: Unilateral = 1, Bilateral =2

Age factor:
0 If < 40 years old
1 If 41–50 years old
2 If 41–50 years old
3 If 61–70 years old
4 If > 70 years old

Smoking Factor: Smoker or Ex smoker - 2

A score of 3–6 = Step 1
A score of 7–10 = Step 2
A score of 11 or above = Step 3

A score of >7 requires referral to the Inpatient (acute) Pain Team and physiotherapy referral

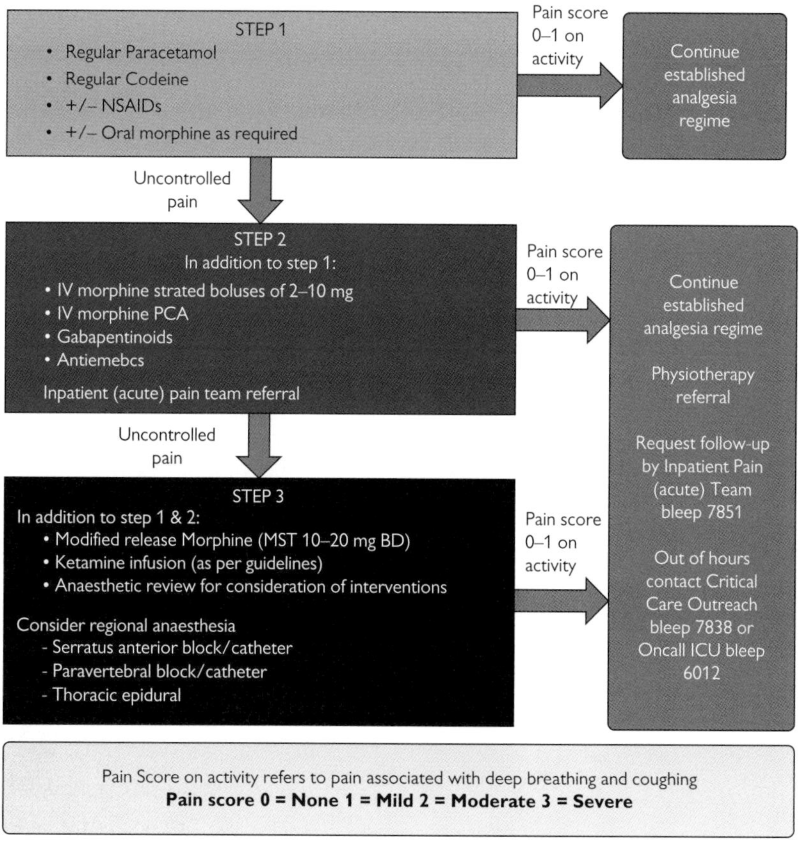

STEP 1
• Regular Paracetamol
• Regular Codeine
• +/– NSAIDs
• +/– Oral morphine as required
Pain score 0–1 on activity
Continue established analgesia regime
Uncontrolled pain
STEP 2
In addition to step 1:
• IV morphine strated boluses of 2–10 mg
• IV morphine PCA
• Gabapentinoids
• Antiemebcs
Inpatient (acute) pain team referral
Pain score 0–1 on activity
Continue established analgesia regime
Physiotherapy referral
Request follow-up by Inpatient Pain (acute) Team bleep 7851
Out of hours contact Critical Care Outreach bleep 7838 or Oncall ICU bleep 6012
Uncontrolled pain
STEP 3
In addition to step 1 & 2:
• Modified release Morphine (MST 10–20 mg BD)
• Ketamine infusion (as per guidelines)
• Anaesthetic review for consideration of interventions
Consider regional anaesthesia
- Serratus anterior block/catheter
- Paravertebral block/catheter
- Thoracic epidural
Pain score 0–1 on activity
Pain Score on activity refers to pain associated with deep breathing and coughing
Pain score 0 = None 1 = Mild 2 = Moderate 3 = Severe

Figure 17.4.4 Sample of rib fracture pain management algorithm

Reproduced courtesy of the Dudley Group NHS Foundation Trust by SR Elaine Roe and Alifia Tameem

Further reading

1. May L, Hillermann C, Patil S. Rib fracture management. BJA Educ 2016;16(1):26–32
2. Chapman BC, Herbert B, Rodil M, et al. RibScore: a novel radiographic score based on fracture pattern that predicts pneumonia, respiratory failure, and tracheostomy. J Trauma Acute Care Surg 2016;80(1):95–101
3. NYSORA. Erector spinae plane block. 2019. https://app.nysora.com/courses/erector-spinae-plane-block/lessons/anatomy-20/

17.5 Abdominal wall blocks

Anatomy—overview and muscles

- The anterior abdominal wall extends from the costal margins and xiphisternum superiorly to the iliac crests, inguinal ligaments and pubic crest, and the symphysis inferiorly
- It comprises three muscle layers antero-laterally: EO, IO, and TA. These taper into a fascial plane medially—the rectus sheath—which encases vertically arranged rectus abdominis muscles
- The fascial plane of the IO and TA converge postero-laterally with the thoracolumbar fascia. This fascia is a complex tubular structure formed by blending of aponeuroses and fascial layers. It divides into anterior, middle, and posterior layers to encase the quadratus lumborum muscle (QLM) and the erector spinae muscles
- The anterior abdominal wall is innervated by the thoraco-abdominal nerves and the ilio-inguinal and ilio-hypogastric nerves
- The QLM inserts on the posterior iliac crest inferiorly and the twelfth rib superiorly and the transverse processes of L1–5. It is located between the psoas major muscle (anteriorly) and the erector spinae muscle group (posteriorly)

Anatomy—innervation

- The thoraco-abdominal nerves are continuations of the intercostal nerves arising from the anterior rami of T6–12. They travel infero-medially in the transverse abdominis plane (TAP). Each gives off a lateral branch, providing cutaneous sensation to the lateral abdominal wall, and an anterior branch, which pierces the rectus sheath laterally to run between the posterior rectus sheath and the posterior aspect of the RA muscle, before piercing it medially to supply the anterior abdominal wall
- The ilio-inguinal and ilio-hypogastric nerves are terminal branches of the L1 nerve roots, with varying contributions from T12 and L2–3. They emerge on the lateral border of the psoas major muscle, run infero-medially, and pierce the TA muscle above the anterior superior iliac crest to run between the IO and TA muscles. The ilio-inguinal nerve supplies the superior medial part of the thigh, the base of the penis/mons pubis, and the anterior scrotum/labia majora. The ilio-hypogastric nerve supplies the skin over the inferior medial anterior abdomen

(a) (b)

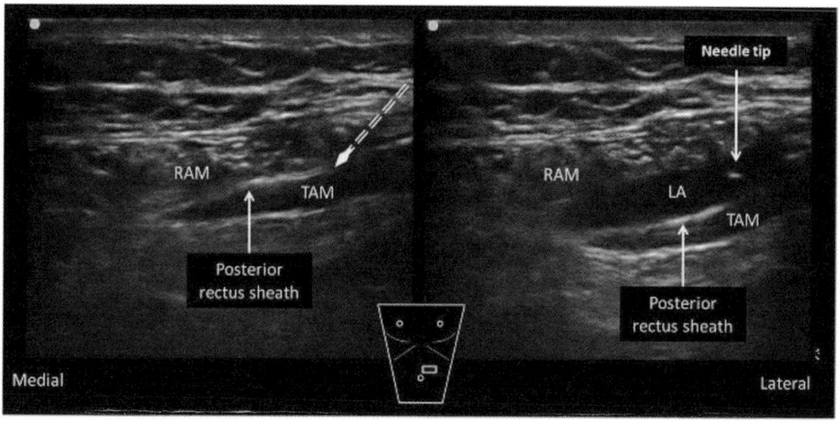

Figure 17.5.1 Ultrasound-guided rectus sheath block

(a) Pre-injection image. The probe is placed in a transverse orientation superior to the umbilicus to visualize the lateral aspect of the rectus abdominis muscle (RAM) and the rectus sheath. The needle is inserted deep to the lateral edge of the RAM but does not penetrate the two layers of the posterior rectus sheath

(b) Post-injection image. Injection here creates a pocket of LA between the RAM and the posterior rectus sheath

LA, local anaesthetic; TAM, transverse abdominis muscle

Posterior rectus sheath block

(See Fig. 17.5.1.)

Indications

- Para- and umbilical hernia repair
- Midline laparotomy (bilateral posterior rectus sheath blocks/catheters in combination with bilateral TAP block or quadratus lumborum block (QLB) for better analgesia)
- Anterior abdominal wall pain syndrome

Patient positioning

- Supine

Technique

- Aims to block the terminal branches of the anterior divisions of the 9th–11th intercostal nerves
- Linear probe transverse and in the midline to identify the rectus muscles on either side of the linea alba and the encasing hyperechoic rectus sheath
- Deposit LA between the rectus muscle and the posterior rectus sheath to separate the muscle from the sheath
- The tendinous intersection of the anterior part of the rectus muscles is absent posteriorly to enable free passage of the LA
- 10–20 mL of LA into each side

Specific complications

- Bowel perforation
- Intravascular injection (inferior epigastric vessels in close proximity)

Tips

- Must block both sides as the midline receives innervation bilaterally
- Can be done by surgeons at abdominal closure under direct vision who can also site LA infiltration catheters

Transverse abdominis plane block

(See Fig. 17.5.2.)

Indications

- Laparotomy (bilaterally for midline incision)
- Pfannenstiel incision in Caesarean section (bilaterally)
- Abdominoplasty (bilaterally)
- Nephrectomy
- Cholecystectomy
- Laparoscopic surgery

Patient positioning

- Supine, with the arms placed anteriorly to expose the lateral abdomen (elevate the ipsilateral hip with sandbag, fluid bag or wedge)

Technique

- Aims to block thoraco-abdominal and ilio-inguinal and ilio-hypogastric nerves prior to their piercing the musculature
- Transducer placed transverse in the mid-axillary line approximately midway between the costal margin and the ASIS. Moving the probe slightly posteriorly from this position often improves the view of the EO, IO, and TA muscle layers with the underlying hyperechoic peritoneum
- Needle inserted in-plane anterior to posterior, and LA deposited in the plane between the IO and TA muscles
- 20–30 mL of LA on each side

Specific complications

- Bowel perforation

Tips

- Must block both sides for midline incisions as innervation is bilateral
- Volume-dependent plane block, so larger volumes of LA needed to cover multiple dermatomes (e.g. 0.6 mL/kg on each side). Therefore, saline can be used to confirm correct needle placement with hydro-dissection of the plane prior to LA administration
- Unilateral subcostal TAP block immediately inferior to the costal margin can be used for upper abdominal surgery (e.g. cholecystectomy)

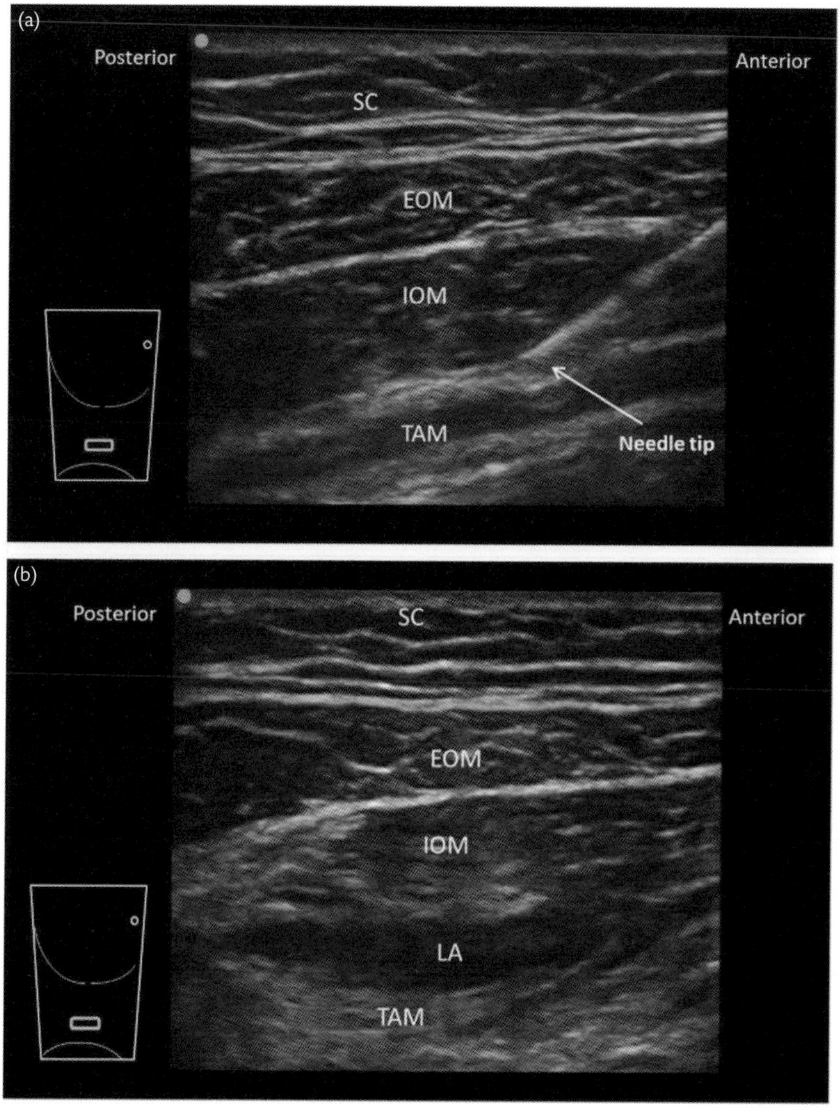

Figure 17.5.2 Ultrasound-guided lateral transverse abdominis plane (TAP) block

(a) Pre-injection image. The US probe is placed in a transverse orientation between the costal margin and the iliac crest in the mid-axillary line. A needle is advanced in an anterior-to-posterior direction through the muscular layers of the abdominal wall to reach the TAP between the internal oblique muscle (IOM) and the transverse abdominis muscle (TAM). The TAM has a characteristic darker hypoechoic appearance and is usually significantly thinner than the IOM

(b) Post-injection image. The local anaesthetic (LA) has distended the TAP, separating the IOM and the TAM

EOM, external oblique muscle; SC, subcutaneous tissue

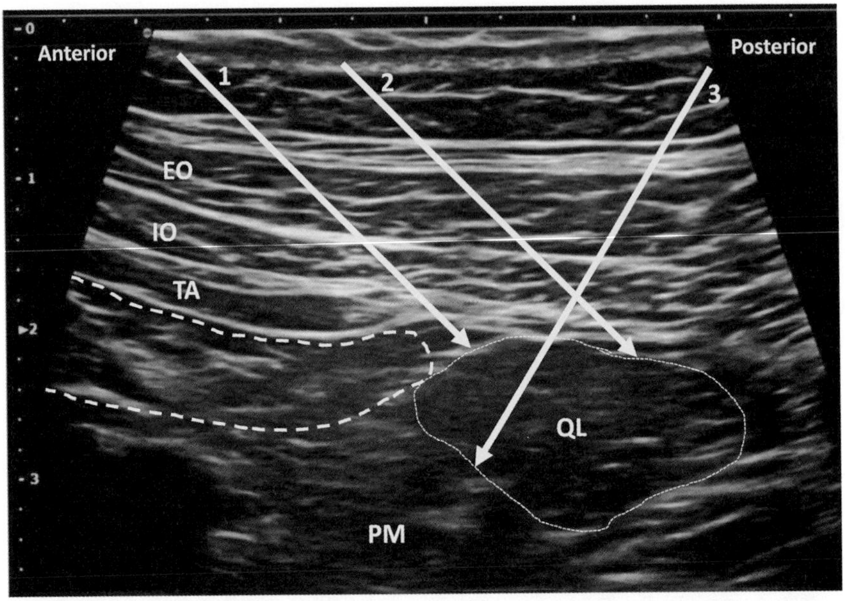

Figure 17.5.3 Three approaches to ultrasound-guided quadratus lumborum block. The ultrasound probe is placed in transverse oblique above the posterior aspect of the iliac crest

1. Anterior approach (QLB-1): the needle is advanced in a lateral-to-medial direction towards the plane between the transversalis fascia (dashed line) and the internal oblique (IO) and transverse abdominis (TA) aponeurosis

2. Lateral approach (QLB-2): the same needle trajectory is used to reach the tissue plane posterior to the quadratus lumborum (QL) muscle

3. Transmuscular or posterior approach (QLB-3): the needle is advanced in a posterior-to-anterior direction to reach the anterior surface of the QL muscle

Muscles: EO, external oblique; IO, internal oblique; PM, psoas major; TA, transverse abdominis

Adapted under a Creative Commons Attribution 4.0 International (CC BY 4.0) from Ueshima, H., Otake, H., Lin, J. A. (2017) Ultrasound-Guided Quadratus Lumborum Block: An Updated Review of Anatomy and Techniques, *BioMed Research International*

Quadratus lumborum block

(See Fig. 17.5.3.)

- Deposition of LA at sites lateral, posterior, and anterior to the QLM have been described as QLB-1, QLB-2, and QLB-3, respectively
- Modality of analgesia incompletely understood, but spread of LA to the paravertebral or epidural space may result in visceral, as well as cutaneous, analgesia

Indications

- Laparotomy
- Pfannenstiel incision in Caesarean section
- Abdominoplasty
- Nephrectomy
- Orchidopexy
- Hip surgery
- Lumbar vertebral surgery

Patient positioning

- Supine with lateral tilt to each side, so that the side to be anaesthetized is uppermost
- Another option is a pillow under the ipsilateral hip

Technique

- A curved probe is placed on the postero-lateral aspect of the abdominal wall in a transverse oblique orientation, between the iliac crest and the costal margin (cranial to the iliac crest)
- The EO, IO, and TA muscle layers are identified and followed posteriorly till the fibres file off into an aponeurosis. The QLM is postero-medial to this
- QLB-1: LA deposited antero-lateral to the QLM (essentially a postero-lateral TAP block)
- QLB-2 block: LA deposited posterior to the QLM between the thoracolumbar fascia, which separates the QLM and the erector spinae muscles (iliocostalis)
- QLB-3 block: AP transmuscular injection (through the QLM) to deposit LA anterior to the QLM
- 20–30 mL of LA (adjust volume if bilateral blocks are needed)

Specific complications

- Retroperitoneal organ injury
- High volumes could theoretically give excessive spread within the epidural space

Further reading

1. Akerman M, Pejčić N, Veličković I. A review of the quadratus lumborum block and ERAS. Front Med (Lausanne) 2018;5:44
2. Chin KJ, McDonnell JG, Carvalho B, et al. Essentials of our current understanding: abdominal wall blocks. Reg Anesth Pain Med 2017;42:133–83
3. Townsley P, Bedforth N, Nicholls B, et al. A Pocket Guide to Ultrasound Guided Regional Anaesthesia. 2nd edition, 2019. London: Regional Anaesthesia UK

CHAPTER 18

Lumbar and Pelvis

Sadiq Bhayani, Yehia Kamel, Yin Yee Ng, Bhavesh Raithatha, Jan Rudiger, and Thomas E Smith

CONTENTS

18.1 Lumbar facet joint/medial branch blocks and radiofrequency denervation

The role of facet joint treatments

- Facet joints ('zygapophyseal joints') are small synovial joints between vertebrae on the postero-lateral aspect of the spine
- They allow a degree of movement of the spine, while stabilizing it against excessive movement
- They are prone to degenerative/osteoarthritic changes (particularly at low lumbar and cervical levels), like other synovial joints that bear a lot of loading in our lives (knees, hips)
- Pain from lumbar facet joints is felt in the lumbar paraspinal area, spreading into the buttocks and often into the posterior thighs (down to the calves)
- Many pain physicians believe that facetogenic pain is worse on loading the joints (e.g. straightening the spine after flexion, extension from neutral, and lateral flexion with extension)
- However, a limited number of studies looking at this have suggested that pain on loading of the joints is not a good discriminator, and that the main positive association is localized paraspinal muscle tenderness
- Muscle tension and tenderness are seen with other drivers of axial back pain
- This leads to the concept of 'back pain for investigation'
- The only way to determine if facet joints are a major driver of low back pain is to treat them and see if the pain considerably diminishes
- Interventional studies suggest that around 15% of cases of axial low back pain may have facet joint arthropathy as the main driver and therefore benefit from facet joint treatments

Facet joint injections

- Facet joint injections with LA and steroid has been a popular treatment for chronic low back pain for decades

- Although described as intra-articular injections, it is likely that in most cases, the injections are periarticular, given the difficult anatomy of degenerative joints and the small volume of the joint
- The efficacy and cost-effectiveness of facet joint injections are controversial
- Patient selection and operator factors are likely to play important roles in determining outcomes
- Past studies reported by interventionalists reported mildly positive outcomes, but in recent years, evidence and opinion have shifted towards the conclusion that facet joint injections have limited efficacy and are not cost-effective in larger populations
- Repeated facet joint injections are no longer recommended for low back pain in the UK
- However, there are some patients who show remarkable and prolonged benefit from traditional facet joint injections, and it may be reasonable to continue to offer these injections to a select group

Facet joint medial branch blocks and rhizolysis leading to facet joint denervation

- An alternative to injecting the facet joint or periarticularly is to block or destroy (lesion) the nerves that supply it
- Each facet joint is supplied by two small branches of the posterior medial branch nerves (from the level above and below the facet joint)
- At the lumbar levels, these nerves run in relatively reliable positions as they approach the joint (see Fig. 18.1.1)
- Using X-ray or US guidance, these nerves can be blocked with small volumes of LA (0.3–0.5 mL) to assess the role of the facet joints in contributing to the pain
- This is known as a **diagnostic block** procedure. The LA effect lasts only for hours, so one is looking for short-lived, but significant pain relief (>50%) to occur
- Patients are required to record their pain and function before and after the blocks
- If a short-lived, but significant reduction in pain occurs, then the patients can be offered RF rhizolysis (burning of the nerves)
- This is a procedure using an RF generator designed for that purpose and needles with special tips and an electrode inside the needle that can be heated to a controlled temperature while delivering a controlled amount of energy
- This creates small burns several millimetres long and wide that 'lesion' the nerves
- This is a day case procedure requires X-ray imaging and operator expertise
- The burning also damages adjacent tissue; therefore, the back tends to be painful for a week or two afterwards
- However, once the post procedural acute pain settles down, benefit from the resulting 'denervation' of the facet joints is expected
- The benefit should last for 9 months or longer—but the destroyed nerves grow back over time
- Facet joint MBBs for pain investigation and, if positive, RF rhizolysis to produce facet joint denervation are supported by current evidence and latest UK guidelines

In April 2020, consensus guidelines were published on interventions for lumbar facet joint pain, with the following recommendations (evidence grades 'A' and 'B' indicate to offer/provide service, 'C' to offer/provide service for some patients, and 'D' to discourage use of service; and 'I' means if offered, patients need to understand the risk–benefit balance):

- **History and examination** did not predict reliably the response to facet joint blocks—paraspinal tenderness had a weak positive correlation; pain pattern and imaging can be useful (C)

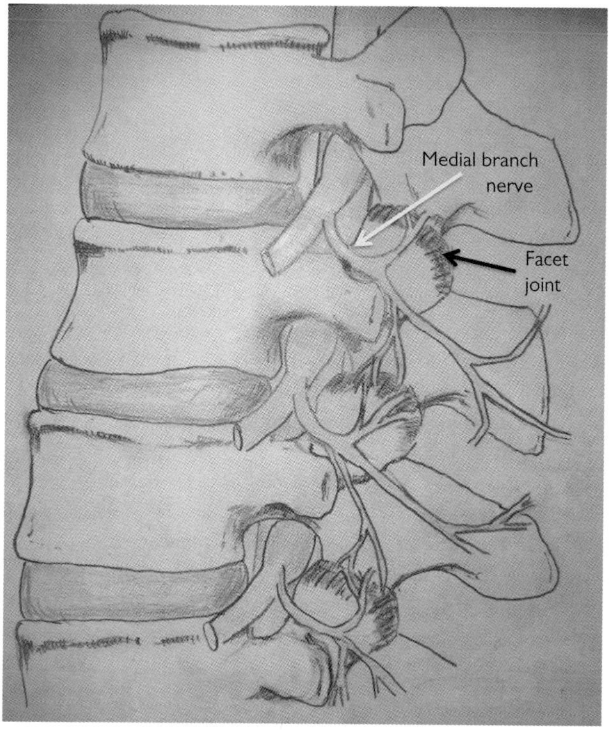

Figure 18.1.1 Illustration of the lumbar spine with facet joints and medial branch nerve

- **Investigations:** weak to moderate evidence for MRI, CT, scintigraphy, and single-photon emission computed tomography (SPECT) before intra-articular blocks (D) and before MBBs (C)
- A 3-month trial of different **conservative treatments** can be offered to some patients (C)
- **CT and fluoroscopy** (US can be considered) are recommended for MBBs or intra-articular facet joint injections (C, D)
- **Intra-articular blocks** seem of higher diagnostic value than **MBBs** (C)
- MBBs and intra-articular injections are better than saline for diagnostic blocks (B)
- MBBs are the prognostic injection of choice prior to RF; intra-articular injections can be used in some patients (C)
- **Sedation** is not routinely recommended (B)
- The ideal volume for MBBs is ≤0.5 mL of LA, and <1.5 mL for intra-articular injections (C)
- Therapeutic use of MBBs and intra-articular injections are only recommended if they produce prolonged pain relief and if RF ablation is contraindicated (D)
- **More than 50% pain relief** is regarded as positive for RF; secondary outcomes should be considered (e.g. activity levels) (B)
- For **prognostic blocks**, a single block is recommended, but multiple blocks (e.g. two) may improve the outcome (C)
- **RF:** larger lesions can improve the outcome (e.g. larger electrode, higher temperatures, longer duration, electrode orientation, fluid modulation) (C, I)
- There is evidence that near-parallel orientation of the electrode is beneficial (B)

- **Sensory stimulation** is recommended for single lesion (C)
- **Motor stimulation** is recommended for safety and effectiveness (B)
- **Complications:**
  - IV uptake is of low validity of MBBs (C)
  - Anticoagulation can be continued for facet blocks and RF ablation (B)
  - There is limited evidence for the use of steroids after RF ablation (C)
  - Multiple views and sensorimotor testing are recommended to lower the risk of nerve root injury (B)
  - There is the possibility of paraspinal muscle degeneration and disc degeneration; therefore, physiotherapy needs to be considered prior to RF denervation (C)
  - Consider interference with implanted electrical devices (turning off neurostimulators, using bipolar RF, grounding pads away from cardiac devices, avoiding excessive sedation) (C)
  - Avoid equipment malfunction or burns (check equipment, dry clean and shave legs for good contact) (B)
  - Lower success rate after spine surgery (avoid contact with metalwork, multiple views to check needle position) (C)
- Different selection and performance criteria can influence the outcome (A)
- **Repeat RF ablation** in patients with >3 or, better, >6 months of pain relief (up to twice per year); the success rate of RF ablation decreases (but pain relief remains above 50%) (B)
- Repeat prognostic blocks are not needed if the pain pattern remains over time (C)

Further reading

1. Cohen SP, Bhaskar A, Bhatia A, et al. Consensus practice guidelines on interventions for lumbar facet joint pain from a multispecialty, international working group. Reg Anesth Pain Med 2020;45(6):424–67
2. Datta S, Lee M, Falco FJ, et al. Systematic assessment of diagnostic accuracy and therapeutic utility of lumbar facet joint interventions. Pain Physician 2009;12(2):437–60
3. National Institute for Health and Care Excellence. Low back pain and sciatica in over 16s: assessment and management. NICE guideline [NG59]. 2016. https://www.nice.org.uk/guidance/ng59
4. Manchikanti L, Datta S, Gupta S, et al. A critical review of the American Pain Society Clinical Practice Guidelines for interventional techniques: Part 2. Therapeutic interventions. Pain Physician 2010;13:E215–64
5. Streitberger K, Müller T, Eichenberger U, et al. Factors determining the success of radiofrequency denervation in lumbar facet joint pain: a prospective study. Eur Spine J 2011;20(12):2160–5
6. Van Kleef M, Vanelderen P, Cohen SP, et al. 12. Pain originating from the lumbar facet joints. In: Van Zundert J, Patijn J, Hartrick CT (eds). Evidence-Based Interventional Pain Medicine. 2012; pp. 87–95. Chichester: Wiley-Blackwell

18.2 Sacroiliac joint block and radiofrequency denervation

Anatomy

- Largest axial joint in the human body with an average surface area of 17.5 cm^2
- A diarthrodial joint between the sacrum and the ilium where only the anterior part is a true synovial joint

- The posterior part is a syndesmosis consisting of both the gluteus medius and minimus muscles, the piriformis muscle, and the sacroiliac ligaments
- Both SIJs move together as a single unit
- Contains hyaline cartilage on the sacral side and fibrocartilage on the iliac side
- SIJ stability depends on both the bony structure and a combination of intrinsic and extrinsic strong ligaments (anterior and posterior SIJ ligament, interosseous SIJ ligament, sacrospinous ligament, sacrotuberous ligaments). These ligaments serve to limit movement in all planes
- Degenerative changes affecting the joint start at puberty and progress throughout life, restricting motion
- Several muscles attach to the SIJ: gluteus maximus and medius, psoas, latissimus dorsi, multifidus, piriformis, biceps femoris, obliquus, transversus abdominis
- Nerve supply:
  - Anterior part: variably by L2–S2, L4–S2, and L5–S2
  - Posterior part: variable from lateral branches of L4–S4 posterior primary rami

Indications

- Intra-articular causes: spondyloarthropathy, OA, malignancies, infections, idiopathic, metabolic
- Extra-articular causes: ligaments, myofascial, fractures, enthesopathy

Contraindications

- Absolute: patient refusal, infection (systemic or local), coagulopathy, profound psychopathology
- Relative: anatomic abnormalities or previous surgeries in the vicinity of the joint

Patient preparation, equipment, and positioning

- In patients with failed back surgery syndrome, a recent MRI scan is a must
- Explanation of the technique and complications, including failure, infection, numbness in the area, and bowel and bladder dysfunction
- A 22G, 88–100 mm needle for the block. Alternatively, for RF procedures, use a 10 cm RF needle with a 5–10 mm active tip. Either needle could have a straight or curved tip
- Prone and full asepsis; place a pillow underneath the iliac crests to neutralize lumbar lordosis

Intra-articular technique

- Having positioned the C-arm in a PA view, angle it to the contralateral oblique side to separate the anterior and the posterior SIJ lines, so as to view the widest gap at the most inferior aspect of the joint. The medial line corresponds to the posterior SIJ line. Tilting the C-arm in a craniocaudal direction may help visualization
- After skin infiltration of the lower part of the joint with lidocaine 1%, introduce the 22G needle until the tip is felt within the joint
- Confirm the position with 0.5–1 mL of contrast. Ideally it should spread within the perimeter of the joint, covering the dorsal and ventral joint lines
- Inject 5 mL of LA ± steroid

Radiofrequency lesioning techniques

Lateral branch sensory-guided radiofrequency neurotomy

- Position as above, aiming to visualize the sacral foramina
- Aim to target the posterior primary ramus of L5 and the lateral branches of the posterior primary rami of S1–S3

- Standard RF needles
- Confirm by sensory stimulation at 50 Hz reproducing concordant pain at <0.5 V. Exclude contact with radicular motor nerves and those controlling sphincters by motor stimulation at 2 Hz between 1.5 V and 2 V (more than twice the voltage needed to achieve sensory stimulation)
- Check the lateral view to exclude needle positions deeper than the sacral cortex
- RF lesion at 85°C for 60 seconds. Some clinicians perform 2–3 lesions per sacral level, 1 cm apart

Bipolar radiofrequency palisade technique

- Position and prepare as above
- Six RF needles with a 10 mm active tip
- Using a postero-anterior view, identify and mark a line between the lateral side of the sacral neural foramina and the SIJ
- In the lateral C-arm view, insert the cannulae perpendicular onto the sacrum along the marked line extending from higher than S1 and ending inferior to S3
- The cannulae should be placed parallel to each other and almost 10mm apart
- Perform motor stimulation between each two adjacent cannulae by 'leap-frogging'. Forgo sensory stimulation
- Perform bipolar RF lesions also between adjacent needles by 'leap-frogging' at 85°C for 60 seconds

Simplicity™ radiofrequency technique

- Simplicity™ is a curved multi-electrode probe
- Position and prepare as above
- A single entry point at 1cm lateral and inferior to the S4 foramen in the lateral inferior sacral border
- Using a 25G, 10 cm needle, infiltrate the skin and the path to be taken by the Simplicity™ probe with lidocaine 1%, avoiding intraforaminal injection
- From the entry point, establish contact with the periosteum
- Advance cranially and laterally, lateral to the foramina and medial to the joint, until it reaches the sacral ala
- Adjust the position to ensure the three independent electrodes are well positioned to lesion the S1–S4 lateral branches
- The L5 posterior ramus will have to be lesioned as usual

SInergy™ cooled radiofrequency technique

- Allows performance of larger lesions with a volume equal to 8–10 thermal RF lesions.
- More predictable ablation that can overcome the anatomical variability of the S1–S3 lateral branches
- The target is the L5 dorsal ramus and the lateral branches of S1–S3
- A special introducer with a stylet is used to be replaced by the RF probe which then extends 4 mm beyond the tip
- The needles should be placed 8–10 mm from the lateral foraminal edge
- The active tip is cooled to −60°C by a water pump
- A total of nine lesions are performed: one at L5, three at S1 and S2, and two at S3

Pulsed radiofrequency technique

- Targets are: L4 medial branch, L5 dorsal ramus, and S1–2 lateral branches
- Two pulsed lesions at 39–42°C at 45 V for 120 seconds

Table 18.2.1 Evidence for interventions for sacroiliac joint pain

Technique	Assessment
Intra-articular steroids and LA	1 B+
Thermal RF of lateral and dorsal rami	2 C+
PRF of lateral and dorsal rami	2 C+
Cooled RF	2 B+

Complications

- Haematoma, nerve damage, sciatic nerve trauma (very rare), temporary flare-up of pain secondary to neuritis, weakness in cases of extra-articular extravasation, vascular particulate embolism, transient perineal numbness, allergic reaction to drugs used

Summary of evidence

(See Table 18.2.1.)

Further reading

1. Gauci C. Manual of Radiofrequency Techniques. 3rd edition, 2011. Ridderkerk: CoMedical BV
2. Raj PP, Erdine S. Pain-Relieving Procedures. 2012. Chichester: Wiley-Blackwell
3. Simpson K, Baranidharan G, Gupta S. Spinal Interventions in Pain Medicine. 2012. Oxford, Oxford University Press
4. Vanelderen P, Szadek K, Cohen SP, et al. Sacroiliac joint pain. In: Van Zundert J, Patijn J, Lataster A, et al. (eds). Evidence-based Interventional Pain Medicine. 2012; pp. 96–102. Oxford: Wiley-Blackwell

18.3 Coccygeal block and ganglion impar block

Anatomy of coccygeal nerve

- Exits the sacral canal from the sacral hiatus at the level of the sacral cornua
- Innervates the coccyx and the skin surrounding the coccyx

Anatomy of ganglion impar

- Most caudal ganglion of the sympathetic trunk located at the sacro-coccygeal junction
- Lies midline in the retroperitoneal space, anterior to the coccyx
- Consists of grey rami communicantes, with grey nerve fibres connecting with the spinal nerves. Lacks white nerve fibres which connect the spinal nerves to the sympathetic ganglia at the thoracolumbar area
- Receives visceral afferent from the anus, distal rectum, perineum, vulva, distal third of the vagina, and distal urethra

Indications

- Coccygeal nerve block: coccygodynia (see 23.12 Coccygodynia, p. 473)
- Ganglion impar block: visceral or sympathetically mediated pain in the perineum, pelvis, genitalia, or coccygodynia

Specific contraindications

- Distorted anatomy

Patient positioning

- Prone position, pillows under the hips and ankles

Technique

Coccygeal nerve block

- Determine the sacro-coccygeal interspace in AP view
- LA infiltration to be injected for needle trajectory to the mid coccyx using a 23G needle
- Insert a 21-23G needle, and advance using a perpendicular needle trajectory technique
- Rotate the C-arm to obtain a lateral view
- Injection of LA/steroid mix should be performed when the needle approaches the coccyx
- The needle should then be walked upwards to the sacro-coccygeal interspace, injecting LA/steroid at this point
- The needle should be walked down to the distal coccyx, injecting LA/steroid at this point
- Contrast should be used before injecting to prevent the risk of any vascular spread and confirm correct positioning

Ganglion impar block

- Determine the sacro-coccygeal interspace in AP view (see Fig. 18.3.1)
- LA infiltration to be injected for needle trajectory to the sacro-coccygeal interspace using a 23G needle

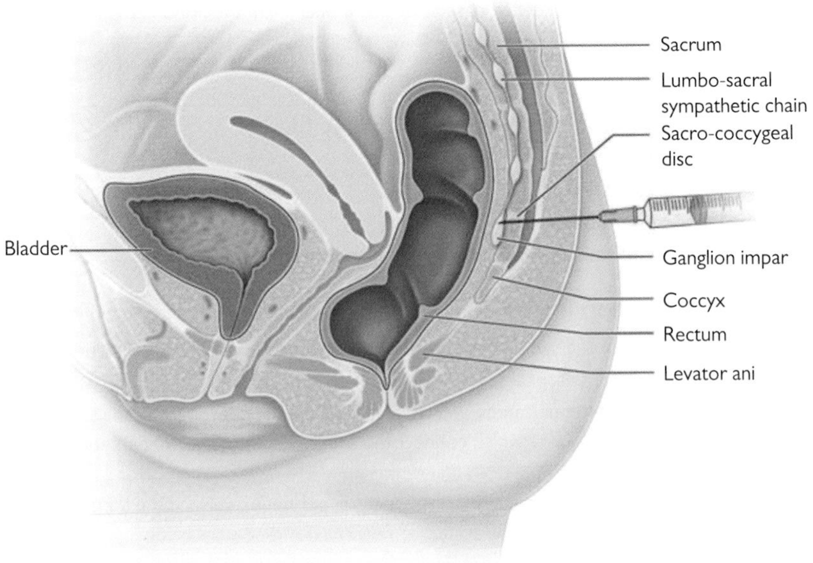

Figure 18.3.1 Ganglion impar block.

Reproduced with permission from Diwan, S., and Staats, P., S. (2015). *Atlas of Pain Medicine Procedures*. New York city, USA: McGraw-Hill Education

- Insert the 21-23G needle, and advance using a perpendicular needle trajectory technique to the C-arm
- Rotate the C-arm to obtain a lateral view, advancing the needle to the anterior aspect of the coccyx
- Inject contrast to determine the position and any vascular spread. Contrast should demonstrate an inferior and superior spread, with a teardrop appearance on fluoroscopy
- Injection of LA/steroids once confirmed

Complications

- Common: sympathetic nerve block causing diarrhoea, hypotension
- Rare: infection, bleeding, nerve injury, LA toxicity, visceral injury (rectum)

Special points

- Remaining in midline to the coccyx (in AP view) and ensuring the needle trajectory is not too anterior to the coccyx to avoid rectal injury
- Can also be performed under US guidance, with use of fluoroscopy to confirm contrast spread and avoid vascular injection

Further reading

1. Toshniwal GR, Dureja GP, Prashanth SM. Transsacrococcygeal approach to ganglion impar block for management of chronic perineal pain: a prospective observational study. Pain Physician 2007;10:661–6
2. Diwan S, Staats PS. Ganglion impar block. In: Diwan S, Staats PS (eds). Atlas of Pain Medicine Procedures. 2015. New York, NY: McGraw-Hill Education

18.4 Caudal epidural

Anatomy

- The dural sac usually terminates in babies at S4 and rises to S2 in adults
- The epidural space extends beyond and is accessible via the sacral hiatus located between the two sacral cornua (unfused S5 vertebral lamina) and the sacro-coccygeal ligament, with extension of the ligamentum flavum overlying it
- Sacral canal contents (average 30–35 mL): filum terminale, termination of the dural sac, Batson's venous plexus, epidural fat, sacral and coccygeal nerves

Indications

- Acute pain in paediatric surgery below the umbilicus (general surgery, urology, orthopaedics)
- Persistent low back pain:
  - Subacute or chronic lumbo-sacral radiculopathy—can provide short-term improvement in pain and disability in patients not responding to conservative or non-surgical management for continued radicular pain
  - Lumbo-sacral spinal stenosis—evidence is limited (careful injection and monitoring of patient)
  - Non-specific low back pain—evidence does not show a strong benefit in pain, disability, or reduction of patients undergoing spinal surgery

Contraindications

- Absolute: patient refusal, bleeding diathesis, infection, allergy
- Relative: spina bifida/anatomical variation

Patient preparation and positioning

- Prone/lateral decubitus

Technique

- Landmark with fluoroscopy/US guidance improves accuracy
- Asepsis, thorough skin disinfection
- Use a line between the posterior superior iliac spines (PSIS) as the base of an equilateral triangle and approximate the apex caudally as the sacral hiatus
- Infiltrate the skin entry point with LA
- Insert a 21–22G, short-bevel needle/20–22G cannula at an angle of approximately 45° to the sacrum, and advance the needle cephalad. If bone is contacted, redirect the needle to reduce the insertion angle relative to the skin
- Following loss of resistance, advance the needle 2 mm/advance the cannula over the needle, and remove the needle
- Allow time for CSF/blood flow out in the event of intradural/intravascular placement
- Aspirate gently as the vessel wall can collapse, producing a false negative
- If fluoroscopy is used, inject radio-opaque contrast (1 mL) to demonstrate spread in the canal
- Inject drug mixture, and observe/palpate for midline swelling (superficial injection)
- Drugs used:
    - LAs: 1–2% lidocaine, 0.1–0.5% bupivacaine, 0.2–1% ropivacaine
    - Adjuvants (extend block duration): clonidine 1 mcg/kg, preservative-free opioids (diamorphine 30 mcg/kg, morphine 50 mcg/kg), steroids (e.g. 40 mg triamcinolone)
    - *Adult dose:*
        - 20–25 mL of 0.125–0.5% bupivacaine
        - Use low concentrations of LA if want to avoid a motor block
    - *Paediatric dose (Armitage formula with 0.25% bupivacaine):*
        - Sacral–lumbar block: 0.5 mL/kg
        - Upper abdominal block: 1 mL/kg
        - Mid-thoracic block: 1.25 mL/kg
        - Duration 4–8 hours

Complications

General

- Failure, bleeding, bruising, infection, nerve injury, medication allergy

Specific

- Superficial/periosteal injection, lower limb motor block (rarer with lower LA concentration), temporary/permanent worse pain, autonomic dysfunction (higher blocks), post-dural puncture headache, intravascular injection

Special points

Differences between adult and paediatric caudal epidurals

- Unpredictable upper abdominal and thoracic spread in adults
- Approximately 5% variability and difficulty in locating the sacral hiatus (complete absence to the bifida of the sacrum) in adults
- Higher paediatric block as less dense and less tightly packed epidural fat, better LA spread with predictable relationship between age, volume of injection, and height of block in pre-adolescent children
- Easier, higher success rate (approximately 95%) in paediatrics

Further reading

1. Chou R, Atlas SJ, Kunins L. Subacute and chronic low back pain: nonsurgical interventional treatment. 2019. UpToDate. https://www.uptodate.com
2. Waldman SD. Caudal epidural nerve block: prone position. In: Waldman SD (ed). Atlas of Interventional Pain Management. 4th edition, 2015; pp. 551–63. Philadelphia, PA: Elsevier

18.5 Piriformis injection

Anatomy

- The piriformis muscle originates from the anterior surface of the S2–S4 sacral vertebrae, the capsule of the SIJ, the anterior sacrospinous, and the sacrotuberous ligament
- It is the only muscle coming out of the greater sciatic foramen and after exiting the foramen, it becomes tendinous and inserts into the upper border of the greater trochanter
- Neurovascular structures that enter the buttock area from the pelvis pass either superior or inferior to the piriformis
- The inferior gluteal artery and nerve, the pudendal artery and nerve, and the sciatic nerve pass below the piriformis muscle although there is significant anatomical variability
- The undivided sciatic nerve most commonly passes below the piriformis muscle. The second most common arrangement is the divided nerve passing through and below the muscle

Indications

- Piriformis syndrome (see 23.13 Piriformis syndrome, p. 475)
- Contracture or spasms of the piriformis muscle secondary to trauma/surgery
- Overuse and hypertrophy of the piriformis muscle
- Abnormal course of the sciatic nerve through the piriformis muscle can lead to sciatic nerve irritation, giving rise to radicular symptoms in the leg

Contraindications

- Patient refusal
- Allergy to LA, steroids, and botulinum toxin
- Relative contraindications: coagulopathy, oral anticoagulants

Patient preparation and positioning

- Patient position: prone
- Full monitoring and consent
- Equipment: curvilinear, low-frequency (2–5 Hz) US probe

Technique

(See Fig. 18.5.1.)

- Scanning is performed in the transverse plane, with the probe placed caudad to the PSIS. The ilium is visualized as a hyperechoic line running across the scan image from medial to lateral
- The probe is then moved caudally to the sciatic notch. When the probe is on the sciatic notch, the hyperechoic line of the ileum is broken into two halves and the shadow of bone (ischium) comes into view in the lateral part of the scan image
- At this level, two layers of muscles—the gluteus maximus muscle dorsally and the piriformis ventrally—will be visualized
- Rotating the hip internally and externally, with the knee flexed, will make the piriformis muscle glide underneath the gluteus maximus muscle
- The origin and insertion of the piriformis muscle can be traced by moving the probe in a medial-to-lateral position
- A 100 mm, short-bevel nerve block needle is usually inserted from medial to lateral, using an in-plane technique
- A total of 2–4 mL of LA and steroid is injected. BTX-A (50–100 Allergan units) with saline can also be used after successful diagnostic block.

Complications

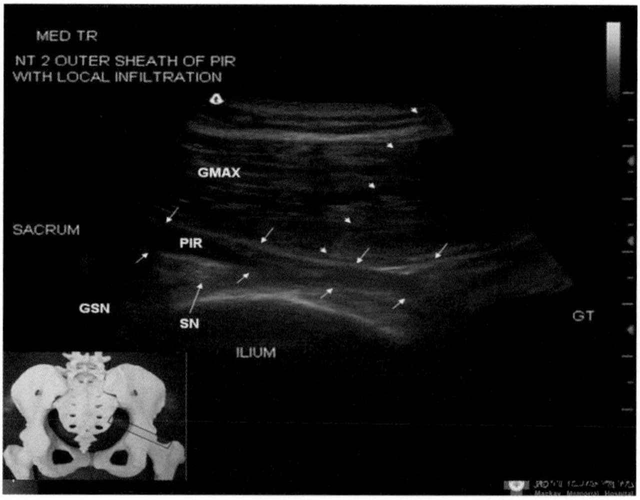

Figure 18.5.1 Anatomy of the piriformis muscle (arrows) and needle path (arrowheads). GMAX, gluteus maximus muscle; GSN, greater sciatic notch; GT, greater trochanter; PIR, piriformis muscle; SN, sciatic nerve

Reproduced courtesy of Dr Sean Lin

- Failure

- Sciatic nerve block—motor weakness
- Sciatic nerve injury

Additional information

- Given the anatomical variation of the sciatic nerve in relation to the piriformis muscle, use of a nerve stimulator and a short-acting LA (lidocaine) is recommended
- Hydro-dissection using 0.9% saline will help to confirm the needle tip position in the muscle
- Other external hip rotators (obturator externus, superior and inferior gemellus muscle) forming the tricipital tendons below the ischial spine may be mistaken for the piriformis. It is important to scan from the ileum and locate the sciatic notch to avoid this misinterpretation

Further reading

1. Chang KV, Wu WT, Lew HL, Özçakar L. Ultrasound imaging and guided injection for the lateral and posterior hip. Am J Phys Med Rehabil 2018;97(4):285–91
2. Simpson G, Krol A, Silver D, Nicholls B. Piriformis. In: Simpson G, Krol A, Silver D, Nicholls B. (eds). Ultrasound-guided Interventions in Chronic Pain Management. 2019; pp. 201–4. UK: European Society of Regional Anaesthesia & Pain Therapy (ESRA)
3. Hopayian K, Song F, Riera R, Sabandam S. The piriformis syndrome: a report of a systematic review of its clinical features and the methodology developed for a review of case studies—Lecture Notes for GPs. Epub, 2010. https://ueaeprints.uea.ac.uk/id/eprint/34961/1/PS_SR_Full_report.pdf
4. Peng PWH, Narouze S. Ultrasound-guided interventional procedures in pain medicine: a review of anatomy, sonoanatomy, and procedures, Part I: nonaxial structures. Reg Anesth Pain Med 2009;34:458–74

Autonomic Nervous System

Ann-Katrin Fritz, Rahul Guru, Gustav Jirikowski, Bhavesh Raithatha, Subramanian Ramani, and Jan Rudiger

CONTENTS

19.1 Anatomy of the sympathetic and parasympathetic nervous systems

Introduction

- The autonomic nervous system (ANS) is divided into two antagonistic systems—the sympathetic and the parasympathetic systems, which are separate entities. These provide innervation to visceral organs, the circulatory system, and their smooth muscle cells. Myofibroblasts and myoepithelial cells require a specific system of motor neurons as part of the ANS
- Most activities of the ANS are involuntary—the ANS is distinct from the somatic motor system that innervates skeletal muscles which are subject to voluntary control.
- ANS activity is usually regulated by the reflex arc with an afferent limb (visceral and/or somatic) and an efferent limb (autonomic and/or somatic). Afferent fibres convey stimuli from the skin (nociceptive) and from sensors in organs (noci-, mechano-, and chemosensors) such as the lungs, GI tract, bladder, vascular system, and genitals. Efferent fibres convey information to smooth muscle cells in organs such as the eye, lung, heart, blood vessels, digestive tract, bladder, glands, and skin.
- The regulation of visceral functions depends on the ANS, including eye sight, salivation, HR, BP, respiratory functions, digestion, urination, defecation, reproduction, and sweating
- Most organs are innervated by sympathetic and parasympathetic nerve fibres. The organ's response to the sympathetic and parasympathetic systems can be either antagonistic (e.g. in the heart) or complementary (e.g. sex organs).
- Simple reflexes can take place within an organ, while complex reflexes are controlled by the CNS, primarily in the spinal cord

Anatomy of the sympathetic nervous system (thoracolumbar origin)

- Two types of neurons: preganglionic (cholinergic) and post-ganglionic (adrenergic)
- Preganglionic cells originate from the lateral grey column of the spinal cord from segments T1 to L2/3

- They project mostly to a chain of paravertebral ganglia—the sympathetic trunk—where they synapse with post-ganglionic neurons
- Post-ganglionic neurons extend long axons to their visceral target organs
- The paravertebral ganglia are interconnected by white and grey matter (commissura alba and commissura grisea) to form a chain that extends up to the cervical and down to the sacro-coccygeal segments
- Usually, there are three cervical, 11 thoracic, four lumbar, four sacral, and one coccygeal sympathetic ganglia. They do not exactly match the vertebral segments due to the fact that some ganglia fused during development
- Some sympathetic nerves bypass the paravertebral ganglia to innervate the prevertebral ganglia in close proximity to their targets (e.g. thoracic splanchnic nerves)
- There is no lateral column in the cervical portion of the spinal cord, and consequently no part of the ANS. Cervical sympathetic ganglia and their projections to the head therefore receive their innervation from thoracic segments
- Lower lumbar, sacral, and coccygeal sympathetic ganglia receive their innervation from the lateral columns of the lower thoracic and first lumbar segments. They connect to thoracic, abdominal, and pelvic plexuses
- Cervical ganglia innervate smooth muscles of the eye, cranial blood vessels, oral mucosa, and salivary glands (lacrimal, submaxillary, sublingual, and parotid)
- Upper thoracic ganglia (T1–4) innervate the heart, larynx, trachea, and bronchi
- The coeliac ganglion (via the greater and lesser splanchnic nerves, T5/6 to T11/12) innervates the stomach, abdominal blood vessels, liver and bile duct, pancreas, spleen, adrenal gland, and small and large intestines (superior mesenteric ganglion)
- The inferior mesenteric ganglion (T12/L1 to L2/3) innervates the rectum, kidneys, bladder, uterus, gonads, and external genitalia
- The ganglion impar innervates the coccygeal ganglia

Anatomy of the parasympathetic nervous system (cranio-sacral origin)

- Preganglionic neurons (cholinergic) of the parasympathetic nervous system originate from the nuclei of CN III, VII, IX, and X in the brainstem and the lateral grey horn in the lower lumbar and sacral portions of the spinal cord
- Parasympathetic portions of cranial nerves terminate in specific cephalic ganglia. Their post-ganglionic neurons are cholinergic and innervate glands or smooth muscles
- The vagal nerve (X) provides parasympathetic innervation to countless visceral (intramural) ganglia in the neck, thorax, and abdomen, ranging caudally as far as the left flexure of the transverse colon. Post-ganglionic neurons extend short projections
- The lumbo-sacral outflow innervates the visceral ganglia through pelvic splanchnic nerves (S2–4)
- CN III innervates the eyes (via the ciliary ganglion)
- CN VII and IX innervate the mucosa of the nose and mouth, and the lacrimal, submaxillary, and parotid glands (pterygopalatine and otic ganglion)
- CN X (vagal nerve) innervates the heart, larynx, trachea, bronchi, oesophagus, stomach, abdominal vessels, liver, bile duct, pancreas, and small and large intestines (smooth musculature: Auerbach and Meissner plexuses in the gut, intestinal glands)
- Lower lumbar levels to S5 innervate the large intestine, rectum, kidneys, bladder, gonads, and external genitalia

Physiology and neurotransmitters

- The **sympathetic nervous system** facilitates the body's response to stressors by utilizing energy and enhancing metabolic activity (fight-or-flight response). Preganglionic neurons release ACh which activates post-ganglionic cells via specific receptors. Post-ganglionic neurons release noradrenaline which acts through adrenergic receptors
- The **parasympathetic nervous system** is dedicated to energy conservation and regeneration, e.g. through digestion, decrease in BP, and/or decrease in HR. Both preganglionic and post-ganglionic neurons of the parasympathetic nervous system are cholinergic, hence utilize ACh for activation of their targets

Clinical significance

- The different neurotransmitters involved in the control of the ANS allow for pharmacological therapy with either sympatholytic or sympathomimetic effects. Pharmacotherapy of hypertension utilizes these effects
- Autonomic neuropathy as a complication of diabetes may be caused by damage to autonomic nerves, resulting in the patient´s inability to control HR, BP, or blood sugar levels
- In heart failure, the sympathetic nervous system increases its activity, leading to increased force of muscular contractions that, in turn, increases the stroke volume, as well as peripheral vasoconstriction. These effects accelerate disease progression
- Sympathicotonia is a stimulated condition of the sympathetic nervous system, marked by vascular spasm and elevated BP

Further reading

1. Marieb EN, Wilhelm PB, Mallatt J. In: Human Anatomy. 5th edition, 2008; pp. 460–72. London: Pearson
2. Pocock G, Richards CD, Richards DA. Human Physiology. 5th edition, 2017. Oxford: Oxford University Press
3. Despopoulus A, Silbernagl S. Autonomic nervous. In: Despopoulus A, Silbernagl S (eds). Color Atlas of Physiology. 5th edition, 2001; pp. 78–87. Stuttgart: Georg Thieme Verlag
4. Trepel M. Sympathikus and parasympathikus. In: Trepel M (ed). Neuroanatomie - Struktur und Funktion. 6th edition, 2015; pp. 297–313. München: Urban & Fischer

19.2 Stellate ganglion block

Anatomy

- Formed by fusion of inferior cervical and first thoracic ganglia at level of C7–T1
- Loose anatomical relationship with the lower sympathetic chain
- Lies anteriorly or immediately lateral to the longus colli muscle, the C7 and T8 nerve roots, and the C7 body at the base of the C7 transverse process
- Lies postero-lateral to the carotid artery, posterior to the vertebral artery, and cranial to the dome of the pleura

Indications

- Neuropathic pain, including acute herpes zoster, PHN, and phantom limb pain
- CRPS—upper limb

- Ischaemic conditions, including vascular insufficiency, Raynaud's disease, reimplantation surgery, upper limb arterial embolism, and treatment of accidental intra-arterial drug injection with thiopentone
- Chronic refractory angina
- Sympathetically mediated cancer pain of the head and neck
- Cluster headache
- Differentiation of sympathetically maintained pain syndromes of the head and upper extremity versus sympathetically independent ones
- PTSD
- Refractory ventricular tachycardia

Contraindications

- Patient refusal
- Localized or systemic infection
- Coagulopathy or thrombocytopenia
- Distorted or complicated anatomy
- Contralateral phrenic nerve palsy or advanced respiratory disease
- Previous lower anterior cervical surgery

Patient preparation and positioning

- General principles of interventions (appropriate indication, including written consent and all potential complications, ruling out anticoagulation, allergies, and local or systemic infection, IV access, full monitoring, trained assistant, and resuscitation equipment)
- Position supine on tipping trolley with head ring
- Preferably no sedation
- Patient should breathe through their mouth and not talk, to prevent swallowing

Technique

Fluoroscopy-guided (anterior approach)

- Target is between the vertebral body and the TP (opaque triangle) of C6
- Angle the image intensifier slightly caudally to visualize C6 junction
- Oblique view to visualize the foramen—needle position away from the vertebral artery and nerve root
- Strict tunnel vision for precise needle placement
- Contrast is mandatory (live screening)
- A total of 5 mL of 0.25% levobupivacaine, preferably with adrenaline, is injected slowly after a 0.5 mL test dose
- Sit up the patient to encourage caudal spread
- Check successful block—ipsilateral temperature rise of at least 2°C
- Horner's syndrome (miosis, ptosis, enophthalmos, conjunctival injection, anhydrosis)
- Monitor the patient for at least 30 minutes
- Identify if motor or sensory block is present versus selective sympathetic block
- Document changes in post-procedure pain score prior to discharge

Ultrasound-guided

- Linear, high-frequency US probe
- Use of sterile gel, probe cover, and primed needle with injection tubing (Stimuplex®)

- Identification of the anterior tubercle of C6 (Chassaignac's tubercle)
- Ideal placement of the needle tip should be antero-lateral to the longus colli muscle, deep to the prevertebral fascia (to avoid spread along the carotid sheath), but superficial to the fascia investing the longus colli muscle (to avoid injecting into the muscle substance)
- More precise injection of a smaller volume of around 4 mL after a 0.5 mL test dose
- Assessment of block as under fluoroscopy

CT-guided

- Not routinely performed

Complications

- Arrhythmias (vagal block = bradycardia)
- Hypotension
- Inadvertent intravascular injection (carotid, vertebral, and inferior thyroid artery), vascular puncture, and haematoma
- LA toxicity (seizure)
- Hoarseness (recurrent laryngeal nerve—more likely if injected near the carotid sheath)
- Horner's syndrome (miosis, ptosis, ipsilateral anhydrosis)
- Blocked nose (Guttman's sign)
- Motor/sensory deficits (cervical/brachial plexus block)
- Phrenic nerve palsy
- High spinal (intrathecal injection)
- Damage to vagal nerve or parts of the brachial plexus
- Pneumothorax
- Oesophageal puncture and mediastinitis
- Infection—abscesses, meningitis, osteitis
- Reaction to drugs or skin prep
- Thoracic duct injury

Additional information

- The vertebral artery at C7 is unprotected; however, in up to 10% of cases, it may enter the foramen of the transverse process at C5 or higher
- Prevent intra-arterial injection with oblique views, gentle aspiration, and contrast media (continuous imaging during injection)—as little as 0.25 mL of LA in the vertebral artery may cause seizure
- Stellate ganglion block may not reliably block all sympathetic fibres to the hands due to varying contributions of T2 and T3 (Kuntz fibres)

Further reading

1. Cepeda MS, Lau J, Carr DB. Defining the therapeutic role of local anaesthetic sympathetic blockade in complex regional pain syndrome: a narrative and systematic review. Clin J Pain 2002;18(4):216–33
2. Chester M, Hammond C, Leach A. Long-term benefits of stellate ganglion block in severe chronic refractory angina. Pain 2000;87:103–5
3. Makharita MY, Amr YM, El-Bayoumy Y. Effect of early stellate ganglion blockade for facial pain from acute herpes zoster and incidence of postherpetic neuralgia. Pain Physician 2012;15:467–74

4. Moore R, Groves D, Hammond C, et al. Temporary sympathectomy in the treatment of chronic refractory angina. J Pain Symptom Manage 2005;30(2):183–91
5. Narouze S. Ultrasound-guided stellate ganglion block: safety and efficacy. Curr Pain Headache Rep 2014;18(6):424
6. Price DD, Long S, Wilsey B, Rafii A. Analysis of peak magnitude and duration of analgesia produced by local anaesthetics injected into sympathetic ganglia of complex regional pain syndrome patients. Clin J Pain 1998;14(3):216–26
7. Schott GD. Interrupting the sympathetic outflow in causalgia and reflex sympathetic dystrophy. BMJ 1998;316(7134):792–3
8. Simpson G, Krol A, Silver D, Nicholls B. Stellate ganglion block. In: Simpson G, Krol A, Silver D, Nicholls B (eds). Ultrasound-guided Interventions in Chronic Pain Management. 2019; pp. 174–7. UK: European Society of Regional Anaesthesia & Pain Therapy (ESRA)

19.3 Splanchnic and coeliac plexus block and neurolysis

Anatomy

Coeliac plexus

- The coeliac plexus is one of the three major divisions of the abdominal prevertebral plexus. It is a network of nerves situated retroperitoneally in the upper abdomen anterior to T12–L1 vertebrae
- The coeliac plexus lies anterior to the crura of the diaphragm and antero-laterally to the abdominal aorta
- The coeliac plexus is composed of a network of nerve fibres, from both the sympathetic and parasympathetic systems, including the vagal nerve and contributions from the phrenic nerve and the upper two lumbar sympathetic nerves
- Post-ganglionic fibres arise from the coeliac plexus and supply the distal oesophagus, stomach, duodenum, small intestine, ascending and proximal transverse colon, adrenal glands, pancreas, spleen, liver, and biliary system

Splanchnic plexus

- The sympathetic preganglionic fibres from T5 to T12 arise from the infero-medio-lateral grey column of the spinal cord
- They travel via the greater (T5–9 spinal roots), lesser (T10, T11), and least (T11, T12) splanchnic nerves, passing over the antero-lateral aspect of the lower thoracic vertebrae (T10–12), to synapse with their post-ganglionic fibres in the coeliac plexus
- The three splanchnic nerves pass over the lateral border of T11 and T12 vertebrae and carry the majority of nociceptive stimuli from the upper abdominal viscera
- *They are contained in a narrow compartment defined by:*
    - Vertebral bodies—medial
    - Pleura—lateral
    - Posterior mediastinum—ventral
    - Pleura attachment to the vertebra—dorsal
    - Crura of the diaphragm—caudal

Indications

- To treat visceral pain from the upper part of the abdomen either due to cancer or non-cancer causes

- Diagnostic block with LA is used to determine whether the pain is arising from the organs supplied by the coeliac plexus. If adequate relief is obtained after a diagnostic block, neuroablation is then done to provide longer-lasting pain relief
- Conditions for these blocks:
    - Malignancies of the upper abdomen, e.g. pancreatic carcinoma (most common indication)
    - Chronic pancreatitis
    - Abdominal angina due to arterial insufficiency
    - Pain due to arterial embolization of the liver for cancer therapy
    - Acute pancreatitis (LA block only)
- A splanchnic nerve block can be tried for non-cancer procedures and when coeliac plexus block (CPB) has failed to provide pain relief

Contraindications

- Similar to other interventions
- Respiratory insufficiency or pleural adhesions (due to risk of pneumothorax)
- Abdominal or thoracic aneurysm

Technique

- CPB has been traditionally performed using fluoroscopy; however, CT- and US-guided approaches are now being used successfully
- Here the transcrural fluoroscopic approach for CPB is described

Patient preparation and positioning

- The patient is positioned prone, with a pillow under the abdomen

Transcrural approach for CPB

- The C-arm is aligned to obtain an AP view of the thoracolumbar region. It is then rotated obliquely to the left, until the tip of the TP of L1 overlies the antero-lateral margin of the L1 vertebral body. LA is infiltrated into the skin corresponding to the superolateral margin of the L1 vertebra
- A 22G, 15 cm needle is inserted at the left superolateral margin of the L1 vertebra
- It is advanced under fluoroscopic guidance, 0.5 cm at a time, towards the antero-lateral and superior margin of the L1 vertebra, aiming for bone contact
- Once bone contact has been established, a lateral view is taken to confirm the position of the needle. The needle is advanced a further 2–3 cm anterior to the L1 vertebra
- There is a risk of puncture of the aorta at this stage, in which case the needle is either withdrawn and redirected to lie slightly more laterally or continued through the anterior wall of the aorta (**trans-aortic approach**)
- In the AP view, the needle should lie medial to the lateral border of the L1 vertebra. The position is confirmed with 1–2 mL of radio-opaque contrast, which should spread towards the midline, and not beyond the lateral margin of the vertebra in the AP view (see Fig. 19.3.1)
- In the lateral view, the contrast should lie anterior to the aorta and must not spread posteriorly towards the nerve roots (see Fig. 19.3.1)
- The same procedure is followed on the right side
- Amount of drug injected:
    - Diagnostic block—10–12 mL of levo-bupivacaine per side
    - Neurolytic block—10–12 mL of phenol or alcohol per side

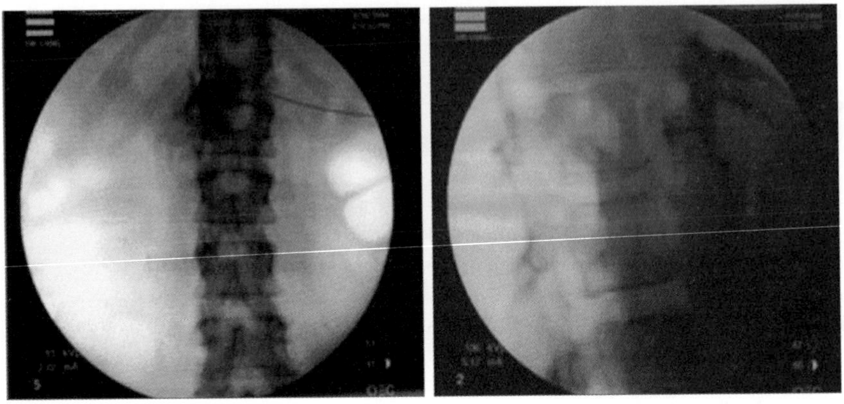

Figure 19.3.1 Coeliac plexus block. Left: in the anteroposterior view, the contrast medium extends across the midline. The right needle is inserted superior to the transverse process of L1 towards the T12/L1 interspace. Right: in the lateral view, contrast is flowing along the anterolateral border of the aorta and silhouetting the coeliac trunk run-off

Reproduced with permission from Waldman, S. (2014). *Atlas of Interventional Pain Management*, Fourth Edition. Amsterdam, Netherlands: Saunders, an imprint of Elsevier

Retrocrural technique for splanchnic nerve block

- The T11 or T12 vertebra is identified and the endplates are squared in the AP view
- The fluoroscope is turned oblique about 15° to the side to be blocked
- A 22G, 15 cm needle is inserted a little below the rib at the costovertebral junction and advanced to reach the junction of the anterior and middle third of the vertebral body, confirmed in the lateral view
- The final position of the needle is on the antero-lateral margin of the T11 or T12 vertebra, just medial to its lateral border
- Radio-opaque contrast is injected to confirm correct needle placement. Spread should be towards the midline, and not beyond the lateral margin of the body of the vertebrae in the AP view (see Fig. 19.3.2)
- The same technique is repeated on the opposite side
- Amount of drug injected:
    - Diagnostic block—5–8 mL of levo-bupivacaine per side
    - Neurolytic block—5–8 mL of phenol or alcohol per side

Radiofrequency denervation of the splanchnic nerves

- The technique of needle placement for RF denervation is similar to the techniques described above
- 15 cm RF needles with a 10 mm active tip are used
- Sensory stimulation should elicit pain and discomfort in the epigastric region of the abdomen
- No contractions should be seen on motor stimulation up to 2 V (RF needle at a safe distance from the intercostal nerve)
- If the patient reports a band-like stimulation pattern, the intercostal nerve has been stimulated and the needle should be advanced slightly
- Neuroablative lesion procedure is similar for all RFs

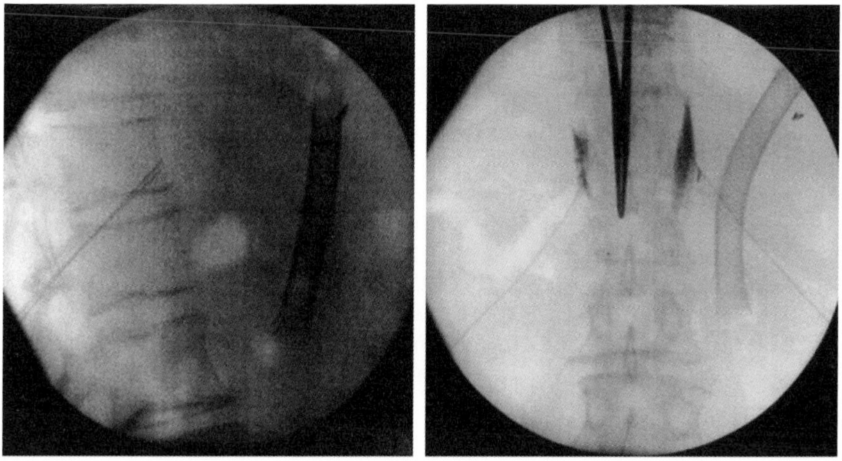

Figure 19.3.2 Splanchnic nerve block. Classic two-needle technique in the lateral view (left) showing the final needle tip position. Note the spread of contrast is limited to the lateral portion of T12 on the right image

Reproduced with permission from Waldman, S. (2014). *Atlas of Interventional Pain Management*, Fourth Edition. Amsterdam, Netherlands: Saunders, an imprint of Elsevier

Complications

- Orthostatic hypotension (50% with splanchnic nerve block; 10% with transcrural approach). This is due to blockade of sympathetic innervation
- Transient diarrhoea (65% with transcrural approach; 5% with splanchnic nerve block), also due to sympathetic blockade
- Pneumothorax is rare, but more likely with splanchnic nerve block than with CPB
- Paraplegia, bowel and bladder dysfunction (1 in 700 after neurolytic block). These complications are due to alcohol or phenol causing spasm or necrosis of spinal segmental arteries that supply the spinal cord such as the artery of Adamkiewicz
- Intravascular injection. Alcohol injected intravascularly will lead to alcohol levels above the legal limits; however, at the dose it is normally given, it is below severe alcohol toxicity. Intravascular phenol causes features similar to LA toxicity
- Backache due to needle trauma, retroperitoneal haematoma. Haematocrit should be measured at serial intervals, and imaging performed if there is a drop in haematocrit
- Abdominal aortic dissection, as a result of trauma from the needle
- Injury to abdominal organs, gastric perforation, haematuria from kidney injury
- Epidural, subarachnoid injection and injury to the nerve roots

Additional information

- Radiographic guidance in the form of fluoroscopy, CT, or US is of paramount importance, given the nature of risks associated with this block
- Needles should always be directed medially towards the antero-lateral margin of the vertebrae. Lateral placement of the needle could cause complications such as organ damage and pneumothorax

- Splanchnic nerve block has a higher incidence of pneumothorax, compared to CPB. The risk of pneumothorax can be minimized by keeping the needles close to the vertebral body at all times
- A positive diagnostic block is a poor predictor for a negative response to a neurolytic block. The practice of performing a diagnostic block before neurolysis is questionable in patients with terminal malignancy
- A review of three RCTs suggested that CPB provides the best results in pancreatic carcinoma without evidence of disease outside the viscera, rather than in advanced pancreatic carcinoma
- An RCT revealed that splanchnic nerve RF ablation led to significantly better pain relief, QoL, and analgesic consumption, compared to CPB, and may be more suitable for patients with upper abdominal pain from non-malignant causes such as chronic pancreatitis. This is because of the predictable anatomy of the splanchnic nerves, allowing accurate placement of the RF needles

Evidence

- CPB for pain secondary to pancreatic cancer—1A
- CPB for pain secondary to chronic pancreatitis—2C

Further reading

1. Dimitrios Papadopoulos GK. Bilateral thoracic splanchnic nerve radiofrequency thermocoagulation for the management of end-stage pancreatic abdominal cancer pain. Pain Physician 2013;16:125–133
2. Koyyalagunta AB. Sympathectomy for cancer pain. In: Sharma KHM (ed). Practical Management of Complex Cancer Pain. 2014; pp. 147–166. Oxford: Oxford University Press
3. Leon-Casasola OA. Neurolysis of the sympathetic axis for cancer pain management. Techniques in Regional Anesthesia and Pain Management 2005;9:161–166
4. Rathmell JP. Celiac plexus block and neurolysis. In: Rathmell JP (ed). Atlas of Image Guided Intervention in Regional Anesthesia and Pain Medicine. 2006; pp. 162–175. Philadelphia, PA: Lippincott Williams and Wilkins
5. Tordoff GG. Percutaneous splanchnic nerve radiofrequency ablation for chronic abdominal pain. ANZ Journal of Surgery 2005;75(8): 640–644.

19.4 Lumbar sympathetic block and sympathectomy

Anatomy of the lumbar sympathetic ganglia

- The target is L1–5 paravertebral sympathetic ganglia
- The L1 and L2 sympathetic ganglia are often fused; hence, there is often only four paired lumbar sympathetic ganglia
- Anterior to the medial origin of the psoas muscle
- Lie on a craniocaudal line connecting the antero-lateral border of the vertebral body
- The relationship of the ganglion is most consistent at the middle to upper third of the L3 vertebral body in the lateral view
- At L2 level, the ganglion is often at the lower third of the vertebral body in the lateral view
- At L4 and L5 levels, this relationship is more variable
- The vena cava lies anterior to the chain on the right side, and the aorta is antero-medial on the left side

Indications

- Phantom limb pain, neuropathic pain, CRPS, and pain from severe cold exposure in the lower limbs
- Vascular abnormalities such as Raynaud's disease, Berger's disease, and arteriosclerotic peripheral vascular disease
- Miscellaneous: hyperhidrosis, erythromelalgia

Contraindications

- Lack of informed consent, patient refusal
- Infection
- Coagulopathy
- Anatomical anomaly of the lumbar spine

Patient preparation and positioning

- The patient is positioned prone on an X-ray table, with a pillow under the abdomen to neutralize the lumbar lordosis

Technique—general principles

- Lumbar sympathetic ganglion interventions are usually done in two stages
- Initially a diagnostic block is performed
- If effective in symptom management and improving QoL, the following can be considered:
  - The procedure can be repeated
  - RF ablation can be considered
  - Neurolytic injection (alcohol/phenol) in cancer pain or palliative conditions
- The procedure is best done at L3 level

Technique of procedure

- AP view of lumbar vertebrae
- Count up from L5 and identify L2, L3, and L4 vertebrae
- The vertebra in focus is squared by either a caudal or sometimes a cranial tilt of the fluoroscopy tube to eliminate the double edge of the inferior border of the vertebral body, which should be visualized as a largely single line
- An oblique ipsilateral tilt of the fluoroscopy tube to the side of the block is then done. Sufficient tilting to obscure the TP projection within the vertebral body will help achieve an extraforaminal needle path, avoiding nerve root injury and genitofemoral neuralgia during RF ablation
- The final target is the antero-lateral margin in the transverse plane of the lower quarter of the L2 vertebral body, the upper quarter of the L3 vertebral body, or the middle of the L4 vertebral body in the lateral view of fluoroscopy
- The needle entry point is at the lateral border of the vertebral body projection in the oblique view and at the appropriate level of the vertebral body according to the preceding point
- The needle is inserted along the X-ray beam (gun barrel approach)
- The position of the needle should be adjusted to achieve this in the superficial planes
- After insertion of the needle to a few centimetres deep, a lateral view is used to confirm the distance from the foramen (a craniocaudal tilt is best left undisturbed in the lateral view)

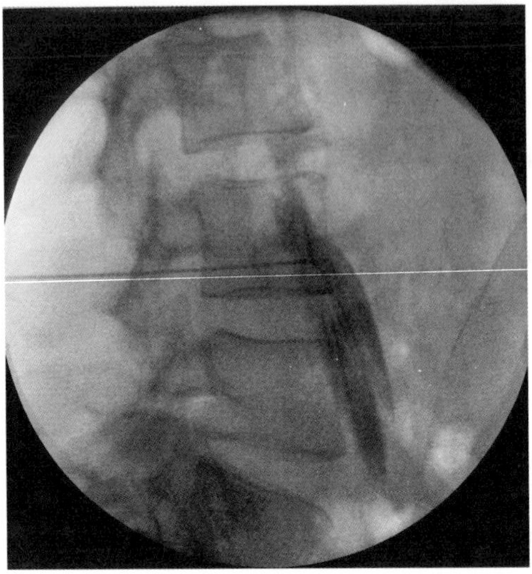

Figure 19.4.1 Final needle position in the lateral view, but contrast delineates the striated myogram of the psoas muscle. The needle is advanced antero-medially

- Once the needle approaches the posterior edge of the foraminal projection, the needle should be advanced carefully, looking for paraesthesiae due to contact with the nerve root. If this is encountered, then the needle should be angled superiorly or inferiorly to pass the nerve root safely
- The needle is then advanced in the lateral view to the anterior edge of the vertebral body
- In the AP view, the needle should be medial to the lateral projection of the vertebral body on the side of the block
- Switching again to the lateral view, a small amount of contrast is injected. This should spread anterior to the vertebral body in the retroperitoneal space and has a typical vacuolated appearance
- If there is posterior spread with a typical striated appearance of muscle, this implies that the needle is within the psoas muscle. The needle should be carefully advanced by a few millimetres to lie anterior to the muscle, to avoid a lumbar plexus block or thermal/chemical injury to the plexus (see Figs. 19.4.1 and 19.4.2)

Diagnostic block

- A total of 10–15 mL of LA (levo bupivacaine or ropivacaine) at L3 level, aiming for LA spread to cover L2–4 levels
- May need multiple-level injections for adequate LA spread

Chemical neurolysis

- 6–10% phenol or alcohol 50–100% with contrast can be used for chemical neurolysis
- It is best done with small volumes at multiple levels

Radiofrequency thermal neurolysis

- A 20G curved, blunt needle with a 5 mm active tip is preferred to minimize vascular puncture and nerve root injury

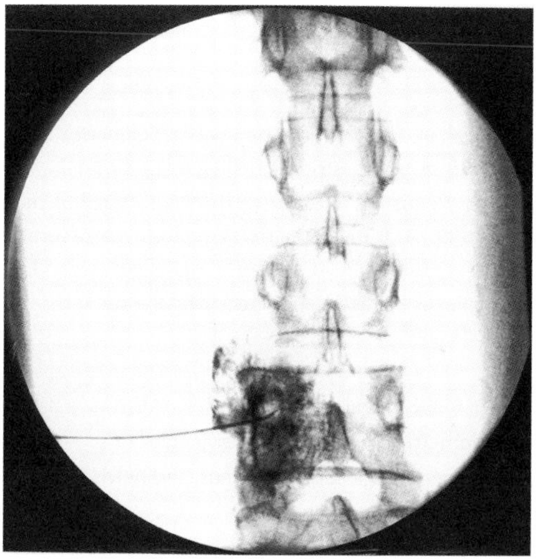

Figure 19.4.2 Final needle position in the AP view. Contrast delineates the correct vacuolated appearance of retroperitoneal tissue

- After needle positioning, as discussed, sensory stimulation at 50 Hz would elicit a deep ache in the abdomen and no paraesthesiae in the lumbar plexus distribution
- Motor stimulation at 2 Hz should not elicit muscle contractions in the lower limb (femoral and obturator nerve supply)
- A total of 5 mL of 0.25% levo-bupivacaine or 0.2% ropivacaine with dexamethasone is injected prior to the lesions
- Lesions at 80°C for 60–90 seconds at L2, L3, and L4 levels

Complications

- Quoted risk of 4–15% of genitofemoral neuralgia after therapeutic chemical or RF sympathectomy (highest risk if procedure performed at L4)
- Disc puncture and discitis
- Radicular artery injury and paraplegia
- Ureteric injury
- Impotence
- Retroperitoneal haematoma
- Hypotension and diarrhoea
- Infection and LA toxicity

Further reading

1. Gauci C. Manual of Radiofrequency Techniques. 3rd edition, 2011. Ridderkerk: CoMedical BV
2. Raj PP, Erdine S. Pain-Relieving Procedures. 2012. Chichester: Wiley-Blackwell
3. Waldman S. Pain Management. 2nd edition, 2011. Philadelphia, PA: Saunders

19.5 Hypogastric plexus block

Anatomy

- The hypogastric plexus is an extension of the sympathetic (superior hypogastric plexus) and parasympathetic ANS (inferior hypogastric plexus) (see Fig. 19.5.1)
- The superior hypogastric plexus lies anterior to the lower third of the L5 vertebral body and the upper third of S1. It mediates most nociceptive visceral stimuli from the pelvic organs
- The inferior hypogastric plexus lies at S2–4, surrounding the rectum

Indications

- Non-gynaecological pain: PHN (sacral region)
- Gynaecological pain: endometriosis, vulvodynia, pelvic tumour
- Pain involving the bladder, penis, vagina, rectum, anus, and pelvis

Patient positioning

- Prone position, pillows under the hips and ankles

Technique—superior hypogastric posterior approach

- Determine the L5/S1 interspace using fluoroscopy guidance in the AP view
- Rotate the C-arm in a cephalad/caudad direction to ensure the vertebral endplates are aligned
- Rotate the C-arm ipsilaterally in the oblique plane to visualize the lateral vertebral body, ensuring the end of the TP is on the anterior aspect of the vertebral body
- Position to aim for: mid/anterior aspect of the lower third of the L5 vertebral body
- LA to skin entry point using a 23G, then 21G needle
- A 20G, 15 cm curved tip to be inserted using the perpendicular needle trajectory technique to the C-arm
- When the vertebral body is struck, visualize in the AP view to confirm needle position
- Rotate the C-arm to the lateral position and rotate the needle, advancing gently
- A 'give' should determine the needle position anterior to the vertebral body
- Confirm the needle position in the lateral and AP views
- Aspirate to ensure no vascular injection; contrast injection should demonstrate spread inferiorly and superiorly to the anterior of the vertebra
- Inject LA/steroids once you have achieved confirmation of spread
- Repeat for the contralateral side

Complications

- Common: sympathetic nerve block causing diarrhoea, hypotension
- Rare: infection, bleeding (aortic/vena cava puncture), nerve injury, LA toxicity, visceral organ injury

Special points

- The procedure can also be performed with:
  - Superior hypogastric plexus block with a postero-medial transdiscal or anterior approach, with the aid of US, fluoroscopy, or CT guidance
  - Inferior hypogastric plexus block with a coccygeal transverse or trans-sacral approach

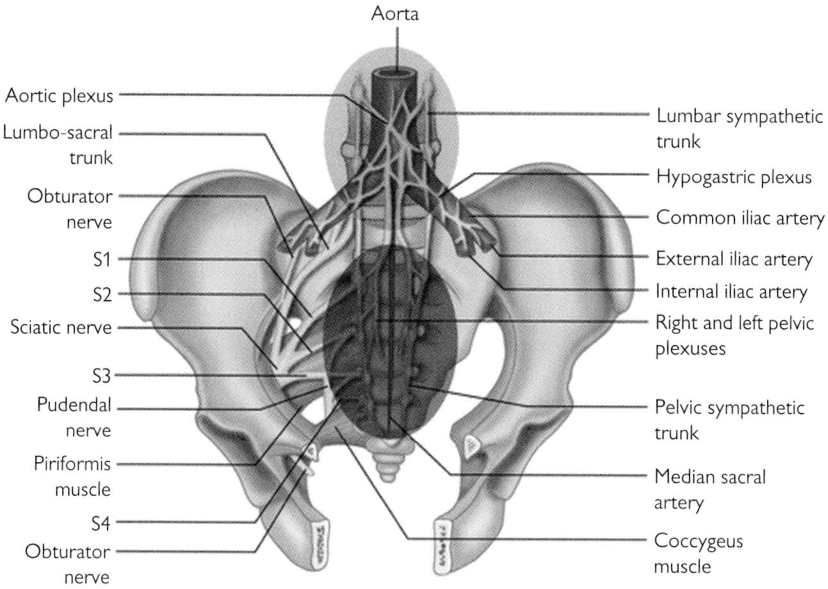

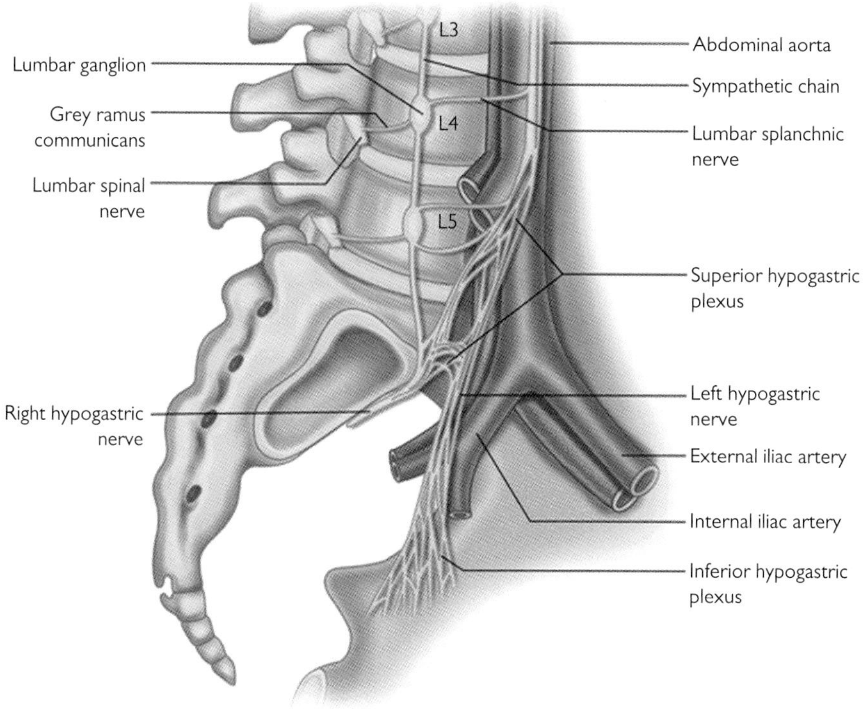

Figure 19.5.1 Hypogastric plexus

Reproduced with permission from Waldman, S. (2014). *Atlas of Interventional Pain Management*, Fourth Edition. Amsterdam, Netherlands: Saunders, an imprint of Elsevier

Further reading

1. Fronk B, Doulatram GR. Hypogastric plexus blocks. In: Manchikanti L, Kaye A, Falco F, Hirsch J (eds). Essentials of Interventional Techniques in Managing Chronic Pain. 2018; pp. 573–580. Cham: Springer
2. Mishra S, Bhatnagar S, Gupta D, Thulkar S. Anterior ultrasound-guided superior hypogastric plexus neurolysis in pelvic cancer pain. Anaesth Intensive Care 2008;36:732–5
3. Gamal G, Helaly M, Labib YM. Superior hypogastric block: transdiscal versus classic posterior approach in pelvic cancer pain. Clin J Pain 2006;22(6):544–7

CHAPTER 20

Spinal Cord and Neuromodulation

Sangeeta Das, Gustav Jirikowski, Yehia Kamel, Deepak Malik, Manish Mittal, Yin Yee Ng, Stefano Palmisani, David Pang, Jan Rudiger, and Athmaja Thottungal

CONTENTS

20.1 Anatomy of the spinal cord

Definition

- The spinal cord is part of the CNS
- Connection between the brain and the peripheral nervous system
- 32 segments: eight cervical, 12 thoracic, five lumbar, five sacral, two coccygeal

Grey matter

(See Figs. 20.1.1 and 20.1.2.)

- Numerous nerve cells and their connections form the core, which shows bilateral symmetry
- It contains cell bodies of second-order sensory afferents in the dorsal horn (DH), autonomic nerves (intermediate column), and motor efferents in the ventral horn (VH)

Dorsal horns (DHs)

- Entry for sensory nerve fibres which originate from DRGs.
- Important for perception of pain, tactile stimuli, proprioception, etc.
- The dorsal horn includes the nucleus dorsalis, nucleus proprius, and stellate ganglion

Lateral horns (LHs)

- Part of the sympathetic nervous system. The LH is absent in cervical segments
- Dorsal LH has viscero-sensory properties, and ventral LH controls viscero-motor functions
- Interneurons control visceral reflexes

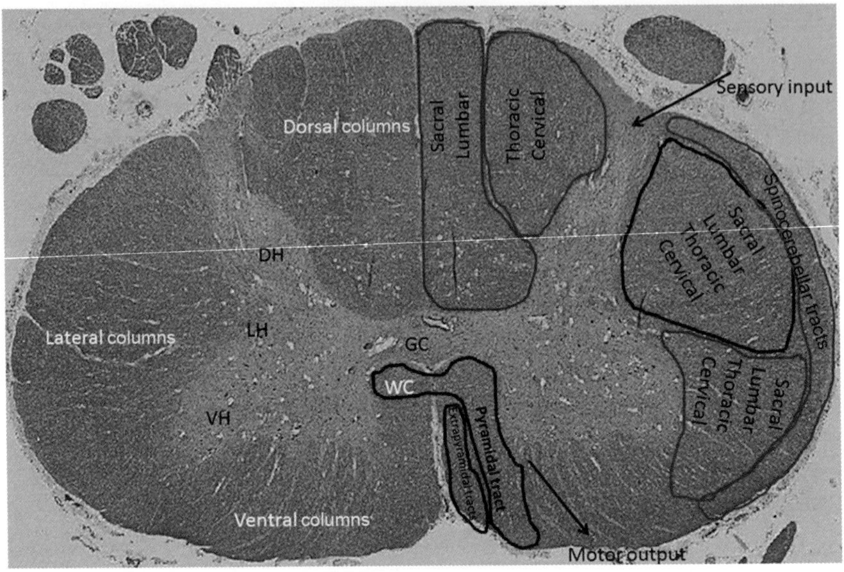

Figure 20.1.1 Histological cross-section of the spinal cord. Grey matter: DH, dorsal horn; GC, grey commissure; LH, lateral horn; VH, ventral horn; WC, white commissure. White matter: ascending tracts in black; descending tracts in grey

Ventral horns (VHs)

- Contain motor nuclei
- Alpha motor neurons innervate skeletal muscles, and gamma motor neurons supply muscle spindles. Their axons form the anterior root as part of the spinal nerves

Monosynaptic and polysynaptic reflexes

- Grey matter neurons are interconnected. Connections between the DH and VH are the basis for **monosynaptic (somato-motor) reflexes**

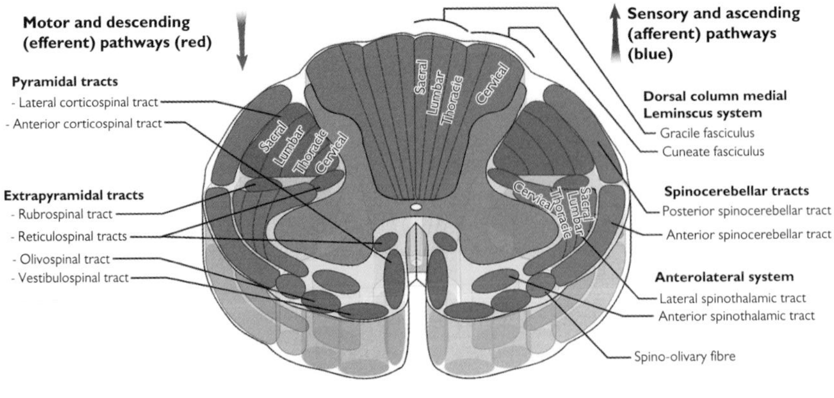

Figure 20.1.2 Spinal cord tracts

- Grey matter of both sides of the spinal cord is interconnected by the **grey commissure (GC)**. This is the basis for **polysynaptic reflexes**. Involvement of the LH controls **visceral reflexes**

Reticular formation

- Connection of all portions and all segments of the grey matter; important for all sensory and motor functions. Highly significant for perception of pain
- The centre of the GC hosts the central canal. Neurons that surround the reticular formation extend processes through the ependyma

White matter

- Bundles of myelinated neuronal fibres leading to blue: dorsal column, spinocerebellar tracts, anterolateral system and from red: pyramidal and extrapyramidal tracts the brain (see Fig. 20.1.2). They surround the grey matter and show somato-topic organization

Dorsal columns

- Contain ascending sensory nerve fibres to the medulla oblongata
- The fasciculus gracilis hosts afferents from sacral, lumbar, and thoracic segments; the fasciculus cuneatus contains upper thoracic and cervical afferents

Lateral columns

- Contain lateral spinocerebellar tracts, and descending corticospinal = pyramidal (red) and ascending spinothalamic tracts (blue)

Ventral columns

- Contain descending fibres of the extrapyramidal system, including rubrospinal, olivospinal, vestibulospinal, and reticulospinal tracts

White commissure

- Only cervical segments have a **white commissure (WC)** which contains fibres of the pyramidal tract prior to crossing to the contralateral side

Blood supply

- One ventral (two-thirds) and two dorsal arteries (one-third) provide oxygen to the entire spinal cord
- The cervical segments are supplied from branches of the vertebral arteries. All other segments are supplied from the aorta via intercostal arteries.
- Numerous anastomoses interconnect spinal arteries
- Spinal veins drain into venous plexuses along spinal nerves

Clinical significance

- Destruction of the grey matter results in permanent motor and/or sensory impairment of the respective segment, depending on the extent of the lesion
- Destruction of the white matter causes paralysis of all segments caudal to the lesion. Due to increased excitability of motor neurons, such paralysis eventually becomes spastic

Further reading

1. Martini F, Tallitsch R, Nath J. In: Human Anatomy. 9th edition, 2017. London: Pearson

2. Martins I, Tavares I. Reticular formation and pain: the past and the future. Front Neuroanat 2017;5:1–14
3. Trepel M. Rückenmark (Medulla spinalis). In: Trepel M (ed). Neuroanatomie – Struktur und Funktion. 6th edition, 2015; pp. 297-313. München: Urban & Fischer

20.2 Anatomy of vertebral bodies

Shape of a typical vertebral body

- Cylindrical body
- Superior and inferior vertebral endplates
- Anterior and posterior longitudinal ligaments
- Horizontal view—convex anteriorly, concave posteriorly
- Sagittal view—concave anteriorly, flat posteriorly

Blood supply

- Paired segmental arteries
- Posterior venous drainage into internal and external vertebral venous plexus, then into regional segmental veins (vertebral, posterior intercostal, lumbar, sacral), then into the central venous system
- Free anastomoses, valveless venous communication to pelvic, renal, and azygos venous systems aid haematogenous disease spread, including infection and malignancy

Innervation

- Sinu-vertebral branches
- Via endplates; also gives some innervation to intervertebral discs
- Interosseous nerves follow the vasculature

Lymphatic drainage

- Details unknown
- Likely deep lymphatic vessels following arteries

Vertebral endplates

- Thin hyaline cartilage layer with supporting cortical bone plate
- Supports intervertebral discs
- Fracture risk centrally as weak, superior more than inferior

Cervical vertebrae

- Seven cervical vertebrae
- Vertebral artery traverses via foramen transversarium, except in C7
- C1/atlas: ring-shaped, no true body or spine, anterior spinal canal facet for dens articulation
- C2/axis: body with dens overlying superiorly, held against C1 'body', allowing rotation of the head
- C3–6: small body, wider in the transverse than in the AP plane, flat lamina, bifid spinous process
- C7/vertebra prominens: more similar to thoracic vertebrae, non-bifid spinous process, foramen transversarium traversed by venous and post-ganglionic sympathetic plexuses

Thoracic vertebrae

- Twelve thoracic vertebrae
- T1: atypical, more similar to C7, longer upper rib facet joint, smaller lower rib facet joint
- T2–T8: heart-shaped body, with small costal demi-facet joint on superolateral border (for rib at same level) and larger costal demi-facet joint infero-laterally (for rib at level below)
- T9–12: single superior costal facets

Lumbar vertebrae

- Five lumbar vertebrae
- Large kidney-shaped body, short pedicles, without foramina transversaria and costal facets
- L5 body wedge-shaped for weight loading; higher anteriorly, forming lumbar lordosis

Sacrum

- Five vertebral bodies fused to form a large triangular sacrum with a concave ventral surface
- Central axis of pelvic girdle between the two iliums, forming the sacroiliac (SI) joints
- Sacral promontory articulates with L5 cranially
- Inferior oval facet for articulation with coccyx

Coccyx

- Small triangular bone/rudimentary tail made of 4–5 fused coccygeal vertebrae
- Directed infero-ventrally from sacral apex
- Orientation may vary and can be mobile

Pathologies in vertebral bodies

- Degenerative, e.g. OA, spondylosis, spondylolisthesis
- Trauma/vertebral fracture
- Malignancy (primary or secondary)
- Infection
- Inflammatory
- Metabolic, including osteoporosis
- Vascular malformations

Radiological investigations

X-ray and computed tomography

- Used for bony changes, including:
  - Misalignment, e.g. scoliosis, antero-/retrolisthesis, pars defect
  - Fracture
  - Sacralization of L5 vertebra
- X-ray less useful as likely normal with high false positive rate; CT useful if MRI contraindicated

Magnetic resonance imaging

- Used for soft tissue changes
- May demonstrate changes of unknown significance, e.g. Schmorl's nodes, Modic changes

Bone scans

- Technetium-99 scan: identifies inflammatory processes in bone which can be from pathologies such as cancers (primary or secondary), infections, and fractures
- SPECT: localizes lesions which can be malignant (e.g. in facet joints, pedicles, spinous processes, vertebral bodies) or secondary to other inflammatory processes

Further reading

1. Standring SB. Back. In: Standring S (ed). Gray's Anatomy. 41st edition, 2015. London: Elsevier
2. Brooks MK, Mazzie JP, Orlando AO. Degenerative disease. In: Haaga J, Boll D (eds). CT and MRI of the Whole Body. 6th edition, 2017; pp. 827–43. Philadelphia, PA: Elsevier

20.3 Discography

Introduction

- Chronic discogenic back pain has a prevalence of 35–40%
- Due to low sensitivity and specificity of clinical diagnosis and the presence of asymptomatic disc changes seen with conventional imaging methods, i.e. MRI, invasive methods such as provocative discography, in combination with post-discography CT, can be used to diagnose discogenic pain

Anatomy

- The intervertebral disc has four distinct regions

Nucleus pulposus

- It forms the gelatinous core of the disc and contains collagen and elastin fibres embedded in proteoglycan matrix
- Main function is to maintain disc hydration

Annulus fibrosus

- Thick outer ring of fibrous cartilage made of 15–25 concentric rings or lamellae, with collagen fibres lying parallel to individual lamellae and elastin fibres in between the lamellae (they assist in preserving the disc shape)

Vertebral endplates

- Thin layer of hyaline cartilage that articulates between the disc and vertebral body

Nerve supply of intervertebral disc

- In a normal disc, only the outer third of the annulus fibrosus and vertebral endplates are innervated, but in discogenic pain, this innervation extends to the inner third and even to the nucleus pulposus via vascular granulation tissue after healing of annular tears
- The anterior and lateral annulus fibrosus is supplied by grey rami of the sympathetic trunk, and the posterior is supplied by the recurrent sinu-vertebral nerve, formed by a branch from the ventral ramus and grey rami

Indications

- Persistent severe symptoms when other diagnostic tests were inconclusive
- Assessment of disc prior to fusion to identify the symptomatic disc and whether the adjacent disc can support the fusion
- Evaluation of abnormal disc or recurrent pain from a disc that was previously operated on
- Failed back surgery or a different source of back pain
- Assessment of candidates for minimally invasive surgery, with confirmed disc herniation

Contraindications

- As with other interventions
- Substantial psychosocial stressors or poorly controlled mood disorders
- Solid bone fusion
- Severe spinal canal compromise

Patient preparation and positioning

- Standard protocol followed
- Strict asepsis, under X-ray fluoroscopy
- The patient is positioned prone, with the C-arm oblique, to align the facet joint in the middle of the fluoroscope screen

Technique—lumbar discography

- LA infiltration (e.g. lidocaine 1%) for skin infiltration; avoid excessive use to prevent anaesthetizing the sinu-vertebral nerve and ramus communicans
- Introduce the needle just above the lateral margin of the superior articular process
- The introducer needle is then advanced just over the lateral edge of the superior articular process or to the margin of the disc
- After confirming the introducer needle position on the lateral view, a 25G, 15cm discogram needle is slowly advanced into the centre of the disc through the introducer needle, while monitoring the lateral view
- The disc is slowly pressurized by injecting 0.5 mL increments of contrast through a syringe attached to a pressure-measuring device, while recording the opening pressure, injection pressure, location of the contrast medium, and evoked pain response

End points

- Intradiscal pressure of 80–100 psi above the opening pressure with a normal-appearing nucleogram
- 3.5 mL of contrast has been injected

Diagnostic criteria (Spine Intervention Society)

- Provocation of the suspect disc induces concordant pain
- The pain is at least 7/10 on NRS
- The pain is provoked by <50 psi above the opening pressure in a disc with a grade 3 annular tear
- Provocation of at least one adjacent disc does not induce concordant pain

Four-type classification by Derby et al. in respect to annular sensitivity

- Discs which are painful at pressures <15 psi above the opening pressure are termed low-pressure positive or 'chemically sensitive' discs
- Discs which are painful at pressures between 15 and 50 psi are termed 'mechanically sensitive' discs
- Indeterminate discs are painful at pressures between 51 and 90 psi
- Normal discs are not painful on provocation

Interpretation of post-discography CT

- Depicts vertebral disc architecture

Modified Dallas discogram scale to classify post-CT findings

- Grade 0 describes contrast contained within the nucleus
- Grades 1–3 describe the degree of fissuring extending to the inner, middle, and outer annulus, respectively
- Grade 4 describes a grade 3 annular fissure with >30° circumferential arc of contrast.
- Grade 5 annular tear indicates rupture or spread of contrast beyond the outer annulus

Complications

- Bacterial discitis (0.25% per patient and <0.14% per disc)
- Meningitis, arachnoiditis, epidural abscess
- Acute disc herniation, spinal headache/CSF leakage, intrathecal (IT) haemorrhage
- Retroperitoneal bleeding, pulmonary embolism from nucleus pulposus material
- Allergic reaction
- Seizure

Special points

- Discography performed in accordance with current standards in appropriately selected patients is a safe and useful diagnostic tool to inform treatment decisions
- Lumbar discography can be a useful tool in assessing chronic back pain
- Weak evidence for cervical, and no evidence for thoracic back pain

Further reading

1. Walker J 3rd, El-Abd O, Isaac Z, et al. Discography in practice: a clinical and historical review. Curr Rev Musculoskelet Med 2008;1(2):69–83
2. McCormick ZL, DeFrancesch F, Loomba V, et al. Diagnostic value, prognostic value, and safety of provocation discography. Pain Med 2018;19(1):3–8
3. Manchikanti L, Soin A, Benyamin RM, et al. An update of the systematic appraisal of the accuracy and utility of discography in chronic spinal pain. Pain Physician 2018;21:91–110 [systematic review]
4. Derby R, Howard MW, Grant JM, et al. The ability of pressure-controlled discography to predict surgical and nonsurgical outcomes. Spine. 1999;24:364–71; discussion 371–2

20.4 Dorsal root ganglion

Definition

- Cluster of nerve cells
- Interface between the peripheral and central nervous system
- Port of entry of peripheral inputs (somato-sensory, proprioceptive, viscero-sensory, nociceptive)
- Contains the cell bodies of the first-order sensory neurons (pseudo-unipolar ganglion cells) which are engulfed by satellite cells
- DRGs are encapsulated by a layer of dense connective tissue that connects with the dura mater of the spinal cord

Localization

(See Figs. 20.4.1 and 20.4.2.)

- DRGs are associated with spinal nerves
- DRGs are part of the peripheral nervous system, derived from the neural crest

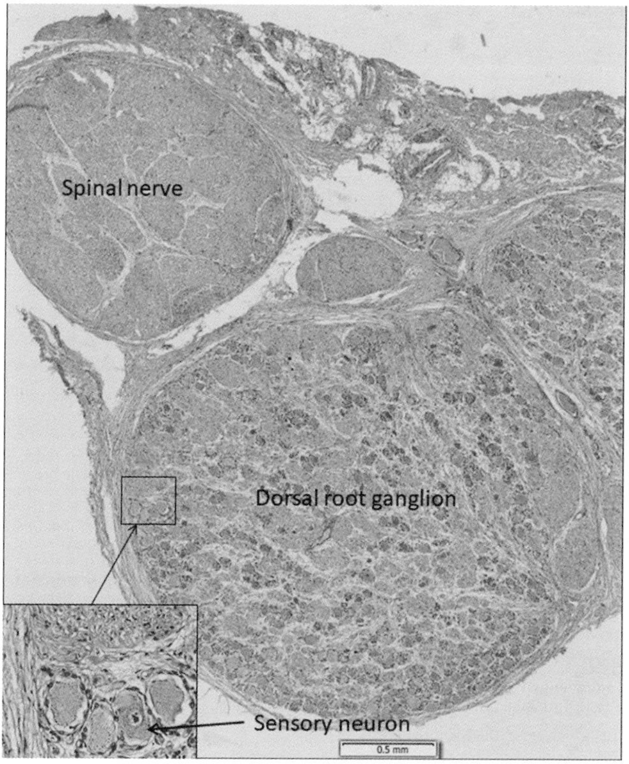

Figure 20.4.1 Histological image of the dorsal root ganglion and spinal nerve root, with subsection demonstrating the sensory input

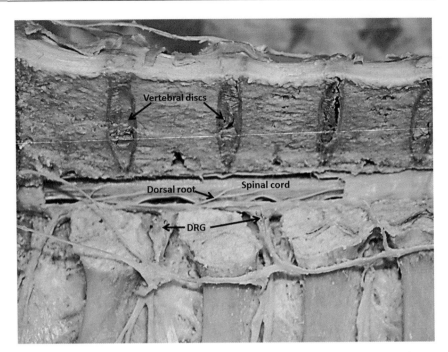

Figure 20.4.2 Macroscopic image of the dorsal root ganglion (DRG) in relation to surrounding structures

- They are located in the intervertebral foramina
- DRG neurons project to 2nd ONs in the DH of the spinal cord
- Afferents connect DRG neurons via myelinated dendrites with either dermatomes or myotomes, or with visceral organs

Function

Somato-sensory perception

- Specific innervation of receptors within dermatomes (Merkel bodies, Vater–Paccini bodies, Ruffini bodies, free nerve endings). Important for perception of pain, heat, cold, pressure, movement, and tactile stimuli

Viscero-sensory perception

- Free nerve endings in visceral organs are sensory dendrites of DRG neurons (intestinal pain, cardiac pain, fullness of urinary bladder or rectum)

Motor control

- DRG neurons innervate proprioceptors (muscle spindles, Golgi tendon organs, kinaesthetic joint receptors)—important for reflexes

Drainage of cerebrospinal fluid

- Peri-ganglionic venous plexuses are important for CSF resorption and CSF current

Functional impact—pathophysiology

- Loss of somatic reflexes: indicative of interrupted neuronal circuits of either peripheral nerves, DRGs, or the spinal cord
- Loss of sensation of specific dermatomes, e.g. as a consequence of a ruptured vertebral disc
- Head zones: somato-sensory and viscero-sensory neurons represent distinct groups of cells within the DRG. Their axons terminate on identical neurons in DH nuclei. Brain circuits can recognize visceral pain as somato-sensory pain. Therefore, visceral pain can be experienced as somatic pain in certain dermatomes (see 26.1. Overview of visceral pain, p. 527)
- Viral infections can specifically affect sensory spinal nerves and DRGs (e.g. herpes zoster)

Diagnostic tests

Sensory tests of dermatomes

- Help to determine the extent of damage to a peripheral nerve

Reflex tests

- Stimulation of proprioceptors
- Axons of DRG neurons terminate on interneurons in the spinal cord which innervate motor neurons to trigger reflexes

Sensory neurography

- Measurement of sensory nerve action potentials (SNAPs)

Histamine test

- Failure to develop redness of skin at the injection site indicates deafferentation

Clinical relevance

- DRG injections block sensory supply of a specific spinal nerve without motor impairment
- Neurostimulation of DRG neurons can be useful in chronic neuropathic pain
- Chronic pain: injuries can cause maladaptive molecular changes in DRG neurons, resulting in hypersensitivity and hyperexcitability

Further reading

1. Berta T, Qadri Y, Tan PH, Ji RR. Targeting dorsal root ganglia and primary sensory neurons for the treatment of chronic pain. Expert Opin Ther Targets 2017;21(7):695–703
2. Liem L, van Dongen E, Huygen FJ, et al. The dorsal root ganglion as a therapeutic target for chronic pain. Reg Anesth Pain Med 2016;41(4):511–19
3. Silav G, Arslan M, Comert A, et al. Relationship of dorsal root ganglion to intervertebral foramen in lumbar region: an anatomical study and review of literature. J Neurosurg Sci 2016;60(3):339–44

20.5 Epidural injections

Introduction

- Epidural injections are used in chronic spinal pain and can be a useful part of multidisciplinary care

- Careful patient selection, and it is important that it is offered as part of a package of care, and not as a stand-alone treatment
- Epidurals do not cure the underlying pathology but are a useful temporary analgesic modality to allow for natural resolution or to facilitate other pain management strategies (e.g. physiotherapy)
- Different approaches are available—the aim is to deposit LA and steroid to the DRG or the nerve root that is affected by spinal pathology (e.g. prolapsed intervertebral disc or foraminal stenosis)

Indications

- Nerve root inflammation or compression with spinal radicular pain that has not responded to conservative management
- Nerve root compression on imaging is common, but there must be a clear clinical correlation with symptoms and signs of nerve root irritation
- A large network meta-analysis did show that ESI was effective in lumbar radicular pain
- However, it is not indicated in axial low back pain without radicular features

Contraindications

- Patient refusal
- Local infection and coagulopathy
- Severe central spinal stenosis
- Adverse reaction to LA or steroids

Applied anatomy

- As the nerve roots and DRG exit the spinal cord, they are initially located in the epidural space
- Therefore, nerve irritation caused by a prolapsed intervertebral disc or spinal OA and degenerative changes can be treated with an injection into the epidural space
- Many trials of ESIs are flawed by poor methodology and by poor reporting on whether the medication was injected in the correct place
- LA and steroids can exert both an analgesic and an anti-inflammatory effect

Technique

- Strict aseptic technique and image guidance with radiographic contrast are mandatory
- The approaches to the epidural space are:
  - Interlaminar
  - Transforaminal
  - Sacral hiatus/caudal
  - Catheter techniques and epidurolysis
- The transforaminal approach has the advantage of depositing LA and steroid in the anterior epidural space, which is closer to the source of pathology
- However, the transforaminal approach is technically more difficult, and there is a risk of nerve injury by direct needle trauma or vascular injury
- If steroids are used, they must be non-particulate since injection in nutrient arteries has been associated with spinal cord infarction
- IV access is secured prior to the procedure, and the skin is disinfected
- Patients are usually positioned prone to allow optimal fluoroscopic imaging
- A lateral approach is sometimes used for lumbar and caudal epidurals

- Full aseptic technique must be used at all times (including sterile gloves and gown, hat, and mask)

Interlaminar

- Loss of resistance technique with Tuohy needle and saline (or air)
- Needle placement is in the space between the vertebral bodies/laminae
- A paramedian approach is preferred to improve steroid deposition in the antero-lateral epidural space
- For the cervical approach, a contralateral oblique approach can be useful

Transforaminal

- Under fluoroscopic imaging, the needle is directed to the intervertebral foramen
- Care must be taken to avoid nerve injury as the needle is placed very close to the nerve root
- Minimal or no sedation is recommended, and a blunt (non-curved) needle is recommended if available
- This approach is recommended for lumbar epidurals
- A transforaminal approach for the cervical area risks nerve and vascular injury and should be performed by experienced operators only

Sacral hiatus/caudal approach

- The lumbar epidural space can be accessed via injection at the sacral hiatus which is where the epidural space terminates inferiorly
- Using a large volume, it is possible to deliver injectate to the lumbar nerve roots
- Usually technically simple, with a low risk of dural puncture

Catheter techniques/epidurolysis

- One of the challenges is to ensure delivery of steroid precisely to the pathological area
- Using a blunt steerable catheter in the epidural space can allow precise targeting of nerve roots (see 20.6 Lumbar epidural adhesiolysis, p. 380)
- In addition, if there is epidural fibrosis or filling defects that may represent obstruction, the injectate may not reach the desired target
- Entry into the epidural space with an introducer needle with a circular cross-section and the catheter placed through with a needle-through-needle technique
- For the lumbar area, the sacral hiatus is used, but for thoracic and cervical areas, the introducer is placed using an interlaminar approach
- The catheter is steered under fluoroscopy to the antero-lateral epidural space at the site of pathology
- It is important not to force the catheter through any obstruction, but to use hydro-dissection if there are any filling defects

Complications

- Dural puncture (approximately 0.5–1%) that may cause post-dural puncture headache
- Nerve injury (make sure that there is contrast run-off outside the spine, so that the injected volume does not compress the spinal cord)
- Epidural haematoma
- Infection and epidural abscess

- Vascular injection (avoid particulate steroids using a translaminar approach—the particulate component causes embolic infarcts into the spinal arteries; that risk is minimized with the use of non-particulate steroid and blunt needles)

Further reading

1. Cohen SP, Bicket MC, Jamison D, et al. Epidural steroids: a comprehensive, evidence based review. Reg Anesth Pain Med 2013;38(3):175–200
2. Lewis RA, Williams NH, Sutton AJ, et al. Comparative clinical effectiveness of management strategies for sciatica: systematic review and network meta-analysis. Spine J 2015;15(6):1461–77
3. Pinto RZ, Maher C, Ferreira ML, et al. Epidural corticosteroid injections in the management of sciatica: a systematic review and meta-analysis. Ann Intern Med 2012;157:865–87
4. Rathmell J, Benzon HT, Dreyfuss P, et al. Safeguards to prevent neurological complications after epidural steroid injections. Anesthesiology 2015;122(5):974–84

20.6 Lumbar epidural adhesiolysis

Anatomy

- Both techniques (percutaneous and endoscopic technique) target the lumbar epidural space
- Basic knowledge of lumbar spine anatomy and its visualization under fluoroscopy is required

Indications

- Chronic lower back pain with or without radiculopathy
- Especially in the context of previous spine surgery, spinal stenosis, and epidural scar tissue (demonstrated with either contrast-enhanced MRI or epidurogram under live fluoroscopy)

Contraindications

- Bleeding disorders
- Antiplatelet/anticoagulation therapy
- Headache disorders not appropriately investigated (*endoscopic adhesiolysis only*)
- Vision disorders (*endoscopic adhesiolysis only*)

Patient preparation and positioning

- Prone position (support in the abdominal area to straighten the lumbar lordosis)
- Full sterile preparation for both the patient and the operator
- Antibiotics are not required
- IV access is mandatory (for safety reasons), even if sedation is not administered

Technique

- Both techniques require cannulation of the sacral hiatus under fluoroscopy (lateral and AP view) to access the posterior epidural space

Percutaneous adhesiolysis

- The original technique involves the identification of epidural filling defects (epidurogram)

- Placement of a spring-tip radio-opaque catheter in the area of the defect and multiple injections of a mixture of drugs to facilitate adhesiolysis:
  - Day 1 (hyaluronidase, bupivacaine, triamcinolone, 10% sodium chloride)
  - Days 2 and 3 (bupivacaine and 10% sodium chloride)
- A modified technique seems to be equally effective despite being a single-day procedure, the use of short-acting LA and non-particulate steroids, and the overall reduction in volume of the injectate
- No strong evidence showing substantial benefits of 10% saline versus 5% or 0.9%
- Benefits of the procedures are believed to be secondary to dissolution of adhesions (unconfirmed), prevention of recurrence through inhibition of fibroblasts, and greater access for analgesic substances in the perineural spaces

Endoscopic adhesiolysis

- The endoscopic technique requires a flexible steerable endoscope to explore the postero-lateral epidural space around the dura, and to visually identify pathological scar tissue and remove it using mechanical (Fogarty-like balloon) or thermal (RF probe) tools that are inserted through one of the working channels of the endoscope
- Most practitioners do not inject drugs at the end of the procedure
- Benefits of the procedures are believed to be secondary to mechanical and/or thermal lysis of adhesions (confirmed under direct vision)

Complications

- Epidural bleeding—very rare
- Dural tear—4% (*percutaneous*) to 8–10% (*endoscopic*)
- Post-procedural headache
- Potential for trauma to the nerve roots, mass effect of the high volume of injectate causing transient or permanent neurological deficits
- Temporary or permanent visual disturbances (*endoscopic adhesiolysis only*)—very rare
- Allergic reaction to any of the drugs used (*percutaneous adhesiolysis only*)—very rare
- Shearing of the catheter (*percutaneous adhesiolysis only*)

Additional information

Percutaneous adhesiolysis

- Use of epidurogram to guide treatment
- Try to inject part of the drug mixture in the lateral epidural space to ensure adequate spread towards the anterior epidural compartment
- Use contrast dye injection under live fluoroscopy prior to injection of any drug, to detect intravascular or subarachnoid spread
- If using hypertonic saline, first inject an LA test dose and assess neurology at 15 and 30 minutes to detect subdural/IT catheter tip positioning

Endoscopic adhesiolysis

- To avoid the risks related to saline over-infusion, monitor carefully the volume injected (usual range 80–300 mL); volumes above 100–150 mL require an awake patient to monitor the onset of neck discomfort, the first sign of over-infusion
- To distinguish between pathological and non-pathological fibrous tissue, it is useful to 'probe' the tissue either with the tip of the scope or with one of the surgical tools available to elicit pain which is concordant with the subject's usual pain

Further reading

1. Pereira P, Severo M, Monteiro P, et al. Results of lumbar endoscopic adhesiolysis using a radiofrequency catheter in patients with postoperative fibrosis and persistent or recurrent symptoms after discectomy. Pain Pract 2016;16:67–79
2. Racz GB, Holubec JT. Lysis of adhesions in the epidural space. In: Racz GB (ed). Techniques of Neurolysis. 1989; pp. 57–72. Boston, MA: Kluwer Academic Publishers
3. Manchikanti L, Singh V, Kloth D. Interventional techniques in the management of chronic pain: part 2.0. Pain Physician 2001;4:24-98

20.7 Percutaneous cordotomy

Introduction

- This involves the use of RF to ablate the sensory fibres of the lateral spinothalamic tract
- It is used in refractory cancer pain that is unilateral and below the fourth cervical dermatomal level
- Although bilateral cordotomy can be performed for bilateral pain, it is associated with a greater risk of complications and is less commonly done
- Recommended if life expectancy is less than 12 months
- Refractory incident and neuropathic pain are good indications, but deafferentation pain responds poorly
- There are no RCTs evaluating its use and evidence is based on case series
- A small proportion of patients with cancer-related pain do not get satisfactory analgesia with systemic medication and cordotomy can provide a useful means of achieving analgesia

Indications

- Chest wall pain from malignant mesothelioma
- Unilateral limb pain
- Other unilateral chest wall pain
- Pain from brachial plexus lesions

Contraindications

- One of the difficulties is that patients are referred late for a cordotomy and the disease may be too advanced
- The patient must be able to lie supine for about 60–90 minutes
- Coagulopathy
- Respiratory distress
- Localized infection

Applied anatomy

- Cordotomy involves an RF lesion in the lateral spinothalamic tracts that correspond to the painful area
- The lateral spinothalamic tracts lie in the antero-lateral quadrant of the spinal cord (they carry contralateral pain and temperature sensation) (See 20.1 Anatomy of the spinal cord, p. 367)
- An important anatomical structure is the dentate ligament that is used to identify the midline of the spinal cord

- Lesions must be placed anterior to this structure as the spinothalamic tract lies just anterior to it
- The lesion is done at C1/2 as it allows needle placement to lesion the lateral spinothalamic tract high enough to result in analgesia from the level of C4 downwards
- Lesioning at the lateral spinothalamic tract reduces pain and temperature sensation, with preservation of motor function, touch, and proprioception

Technique

- The most common approach is the percutaneous approach using LA or conscious sedation
- An open surgical approach is an alternative but requires a laminectomy and is more invasive with the requirement of intraoperative wake-up testing
- CT guidance is another alternative with the advantage of easier needle placement at the expense of a longer procedure duration
- Patient positioning is supine and due to crossover of the sensory pathways, the lesion must be done in the spinothalamic tract contralateral to the painful area
- IV access is mandatory and the head is restrained using either a Pounder or Rosomoff headrest
- An RF needle with a 2 mm tip is placed under fluoroscopic guidance at C1/2 in the lateral view until CSF is encountered
- Radiographic contrast is injected to confirm needle placement anterior to the dentate ligament to ensure correct direction of the needle; then the electrode is inserted through this needle
- Once the electrode is inserted, the RF machine will show a low impedance as the tip is still in the CSF
- Advancing the needle into the spinal cord will result in an increase in impedance, and once in the spinal cord, both motor and sensory testing are performed to check that the electrode is in the correct position to create a lesion in the spinothalamic tract
- Motor stimulation at 2 Hz will elicit local ipsilateral neck muscle twitching, but any contralateral limb movement suggests that the tip is at the corticospinal tract and the needle must be repositioned to avoid damage to the motor fibres (2 Hz stimulation is to confirm that the electrode is not in the motor tracts)
- Stimulation at 50 Hz determines correct electrode positioning (if the tip is correctly positioned, this stimulation will result in pain and a warm or cold sensation on the contralateral side)
- RF lesioning is only done once correct sensory testing is obtained with no limb movement on stimulation testing. Multiple lesioning is performed at 75°C, increasing to 85°C. During lesioning, the patient is asked to move the ipsilateral limbs to check no motor lesioning has occurred
- The effect of cordotomy is immediate, with rapid onset of analgesia upon successful lesioning

Complications

- Headache
- Neuropathic mirror pain can occur on the contralateral side but is commonly mild
- A transient Horner's syndrome can be seen, which resolves spontaneously
- Respiratory impairment is uncommon with unilateral cordotomy and may be as a result of damage to the reticulospinal tract
- Motor weakness (short-term weakness on the ipsilateral side to the lesion is usually self-limiting and due to transient spinal cord oedema)
- Urinary dysfunction

Further reading

1. Bain E, Hugel H, Sharma M. Percutaneous cervical cordotomy for the management of pain from cancer: a prospective review of 45 cases. J Palliat Med 2013;16(8):901–7
2. Deandrea S, Montanari M, Moja L, Apolone G. Prevalence of undertreatment in cancer pain. A review of published literature. Ann Oncol 2008;19:1985–91
3. Poolman M, France B, Lewis R, et al. The use of cordotomy in mesothelioma-related pain: a systematic literature review. Palliat Med 2012;26:459–60
4. Rosomoff HL, Carroll F, Brown J, Sheptak P. Percutaneous radiofrequency cervical cordotomy: technique. J Neurosurg 1965;23:639–44

20.8 Intrathecal drug delivery systems

Introduction

- Intrathecal drug delivery (ITDD) systems provide effective analgesia with smaller doses of analgesics, thereby reducing medication-related S/Es. There is supportive evidence for the use of ITDD for cancer pain, chronic non-malignant pain (CNMP), and painful spasticity.

(See relevant information in Chapters 6 and 7, and in 13.1 Baclofen, p. 229, 13.8 Clonidine, p. 244, and 29.6 Intrathecal drug delivery treatment for cancer pain, p. 602.)

Indications and efficacy

- The polyanalgesic consensus guidelines systematically evaluate the level of evidence and degrees of recommendations for IT therapy. This guideline weighs the risk versus benefits, outlines best practices, patient selection, and medication selection, and educates about the potential for treatment failure and unacceptable adverse effects. The main conclusions include:
  - Complete assessment and management of a patient's physical, psychological, and social characteristics, and can guide practitioners in determining the appropriateness of initiating, and the effectiveness of, IT therapy
  - The evidence for using IT opioid therapy for cancer pain is 1A. There is strong evidence supporting the use ziconotide for active cancer pain. It has been shown to improve QoL and longevity, with lesser toxic effects
  - There is poor evidence for using IT opioid therapy in CNMP. The National Health Service (NHS) England currently does not routinely commission ITDD for CNMP
  - The use of IT baclofen is well established in treating spasticity associated with cerebral palsy, SCI, and MS

Patient selection

- Patient selection is extremely crucial and should ideally be done within a multidisciplinary setup
- History, physical examination, investigations and psychological evaluation supporting a clear organic pain generator without much psychological overlay
- Persistent pain unresponsive to conservative therapy
- Intolerable S/Es from systemic opioid therapy
- Positive IT trial results
- Stable enough medical condition to undergo anaesthesia and surgery
- No risk of spinal cord compression—tumour or metastasis
- Cognitive ability to use patient device present

Patient education

- Risks and benefits of therapy
- Educate on expected signs and symptoms caused by underdosing or overdosing which can be life-threatening
- Avoid high-impact activity and scuba diving at a depth of 2 atmospheres
- If MRI needed, an IT pump that is MRI-compatible is required. The pump needs to be interrogated after MRI to ensure proper functioning

Contraindications

Absolute

- Systemic infection/local infection over insertion site
- Clotting abnormalities
- Failed IT trial
- Allergy to IT drugs used

Relative

- Abnormal behaviour/response during screening trial

Types of systems

External pumps

- Can be tunnelled or non-tunnelled catheters or with an SC port
- Advantages: technically easier, cheaper, suitable for patients with limited life expectancy
- Disadvantages: increased risk of infection, cumbersome pumps hampering patient mobility

Implanted pumps

- Comfortable for patients and useful for long-term use. Life expectancy should be at least 3 months
- *Fixed-rate gas-driven pumps:*
    - Flow at constant rate that cannot be changed; only drug concentration can be changed
    - Advantages: suitable for long-term use, less expensive, have longer refill intervals
    - Disadvantages: lack flexibility in drug prescription; rate cannot be changed; pump and catheter dead space need to be emptied to stop the pump in an emergency
- *Programmable pumps:*
    - Battery-driven pump with battery life of 7–10 years
    - Reservoir volumes usually 20–40 mL
    - Advantages: offer flexibility in changing rate and in using bolus doses
    - Disadvantages: expensive, refill intervals usually every 6 weeks, and bolus facility may also mean shorter refill intervals

Drugs

Cerebrospinal fluid dynamics

- CSF is secreted by the choroid plexus at 0.3–0.4 mL/hour, with a total volume of 90–150 mL
- Current knowledge shows that CSF revolves around the spinal cord in circles with little overall net flow. Instead there is an oscillatory flow determined by HR, BP, and intrathoracic pressure variations

- Morphine concentration has a decreasing rostral-to-caudal gradient as the distance from the catheter tip increases. Therefore, the catheter tip needs to be at least at, or just above, the dermatomal level innervating the painful area
- Lipophilic drugs remain more localized around the site of intrathecal delivery than hydrophilic drugs which have broader spread in the CSF and can diffuse cranially into the respiratory centres

Pharmacotherapy of intrathecal analgesia

(See Table 20.8.1.)

Morphine

- Acts on mu receptors in the DH and PAG
- Only opioid approved by the FDA for IT administration
- Small molecule (285 Da) and very hydrophilic substance, resulting in prolonged duration of action
- t1/2 in CSF is 80 minutes
- 300 mg of PO morphine is equivalent to 1 mg of IT morphine

Hydromorphone

- Semi-synthetic morphine derivative
- Compared to morphine: five times more potent and lesser supraspinal effects as it is more lipophilic

Fentanyl

- Synthetic anilopiperidine
- Highly lipophilic, resulting in segmental analgesia near the catheter tip

Bupivacaine

- Amino amide that binds to the α subunit of voltage-gated Na^+ channels, reducing Na^+ influx, thereby inhibiting nerve conduction in sensory fibres. Needs close monitoring as motor and autonomic nerve fibres are also blocked
- Being highly lipid-soluble, its rostral spread in the IT space is limited
- Rarely used alone; acts synergistically with opioids, decreasing the need for progressive dose escalation of opioids
- Bolus doses of 1–2 mg are more effective than continuous background infusions

Ziconotide

- Also known as SNX-111, it is a novel non-opioid analgesic drug
- It is a ω-conopeptide, derived from the venom of the giant marine snail *Conus magnus*
- N-type Ca^{2+} channel blocker, acting pre-synaptically; decreases the release of the excitatory NTs SP and CGRP
- Completely ionized in the CSF with a high molecular weight of 2659 Da. Therefore, confined to the CSF, and clearance is by CSF bulk flow, not by metabolism
- Can be used for nociceptive and neuropathic pain
- No evidence of granuloma formation, developing tolerance, or respiratory depression
- Common S/Es: dizziness, confusion, nystagmus, amblyopia, nausea/vomiting, urinary retention

Table. 20.8.1 Recommended doses of intrathecal analgesia

Drug	Morphine	Hydromorphone	Fentanyl	Bupivacaine	Clonidine	Ziconotide	Baclofen
IT trial dose	0.1–0.5 mg	0.025–0.1 mg	15–75 mcg	0.5–2.5 mg	5–20 mcg	1–5 mcg	50–100 mcg
Recommended starting daily dose	0.1–0.5 mg	0.01–0.15 mg	25–75 mcg	0.01–4 mg	20–100 mcg	0.5–1.2 mcg (manufacturer suggests up to 2.4 mcg)	50–100 mcg
Maximum concentration	20 mg/mL	15 mg/mL	10 mg/mL	30 mg/mL	1000 mcg/mL	100 mcg/mL	2–3 mg/mL
Suggested maximum daily dose	15 mg	10 mg	1 mg	15–20 mg	600 mcg	19.2 mcg	1.5 mg

Adapted with permission from Deer TR, Pope JE, Hayek SM., *et al.* (2017). The Polyanalgesic Consensus Conference: Recommendations on Intrathecal Drug Infusion Systems Best Practices and Guidelines. *Neuromodulation*, 20: 96–132.

Clonidine

- Selective α-2 adrenergic receptor agonist
- Produces dose-dependent analgesia when delivered intrathecally
- Acts at pre-synaptic and post-synaptic DHs, reducing the preganglionic sympathetic flow and decreasing the release of excitatory neuropeptides such as SP and CGRP
- FDA-approved for epidural use in cancer pain
- Works particularly well for neuropathic pain. Greater efficacy when given intrathecally than systemically
- It is not prone to causing granulomas or development of tolerance

Baclofen

- FDA-approved for IT use as treatment for spasticity
- GABA-B receptor agonist
- Decreases spasm-induced pain and can have a primary analgesic effect mainly in central pain states
- Tolerance and tachyphylaxis can occur with long-term infusions
- Abrupt withdrawal can be a serious life-threatening situation that mimics a serotonin crisis
- Overdose may be a life-threatening situation identified by increased drowsiness, hypotonia, seizures, bradycardia, and respiratory depression

Experimental agents

- Gabapentin, octreotide, adenosine, XEN2174, AM336

Contraindicated drugs

- Ketamine is neurotoxic, causing demyelination and spinal necrosis
- Methadone is neurotoxic
- Diamorphine breakdown products cause the pump to stall

Polyanalgesic Consensus Conference Algorithm for IT analgesia (2016)

Line 1A Morphine/ziconotide

Line 1B Hydromorphone/morphine + bupivacaine

Line 2 Hydromorphone/morphine + clonidine
Hydromorphone/morphine + ziconotide

Line 3 Hydromorphone/morphine/fentanyl + bupivacaine + clonidine
Ziconotide + bupivacaine
Ziconotide + clonidine

Line 4 Sufentanil + ziconotide
Baclofen
Sufentanil + clonidine

Line 5 Sufentanil + bupivacaine + clonidine
Sufentanil + bupivacaine + ziconotide
Sufentanil + clonidine + ziconotide

Line 6 Opioids + bupivacaine + clonidine + adjuvants
(opioids—all known IT opioids)
(adjuvants—midazolam, octreotide)

Implant technique

- Consent
- Procedure can be done under part LA and general anaesthesia versus full general anaesthesia with X-ray guidance
- Antibiotic prophylaxis as per local policy
- Pump side and site need to be marked before the procedure. The pump is usually implanted below the costal margin above the ilium and away from the rectus abdominis
- Position initially prone for IT catheter placement and then lateral, or lateral throughout
- Sterile preparation and draping
- Dural puncture: 15G needle inserted 2–3 vertebral bodies below planned entry to achieve a shallow paramedian entry into IT space. Also ensures catheter stays dorsally
- Catheter is inserted with guidewire to the desired level defined by the area of pain
- The guidewire is extracted, and CSF flow at the end of the catheter confirmed. Required length is cut and the end of the catheter clamped after removing the needle. A V-wing connector is used to anchor the catheter. The remaining segment is kept for calculating the priming bolus
- Prepare the SC pocket for the pump. This should not be >5 cm deep to the skin to ensure interrogation with the patient manager
- Pump is filled with the pre-prepared drug under asepsis and fixed with sutures
- The spinal segment and pump segment are connected via a connector pin that has sutureless squeeze on-and-squeeze off technology. Check for CSF backflow at the pump segment before connecting it to the pump
- Programme the pump for background with or without bolus, as decided by the physician
- Arrange a date for next refill, as calculated by the patient manager

Complications

Complications—immediate post-operative period

- Bleeding: spinal, epidural, or pocket haematoma
- Infection: pump pocket infection or meningitis
- Post-dural puncture headache
- CSF leak and seroma formation

Complications—hardware problems

- Disconnections
- Pump stalling, usually secondary to corrosion
- Leakage of infused drug
- Occlusion, displacement, or kinking of the catheter

Late complications—intrathecal granulomas

- Granulomas are inflammatory masses developing at the tip of the catheter
- Suspected when there is sudden loss of analgesia and new neurological deficits
- More commonly seen with morphine and hydromorphone, and rarely with ziconotide
- Diagnosed with help of MRI or CT myelogram

Complications—drug effects

- *Opioids:*
    - Nausea/vomiting/pruritus
    - Respiratory depression

    - Urinary retention
    - Endocrine suppression. When used for at least >1 year—monitor testosterone and luteinizing hormone (LH) levels in men, and oestrogen, progesterone, LH, and follicle-stimulating hormone (FSH) levels in women
- *Bupivacaine:*
    - Sensory/motor deficits
    - Cardiovascular depression
- *Clonidine:*
    - Bradycardia and hypotension
    - Rebound hypertension on withdrawal

Further reading

1. Deer TR, Leong MS, Buvanendran A, et al. Treatment of Chronic Pain by Interventional Approaches. The American Academy of Pain Medicine Textbook. 2015. New York, NY: Springer
2. Deer TR, Pope JE, Hayek SM, et al. The Polyanalgesic Consensus Conference: recommendations on intrathecal drug infusion systems best practices and guidelines. Neuromodulation 2017;20:96–132
3. Simpson K, Baranidharan G, Gupta S. Oxford Handbook of Spinal Interventions in Pain Management. 1st edition, 2012. Oxford: Oxford University Press

20.9 Percutaneous electrical nerve stimulation

Introduction

- Percutaneous electrical nerve stimulation (PENS) is a non-pharmacological neuromodulation therapy for regional neuropathic pain

Indications

- Refractory neuropathic pain and a wide variety of conditions (see Table 20.9.1)

Contraindications

- Absolute: needle phobia, local or systemic infection, coagulopathy, burns, ulcerations, poorly controlled mental health illness. Not to be applied over the heart, chest wall, and brain
- Relative: pregnancy, cardiac pacemaker, epilepsy, anticoagulation, immunosuppression, infants

Mechanism of action

- Similar to electro-acupuncture
- At 2 Hz stimulation—analgesia is mediated by MOP and DOP receptors
- At 100 Hz stimulation—analgesia is mediated by KOP receptors
- Reduction in SP and increased release of endogenous corticosteroids, endorphins, and enkephalins
- Rebalancing of the mesolimbic loop
- Electrical stimulation leading to self-sustaining reverberation and causing resetting of the pain modulation pathways

Table 20.9.1 Indications for percutaneous electrical nerve stimulation

Pain conditions	Level of evidence – number of RCTs
Headache disorders • Migraine, tension-type headache, post-traumatic headache	1
Trigeminal neuralgia	–
Peripheral neuropathic pain	
• Sciatica	1
• Diabetic neuropathic pain	1
• Surface hyperalgesia associated with various neuropathic pain (post-herpetic neuralgia)	1
Other chronic pain	
• Chronic neck pain	1
• Chronic low back pain	9
• Osteoarthritis of the hip	1
• Interstitial cystitis (posterior tibial nerve stimulation)	–
• Chronic pelvic pain	–
• Class IIIB chronic prostatitis/chronic pelvic pain (posterior tibial nerve stimulation)	1

RCT, randomized controlled trial.

Source: data from Interventional procedures guidance [IPG450]. London, United Kingdom: National Institute of Clinical Excellence.

Technique

- Acupuncture needles (32–36G) or PENS needles
- Single-lead probe with grounding pad or fine-gauge needle probes
- Asepsis
- Insertion of needle in fatty tissue under the skin, close to the relevant nerve or the regional distribution of the pain
- Needles are connected to a low-voltage pulse generator
- Electric current passed through the needles
- Alternating frequency: 15/30 Hz (effective for 58%) have been found more effective than 4 or 100 Hz (49%)
- Stimulation duration: between 15 and 60 minutes (30 minutes were more effective than 15 minutes and nearly equally as effective as 45 minutes)
- Montage providing stimulation along the involved nerve root is better than diffuse placement
- Recommended 3-weekly sessions of 30 minutes for 2 weeks
- Sensations perceived: paraesthesiae and/or muscle twitch or contractions in the stimulated myotome

Complications

- NICE did not demonstrate any adverse events, but evidence on safety is limited

- Potential adverse events: bleeding, local bruising, swelling and haematoma, flare-up of pain, neurovascular damage, local nerve damage, pneumothorax (over chest wall), cardiac tamponade (over heart), dislodgement (with loss of effect), unpleasant paraesthesiae

Advantages of percutaneous electrical nerve stimulation versus transcutaneous electrical nerve stimulation

- Reduction in pain
- Reduction in oral analgesic medication requirement
- Improved physical activity, sleep, and QoL
- Satisfaction with treatment

Further reading

1. National Institute for Health and Care Excellence. Percutaneous electrical nerve stimulation for refractory neuropathic pain. Interventional procedures guidance [IPG450]. 2013. https://www.nice.org.uk/guidance/ipg450
2. Wilkinson J, Faleiro R. Acupuncture in pain management. Contin Educ Anaesth Crit Care Pain 2007;7(4):135–8

20.10 Peripheral nerve stimulation

Definition

- Use of electrical stimulation along peripheral nerves as a neuromodulatory technique to deliver pain relief

Application

- To treat persistent pain that has failed conservative therapy
- There are specific devices, including those using wireless technology
- Many techniques and targets are under extensive investigations to treat a wide range of conditions
- Success of peripheral nerve stimulation (PNS) depends upon patient selection, method used, selection of electrodes, placement of batteries, surgeon's experience, and identification of targets
- US-guided percutaneous approaches are simple, easy to use, and widely applicable for many neuropathic pain problems

History

- Use of PNS began in the mid 1960s (earlier than spinal cord stimulators)
- Originally the technology was the same as that of spinal cord stimulators
- The first percutaneous PNS was reported in 1999
- Becoming more popular recently due to developments in ultrasound-guided pain interventions and technology advancements in electrical leads and wireless technology

Descriptions of PNS

- External peripheral nerve stimulation (EN-PNS)
- Internal peripheral nerve stimulation (IN-PNS)
- There is an overlap of described terminologies and how the stimulation is applied

Types of PNS

- Transcutaneous electrical nerve stimulation (TENS)
- Percutaneous electrical nerve stimulation (PENS)
- Peripheral nerve field stimulation (PNFS)
- Subcutaneous peripheral nerve stimulation (SENS)

Indications/conditions treated using PNS

- Any peripheral nerve entrapment or neuropathy that is accessible for implantation could be treated with PNS
- Neuropathic pain (all types, including persistent post-surgical neuropathic pain, entrapment symptoms, CRPS, post-infection, and post-chemo-/radiotherapy)
- Visceral pain
- Abdominal pain
- Back pain
- Cardiac pain
- Epilepsy
- Facial pain
- Headache
- Incontinence
- Obesity

Conditions treated—targets/areas

- This is an expanding area; many research projects are ongoing, and new targets identified
- Headache, occipital neuralgia—occipital nerve stimulation (ONS) and sphenopalatine ganglion stimulation
- Trigeminal neuralgia (trigeminal nerve branches stimulation)
- Migraines—vagus nerve stimulation (VNS) (ongoing trials for epilepsy and depression)
- Obesity—gastric stimulation
- Brachial plexus injury—brachial plexus stimulation
- Upper limb neuropathic pain—radial, median, or ulnar nerve stimulation
- Shoulder pain—suprascapular nerve, axillary nerve, deltoid muscle (IM stimulation)
- Thoracic wall pain—paravertebral plexus stimulation
- Intercostal neuralgia—intercostal nerve stimulation
- Post-hernia repair pain—ilio-inguinal/ilio-hypogastric nerve, genitofemoral nerve stimulation
- Post-surgical scar pain—cutaneous nerve stimulation
- Post-radiotherapy pain—cutaneous nerve stimulation
- Low back pain—percutaneous stimulation, medial branches stimulation, cluneal nerve stimulation
- Chronic pancreatitis pain—splanchnic nerve
- Stump pain after amputation—cuff electrodes/specific nerve stimulation
- Percutaneous posterior tibial nerve stimulation (PTNS) for urinary incontinence (overactive bladder)
- Pudendal nerve
- Sacral stimulation—pelvic pain, urinary incontinence, faecal incontinence
- Peripheral nerves of upper and lower limbs—plexus and individual nerves
- Patchy area of neuropathic pain anywhere in the skin of most of the body area (PENS)

Techniques

- Either landmark, nerve stimulator, or US-guided techniques are used
- The leads are placed percutaneously or surgically (open)
- Some centres do a trial period similar to spinal cord stimulation (SCS)

Complications

- Mainly related to hardware
- The most common hardware-related complication is lead migration; the largest case series of PNS showed 2–13% of PNFS leads were affected
- Biological complications include infection or pain over implant site
- Serious complications, such as neurological damage, have not been reported

Current evidence

- Most RCTs currently available are on sacral stimulators (seven RCTs) and ONS (one RCT)
- Other studies—mostly retrospective analyses, case series, anecdotal reports, and small studies

Future

- There will be further developments in technology (especially leads and batteries specifically designed for PNS)
- Use of US for identifying and targeting peripheral nerves will widen the application of PNS
- More evidence is required (RCTs and multicentre studies)

Further reading

1. Al-Jehani H, Jacques L. Peripheral nerve stimulation for chronic neurogenic pain. Prog Neurol Surg 2011;24:27–40 [review]
2. Goroszeniuk T, Pang D. Peripheral neuromodulation: a review. Curr Pain Headache Rep 2014;18(5):412
3. Gupta P, Ehlert MJ, Sirls LT, Peters KM. Percutaneous tibial nerve stimulation and sacral neuromodulation: an update. Curr Urol Rep 2015;16(2):4 [review]
4. Rasskazoff SY, Slavin KV. An update on peripheral nerve stimulation. J Neurosurg Sci 2012;56(4):279–85 [review]
5. Stevanato G, Devigili G, Eleopra R, et al. Chronic post-traumatic neuropathic pain of brachial plexus and upper limb: a new technique of peripheral nerve stimulation. Neurosurg Rev 2014;37(3):473–9; discussion: 479–80

20.11 Spinal cord stimulation

Introduction

- Spinal cord stimulation (SCS) is an interventional pain procedure that involves placement of electrodes in the posterior epidural space to stimulate components of the spinal cord to relieve pain
- Currently reserved for treatment of refractory neuropathic pain and pain of ischaemic origin
- Unlike most medical procedures, it is possible to perform a temporary trial of therapy (e.g. for 7–10 days) before committing to permanent implantation
- It has the advantage of reversibility and safety

Mode of action

- Initially based on Wall and Melzack's gate control theory of pain
  - The electrodes emit an electric field that stimulates the dorsal column of the spinal cord at frequencies typically between 40 and 70 Hz (higher frequencies are also available)
  - This activates Aβ afferents that produce pleasant paraesthesiae over specific anatomical areas
  - Overlapping the painful areas with this paraesthesiae produces analgesia as Aβ stimulation inhibits A-delta or C-fibre transmission
- Although the gate control theory is a useful concept, the exact mechanism of action has not been fully elucidated and its mechanism of action is likely to involve:
  - Ortho- and anti-dromic activation of sensory afferents
  - Modulation of DH cells and WDR neurons at the spinal cord
  - Activation of GABA transmission
  - Activation of higher inhibitory pathways

Indications

- SCS is primarily effective for pain of neuropathic origin
- Some evidence of its efficacy in pain of ischaemic origin exists
- Nociceptive pain is not affected by SCS
- SCS is commonly used in:
  - Lumbar radicular pain as a result of previous spinal surgery
  - CRPS
  - Chronic post-surgical neuropathic pain

Contraindications

- Pain that is predominantly nociceptive
- Allergies to certain metals (most of the devices include metallic parts)
- Significant psychosocial comorbidity
- Widespread chronic pain syndromes
- Central pain syndromes
- Insufficient cognitive function to use and self-adjust stimulation

Electrode placement

- Success of SCS is determined by stimulation of dorsal column nerves to produce overlapping paraesthesiae
- Correct electrode placement is critical to its success (see Table 20.11.1)

Table 20.11.1 Electrode placement

Painful area	Electrode placement
Neck and arm	C2–5
Chest	C7–T1
Low back	T7–9
Legs	T9–12

Patient preparation and electrode positioning

- Strict aseptic technique is mandatory
- Image guidance using fluoroscopy is essential
- Electrode placement depends on the anatomical area of pain
- This procedure is done under LA and/or sedation, as intraoperative stimulation is performed to ensure correct placement of the electrode(s) unless high-frequency stimulation is used

Types of electrodes

- Cylindrical electrodes can be used for both trial and permanent implants
- Surgical paddle electrodes are only for permanent implants (lower power consumption and less migration, but a laminotomy is required for insertion and removal is technically more difficult)

Temporary percutaneous trial

- Placement of the lead percutaneously under image guidance:
  - Patient in prone position
  - A 14G modified Tuohy needle is used to access the epidural space using a loss of resistance technique (the Tuohy needle is placed at a shallow angle, and skin entry is usually two vertebral levels below the desired area for loss of resistance)
  - Once the epidural space is accessed, a cylindrical electrode is inserted and steered under fluoroscopic guidance to the desired anatomical area
  - The patient is then woken up, and intraoperative activation of the electrode is performed to ensure correct coverage unless high frequency is used
- A second electrode can be placed if further anatomical areas are needed to be stimulated
- The electrode is left *in situ* and anchored to the skin with a suture
- The trial period is typically 7–10 days and the patient can then determine both the analgesic effect of spinal stimulation and its tolerability

Full permanent implant

- An incision over the back is made prior to placement of the electrode in the epidural space (as described earlier)
- This allows the electrode and connector to be implanted under the SC tissue
- A battery is placed in the buttock area or loin
- Intraoperative testing is performed (as described earlier)

Complications

Although minor complications are common, major or serious complications are rare (see Table 20.11.2).

Table 20.11.2 Common complications of spinal cord stimulation

Hardware-related	
• Electrode migration	13.4%
• Electrode damage *in situ*	9.1%
• Battery failure	1.6%
• Battery-related discomfort	6%
Infection	3.4%

- Electrode migration can frequently be compensated for by reprogramming and/or using an alternative electrode configuration
- Infections require removal of the system and the use of systemic antibiotics
- Most of the current systems used are now MRI-compatible and newer devices are available that are safe to use at up to 1.5 Tesla

Post-procedure management

- Patients are encouraged to restrict excessive spinal movements for 3 months to minimize the risk of electrode migration (a small degree of electrode migration can be compensated for by reprogramming the stimulation)
- Non-rechargeable batteries can last for 5–6 years, depending on how much stimulation is used
- Rechargeable batteries have the advantage of being smaller and able to accommodate higher energy requirements, but they will require changing every 8–10 years
- The procedure to change the battery is straightforward and done as a day case
- If the patient needs an MRI scan, check if the implanted device is MRI-safe

Special points

- The most important factor associated with success is careful patient selection
- It is important that patients undergoing this procedure understand that stimulation only works as part of a pain management approach and be aware of the biopsychosocial factors that affect chronic pain
- Newer modalities of stimulation have the potential to expand on both the indications for use and treating areas of pain that were previously difficult

Newer modalities of stimulation

- High-frequency and burst stimulation (these are paraesthesiae-free systems and can target axial back pain better than conventional systems; another advantage is that intraoperative testing is not required and the electrode is placed anatomically)
- DRG stimulation (this can improve stimulation in more localized areas such as the foot)

Further reading

1. Al-Kaisy A, Van Buyten JP, Smet I, et al. Sustained effectiveness of 10 kHz high-frequency spinal cord stimulation for patients with chronic, low back pain: 24-month results of a prospective multicenter study. Pain Med 2014;15:347–54
2. Cameron T. Safety and efficacy of spinal cord stimulation for the treatment of chronic pain: a 20-year literature review. J Neurosurg 2004;100:254–67
3. Deer T, Pope J, Hayek S, et al. Neurostimulation for the treatment of axial back pain: a review of mechanisms, techniques, outcomes, and future advances. Neuromodulation 2014;17:52–68
4. Linderoth B, Foreman RD. Mechanisms of spinal cord stimulation in painful syndromes: role of animal models. Pain Med 2006;7:S14–26

20.12 Transcutaneous electrical nerve stimulation

Background

- Defined as 'the application of electrical stimulation to the skin for pain control'

- Accepted by the medical community following the publication in 1967 of a paper which showed a reduction in neuropathic pain in eight patients who were stimulated at 100 Hz with an intensity sufficient to stimulate large afferent fibres
- Inexpensive
- Non-invasive
- Easy and safe to use
- Clinical evidence of effectiveness controversial

Mechanism of action (several theories)

- Gate control theory
- Interruption of the transmission of noxious signals through stimulation proximal to the injury site, resulting in anti-dromic conduction along the nerve
- Production and release of endogenous opioids in the PAG area and reticular activating system

Components

- Device with internal electronics that allow variable programming
- Dials on the device to allow selection of the intensity for each channel, pulse duration, and frequency and pattern of stimulation
- Connecting wires
- Two or four electrodes/pads

Method of application

Application site

- Over healthy skin (not broken)
- Close to the painful area
- Within the same myotome, dermatome, or sclerotome
- Choose acupuncture points, trigger points, or over the peripheral nerve in neuropathic pain
- Close to the spinal nerves next to the vertebral column
- When not feasible or accessible, opt for the corresponding position on the contralateral side

Avoid application over

- Front of the neck near the carotid sinus (precipitation of arrhythmias)
- Skin without cutaneous sensation
- Pharyngeal area (it could theoretically affect breathing)
- Pregnant uterus

Contraindications

- Pacemakers and implantable defibrillators
- Epilepsy
- Arrhythmias
- Over malignancy
- Over broken skin
- Over metalwork

Table 20.12.1 Stimulation patterns of TENS

	High-frequency stimulation (>50 Hz) (conventional)	Low-frequency stimulation (2–4 Hz)
Employed	Standard	Acupuncture-like TENS (ALTENS)
Onset	Immediate	Delayed for hours or days
Presumed mode of action	Stimulation of large A-beta fibres: Gate mechanism Anti-dromic conduction Release of dynorphin at the dorsal horn	Release of β-endorphins at the dorsal horn through stimulation of high-threshold A-delta and C-fibres
Duration of action	Short	Prolonged
Other types		
Modulation TENS	Automatic variation of pulse width, frequency, and duration	Dual benefit of both conventional and ALTENS
Burst TENS	Bursts of conventional, high-frequency stimulation of increasing intensity	Useful, especially over prolonged use, due to prevention of adaptation of nerve fibres

Clinical use

(See Table 20.12.1.)

- Has been used for decades in various chronic pain conditions, primarily low back pain, and in acute pain such as labour
- Effectiveness remains controversial in view of the relative paucity of evidence from high-quality, rigorously conducted RCTs until recently
- Currently, it is used as part of a multimodal approach in an attempt to reduce use of other analgesia in the following.

Acute pain

- *Labour pain:* the electrodes are applied over the spinal nerve roots of T10–L1 and S2–S4, using either conventional or burst modes
- *Acute post-operative pain:* application of sterile electrodes parallel to the incision, in addition to possible occasional application close to the corresponding spinal segments

Chronic pain

- Knee OA: using both conventional TENS (incl. conductive silver garments for the knee, elbow, hands, and feet) and acupuncture like TENS
- Primary dysmenorrhoea: electrodes applied either to the abdomen or close to thoracic segments that receive input from nociception in the uterus (occasionally, they have been placed on classical acupuncture points)
- Neuropathic pain
- Post-stroke shoulder pain: based on anecdotal case reports
- Although it had been traditionally used for chronic low back pain, current guidance in UK advises **against** its use for this indication

Further reading

1. Kotzé A, Simpson KH. Stimulation-produced analgesia: acupuncture, TENS and related techniques. Anaesth Intensive Care Med 2008;9(1):29–32
2. Peacock J. Tens and acupuncture therapy for soft tissue pain. Anaesth Intensive Care Med 2013;14(11):502–4.
3. Sluka KA, Walsh D. Transcutaneous electrical nerve stimulation: basic science mechanisms and clinical effectiveness. J Pain 2003;4(3):109–21
4. Wright A. Exploring the evidence for using TENS to relieve pain. Nurs Times 2012;108(11):20–3
5. Wall PD, Sweet WH. Temporary abolition of pain. Science 1967;155:108
6. Melzack R, Wall PD. Pain mechanisms: a new theory. Science 1965;150:971–9

CHAPTER 21

Surgical Techniques

Erlick Pereira

CONTENTS

21.1 Spinal decompressive surgery

Anatomy

- The spinal cord travels in the spinal canal from C1 to L1 vertebrae where it becomes the conus medullaris, then the theca containing the cauda equina of lumbo-sacral nerves from L2 to S4
- Nerves can be trapped in lateral recesses of the spinal canal or foramina by stenosis from ligamentum flavum hypertrophy, bony osteophytes, or disc prolapses. Postero-lateral disc prolapses compress traversing nerves, and lateral disc prolapses compress exiting nerves
- Cervical nerves exit at the foramina above the vertebral level (e.g. C7 nerve at C6–7). Thoracic and lumbar nerves exit below the vertebral level (e.g. a far lateral L2–3 disc prolapse will compress the exiting L2 nerve root)

Indications

- Pain, weakness, altered sensation, loss of function causing significant disability and impairment of QoL, persisting for >3 months with focal neural compression unrelieved by analgesia ± injections
- Cervical myelopathy (cord compression from canal stenosis)—anterior cervical discectomy and fusion if 1–2 levels, cervical laminectomy ± fusion if ≥3 levels
- Cervical radiculopathy (nerve compression)—cervical foraminotomy if foraminal stenosis, anterior cervical discectomy, and fusion if vertebral osteophytes and disc prolapse
- Thoracic myelopathy—thoracic laminectomy if canal stenosis or thoracotomy and discectomy if central disc prolapse
- Neurogenic claudication—lumbar laminectomy
- Sciatica—lumbar discectomy if disc prolapse, foraminotomy if foraminal stenosis, undercutting facetectomy if lateral recess stenosis (not always possible without fusion)

Contraindications

- Deformity (scoliosis, kyphosis, spondylolisthesis) requiring fusion
- Coagulopathy (anticoagulation should be reversed/stopped before surgery)

- Unfit for general anaesthesia (cardiovascular, renal, pulmonary impairment)
- Multiple past spinal surgeries (may require fusion or spinal cord stimulation)
- Trauma, malignancy (may require fixation)

Technique

- Most decompressions are open midline longitudinal incisions, with the paravertebral muscles stripped to expose the posterior spine. Anterior cervical decompressions are approached in a plane of deep investing cervical fascia between the sternocleidomastoid and the carotid sheath laterally and the oesophagus, trachea, and recurrent laryngeal nerve medially
- Radiographs before and during decompression mandatory to confirm the spinal level decompressed

Complications

- Infection (1%)
- Bleeding requiring blood transfusion (1%)
- Paralysis or focal weakness and loss of function (0.1%)
- CSF leak and potential meningitis (1%)
- Recurrent disc prolapse/stenosis
- Adjacent level disc prolapse/stenosis
- For anterior cervical approach—injury to oesophagus, trachea, recurrent laryngeal nerve (difficulty with speaking, breathing, or swallowing), stroke
- General anaesthetic risks (deep vein thrombosis (DVT), pulmonary embolus (PE), pneumonia, stroke, death)

Special points

- Open approach is standard of care. X-ray-guided percutaneous decompressions are less reliable. Microscopes and, more rarely, loupes and endoscopes are used to improve visualization of neural compression
- Most surgery has post-operative wound pain for several days and necessitates overnight hospital stay
- Most surgeons advocate a wound drain for a day after surgery and 2 days of bed rest if CSF leak occurs at surgery
- Best outcomes arise from focal nerve root compression that is anatomically consistent with the dermatomal pain, with >80% of patients improving. In contrast, the aim of surgery in myelopathy is to prevent symptom progression
- Early discectomy for sciatica promotes early mobilization, but 1-year outcomes are similar to conservatively managed sciatica

Further reading

1. Peul WC, van Houwelingen HC, van den Hout WB, et al. Surgery versus prolonged conservative treatment for sciatica. N Engl J Med 2007;356(22):2245–56

21.2 Spinal fusion surgery

Introduction

- Spinal stability is conferred by ligaments, bones, and intervertebral discs. Movement or damage to any of these elements can result in pain, deformity, or loss of function
- Spinal fusion surgery fuses two or more vertebral bodies to correct abnormal spinal movement as a cause of pain, remove the intervertebral disc (the presumed pain generator), and provide spinal stability. Best outcomes are normally found when:
    - History, examination, and investigations suggest that the pain generator is most likely a single intervertebral disc
    - Patients are motivated and fit, with realistic expectations, who understand the surgical risks
    - Patients have no profound dysfunctional lives or severe pain-related disabilities
- Spinal fusions can be combined with neural decompression surgery (e.g. discectomy, laminectomy) when neural compression is also a pain generator
- Patients who have had a spinal fusion can develop degenerative changes in adjacent spinal vertebrae due to changes in spinal mechanics from the surgery

Surgical techniques

- Spinal fusions involve placing a bone graft between adjacent vertebrae
- There are multiple techniques and different hardware that can be used to provide spinal stability (cages, screws, plates) until the bone graft heals

Posterior interbody fusion

- A lateral mass screw is inserted in the cervical spine
- A pedicle screw is inserted in the thoracic, lumbar, or sacral spine
- A lateral gutter bone graft or bone substitute is inserted

Lumbar spine posterior interbody fusion

- Intervertebral disc is replaced with a titanium or polyethyletherketone cage and bone graft/substitute
- Commonly performed posteriorly or transforaminally through open or minimally invasive approaches

Anterior lumbar and extreme lateral interbody fusion

- Confers the advantages of implanting cages that cover a greater surface area of the vertebral body endplates, thus creating a stronger construct. This may effectively restore lordosis or correct scoliosis, and indirectly decompress neural elements
- Stability may be augmented by an overlying plate and pedicle screws

Anterior cervical discectomy and fusion

- Can be stand-alone or augmented by a plate if over multiple levels
- Can directly decompress neural elements

Cervical corpectomy

- Indicated for vertebral body disease/neural compression
- Preformed with a cage and plate or a fibular/iliac crest strut graft

Transcervical odontoid screw, posterior C1–2, or occipito-cervical fusion

- Indicated for cranio-cervical junction pathologies

Indications

- Spondylolisthesis
- Multi-level cervical canal stenosis
- Degenerative disc disease with vertebral body Modic changes and positive discography
- Deformity (kyphosis, scoliosis)
- Trauma (often fixed, rather than fusion, as screws can be removed after fracture union)
- Metastatic spinal cord compression
- Other causes of spinal instability (e.g. spondylodiscitis, osteomyelitis, chordoma or other tumour, osteoporotic collapse, RA at cranio-cervical junction)

Contraindications

- Osteoporosis, osteopenia
- Coagulopathy
- Some metal allergies
- Deformity is a contraindication to short spinal segment fusions, as longer constructs respecting sagittal and coronal balance should be considered by trained deformity surgeons
- Paraspinal myopathies and movement disorders (e.g. Parkinson's disease, dystonia) require caution as outcomes are often worse

Technique

- Extreme care with infection control. Vancomycin powder is commonly used in wounds
- Usually open midline incisions. Small flank or larger thoraco-abdominal incision for extreme lateral interbody fusions. Mini-laparotomy or Pfannenstiel incision in the abdomen for an anterior lumbar fusion. Transverse anterior neck incision for an anterior cervical discectomy and fusions
- Can be minimally invasive or image-guided by intraoperative CT, which reduces surgeon intraoperative radiation exposure and can reduce screw misplacement risk

Complications

- Standard risks of spinal surgery: paralysis, focal weakness, pain or numbness from nerve injury, CSF leak, meningitis, infection, and bleeding
- Instrumented fusion confers additional risks of screw misplacement, cage misplacement or migration, non-union, adjacent spinal segment failure, and instrumentation failure
- Anterior and extreme lateral interbody fusions have specific risks related to their approaches, both including aortic, iliac vessel, or inferior vena cava injury
- Specific complications include:
  - Lateral interbody fusions: lumbo-sacral plexopathy
  - Anterior lumbar fusion: ureteric damage, hypogastric plexus injury resulting in retrograde ejaculation or vaginal dryness

Special points

- Lumbar fusion for back pain in degenerative disc disease without spondylolisthesis is controversial with little strong RCT evidence and preliminary data suggesting such patients if otherwise refractory may benefit from non-surgical treatment strategies

Further reading

1. Weinstein JN, Lurie JD, Tosteson TD, et al. Surgical versus nonsurgical treatment for lumbar degenerative spondylolisthesis. N Engl J Med 2007;356(22):2257–70
2. Fairbank J, Frost H, Wilson-MacDonald J, et al. Randomised controlled trial to compare surgical stabilisation of the lumbar spine with an intensive rehabilitation programme for patients with chronic low back pain: the MRC spine stabilisation trial. BMJ 2005;330(7502):1233

21.3 Dorsal root entry zone lesioning

Introduction

- The dorsal root entry zone is a region comprising the central portion of the dorsal rootlet, the medial part of Lissauer's tract, and the first five layers of Rexed's laminae in the dorsal horn where the afferent fibres synapse (see Fig. 21.3.1)
- Each dorsal root divides into 4–10 rootlets, each 0.25–1.5 mm in diameter and each with a peripheral and a central segment. The transitional zone between the two segments is at the pial ring approximately 1 mm outside where the root penetrates the dorsolateral sulcus. Fine pain fibre group in the lateral dorsal root entry zone, and large tactile fibre group medially towards the dorsal columns

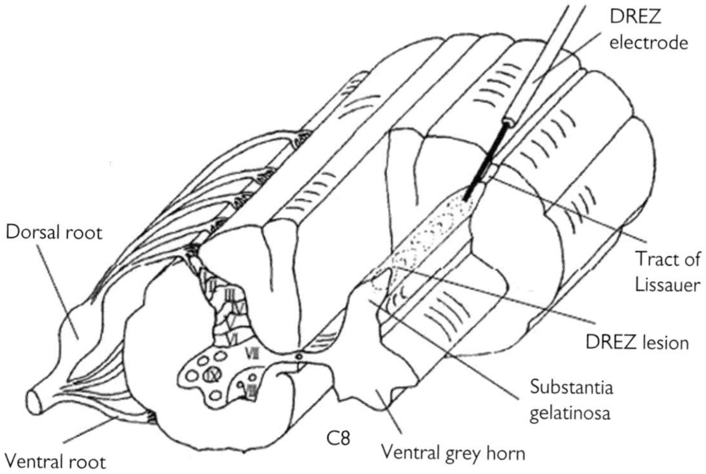

Figure 21.3.1 Anatomy of the dorsal root entry zone (DREZ)

Indications

- Deafferentation pain after nerve root avulsion
- Brachial plexus avulsion
- SCI restricted to a few dermatomes
- PHN
- Amputation pain (phantom limb or stump)

Contraindications

- Coagulopathy
- Whole or hemi-body pain
- Non-dermatomal SCI pain

Technique

- Prone patient
- Laminectomies over affected nerve roots
- Dural opening longitudinal and paramedian over affected nerve roots and microscopic identification of dorsal root entry zone by viewing intact rootlets above and below the injured area
- RF thermocoagulation at 80°C for 15 seconds (Nashold technique) or sharp microincision (Sindou technique) ipsilateral to avulsed nerve roots from caudal to superior intact rootlet to rostral to inferior intact rootlet if over several segments; 30–45° angulation of implement and depth of 2–3 mm. In paraplegic patients, it can be combined with a cordotomy
- Standard dural closure with 2 days of bed rest after surgery

Complications

- Ipsilateral weakness (transient 10%, permanent 5%)
- Ipsilateral loss of proprioception (transient 10%, permanent 5%)
- Usual risks of intradural spinal surgery (infection, bleeding, pain, CSF leak, meningitis)

Special points

- Best outcomes from brachial plexus avulsion (>80% long-term significant improvement) and SCI with limited dermatomal involvement
- Destructive surgery, so neuromodulation (e.g. deep brain stimulation (DBS), spinal cord or DRG stimulation) may be favoured as first-line therapy

Further reading

1. Sampson JH, Cashman RE, Nashold BS Jr, Friedman AH. Dorsal root entry zone lesions for intractable pain after trauma to the conus medullaris and cauda equina. J Neurosurg 1995;82(1):28–34
2. Sindou MP, Blondet E, Emery E, Mertens P. Microsurgical lesioning in the dorsal root entry zone for pain due to brachial plexus avulsion: a prospective series of 55 patients. J Neurosurg 2005;102(6):1018–28

21.4 Deep brain stimulation

Introduction

- Spinothalamic pain processing tracts in the spinal cord are modulated in the midbrain periaqueductal grey (PAG) and the sensory thalamus en route to cortical pain processing brain areas such as the insula and anterior cingulate cortex
- Midbrain PAG (see Fig. 21.4.1) is superior and anterior to the superior colliculi (thus, deep electrode stimulation can cause oscillopia), and posterior to the red nuclei and reticular thalamus. It has a rostrocaudally inverted homunculus, with the face represented most caudally and the legs most rostrally
- The sensory thalamus consists of the ventral posterior medial and lateral nuclei, 6–14 mm lateral to the posterior commissure. The ventral posterior thalamus has a mediolaterally oriented somato-sensory homunculus, with the face represented in the ventral postero-medial and the legs in the ventral postero-lateral thalamus
- The anterior cingulate cortex is involved in emotional and pain valency processing. Its rostral, supragenual component is a target for DBS
- Entry points for DBS surgery are usually frontal and anterior to the coronal suture, to avoid passing through the primary motor cortex more posteriorly, and ipsilateral and extra-ventricular to minimize the bleeding risk and inaccuracy

Indications

- Refractory pain not responding to conventional treatments from the following:
  - Post-stroke pain (also amenable to motor cortex stimulation)
  - Cranial/facial pain (e.g. post-craniotomy or anaesthesia dolorosa)
  - Post-amputation (phantom limb or stump) pain

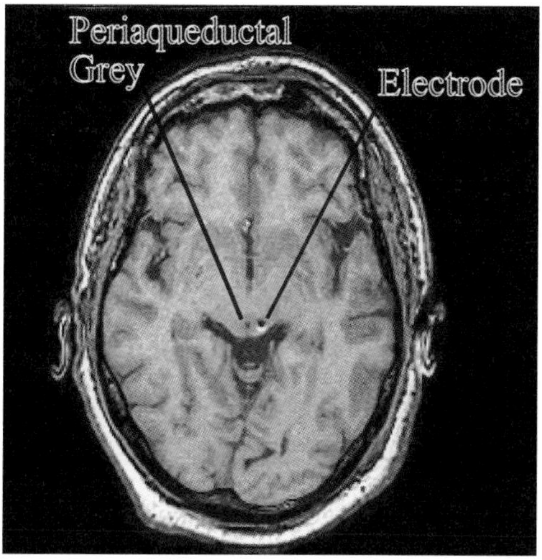

Figure 21.4.1 Deep brain stimulation electrode placement

    - Brachial plexus avulsion
    - SCI
    - Low back pain refractory to spinal cord stimulation and spinal surgery
    - Hemi- or whole-body neuropathic pain
    - Trigeminal autonomic cephalgia (the posterior hypothalamus is the target)

Contraindications

- Coagulopathy
- Hydrocephalus
- Dementia
- Functional pain syndromes

Technique

- Awake surgery desirable to assess intraoperative response to DBS
- Stereotactic frame placed on the head and used to calculate the coordinates of the brain target
- Brain targets include contralateral ventral posterior thalamus (medial—face, lateral body), contralateral midbrain PAG (see Fig. 21.4.1), and bilateral rACC (for hemi- or whole-body pain)
- After awake electrode placement and subsequent CT brain confirming correct placement of the electrodes, the stereotactic head ring is removed and wires externalized for a week of trialling
- If trialling successful, then brain electrode wires are tunnelled to a subclavicular implanted pulse generator under general anaesthesia

Complications

- Risks of brain surgery, including infection, bleeding causing stroke or death, and seizures (higher risk with anterior cingulate DBS)
- Chest area site with implanted pacemaker—highest risk of infection (2%)
- Electrode malposition requiring revision surgery
- Implanted hardware failure or breakage
- Stimulation S/Es (e.g. twitching, visual problems, unpleasant sensation)

Special points

- Safer forms of neuromodulation (e.g. DRG stimulation for amputation pain, ONS for cluster headache) can be trialled before DBS
- No strong RCT evidence. Large case series suggest initial 80% efficacy, dropping to two-thirds at 2 years and to 50% at half a decade

Further reading

1. Boccard SG, Pereira EA, Moir L, Aziz TZ, Green AL. Long-term outcomes of deep brain stimulation for neuropathic pain. Neurosurgery 2013;72(2):221–30
2. Pereira EA, Aziz TZ. Neuropathic pain and deep brain stimulation. Neurotherapeutics 2014;11(3):496–507

Miscellaneous Interventions

Hadi Bedran, Sadiq Bhayani, Bill Clark, Ilya Kantsedikas, Andrzej Krol, Attam Jeet Singh, and John Tanner

CONTENTS

22.1 Bier's block

Introduction

- Bier's block is a peripheral IV regional technique that may be used for chronic pain management of the limbs
- Evidence to support its efficacy is limited

Anatomy

- Arteries and peripheral veins of the limbs

Indications

- CRPS
- Ischaemic limb pain
- Neuropathic limb pain

Contraindications

- Patient refusal
- Allergy to LA
- Cannulation site infection
- Crush injuries
- Compound fractures
- Arterio-venous shunt or fistula
- Severe peripheral vascular disease
- Disrupted venous drainage of the limb
- Difficult venous access
- Severe liver disease

- Sickle cell disease

Patient preparation and positioning

- Supine with standard monitoring
- IV access established away from limb to be blocked
- Ensure tourniquet is functional and checked for air leaks

Technique

- Place a double-cuffed pneumatic tourniquet on the block limb over a stockinette bandage
- Cannulate the most distal vein possible in the block limb
- Elevate the limb above the level of the heart for 1–2 minutes for passive exsanguination
- Apply a compression bandage to the elevated limb spirally up to the tourniquet cuff
- Occlude the artery proximal to the tourniquet; inflate the distal cuff of the tourniquet to 50–100 mmHg above systolic BP, then inflate the proximal cuff. Once the proximal cuff is inflated, deflate the distal cuff and remove the compression bandage
- Slowly inject LA into the IV cannula in the block limb—typical volume of 40–60 mL of 0.5% lidocaine (up to 3 mg/kg) or 0.5% prilocaine (up to 6 mg/kg)
- Onset of anaesthesia takes up to 5 minutes. Progressive numbness and limb insensitivity, followed by motor paralysis and skin discoloration
- The distal tourniquet is inflated and the proximal one deflated when tourniquet pain occurs (usually 30–45 minutes)—allowing 15–20 minutes of tourniquet tolerance
- Gradually release the tourniquet in two steps at the end of the procedure

Complications

- Complications are rare and often due to equipment malfunction or not following the correct procedure for performing the block
- LA toxicity—often from equipment failure/poor tourniquet inflation
- Haematoma at cannula site
- Engorgement of the limb—more common in patients with arteriosclerosis
- Ecchymosis/SC haemorrhage
- Tourniquet complications

Special points

- Exact mechanism of action is subject to debate. LA is thought to diffuse to nerve trunks, peripheral nerves, and nerve endings. Nerve fibre compression and ischaemia from the tourniquet may also contribute to the block
- The following can be added, which may improve the efficacy of Bier's blocks:
  - Mg^{2+}—possible direct analgesic effect, NO release, and Ca^{2+} channel and NMDA receptor blockade
  - α-2 adrenoreceptor agonists—likely decrease in AP conduction along A-delta and C-fibres and hyperpolarization of cation channels
  - NSAIDs (e.g. ketorolac)—effect on PGE2 and PGI2 release may be of relevance in CRPS, along with reduction in inflammation
  - Corticosteroids—attenuation of inflammation in CRPS (also may prolong LA action)
  - Ketamine—NMDA antagonism
  - Ondansetron—serotonergic nociceptive pathways, action on Na^{+} channels

Further reading

1. Harden RN, Oaklander AL, Burton AW, et al. Complex regional pain syndrome: practical diagnostic and treatment guidelines. Pain Medicine 2013;14(2):180–229
2. New York School of Regional Anaesthesia. Intravenous regional block for upper and lower extremity surgery. https://www.nysora.com/techniques/intravenous-regional-anesthesia/intravenous-regional-block-upper-lower-extremity-surgery

22.2 Bursa injection

Introduction

- Bursitis is inflammation of fluid-filled sacs which are normally positioned between two muscles or between a muscle and its tendon or bone
- Bursa injections can be performed in patients with bursitis who fail to respond to conservative therapy. Evidence to support its efficacy is limited
- Contraindicated if there is an infected bursa (needs aspiration and antibiotics)
- Bursa injections are normally done with LA (e.g. 5 mL of 0.5% bupivacaine) and steroid (e.g. 40 mg triamcinolone)
- Refer to Chapter 15 on overview of interventions in Section 4 for standard clinical practice before, during, and after interventions in pain management

Subacromial bursa injection

Anatomy

- Subacromial space noted to be above the supraspinatus muscle and below the acromion
- Bursa extends from the subdeltoid to the subacromial space
- It is the largest bursa in the body (up to 20 mL of fluid)

Indications

- Subacute and chronic shoulder pain from subacromial bursitis

Technique

- Sitting position and shoulder in neutral position
- Linear transducer placed over the distal acromion in a perpendicular position
- Important to obtain a 'bird's beak view' of the supraspinatus tendon
- Needle is inserted in an in-plane orientation into the thin, double hyperechoic capsule. May be enlarged in bursitis
- Inject LA and steroid under direct vision to avoid disruption of the supraspinatus tendon

Special points

- Aim bevel away from the supraspinatus—avoid damaging the tendon
- Double-lined capsule may be seen as a fluid-filled sac
- Slight anterior orientation may deliver a better view

Greater trochanter bursa injection

(See 23.14. Greater trochanteric pain syndrome, p. 477.)

Anatomy

- The greater trochanter bursa is situated over the most prominent and lateral part of the hip at the insertion of the gluteus muscles
- Symptoms include pain along the outer surface of the leg/hip towards the knee

Indications

- Acute or chronic inflammation of the greater trochanter bursa due to OA, RA, repetitive use, trauma, or other causes

Ultrasound-guided injection

- Linear probe
- Lateral position with the hip gently flexed
- Imaging of the greater trochanter in a transverse plane (short axis)
- Approach from a posterior to anterior position in plane with the transducer
- LA and steroid injected within the peritendinous soft tissues of the greater trochanter

Fluoroscopic-guided injection

- Supine position with the knees straightened
- Locate the greater trochanter and the point of maximal tenderness in AP view
- Needle inserted perpendicular to the skin
- Pass down directly onto bone contact and then withdraw before injecting
- Inject LA with steroid

Further reading

1. Canoso J, Isaac Z, Curtis MR. Greater trochanteric pain syndrome. 2018. https://www.uptodate.com
2. Todd DJ, Isaac Z, Ramirez-Curtis M. Bursitis: an overview of clinical manifestations, diagnosis, and management. 2018. https://www.uptodate.com
3. Simpson G, Krol A, Silver D, et al. Subacromial bursa. In: Simpson G et al. Ultrasound-guided Interventions in Chronic Pain Management. 2019; pp. 188–90. Geneva: European Society of Regional Anaesthesia & Pain Therapy

22.3 Ilio-inguinal nerve, ilio-hypogastric nerve, and genitofemoral nerve block

Anatomy of the ilio-inguinal nerve (IIN) and ilio-hypogastric nerve (IHN)

- The IIN and IHN arise from the anterior rami of L1, with contribution from T12
- Both nerves run between the lateral border of the psoas major muscle and the quadratus lumborum muscle
- Above the iliac crest, both nerves pierce the TA muscle and continue anteriorly, medial to the ASIS
- The IHN pierces the IO muscle medial to the ASIS, and then travels between the IO and the EO muscles
- One inch above the superficial inguinal ring, the IHN pierces the aponeurosis of the EO muscle

- The IIN nerve runs parallel to and below the IHN, and it pierces the lower border of the IO muscle and passes between the crura of the superficial inguinal ring in front of the spermatic cord
- The IHN nerve provides sensory fibres to the skin over the lower part of the RA muscle (ipsilateral to the midline) and above the inguinal ligament (see Fig. 23.3.1)
- The IIN supplies the skin over the supero-medial area of the thigh and the skin over the root of the penis and anterior scrotum (in women: mons pubis and labia majora)

Anatomy of the genitofemoral nerve (GFN)

- It originates from the L1 and L2 nerve roots
- At the level of the L3–4 intervertebral disc, it pierces the psoas muscle
- On the anterior surface of the psoas muscle, it either runs as a single trunk or as separate genital and femoral branches
- The femoral branch follows the external iliac artery and passes with it under the inguinal ligament. It supplies the skin overlying the femoral triangle
- The genital branch passes through the internal inguinal ring of the transversalis fascia and continues in the inguinal canal
- The GFN runs either outside the spermatic cord or in ventral, dorsal, and inferior locations or within the cremaster muscle
- The genital branch supplies the cremaster muscle and the anterior scrotal skin in males, and the skin of the mons pubis and labia majora in females (see Fig. 23.3.1)

Indications

- Chronic post-surgical pain—after hernia repair, Caesarean section, laparoscopy, and lower abdominal surgery
- Post-vasectomy pain

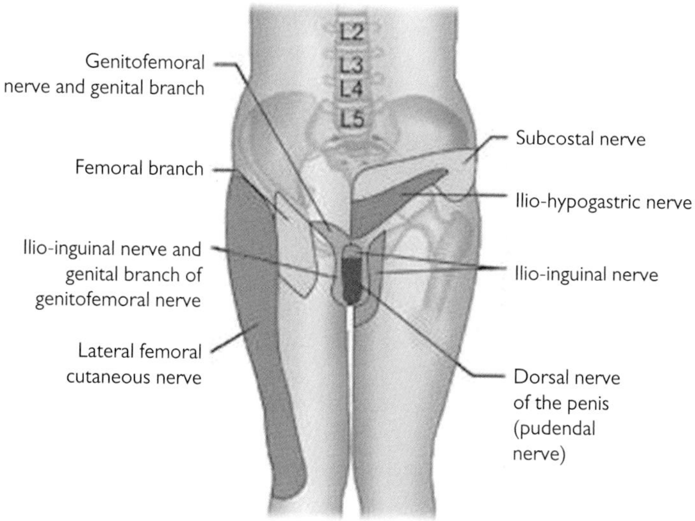

Figure 22.3.1 Territory of supply of the ilio-inguinal, ilio-hypogastric, and genitofemoral nerves

Reproduced with permission from Thomas, P., and Das, G. (2015). The diagnostic dilemma of a genitofemoral-ilioinguinal overlap syndrome, *Journal on Recent Advances in Pain*, 1(1): 28–30. DOI: 10.5005/jp-journals-10046-0009

- Genitofemoral neuralgia
- Chronic testicular pain

Contraindications

- Patient refusal
- Localized infection
- Allergy to LA and steroids

Patient preparation and positioning

- Patient in supine position
- Equipment: linear US probe (6–13 MHZ)

Complications

- Failure
- Infection, bleeding, bruising
- Injury to bowel
- Nerve injury and persistent pain

Technique for IIN and IHN block

- The US probe is positioned 3–4 cm cephalad and lateral (posterior) to the ASIS, perpendicular to the inguinal line joining the ASIS and the pubic tubercle, with the lateral end of the probe just above/posterior to the ASIS. The probe is then tilted until all three layers of muscles (TA, IO, and EO) are visualized (see Fig. 22.3.2)

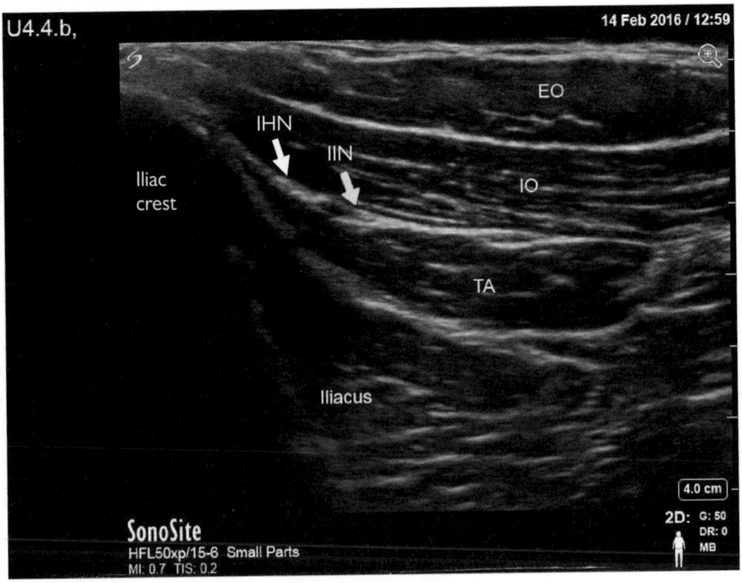

Figure 22.3.2 Ultrasound image of the ilioinguinal (IIN) and iliohyogastric (IHN) nerve block (arrows). EO, external oblique muscle; IO, internal obliques muscle; TA, transverse abdominis muscle; Iliacus, iliacus muscle

- Splitting of the fascial layer between the IO and TA muscle is observed and targeted. Both nerves can run together or approximately 1 cm apart. Colour Doppler is used to locate the deep circumflex iliac artery that frequently accompanies the IIN and IHN
- Either in-plane or out-of-plane technique. Use of a short bevel nerve block needle with 5 mL of LA (and steroid) is recommended

Additional information

- Previous surgical scarring can alter the sono-anatomy; in such cases, a nerve stimulator can be used to locate the nerves
- For the out-of-plane approach, use of hydro-dissection is recommended to identify the needle tip position and avoid localized IM injection

Technique for GFN block

- The US probe is placed in the inguinal crease to visualize the femoral artery in short axis; it is then turned by 90° at the level of the internal inguinal ring to visualize the femoral artery in long axis
- Moving in a cephalad direction, the artery is seen as diving deep towards the inguinal ligament as it becomes the external iliac artery
- At this point, an oval structure can easily be seen superficial to the external iliac artery, opposite the internal inguinal ring (this is the spermatic cord or the round ligament of the uterus)
- The final position of the probe is about two finger-breadths lateral to the pubic tubercle, with the orientation perpendicular to the inguinal line
- The GFN cannot be visualized directly
- The key structure is the spermatic cord (round ligament of the uterus), which is oval, with one or two arteries within it (the testicular artery and the artery to the vas deferens)
- An in-plane or out-of-plane approach with 8 mL of LA and steroids is used

Additional information

- Due to the variable location of the genital branch in the GFN, it is recommended to deposit 4 mL of LA inside and another 4 mL outside the spermatic cord

Further reading

1. Cesmebasi A, Yadav A, Geilecki J, et al. Genitofemoral neuralgia: a review. Clin Anat 2015;28:128–35
2. Peng PWH, Narouze S. Ultrasound-guided interventional procedures in pain medicine: a review of anatomy, sonoanatomy, and procedures: Part I: nonaxial structures. Reg Anesth Pain Med 2009;34:458–74
3. Shanthanna H. Successful treatment of genitofemoral neuralgia using ultrasound guided injection: a case report and short review of literature. Case Rep Anesthesiol 2014;2014:371703
4. Simpson G, Krol A, Silver D, Nicholls B. Ilioinguinal, iliohypogastric and subcostal nerve blocks. In: Simpson, G, Krol A, Silver D, Nicholls B (eds). Ultrasound-guided Interventions in Chronic Pain Management. 2019; pp. 139–42. UK: European Society of Regional Anaesthesia & Pain Therapy (ESRA)
5. Simpson G, Krol A, Silver D, Nicholls B. Genitofemoral nerve block. In: Simpson G, Krol A, Silver D, Nicholls B (eds). Ultrasound-guided Interventions in Chronic Pain Management. 2019; pp.143–6. UK: European Society of Regional Anaesthesia & Pain Therapy (ESRA)

22.4 Shoulder, knee, and hip joint—blocks and denervation procedures

Shoulder joint

Anatomy—innervation

- Brachial plexus via the suprascapular nerve (SSN) and axillary nerve
- Other contributing nerves: lateral pectoral nerve, subscapular nerves, and musculocutaneous nerve
- Majority of innervation is from the suprascapular nerve (posterior shoulder joint capsule, acromioclavicular joint (ACJ), coracoclavicular ligaments, coracoacromial ligament, and subacromial–subdeltoid bursa)
- The SSN arises from the upper trunk of the brachial plexus and runs laterally beneath the trapezius and omohyoid muscle and enters in the supraspinous fossa via the suprascapular notch beneath the suprascapular ligament (accompanied by the neuro-vascular bundle)

Suprascapular nerve block

Indications

- Chronic shoulder pain secondary to rotator cuff tear, arthropathy
- Adhesive capsulitis
- OA, RA
- Chronic post-surgical pain after shoulder surgery
- Post-operative analgesia following shoulder arthroplasty

Contraindications

- Patient refusal
- Localized infection
- Allergy (LA, steroids)

Patient preparation and positioning

- Patient position: sitting, lateral
- Equipment: high-frequency linear US probe (6–13 MHz)

Technique

- A linear probe is recommended, given that the nerve is quite superficial (<5 cm), with the patient in sitting or lateral position
- The US probe is positioned parallel to the scapular spine and then moved anteriorly to visualize the suprascapular fossa and the trapezius and supraspinatus muscles (see Fig. 22.4.1)
- The suprascapular artery can be visualized with colour Doppler
- A volume of 5 mL of LA and steroid is injected under real-time guidance using an in-plane or out-of-plane approach

Complications

- Failure
- Infection, bleeding, bruising
- Pneumothorax
- Nerve injury and injury to blood vessels

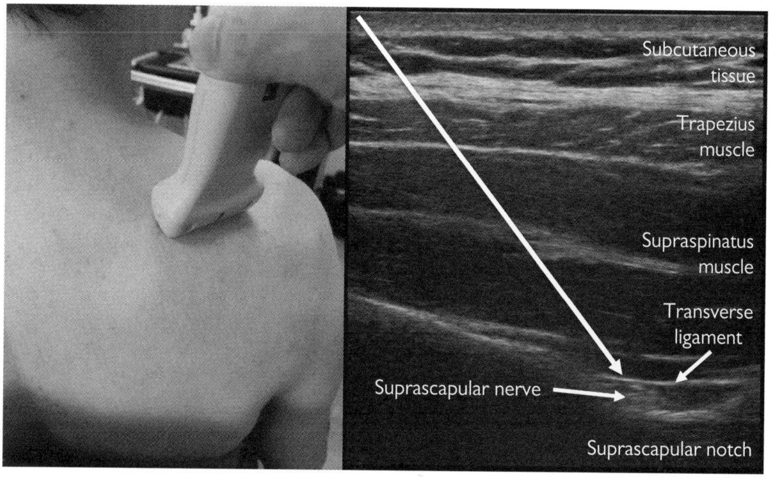

Figure 22.4.1 Ultrasound image of the suprascapular notch with the suprascapular nerve, white arrow = needle path (Right), Ultrasound probe position (Left)
Reproduced with permission of Dr Debajit Phukan (Surrey and Sussex Healthcare NHS Trust, Redhill)

Additional information

- The SSN can be targeted either at the suprascapular notch or in the supraclavicular fossa
- Targeting the SSN at the notch using a blind or landmark approach increases the risk of pneumothorax, intravascular injections, and nerve injury
- This risk can be minimized by placing the needle in the supraclavicular fossa and placing 1–2 ml of LA to block the SSN.

Knee joint

Anatomy—innervation

- The knee capsule innervation can be simplified into an anterior and a posterior group of nerves called genicular nerves (supero-medial, superolateral, infero-medial, infero-lateral) (see Fig. 22.4.2)
- Anterior group of genicular nerve branches:
  - Femoral nerve (muscular branches to vasti muscles, saphenous nerve)
  - Sciatic nerve (common peroneal nerve: recurrent and lateral retinacular branches)
- Posterior group of genicular nerve branches:
  - Sciatic nerve (tibial branch)
  - Obturator nerve (branches of the posterior division)

Knee genicular nerve blocks and radiofrequency treatment

Indications

- Alternative treatment modality for patients who are not suitable for knee replacements due to comorbidities
- Very obese patients
- Patients unwilling to undergo surgery
- Chronic post-surgical pain after knee replacement

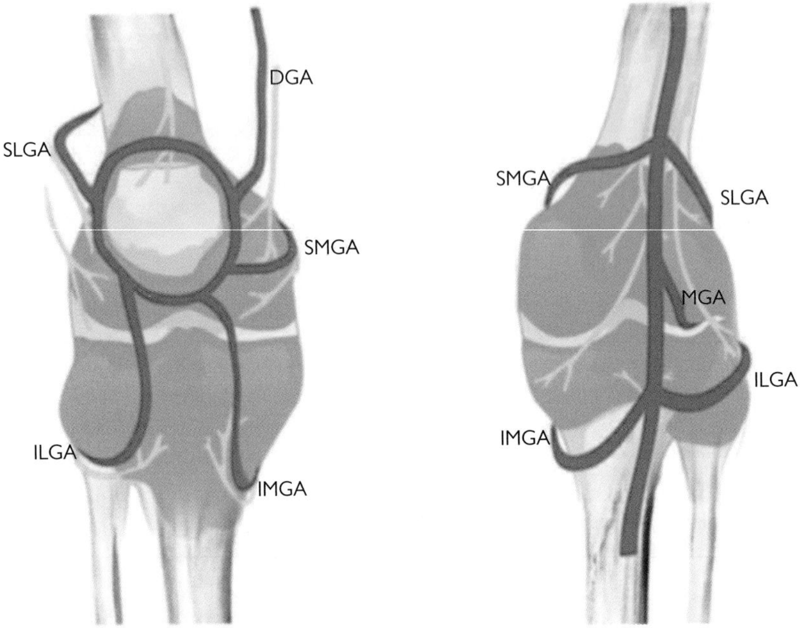

Figure 22.4.2 Genicular arteries accompanied by genicular nerves. DGA, descending genicular artery; ILGA, inferior lateral genicular artery; IMGA, inferior medial genicular artery; MGA, middle genicular artery; SLGA, superior lateral genicular artery; SMGA, superior medial genicular artery
Reproduced with permission of Dr Vicente Roqués

Contraindications

- Patient refusal
- Localized infection
- Allergy to LA and steroids
- Pacemaker and other implantable devices (relative contraindication for RF)

Patient preparation and positioning

- Patient position: supine
- Equipment:
  - Linear US probe (6–13 MHZ)
  - X-ray and RF generator with 16G or 18G RF needles with 10 mm exposed tips
  - A larger needle gauge will provide a bigger lesion size and is recommended

Technique

- The patient is in supine position, with the knee slightly elevated/flexed
- Three genicular branches—superolateral, supero-medial, and infero-medial—are targeted for both diagnostic blocks and RF treatment
- For diagnostic blocks, the linear US probe is placed parallel to the femoral shaft and moved caudally to locate the junction between the shaft and the condyle, both medially and laterally, to visualize the supero-medial and superolateral genicular nerves
- The US probe is placed parallel to the tibial shaft medially to locate the junction between the tibial shaft and the medial condyle to visualize the infero-medial genicular nerve
- The nerves are usually accompanied by arteries

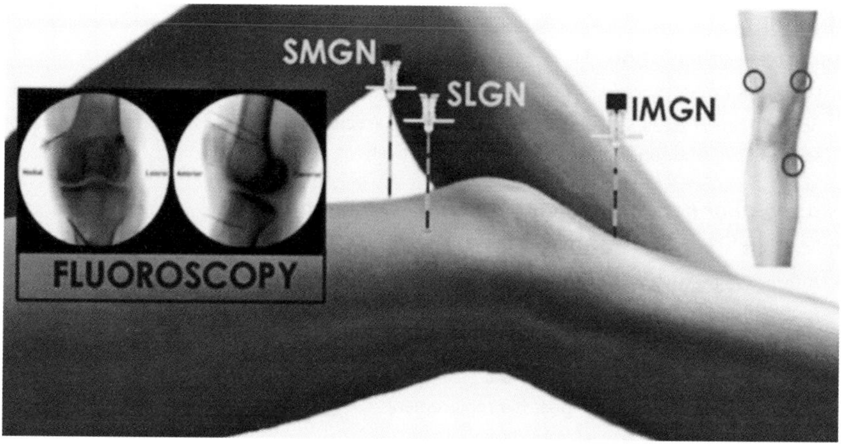

Figure 22.4.3 RF treatment of genicular nerves of the knee under fluoroscopy guidance. IMGN, inferior medial genicular nerve; SLGN, superior lateral genicular nerve; SMGN, superior medial genicular nerve
Reproduced with permission of Dr Vicente Roqués

- Diagnostic blocks are performed using a 25G, 35 mm needle with an out-of-plane approach using 2–5 mL of LA
- The genicular nerves are ablated at the junction of the lateral femoral shaft and the epicondyle, the junction of the medial femoral shaft and the epicondyle, and the junction of the medial tibial shaft and the epicondyle, correspondingly
- In addition to the above three nerves, lesioning to the medial (retinacular) genicular branch from the vastus intermedius can be performed at the midline of the femoral shaft just above the patella
- AP view and lateral fluoroscopy guidance are used to advance the RF needles to meet bony end points
- Each nerve is treated with RF lesion of 80°C for 90 seconds, with 25 seconds of ramp time (see Figs. 22.4.3 and 22.4.4)

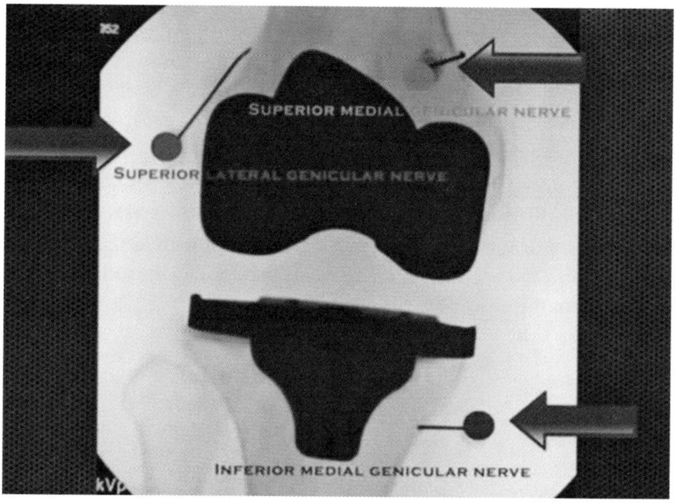

Figure 22.4.4 Supero-medial, superolateral, and infero-medial genicular nerves—radiofrequency needle positioning using fluoroscopy guidance
Reproduced with permission of Dr Vicente Roqués

Hip joint

Anatomy—innervation

- Innervation to the hip joint capsule is divided into anterior, antero-medial, postero-medial, and postero-lateral areas, which are innervated by the articular branches of the femoral, obturator, sciatic nerve, and superior gluteal nerve, respectively

Hip genicular nerve blocks and radiofrequency treatment

Indications

- Alternative treatment modality for patients who are not surgical candidates to undergo hip replacement secondary to comorbidities
- Obese patients
- Patients unwilling to undergo surgery
- Chronic post-surgical pain—post-hip replacement

Contraindications

- Patient refusal
- Localized infection
- Allergy to LA and steroids
- Pacemaker and other implantable devices

Patient preparation and positioning

- Patient position—supine
- X-ray and RF generator with 18G RF needles with 10 mm exposed tips

Technique

- To target the sensory branch of the obturator nerve, the tip of the needle is placed under fluoroscopy at the site below the inferior junction between the ischium and the pubis. This is a radiological target and is referred to as a teardrop on X-ray. For diagnostic blocks, 1–2 mL of LA is injected after negative aspiration
- For RF treatment, sensory stimulation is performed to cause paraesthesiae and elicit groin and thigh pain. Motor stimulation is performed to exclude muscle contractions before performing the RF lesion
- Femoral nerve articular branches are targeted by inserting the needle using an antero-lateral approach, aiming for the tip of the needle to be placed below the anterior inferior iliac spine near the antero-lateral margin of the hip joint (see Fig 22.4.5). For diagnostic block, 1–2 mL of LA is injected after negative aspiration
- Sensory and motor testing is performed to exclude quadriceps muscle contraction
- After injection of LA, RF lesion is performed at 80°C for 60–90 seconds
- Use of US has been described to block both femoral and obturator articular branches to the hip joint. US can allow the operator to safely avoid critical structures such as blood vessels and increase the safety of the procedure

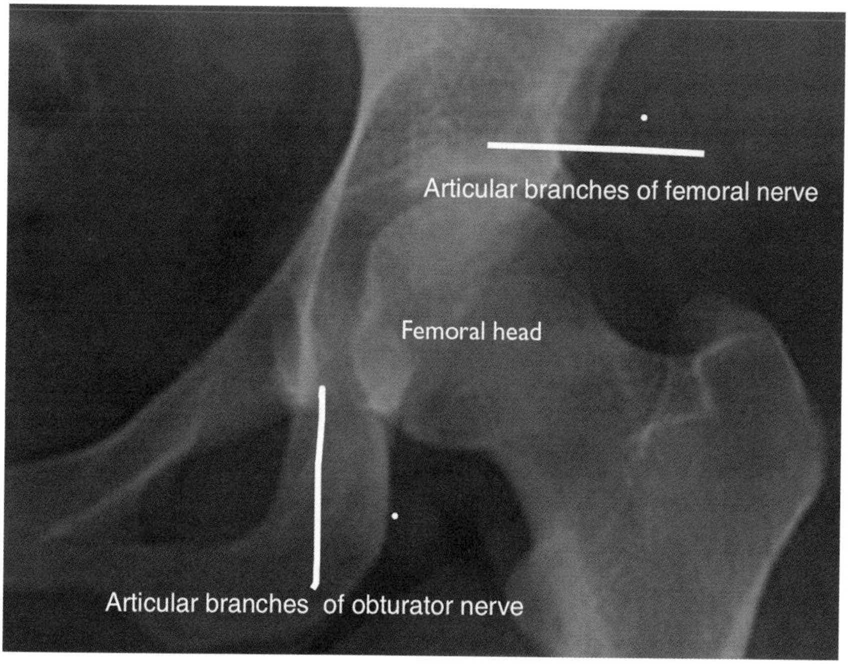

Figure 22.4.5 Targets for needle positioning for radiofrequency lesioning of articular branches (genicular nerves) of the femoral and obturator nerves

Further reading

1. Peng PW, Narouze S. Ultrasound-guided interventional procedures in pain medicine: a review of anatomy, sonoanatomy, and procedures: part I: nonaxial structures. Reg Anesth Pain Med 2009;34(5):458–74
2. Franco CD, Buvanendran A, Petersohn JD, et al. Innervation of the anterior capsule of the human knee: implications for radiofrequency ablation. Reg Anesth Pain Med 2015;40(4):363–8
3. Choi WJ, Hwang SJ, Song JG, et al. Radiofrequency treatment relieves chronic knee osteoarthritis pain: a double-blind randomized controlled trial. Pain 2011;152(3):481–7
4. Kawaguchi M, Hashizume K, Iwata T, Furuya H. Percutaneous radiofrequency lesioning of the sensory branches of obturator and femoral nerve for the treatment of hip joint pain. Reg Anesth Pain Med 2001;26:576–81
5. Chaiban G, Paradis T, Atallah J. Use of ultrasound and fluoroscopy guidance in percutaneous radiofrequency lesioning of the sensory branches of the femoral and obturator nerves. Pain Pract 2014;14(4):343–5
6. Simpson G, Krol A, Silver D, Nicholls B. Genicular nerves. In: Simpson G, Krol A, Silver D, Nicholls B (eds). Ultrasound-guided Interventions in Chronic Pain Management. 2019; pp. 163–7. UK: European Society of Regional Anaesthesia & Pain Therapy (ESRA)
7. Escolar VR. Ultrasound guided genicular nerve block. 2014. https://www.youtube.com/watch?v=uY93Oekl2j8

22.5 Myofascial trigger point injections

Introduction

- Myofascial pain is caused by a complex combination of sensory and motor abnormalities involving the peripheral and central nervous systems. It is characterized by regional pain, muscular tenderness, and the presence of myofascial trigger points (MTrPs)
- MTrPs are focally hypersensitive taut bands in muscles. Palpation produces a painful local twitch response or a 'jump sign', characterized by a jump or involuntary reflex-like; reproducible movement of the patient that is disproportionate to the amount of pressure exerted on an MTrP
- Palpation of MTrPs normally produces a typical referral pattern
- It is not understood why MTrPs occur, but some postulated mechanisms include:
    - Focal inflammation leading to sensitization, spontaneous discharge, and mechanical sensitivity of peripheral nerves. There is secondary hyperalgesia and sensitization in the muscles in close proximity to these inflamed nerves
    - Nociception in deep tissues that can lead to remote localized pain and alteration in central nociceptive processes. This may relegate the MTrPs as sites of secondary allodynia
- MTrPs are commonly treated by manipulation with manual pressure or injections

Indications

- Symptoms and examination findings consistent with active MTrPs
- Most studies of the evidence/studies are very heterogenous:
    - TPIs can be helpful to reduce pain associated with MTrPs
    - Majority of the studies have not found strong evidence to support the use of steroids or botulinum toxin
    - Some studies have found dry needling as effective as needling with LA

Contraindications

- Systemic or local infection, bleeding disorders or anticoagulation, pregnancy, allergy to LA agents, acute muscle trauma, needle phobia

Mechanism of action

- Uncertain, but some of the mechanisms involved in inactivation of the neural feedback mechanisms include:
    - Needling-mediated local release of intracellular K^+-disrupting nerve conduction
    - Dilution of nerve-sensitizing substances
    - Vasodilatation enhancing local removal of metabolites and increasing local energy supply
    - Focal necrosis of the trigger point
    - Counterirritation or application of a competing noxious stimulus which leads to activation of regions in the brain responsible for anti-nociception
    - Placebo effect

Patient preparation and positioning

- Position: prone, supine, or seated position
- Solutions: lidocaine or procaine (least myotoxic of all local injectable anaesthetics). Do not use adrenaline

- Isotonic saline or dry needling may be used in patients allergic to LAs
- Steroids may be considered for ligamentous trigger points

Technique

- Digital examination of muscles may exhibit a palpable taut band or cord of tense muscle fibres approximately 1–4 mm in diameter. Palpate along this band to locate the point of maximum tenderness. Pressure is held firmly to elicit the referred pain pattern
- Once a trigger point has been located and the overlying skin has been cleansed with alcohol, the clinician should isolate the trigger point with a pinch between two fingers, with stabilizing pressure to prevent it from rolling away from the advancing needle. The needle is inserted 1–2 cm away from the trigger point and then advanced into the trigger point at an acute angle of 30° to the skin. Aspirate before injection to avoid intravascular injection
- Once the needle is inside the trigger point, a small amount (0.2 mL) of LA is injected. The needle is withdrawn to the level of the SC tissue, then redirected superiorly, inferiorly, laterally, and medially. The needling and injection process is repeated in each direction without withdrawal of the needle, until the local twitch response is extinguished or until the muscle relaxes. Pressure should be applied over injection sites

Complications

- Vasovagal syncope, skin infection, pneumothorax (when performed in thorax), needle breakage, haematoma

Special points

- The priority is to correct the causative underlying aetiology
- It is important to correct other biopsychosocial perpetuating factors such as chronic infections, abnormal postures, nutritional deficits, stress, and sleep disturbances
- Stretching and exercise are critical part of the treatment programme in patients that receive a TPI

Further reading

1. Kishner S, Treuting. Trigger point injection. Medscape, 2018. https://emedicine.medscape.com/article/1997731-overview
2. Travell J, Simons D, Simons L. Myofascial Pain and Dysfunction. 2nd edition, 1999. Philadelphia, PA: Lippincott Williams & Williams
3. Wong CSM, Wong SHS. A new look at trigger point injections. Anesthesiol Res Pract 2012;2012:492452

22.6 Upper limb blocks

Introduction

- This chapter describes blocks for the brachial plexus and peripheral nerves in the arm
- Contraindications for these blocks include:
  - Absolute: patient refusal, local infection, LA allergy
  - Relative: coagulopathy, systemic infection
- Complications that can occur include infection, haematoma, vascular puncture, and nerve injury

- The typical volume of LA normally used for brachial plexus blocks is 10-20mls with intermittent aspiration during administration. The specific LA used depends on the onset and duration of action (maximum dose is calculated per body weight). Other agents that can be used to improve the efficacy of blocks are steroids, adrenaline, bicarbonate, magnesium, clonidine, dexmedetomidine and in palliative procedures neurolytic agents (please refer to Chapter 6, 15 and 29 for further information)
- A peripheral nerve stimulator is a useful aid to locate nerves and can improve safety when nerve blocks are performed

Blocks of the brachial plexus

- The neck is a highly vascular area, and care must be exercised to avoid intravascular injection, in particular the vertebral, inferior thyroid, suprascapular, and transverse cervical arteries
- Visualization is normally best with a high-frequency US linear probe
- Most blocks done with a 21G and 5/8/10 cm needle

Anatomy of the brachial plexus

- The brachial plexus innervates the shoulders, arms, and hands. It consists of:
  - Roots: originate from the anterior primary rami of the spinal nerves, C5–T1, that leave through the intervertebral foramina
  - Trunks: C5–T1 spinal nerves that form the upper (C5–6), middle (C7), and lower (C8–T1) trunks of the brachial plexus
  - Divisions: each trunk splits into an anterior and posterior division, generally respectively supplying the flexor and extensor muscles of the upper limb
  - Cords: the cords are divided into lateral, median, and posterior, according to their relation to the mid-axillary artery
  - Terminal branches arise from the cords:
    - musculocutaneous nerve – lateral cord
    - ulnar nerve – medial cord
    - median nerve – lateral & medial cord
    - axillary nerve – posterior cord
    - radial nerve – posterior cord
  - Additional branches are dorsal scapular, long thoracic, phrenic, suprascapular, long thoracic, lateral & medial pectoral, medial brachial cutaneous, medial antebrachial cutaneous nerves, and the nerve to the subclavius muscle

Interscalene block

Indications

- Analgesia and anaesthesia of the shoulder and upper arm

Specific contraindications

- Contralateral block to avoid bilateral phrenic nerve and recurrent paresis
- Moderate/severe COPD or limited respiratory reserve

Patient preparation and positioning

- Supine, with head slightly rotated to the contralateral side. Ipsilateral arm resting on the patient's thigh

Technique

- Block performed at the root or trunk level. The plexus at this level is seen antero-lateral to the carotid artery, between the anterior and middle scalene muscles—typically at 1–3 cm depth (see Fig. 22.6.1)

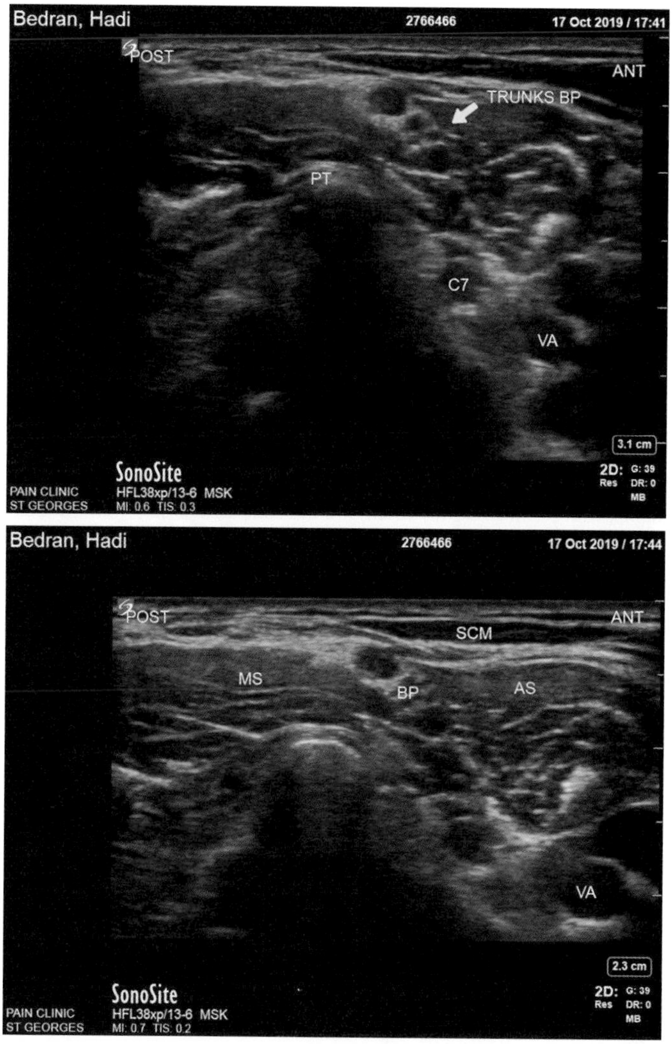

Figure 22.6.1 Interscalene views of the brachial plexus. AS, anterior scalene muscle; BP, brachial plexus; MS, musculocutaneous nerve; PT, posterior tubercle of C7; SCM, sternocleidomastoid muscle; TRUNKS BP, trunks of the brachial plexus; VA, vertebral artery

- From the supraclavicular position, the US probe is moved superiorly to an optimal point where the nerve roots can be visualized as round hypoechoic structures between the anterior and medial scalene muscles, but away from the subclavian artery and lung
- In-plane or out-of-plane approach. Deposit 15–20 ml LA below C6 and between C5 and C6 under real-time guidance

Disadvantages

- May miss C7–T1 (ulnar)—often difficult to visualize as located deeply
- 80% chance of phrenic nerve palsy—avoid in limited respiratory reserve

- Inadvertent epidural/subarachnoid injection, Horner's syndrome (miosis, partial ptosis, apparent anhidrosis, and enophthalmos), unilateral vocal cord palsy, vertebral artery injection, pneumothorax

Advantages

- Superficial anatomy
- Rapid onset

Supraclavicular block

Indications

- Analgesia and anaesthesia of the arm and hand

Specific contraindications

- Severe COPD

Patient preparation and positioning

- Patient supine, with the head slightly rotated to the contralateral side. Arm abducted with the hand resting on the abdomen

Technique

- US probe is placed above and parallel to the clavicle. In the optimal image, the subclavian artery, plexus, and first rib can be seen. The brachial plexus is normally postero-lateral to the subclavian artery. 15 – 20ml LA can be infiltrated by an in-plane approach at 12, 3, and 5 o'clock to the subclavian artery (see Fig. 22.6.2)

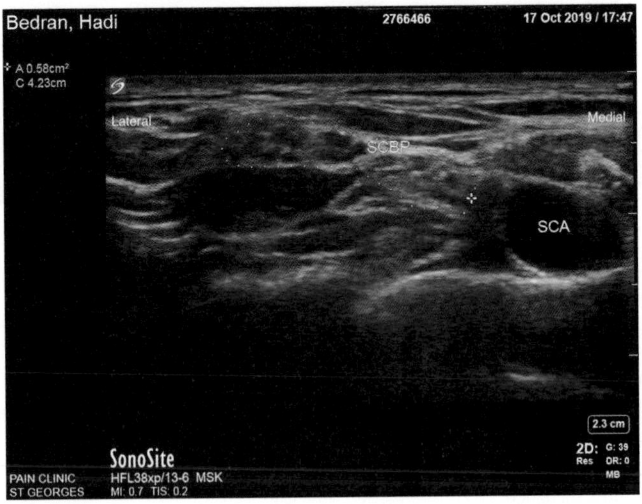

Figure 22.6.2 Supraclavicular view of the brachial plexus. SCA, subclavian artery; SCBP, supraclavicular brachial plexus

Disadvantages

- Pneumothorax—high risk as it is close to the pleura
- Phrenic nerve block (around 50–60% risk)
- Subclavian artery puncture—avoid in coagulopathic patients as bleeding is non-compressible

Advantages

- Anatomy is usually consistent
- Normally easy to visualize—the plexus is clumped together

Infraclavicular block

Indications

- Analgesia and anaesthesia of the arm and hand

Specific contraindications

- Clavicle/thorax deformities
- Devices in thorax (e.g. cardiac pacemaker)
- Coagulopathy (relative) as subclavian vessels are non-compressible

Patient preparation and positioning

- Patient supine, with the head slightly rotated to the contralateral side. Elbow flexed and shoulder abducted

Technique

- Aim to block the cords, which are arranged around the proximal part of the axillary artery
- Place US probe parasagittal, just medial to the coracoid process, to visualize the axillary artery ± vein (see Fig. 22.6.3)
- Inject 15 – 20ml LA around the artery via an in-plane approach under real-time guidance

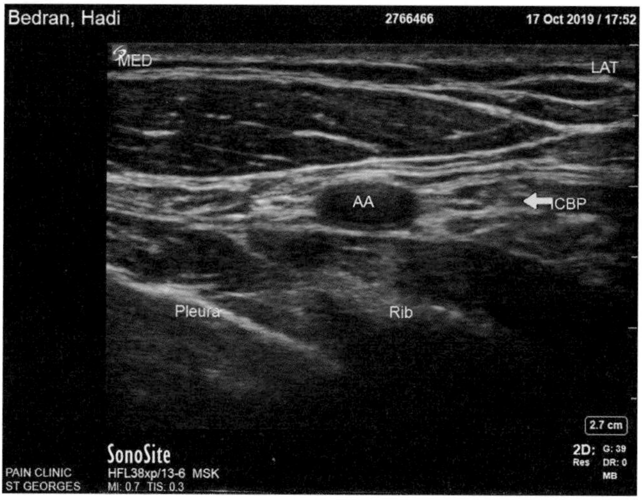

Figure 22.6.3 Infraclavicular view of the brachial plexus. AA, axillary artery; ICBP, infraclavicular brachial plexus

Disadvantages

- Pneumothorax—retro-clavicular or modified classical approach can decrease the risk of puncturing the pleura
- Difficult needling technique—can be more difficult in patients with large breasts or who are very muscular. Retro-clavicular and costoclavicular techniques can improve needle visualization
- Avoid in coagulopathic patients

Advantages

- Anatomy is usually consistent
- In patients with limited respiratory reserve an infraclavicular block is better to a supraclavicular/interscalene nerve blocks

Axillary block

Indications

- Analgesia and anaesthesia in the forearm and hand

Patient preparation and positioning

- Patient supine, with the head slightly rotated to the contralateral side. Arm abducted with elbow flexed

Technique

- Aim to block the terminal nerve branches as they pass through the base of the axilla in close proximity to the axillary artery (see Fig. 22.6.4)
- The probe across the axilla, aiming to visualize the axillary artery and vein, the coracobrachialis muscle, and the two heads of the biceps
- The musculoskeletal nerve is a bright structure between the muscles between the biceps and coracobrachialis muscle and normally above the axillary artery

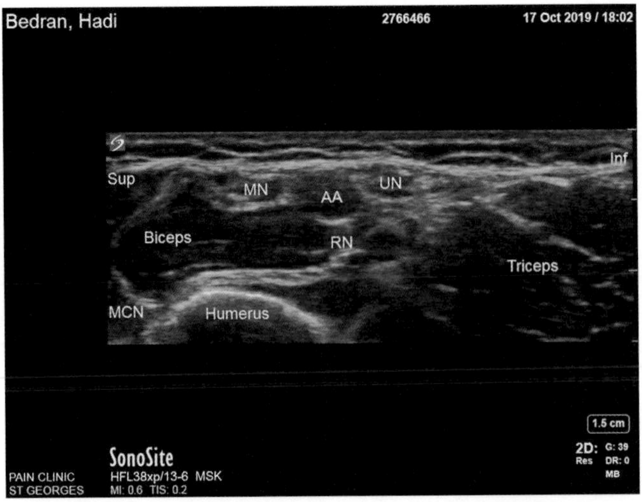

Figure 22.6.4 Axillary view of the brachial plexus. AA, axillary artery; MCN, musculocutaneous nerve; MN, medial nerve; RN, radial nerve; UN, ulnar nerve

- The median, ulnar, and radial nerves are seen around the axillary artery (median nerve is above, ulnar nerve is below and radial nerve is below or behind)
- Inject 15 – 20ml LA via an in-plane or out-of-plane approach under real-time guidance

Disadvantages

- High anatomical variation of the nerves and nerves located in several areas
- Sometimes it is difficult to find the musculocutaneous nerve

Advantages

- Compressible if there is any bleeding
- Safest approach to the brachial plexus blocks

Additional information

- Intercostobrachial nerve block needed in surgery in the axilla/medial aspect of the arm or if a tourniquet is applied on the upper arm. Frequently done with the landmark technique as difficult to see with USS

Peripheral upper limb blocks

Anatomy relevant to blocks

- Radial nerve: found in the groove between the lateral border of the biceps tendon and the brachioradialis, 1.5–2 cm proximal to the elbow crease
- Median nerve: lies medial to the brachial artery in the antecubital fossa. Enters the hand via the carpal tunnel
- Ulnar nerve: enters the forearm beneath the two heads of the flexor carpi ulnaris. It joins the ulnar artery along the forearm and runs to the wrist posterior to the artery and deep to the flexor carpi ulnaris

Indications

- Surgical anaesthesia along the course of the individual nerve
- Supplement to brachial plexus block
- Radial tunnel syndrome; Cheiralgia paresthetica (Wartenberg's syndrome)

Patient preparation and positioning

- The preferred position is supine, with the arm supported on the side
- Visualization is best with a high-frequency US linear probe
- The forearm should be held in supination for blocking the median nerve. For easy access to the ulnar nerve, the arm can be abducted and the elbow flexed. Access to the radial nerve above the elbow is best when the hand is rested over the patient's abdomen

Technique

- The typical volume of LA used to block a peripheral nerve is 5-8mls (LA maximum dose is calculated per body weight as outlined in Chapter 6)
- *Radial nerve:*
    - Place the transducer a few centimetres proximal to the lateral epicondyle of the humerus, transversely across the upper arm
    - Identify the nerve as a hyperechoic triangular or ovoid structure, which can separate into two branches with distal movement of the transducer
    - In- or out-of-plane approach is acceptable

- *Median nerve:*
  - Place the transducer transversely across at the antecubital fossa at the level of the elbow crease
  - The nerve lies medial to the brachial artery as a distinct hyperechoic structure, either lateral or deep to the pronator teres muscle
  - Approach in-plane or out-of-plane, preferably injecting on the medial side of the nerve
- *Ulnar nerve:*
  - Place the transducer transversely across the ulnar border of the proximal mid forearm, scanning distally to identify the ulnar nerve and artery as they come closer to each other
  - The nerve stays in close proximity to the flexor carpi ulnaris
  - The needle can come from either side of the nerve, aiming to avoid the artery

Further reading

1. Kishner S. Brachial Plexus Anatomy. Medscape. 2015.https://emedicine.medscape.com/article/1877731-overview#a2
2. Juels AN, Raghavendra M. Infraclavicular Nerve Block. 2018. https://emedicine.medscape.com/article/2000107-overview
3. Upper Extremity Blocks. NYSORA. https://www.nysora.com/techniques/upper-extremity/

22.7 Lower limb blocks

Introduction

- High-frequency linear US probe is suitable for all, except in the very obese
- Most blocks are done with 21G and 8/10 cm needle
- The typical volume of LA normally used for lower limb blocks is 10-20mls for proximal blocks and 5-10mls for distal individual peripheral lower limb nerves. The specific agent used depends on the onset and duration of action of the LA (maximum dose is calculated per body weight). Other agents can be used to improve the efficacy of blocks such as steroids, adrenaline, bicarbonate, magnesium, clonidine, dexmedetomidine and neurolytic agents in palliative procedures (please refer to Chapter 6, 15, 29 and 13.8 Clonodine, p. 244 for further information)
- A peripheral nerve stimulator is a useful aid to locate the nerve and can improve safety when these nerve blocks are performed

Anatomy

Femoral nerve

- The femoral nerve originates from the anterior rami of the L2, L3 and L4 nerve roots
- Enters the thigh under the ilio-inguinal ligament lateral to the femoral artery
- Divides into anterior and posterior divisions, with the latter giving rise to the saphenous nerve
- Supplies all the muscles in the anterior compartment of the thigh
- Gives sensory innervation to the antero-medial thigh and medial side of the leg and foot
- Contributes articular branches to the knee joint

Obturator nerve

- Formed by the anterior primary rami of the L2, L3, and L4 nerves
- Runs within the psoas muscle and exits the pelvis via the obturator foramen, dividing into anterior and posterior branches
- Both branches give sensory innervation to the hip capsule, a small area in the medial thigh and posterior aspect of the knee joint, respectively
- Both branches supply motor fibres to the hip adductors

Saphenous nerve

- A terminal sensory branch of the femoral nerve
- Accompanies the superficial femoral artery in the subsartorial canal
- Exits at the adductor hiatus between the sartorius and gracilis muscles, giving off an infrapatellar branch
- Continues to lie subcutaneously to supply the pre-patellar skin and the medial side of the ankle and foot

Sciatic nerve

- Formed by the anterior divisions of L4, L5, and S1–S3 nerve roots
- Exits the pelvis via the greater sciatic foramen, mostly anterior to the piriformis muscle
- Passes between the ischial tuberosity and the greater trochanter, and enters the posterior thigh by passing deep to the long head of the biceps femoris
- Usually divides at the apex of the popliteal fossa into the tibial and common perineal nerves
- Innervates the muscles of the posterior thigh, entire leg, and foot
- The tibial nerve gives sensory branches to the postero- and antero-lateral sides of the leg, and the sole of the foot
- The common fibular nerve gives sensory branches to the lateral leg and the dorsum of the foot

Indications

- Femoral nerve: analgesia to anterior thigh, hip, and knee surgery
- Obturator nerve: analgesia to the hip and medial aspect of the knee
- Saphenous nerve: analgesia to the antero-medial aspect of the knee, medial aspect of the lower leg and medial border of the foot
- Sciatic nerve block: in combination with a saphenous nerve block, it provides anaesthesia for ankle and foot surgery. Analgesia for hip, knee, and distal surgery on the lower limb

Contraindications

- Absolute: patient refusal, local infection, LA allergy
- Relative: coagulopathy, systemic infection, pre-existing peripheral neuropathies

Patient preparation and positioning

- Femoral/saphenous nerve: patient supine, with the leg slightly abducted (externally rotated for the obturator nerve)
- Sciatic/popliteal nerve: commonly prone or lateral position; supine, with the hip and knee flexed if possible

Technique

Femoral nerve block

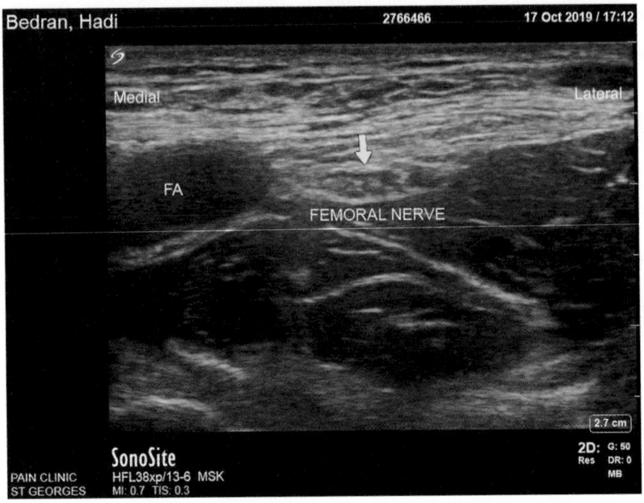

Figure 22.7.1 Femoral nerve. FA, femoral artery

- Place the linear US probe perpendicular to the course of the femoral nerve in the groin, and identify the femoral artery and vein medially just below the inguinal ligament (see Fig. 22.7.1)
- Scan laterally to identify the iliacus muscle and fascia iliaca
- The nerve is located between the artery and the muscle under the fascia
- Inject 15 – 20ml LA via an in-plane or out-of-plane approach under real-time guidance. Position the needle lateral to the femoral nerve and below the fascia iliaca

Obturator nerve block

- Place the US probe transversely over the inner thigh to identify the femoral artery and vein (see Fig. 22.7.2)

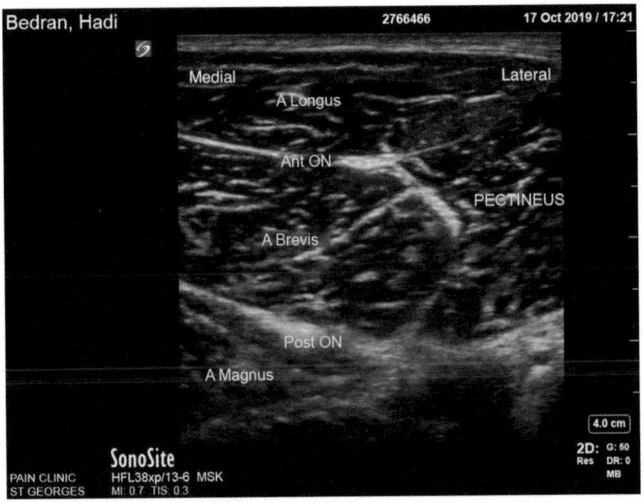

Figure 22.7.2 Posterior and anterior obturator nerve branches. A Brevis, adductor brevis; A Longus, adductor longus; A Magnus, adductor magnus; Ant ON, anterior obturator nerve; Post ON, posterior obturator nerve

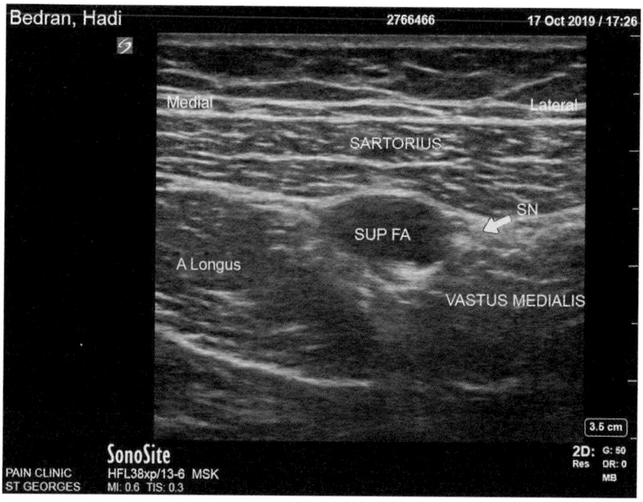

Figure 22.7.3 Saphenous nerve. A Longus, adductor longus; SUP FA, superficial femoral artery; SN, saphenous nerve

- Scan medially until the pectineus muscle belly is seen
- Continue medially until three muscle layers are visible
- From superficial to deep: adductor longus, brevis, and magnus
- The anterior and posterior branches of the obturator nerve pass in the planes between the longus and brevis, and the brevis and magnus muscles, respectively
- Inject a total of 10 ml LA with an in-plane approach at each branch

Saphenous nerve block

- Place the US probe over the mid-thigh (or upper thigh) antero-medially and transversely to view the common femoral artery (see Fig. 22.7.3)
- Follow the artery distally until it passes under the sartorius to enter the adductor canal
- The femoral vein is seen underneath the muscle and the nerve is lateral to the artery. Saphenous nerve block can be performed either at the distal femoral triangle where the medial vastus nerve is blocked leading to some muscle weakness or at the mid-thigh level where the vastus medialis nerve may be spared. Blocking the vastus medialis nerve can be beneficial for analgesia to the knee
- Inject 10 ml LA via an in-plane or out-of-plane approach under real-time guidance

Sciatic (popliteal and mid-thigh) nerve block

- Place the transducer transversely over the popliteal fossa, and identify the popliteal artery and vein. The probe may need to be tilted distally and perpendicular to the popliteal sciatic nerve. The tibial nerve is seen superficial to the vein and artery (see Fig. 22.7.4)
- Scanning laterally, the common peroneal nerve can be found underneath the medial border of the biceps femoris. At this level, popliteal block can be performed by inserting the needle in-plane from the lateral side and depositing LA to surround each nerve
- To perform a sciatic nerve (mid-thigh) block, scan proximally to the point before the sciatic nerve divides into the femoral and peroneal branches (see Figs. 22.7.5, 22.7.6 and 22.7.7)
- Inject 5 – 20ml LA via an in-plane or out-of-plane approach under real-time guidance. During the injection the perineural sheath needs to be penetrated carefully (without injuring the

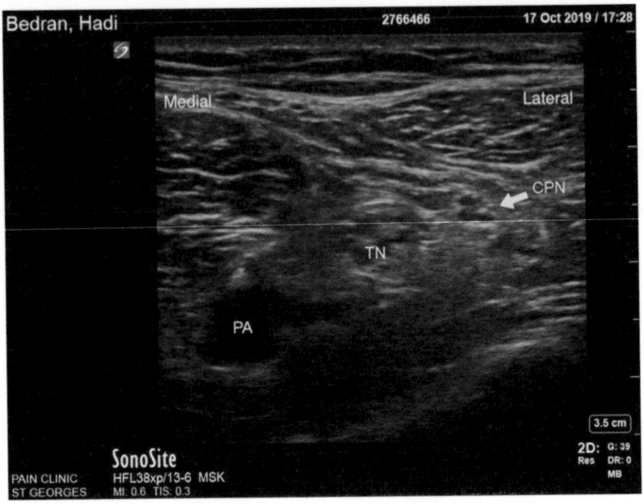

Figure 22.7.4 Common peroneal and tibial nerves. CPN, common peroneal nerve; PA, popliteal artery; TN, tibial nerve

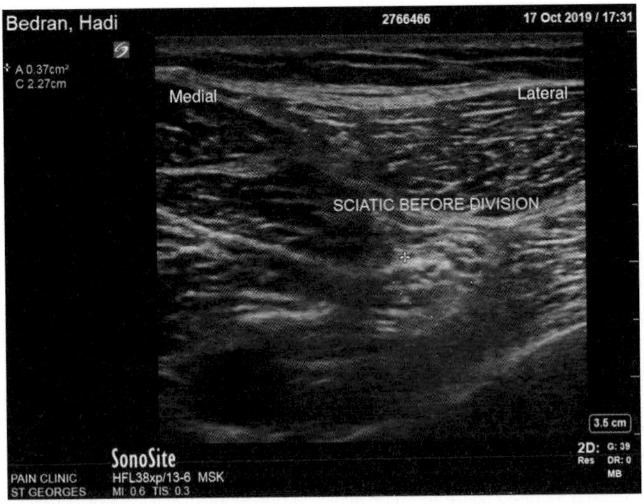

Figure 22.7.5 Sciatic nerve before division

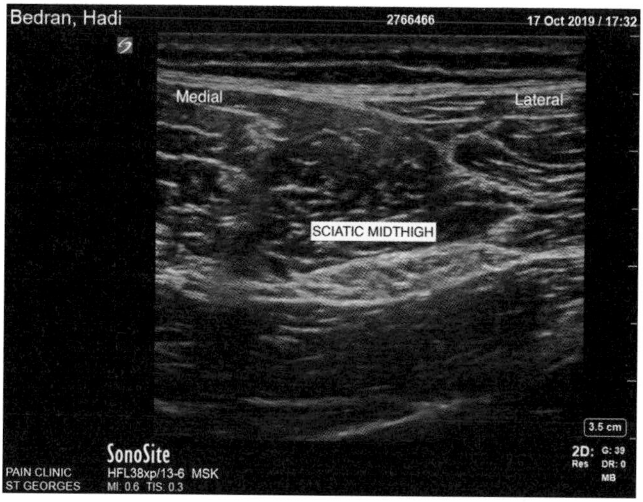

Figure 22.7.6 Sciatic nerve in the mid-thigh region

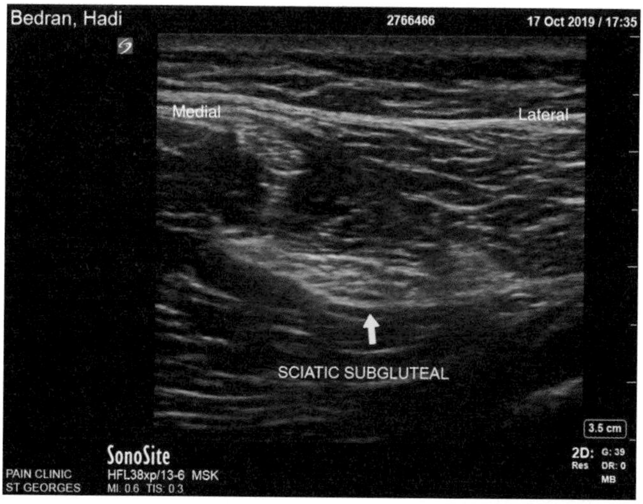

Figure 22.7.7 Sciatic nerve in subgluteal region

nerve). The local anaesthetic is deposited either at the junction or distal to the division of the sciatic nerve into femoral and peroneal divisions. The division of the sciatic nerve is variable but normally occurs above the poplitea or between poplitea and mid-thigh

Special points

- Whenever in doubt, the colour flow Doppler mode should be used to identify vascular structures

Further reading

1. Ultrasound for Regional Anesthesia (USRA). Advancing the science of ultrasound guided regional anesthesia and pain medicine. http://www.usra.ca
2. NYSORA (New York School of Regional Anesthesia). https://www.nysora.com

22.8 Suprascapular nerve block

Anatomy

- The suprascapular nerve is a mixed nerve
- Originates from the superior trunk of the brachial plexus (C5 and C6 nerve roots)
- Passes underneath the omohyoid muscle in the posterior triangle of the neck, aiming posteriorly towards the suprascapular notch. It continues deep to the superior transverse scapular ligament through the scapular notch into the supraspinous fossa. After travelling through the supraspinous fossa, the SSN reaches the spinoglenoid notch laterally and exits into the infraspinous fossa
- Structures innervated:
    - Supraspinatus and infraspinatus muscles
    - Sensory innervation to the glenohumeral and acromioclavicular joints, coracohumeral ligament, subacromial bursa, and scapula
- At the suprascapular notch, the nerve is next to the suprascapular artery and vein, but the vessels pass above the ligament. From an anatomical perspective, it is best to block the nerve over the supraspinous fossa halfway between the suprascapular notch and the spinoglenoid notch

Indications

- Acute shoulder pain
- Chronic shoulder pain secondary to bursitis, arthritis, degenerative joint, and rotator cuff disease

Contraindications

- Absolute: patient refusal, local infection, LA allergy
- Relative: coagulopathy, systemic infection

Patient preparation and positioning

- Position: sitting, ideally placing their hand over to the contralateral shoulder
- US probe: 10–12 MHz, linear
- Other equipment: 22G, 80–100 mm nerve block/RF needle, peripheral nerve stimulator

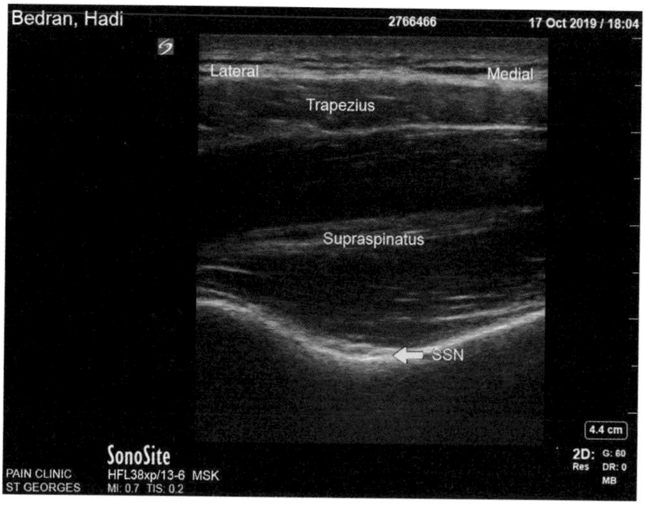

Figure 22.8.1 Suprascapular nerve block. SSN, suprascapular nerve

Technique

- Probe position: place one end of the transducer over the scapular spine and the other end directing towards the coracoid process (see Fig. 22.8.1)
- Aim: view of the suprascapular nerve and vessels
- US landmarks: supraspinous fossa, suprascapular and spinoglenoid notches, suprascapular muscle, superior transverse scapular ligament
- Needle approach: preferably in-plane, aiming from postero-medial to antero-lateral; out-of-plane is also possible. Motor stimulation is recommended
- Proposed injectates:
  - For anaesthesia/acute pain: 5–8 mL of bupivacaine or levobupivacaine 0.5%
  - In patients with chronic pain, a long-acting steroid, such as 40 mg methylprednisolone, can be added to the above mixture and PRF treatment may be performed at the same time

Complications

- Nerve injury, pneumothorax, haematoma, LA toxicity, infection, steroid S/Es if steroids are used

Special points

- The optimal needle end point is reached when the needle tip is positioned underneath the fascia of the supraspinatus muscle
- Avoid targeting the suprascapular nerve in the suprascapular notch because accidental anterior needle advancement can puncture the pleura anteriorly

Further reading

1. Ultrasound for Regional Anesthesia (USRA). Suprascapular nerve block. http://www.usra.ca/pain-medicine/specific-blocks/peripheral-nerves/suprascapular.php
2. Chang KV, Hung CY, Wang TG, et al. Ultrasound-guided proximal suprascapular nerve block with radiofrequency lesioning for patients with malignancy-associated recalcitrant shoulder pain. J Ultrasound Med 2015;34:2099–105

3. Siegenthaler A, Moriggl B, Mlekusch S, et al. Ultrasound-guided suprascapular nerve block, description of a novel supraclavicular approach. Reg Anaesth Pain Medicine 2012;37(3):325–8
4. Simpson G, Krol A, Silver D, Nicholls B. 5.2 Suprascapular nerve block. In: Simpson G et al. Ultrasund-guided interventions in chronic pain management. 2019; pp. 130–135. UK: The European Society of Regional Anaesthesia & Pain Therapy (ESRA)

22.9 Vertebroplasty

Introduction

- Vertebroplasty and kyphoplasty can be effective for the management of pain from vertebral fractures from cancer (primary or metastatic), osteoporosis, and trauma. This topic will focus on the role of vertebroplasty in osteoporotic vertebral fractures
- Osteoporotic compression fractures (OCFs) are the most common vertebral fractures. Most cause minimal symptoms, but a subset of patients develop severe pain and lose their functional independence. Vertebroplasty has been used to reduce pain and enhance earlier recovery in these patients
- The vertebral body comprises trabecular bone surrounded by a thin shell of cortical bone. Osteoporosis reduces the quantity of trabecular bone, causing loss of vertebral body strength. This can result in vertebral fractures secondary to a fall, a lifting or twisting action, or without obvious trigger
- Fractures can be divided into three anatomical regions: thoracic (T4–10), thoracolumbar (T11–L2), and lumbar (L3–5). Thoracolumbar fractures comprise 60–80% of severely painful vertebral fractures. These different regions are exposed to different forces. Thoracic vertebrae are braced against flexion forces by the rib cage. The thoracolumbar segment lies below the inflexible thoracic spine and is subjected to magnified compressive flexion forces
- Osteoporotic vertebral fractures behave differently to traumatic fractures of healthy bone. Osteoporotic fractures may continue to collapse and change morphology, sometimes developing osteonecrotic clefts and further fracture lines. Such deterioration in fracture morphology occurs in old patients with severe osteoporosis and causes severe fracture pain. Early vertebroplasty in these patients can stop collapse of the bone, stabilize fracture motion, and relieve pain

Evidence

- Vertebroplasty evidence remains controversial. A systematic review identified 13 randomized trials of vertebroplasty. Five were blinded trials comparing vertebroplasty to placebo, and eight were open comparing vertebroplasty to conservative therapy. A meta-analysis of open randomized trials showed vertebroplasty superior to conservative care.
- The VAPOUR trial is the only blinded trial to show superior pain relief from vertebroplasty over placebo. Major differences in patient selection between the VAPOUR trial and other placebo trials include earlier time of vertebroplasty (see Fig. 22.9.1), more severely affected patients, and inclusion of inpatients—excluded in the other blinded trials.
- Kyphoplasty is used interchangeably with vertebroplasty, depending upon operator preference. There are no blinded randomized data for kyphoplasty. Three randomized trials comparing kyphoplasty to vertebroplasty have found equivalent clinical outcomes with both techniques. This topic will focus on vertebroplasty.

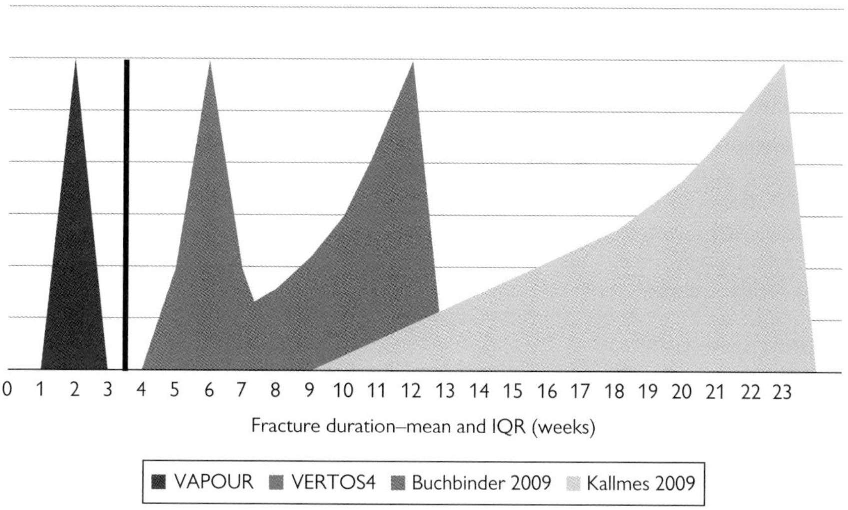

Figure 22.9.1 Fracture duration (mean and interquartile range) in blinded trials of vertebroplasty versus placebo. Note: the mean (triangle apex) and interquartile range (triangle base) of fracture duration is shown for each trial. VAPOUR was the only trial where most patients had fracture duration of <4 weeks. VAPOUR showed vertebroplasty produced superior pain relief to placebo. The other three trials found vertebroplasty and placebo provided equivalent pain relief in older fractures and had different patient groups

Reproduced with permission from Diamond, T., Clark, W., Bird, P. *et al.* (2020). Early vertebroplasty within 3 weeks of fracture for acute painful vertebral osteoporotic fractures: subgroup analysis of the VAPOUR trial and review of the literature. *Eur Spine J*, 29: 1606–1613. https://doi.org/10.1007/s00586-020-06362-2

Anatomy of vertebral body

- OCFs occur from T4 to L5
- Vertebral bodies increase in size from T4 to L5
- Average volume of T6 is 12 cc^3 and L5 is 45 cc^3
- Vertebral bodies comprise a shell of cortical bone surrounding trabecular bone
- The trabecular bone is the component that fractures

Natural history of OCFs

- Most cause mild symptoms and have a favourable natural history
- A subset of patients with increased age (mean 80 years old), severe osteoporosis, and comorbidities experience uncontrolled severe pain and progressive collapse of the fracture—sometimes with retropulsion into the spinal canal
- 'Dynamic mobility' describes a change in fractured vertebral body height in supine and upright postures. This causes severe pain when attempting to get out of bed
- Patients with severe pain, osteoporosis, and early fractures, including hospitalized patients, do poorly with conservative care

Symptoms

- Pain is typically felt four levels below the anatomical site of fracture. For example, L1 fracture typically causes pain in the buttocks
- Pain has a midline component

- Pain is normally described as worse when getting out of bed
- Loss of functional independence may necessitate hospitalization

Mechanics of vertebroplasty

- Vertebroplasty can stabilize soft, non-healed fractures which have not sclerosed. The best predictor of the degree of fracture healing is fracture duration. The next best indicator is MRI. During vertebroplasty, the injected polymethylmethacrylate (PMMA) cement distributes from top to bottom, side to side, and the anterior 70% of the vertebral body. The distribution of the cement provides stability against flexion and compression forces on the vertebral body

Patient selection

- Severe pain not responding to medical therapy
- Intolerance of opioid medications
- Pain duration <4 weeks at time of vertebroplasty
- Established osteoporosis—quantitative CT lumbar T-score <−2.5
- MRI confirms acute fracture
- Thoracolumbar segment responds best to vertebroplasty (T11, T12, L1, L2)

Vertebroplasty procedure

- High-viscosity PMMA
- Patient prone
- Conscious sedation—IV midazolam, fentanyl
- Oxygen mask/pulse oximetry monitor
- High-quality interventional fluoroscope
- Tilt cranio-caudad until the pedicles project midway between the superior and inferior endplates
- Tilt side-to-side until the spinous process is midway between the pedicles
- From this 'neutral' point, angle an additional 20° right posterior oblique
- LA into the posterior pedicle
- Pass an 11G or 13G needle through the pedicle in this projection
- Check the frontal and lateral projections intermittently—ensure the needle does not pass medial to the pedicle (frontal plane) before reaching the posterior cortex of the vertebral body (lateral plane)
- Advance the needle to the anterior third of the vertebral body—so the tip is in the midline
- Repeat needle insertion on the contralateral pedicle
- Inject a small aliquot of PMMA out of the tip of each needle and then wait 60 seconds. This helps prevent venous extravasation
- Adjust the technique, depending on fracture morphology
- The fracture cleft will be the space of least resistance. Once PMMA finds its way to this cavity, it will preferentially fill it rather than the trabecular bone. To stabilize the whole bone, place at least one needle into normal trabecular bone (away from the cleft). Fill trabecular bone first—PMMA will find a way to the cavity and then try to fill both components sufficiently to bond them
- If necessary, needles can be progressively withdrawn into the posterior half of the vertebral body to allow filling of at least the anterior two-thirds of the vertebral body
- If PMMA begins to extravasate, cease the injection; check the position of extravasation in both frontal and lateral projections and wait 30 seconds. Gently recommence injection, initially from

the contralateral needle, and watch for extravasation closely. If extravasation continues, cease the injection.

Recovery

- Wait for 5 minutes after completion of the injection before transferring the patient
- Allow 1–2 hours for recovery before mobilizing as needed

Medical therapy

- Medical osteoporosis management should be optimized
- Best indicator of the degree of osteoporosis is the quantitative CT score of the lumbar spine
- Patient education on how to avoid bending and lifting is important

Further reading

1. Boszczyk B. Volume matters: a review of procedural details of two randomised controlled vertebroplasty trials of 2009. Eur Spine J 2010;19(11):1837–40
2. Clark W, Bird P, Diamond T, et al. Cochrane vertebroplasty review misrepresented evidence for vertebroplasty with early intervention in severely affected patients. BMJ Evidence-Based Medicine 2020;25:85–9
3. Clark W, Bird P, Gonski P, et al. Safety and efficacy of vertebroplasty for acute painful osteoporotic fractures (VAPOUR): a multicentre, randomised, double blind, placebo-controlled trial. Lancet 2016;388:1408–16
4. Lou S, Shi X, Zhang X, et al. Percutaneous vertebroplasty versus non-operative treatment for osteoporotic vertebral compression fractures: a meta-analysis of randomized controlled trials. Osteoporos Int 2019;30:2369–80
5. McKiernan F, Jensen R, Faciszewski T. The dynamic mobility of vertebral compression fractures. J Bone Miner Res 2003;18:24–9.
6. Ong T, Kantachuvesiri P, Sahota O, et al. Characteristics and outcomes of hospitalised patients with vertebral fragility fractures: a systematic review. Age Ageing 2018;47(1):17–25
7. Yang E-Z, Xu J-G, Huang G-Z, et al. Percutaneous vertebroplasty versus conservative treatment in aged patients with acute osteoporotic vertebral compression fractures. Spine 2016;41:653–60

22.10 Prolotherapy

History

- First description of joint stabilization by Hippocrates who recorded the use of cautery in the axillary flesh to stabilize recurrent shoulder dislocation
- Injection of fibroproliferants to strengthen connective tissue has been in use since 1832 (sclerosants for inguinal hernias by Jaynes and Velpeau)
- Mayer (1900) reported on the use of zinc sulphate/phenol for hernia repair
- In 1935, Mayer showed fibroproliferation in mammalian connective tissue
- The first modern record was by G Hackett in 1955 who described joint stabilization in rats
- In 1956, Hackett published his monograph on 1600 cases of back and neck pain caused by incompetent ligamentous tissue (whiplash and industrial accidents in Ohio), claiming a cure rate of 82% in 1600 patients with low back pain
- Progress was delayed by reports of three cases of paralysis and two deaths after inadvertent injection of psyllium seed and zinc sulphate into the subarachnoid space by other practitioners

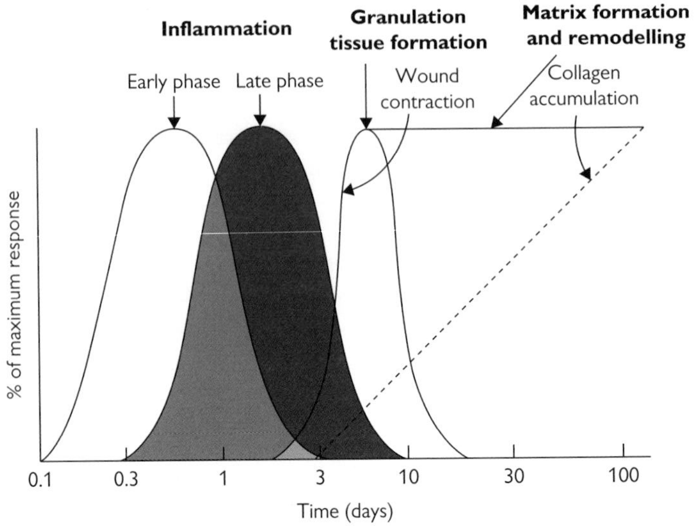

Figure 22.10.1 Inflammatory repair response

- In 1960, MJ Ongley developed a safer solution—vein sclerosant 2% phenol, 25% glucose, 25% glycerol (no serious complications since)
- Since then, several RCTs have been undertaken on heterogenous samples of low back pain patients, with mixed results
- However, use of prolotherapy in sports and exercise medicine has grown and several studies have shown benefit in peripheral joints and conditions

Mechanisms

(See Fig. 22.10.1.)

- Fibroproliferative injection of hypertonic glucose (now more often without phenol) has been shown in animal studies to induce fibroplasia and collagen stimulation and formation, resulting in thicker stronger tissue
- Sample human biopsy tissue from the sacroiliac ligaments pre- and post-injection demonstrated increased fibre density and fibroblast population

Current evidence

- There is level A–C evidence for prolotherapy in various peripheral structures
- Cusi demonstrated benefit for chronic SIJ dysfunction and showed SPECT scan hybrid sequences could accurately identify patients with chronic ligamentous changes in the posterior SIJ ligaments
- Problems with studies on low back pain are numerous: no subgroups were defined; volume, number, and type of proliferant solution varied; confounding existed; some samples were extremely chronic; and no image guidance was used. As a result, it is not recommended by guidelines in the UK at the moment.

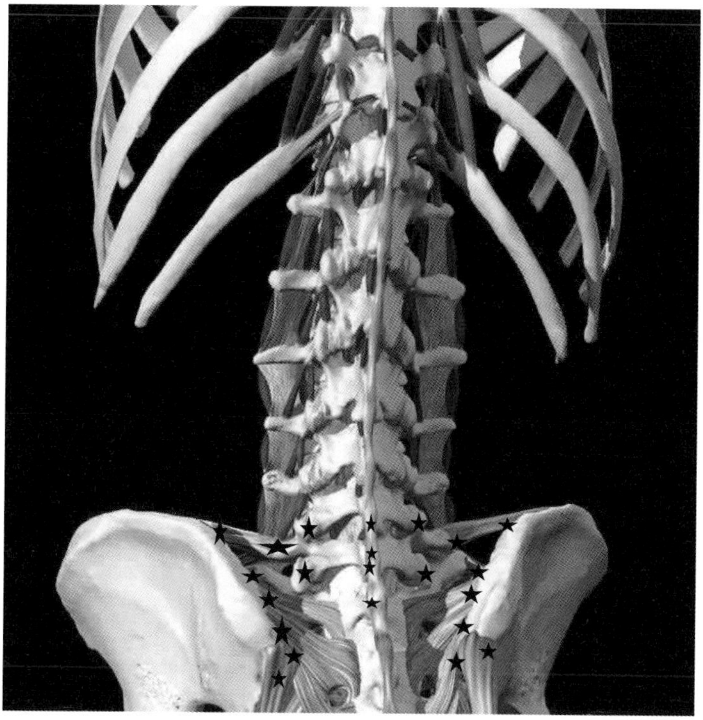

Figure 22.10.2 Injection sites for lumbar/sacroiliac instability syndrome

- This author's experience of over 25 years in 'clinical instability' disorders, sacroiliac dysfunction, whiplash symptoms, and discogenic pain, as well as chronic ankle ligament laxity and ACJ disruption, is rewarding
- Clinical audits over the last decade have found that between 70% and 90% show a 'good to excellent' response on a global perceived benefit scale

Technique

- Mix P2G solution (2% phenol, 25% glucose, and 25% glycerol), with equal volume of 1% lidocaine
- Inject 0.5 mL at either end of enthesis or ligament. Inject as many accessible ligamentous attachments as possible
- Repeat at least three times or more at intervals of 1–6 weeks apart to accumulate the effect
- Restoration and remodelling follow the normal pathway of connective tissue healing

Use in low back pain

(See Fig. 22.10.2.)

- The benefit may not be felt for 1–3 months after the course since full restoration of collagen matrix takes 120 days or more, but can last longer than other current pain intervention for the low back, except spinal or SIJ fusion. Average relief can range for up to 5–10 years

Further reading

1. Cusi M, Saunders J, Hungerford B, et al. The use of prolotherapy in the sacroiliac joint. Br J Sports Med 2010;44(2):100–4
2. Cusi M, Saunders J, Van der Wall H, Fogelman I. Metabolic disturbances identified by SPECT-CT in patients with a clinical diagnosis of sacroiliac incompetence. Eur Spine J 2013;22:1674–82
3. Dagenais S, Yelland MJ, Del Mar C, Schoene ML. Prolotherapy injections for chronic low back pain. Cochrane Database Syst Rev 2007;2:CD004059
4. Hackett GS. Ligament and Tendon Relaxation Treated by Prolotherapy. 3rd edition, 1958. Springfield, IL: Charles Thomas
5. Hauser RA, Lackner JB, Steilen-Matias D, Harris DK. A systematic review of dextrose prolotherapy for chronic musculoskeletal pain. Clin Med Insights Arthritis Musculoskelet Disord 2016;7(9):139–59
6. Liu YK, Tipton CM, Matthes RD, et al. An in situ study of the influence of sclerosing solution in rabbit medial collateral ligaments and its junction strength. Connect Tissue Res 1983;11(2–3):95–102

SECTION 5

CLINICAL

Musculoskeletal Pain Conditions

Owen Bodycombe, Enrique Collantes, Mohamed Dorgham, Bethany Fitzmaurice, Rahul Guru, Yehia Kamel, Sandeep Kapur, Nofil Mulla, Paolo Pais, Arumugam Pitchiah, Shankar Ramaswamy, Jan Rudiger, Thomas E Smith, Alifia Tameem, Athmaja Thottungal, and Ivan Wong

CONTENTS

23.1 Osteoarthritis

Definition

- A disease of synovial joints characterized by cartilage loss with an accompanying periarticular bone response. All joints can be affected, but more common in the hips, knees, and lumbar spine, compared to mobile joints of the hands or neck

Incidence

- 8.75 million people in the UK have sought treatment for OA. Women are more likely to seek help than men. The incidence increases with age, from 33% of people over the age of 45 to 49% of women and 42% of men at ages over 75. The most common joints are the knee (18% of the population) and hip (11%)
- More prevalent in European countries than in America
- OA of the knee is more common than hip OA in African-Americans, South-Asian Indians, and Chinese

Pathophysiology

- Progressive loss of synovial cartilage with failure of replacement with new cartilage. Instead there is increased subchondral plate thickness, development of subchondral cysts, and new bone formation. Further structural bone changes alter the articular surface, creating abnormal biomechanical stresses, further aggravating the problems

Aetiology/risk factors

- Increasing age, female sex, family history, injury, infection, occupation, obesity, congenital deformities
- Trauma to the local joint speeds up the degenerative process
- Athletes suffer more from OA due to severe and recurrent stress/injury to the joint

Diagnosis

- History and examination—pain which worsens on activity, stiffness of the joint in the morning or after inactivity, may be associated with redness and swelling
- Investigations—blood tests to rule out infection and inflammatory arthropathies
- No radiological imaging is needed if the patient fulfils the following criteria: age over 45, pain on movement or use, stiffness after use, and no evidence of infection
- Early radiological changes are of uneven joint space narrowing, progressing to osteophyte and cyst formation, subchondral sclerosis, and subluxations in more severe disease

Differential diagnosis

- Infection, inflammation, trauma, damage to nearby structure (ligaments, etc.), chronic widespread pain, malignancy

Treatment

- Goals are pain management and optimizing function

Education and physical therapy

- Multidisciplinary approach providing patient with information regarding activity, exercise (local muscle strengthening and general aerobic fitness), manipulation and stretching therapy, weight loss, and educational material to enhance understanding and self-management

Non-pharmacological

- TENS, heat, and cold topical applications could be considered. Adjuncts such as braces, joint supports, insoles, and assisting devices, such as walking aids, can be offered. Acupuncture for OA is not recommended.

Pharmacological

- First-line management—paracetamol and topical NSAIDs and topical capsaicin can be considered as adjuncts
- Oral NSAIDs or COX-2 inhibitors (with a proton pump inhibitor) are also recommended as second-line treatment
- NICE 2008 guidance recommends consideration of opiates as second line, and more recent guidance suggests caution and should be reserved for acute flare-ups only
- Oral/parenteral steroids should not be used as treatment for OA, but injection into the joint can be helpful for symptomatic relief
- Glucosamine and chondroitin sulphate supplements have been trialled, with conflicting evidence. It slows down degeneration in OA of the knee by stimulating the synthesis of proteoglycans. Not recommended by NICE

Surgery

- Joint replacement should be considered when pain limits QoL, but after basic conservative therapies have been tried

- Outcome is better in knee OA than with conservative treatment
- Outcome of surgery is multifactorial; predictors include preoperative pain and function (the worse the level, the worse the outcome), the presence of anxiety or depression, and social deprivation (poorer patients did less well)
- Arthroscopic surgery has been shown to be ineffective for knee OA

Pain interventions

- Intra-articular steroid can also be used as an adjunct, although evidence of sustained benefits for some joints remains poor. Frequent steroid injections can worsen cartilage damage
- Hyaluronic acid (not recommended by NICE) and platelet-rich plasma (PRP) have also been used for joint injections
- For refractory pains, other interventions, such as suprascapular nerve blocks for shoulder pain or genicular nerve blocks for knee pain, have been used, although the evidence base is still evolving

Further reading

1. Skou ST, Roos EM, Laursen MB, et al. A randomized, controlled trial of total knee replacement. N Engl J Med 2015;373(17):1597–606
2. Felson DT. Clinical practice. Osteoarthritis of the knee. N Engl J Med 2006;354:841–8
3. National Institute for Health and Care Excellence. Management of osteoarthritis. 2019. http://pathways.nice.org.uk/pathways/osteoarthritis

23.2 Cervicogenic headache

Introduction

- Syndrome characterized by chronic hemicranial pain that is referred to the head from either bony or soft tissue structures in the neck (see Table 23.2.1)
- Cervicogenic headache is often misdiagnosed and mistreated. Early diagnosis and multidisciplinary management can reduce disability

Pathophysiology

- Pain arising from structures in the neck (facet joints, intervertebral discs, muscles and ligaments) innervated by the trigeminocervical nucleus
- The trigeminocervical nucleus is made from:
  - Functional convergence of upper cervical (C1–C3) and trigeminal sensory pathways
  - The spinal nucleus of the trigeminal nerve extending caudally to the outer lamina of the DH of C1–C3 or C4 spinal segments
  - Functional sensorimotor convergence of CN XI (spinal accessory nerve) and the upper cervical nerve roots
- Common sources of pain include:
  - Atlanto-axial joints
  - C2–C3 zygo-apophyseal joints and intervertebral disc
  - Upper cervical spinal nerves and roots

Table 23.2.1 Diagnosis of cervicogenic headache

Features	Pain referred from a source in the neck and perceived in one or more regions of the head and/or face
Evidence	Clinical, laboratory, and imaging evidence of a disorder or lesion within the cervical spine or soft tissues of the neck Demonstration of clinical signs that imply the source of the pain is in the neck (must have demonstrable validity and reliability)
Response to treatment	Abolition of headache following a diagnostic block of a cervical structure or its nerve supply using placebo or other adequate controls. Abolition of headache means complete relief of headache, indicated by a score of 0 on a visual analogue scale Pain resolves within 3 months after successful treatment of the causative disorder or lesion

Source: Data from *The International Classification of Headache Disorders*, Third Edition. London, United Kingdom: International Headache Society.

Differential diagnosis

- Posterior cranial fossa lesions, vertebral artery aneurysm, sinus thrombosis, tumours/fractures/infections of upper cervical spine
- Cervical spondylosis, osteochondritis, RA, myofascial neck pain
- Migraine (without aura), tension headache, cluster headache, hemicrania continua, chronic paroxysmal hemicrania
- Functional headache disorder, somatoform disorder

Treatment

- Multidisciplinary and multimodal treatments:
  - Education on pain management
  - Physiotherapy, OT, psychological treatments as per standard chronic pain medicine management
  - TENS—limited efficacy
  - Medications (anticonvulsants, antidepressants, gabapentinoids)—limited efficacy
  - Pain medicine interventions (see Chapter 15):
    - GON block ± PRF
    - LON block ± PRF
    - TON block ± PRF
    - C2–4 facet injections, MBB ± thermal RF (bear in mind C3 supplies C2–3 facet joints)
    - Cervical epidural, DRG block
    - ONS

Surgery

- Performed in highly selected patients:
  - Transection of GON—beware of S/Es as *anaesthesia dolorosa*
  - Microvascular decompression of the C1–3 DRG
  - Neurectomy
  - Dorsal rhizotomy

Further reading

1. Blau JN, MacGregor EA. Migraine and the neck. Headache 1994;34:88–90
2. Headache Classification Committee of the International Headache Society. The International Classification of Headache Disorders, 3rd edition. Cephalalgia 2018;38(1):1–211

23.3 Neck pain

Introduction

- About half of patients with neck pain have predominantly neuropathic or mixed neuropathic–nociceptive symptoms. Patients with neuropathic pain have higher levels of functional impairment and psychological issues

Incidence

- Annual prevalence 37.2%; lifetime prevalence 48.5%
- Peak prevalence = middle age

Clinical course

- Most acute episodes resolve spontaneously within 2 months. Half have low-grade symptoms or recurrence >1 year later
- Prediction of pain persistence: genetic and psychosocial factors, female, older age, higher baseline intensity, multiple sites
- Prognosis: not impacted on by early treatment or image-proven degeneration

General risk factors

- Trauma:
  - Sporting injuries: highest incidence in race car driving, wrestling, and ice hockey
  - Work-related: office workers, manual labour, health care, occupational drivers. Exacerbated by low job satisfaction and poor perception of occupational support
- Poor general health

Classification

- Acute versus chronic
- Associated with occipital headaches or not
- *Neuropathic versus non-neuropathic:*
  - 43% non-neuropathic pain (nociceptive), 7% neuropathic pain (defined as neck and arm pain, not arm pain alone), 50% mixed pain

History

- Suspected neuropathic pain:
  - *Intervertebral disc herniation:*
    - Nerve root compression due to acute disc herniation will initially produce neck pain, then arm pain
    - Typical dermatomal pattern, considerable overlap in >50% owing to multiple nerve root involvement

- *Foraminal stenosis:*
  - Root compression here tends to have an insidious onset
  - Exacerbated by activities that ↑ subarachnoid pressure, e.g. coughing
- *Cervical spinal stenosis:*
  - Neck pain, stiffness, upper limb radicular pain
  - Upper motor neuron (UMN) impairment secondary to consequential cervical myelopathy
  - If associated with fasciculations and bulbar signs, suspect amyotrophic lateral stenosis
- Mechanical non-radicular neck pain:
  - Insidious onset
  - *Facet arthrosis:*
    - Referral patterns helpful in diagnosis:
      - Atlanto-occipital, atlanto-axial → occipital, posterior auricular
      - C2/3, C3/4 → occipital, suboccipital
      - C4/5, C5/6 → shoulder
      - C6/7, C7/T1 → mid back, scapula
    - Does not extend distal to shoulder; no associated neurological deficit
  - *Discogenic:*
    - Axial neck pain associated with headaches, uni-/bilateral shoulder pain, non-radicular arm pain, ocular and vestibular dysfunction, anterior chest wall pain
    - Provoked by coughing, lifting, and applying pressure over cervical spinous processes. Relieved by lying supine

Examination

- Signs of nerve root compression may be obscured by MTrPs (coexisting in >50%)
- Inspection:
  - Atrophy of upper extremity muscles; indicator of chronicity and nerve root dysfunction
  - Numbness in hands is not specific; can be indicative of carpal and cubital tunnel syndrome
- Manoeuvres:
  - Shoulder pain during rotation and abduction of the upper limb suggests a primary shoulder problem
  - Specific tests more accurate for acute > chronic radiculopathy and disc herniation > stenosis

Red flags

- Age <20 years: rule out congenital abnormalities, infections
- Age >50 years: history of cancer, vascular disease
- Fever, neck stiffness, nausea or vomiting, unexplained weight loss, torticollis, limited neck mobility, erythema or exudate, severe neck tenderness
- Neurological signs such as Hoffmann's and Babinski's sign, hyperreflexia, altered muscle tone, incontinence, altered cognitive status, ataxia, visual loss, severe headache, and photophobia
- Raised inflammatory markers

Investigations

- Diagnostic imaging recommended for neuropathic neck pain
- MRI superior, needs to be interpreted in clinical context

- Consider brachial plexopathy in patients with non-diagnostic imaging, in association with upper extremity pain, weakness, and sensory loss
- EMG and NCS (note: sensitivity is 50–71%):
  - To confirm existence of nerve root dysfunction
  - To exclude other peripheral nerve disorders
  - To identify which nerve root(s) are involved and the type of dysfunction (demyelination, axonal loss, conduction block)
- Provocation discography (limited evidence)

Mechanical (non-neuropathic) neck pain causes

Non-specific neck pain

- Transformation of neck flexors from type I → type II fibres, effects on endurance and strength → fatigue and discomfort
- Deep neck muscles (longus colli, longus capitus, rectus capitus) are found to be dysfunctional

Myofascial pain

- Involves discrete or diffuse areas of sensitivity within ≥1 muscle
- May be secondary to biochemical imbalance, trauma, emotional stress, and endocrine and hormonal abnormalities
- Palpable trigger points—taut muscle bands that refer pain in a defined pattern. Primary trigger points often elicit remote trigger points → stiffness, spasms, muscle fibre shortening, and reduced strength
- Acute or insidious onset, axial neck pain, possibly referred to the shoulders and mid back
- Paraspinal tenderness and guarding, reduced range of movement (ROM), no neurological deficit
- Treatment:
  - Correct underlying structural and postural imbalance
  - Physical therapy, including massage, laser, and US, can be effective
  - Pharmacotherapy
  - Psychotherapy, including CBT and biofeedback
  - TPIs can be considered as adjunct—weak evidence

Cervical facet joint pain

- Risk factors: Road traffic accident, trauma, whiplash
- Prevalence: 40–55%
- Insidious onset of axial neck pain, referred to the occiput, shoulder, mid back
- Reduced ROM, paraspinal tenderness, no neurological deficit
- Plain films: weak association with arthrosis

Cervical discogenic pain

- Risk factors: smoking, older age, trauma, repetitive neck motions
- Prevalence: >70% of patients without pain have significant disc degeneration by their mid-forties, and >85% by 60 years
- Disc degeneration increases the likelihood of herniation
- Insidious onset
- Axial neck and shoulder pain, arm pain (non-radicular), vestibular findings
- Reduced ROM (extension > flexion, lateral flexion > rotation), midline tenderness

- Plain films: reduced disc height. MRI: annular tears or fissures
- Treatment:
  - Surgery is often the mainstay; options include cervical disc arthroplasty (CDA) and fusion
  - Evidence for epidural injections, intradiscal injections, and thermal ablation is weak and inconsistent

Neuropathic neck pain causes

Cervical disc herniation

- Annual incidence: 1–3.5/1000; most common in 60-year olds; male = female; C7 (45–60%), C6 (20–25%), C5 and C8 (10%)
- Acute onset. Not all symptoms are related to nerve root compression. Cytokines and other inflammatory mediators play a crucial role in radicular pain
- Approximately 50% of cervical disc herniations will decrease within 6 months; 75% will decrease by >50% within 2 years
- Neck pain, myotomal pattern weakness, dermatomal sensory changes
- Spurling's test: 40–50% sensitive, 85–95% specific
- Shoulder abduction: 40–50% sensitive, 80–90% specific
- Neck distraction: 40–50% sensitive, 90% specific
- Upper limb tension: 70–90% sensitive, 15–30% specific
- Valsalva: 22% sensitive, 94% specific
- MRI for nerve root compression: false positive 45%, false negative 26%. CT/CT myelogram: to differentiate between osteophytes and soft tissue changes. EMG: 50–71% sensitive, 85% specific
- Treatment:
  - Evidence in favour of transforaminal ESIs
  - Anti-neuropathic medication

Cervical spinal stenosis

- Central, involvement of lateral recesses and/or foramina
- Risk factors: advancing age, congenitally small spinal canal, genetics, possibly occupation (e.g. porters, aviation, rugby players)
- Incidence: 1:100 000 (for central stenosis where spinal canal diameter <10 mm). Significant ↑ >50 years, does not regress with time
- Most common cause in adults = degenerative spondylosis
- Insidious onset of neck pain and stiffness, radicular pain
- Non-specific, but include reduced ROM and paraspinal tenderness
- Often → multi-level neuropathic symptoms
- MRI: soft tissue evaluation. CT: osseous diameter of spinal canal. EMG: for radiculopathy

Cervical myelopathy

- Spinal stenosis associated with spinal cord compression resulting from disease (e.g. myelitis) or injury (e.g. trauma, syrinx), or in older patients = spondylosis
- Proposed pathogenesis: chronic neurogenic compression, spinal cord and nerve root ischaemia secondary to venous congestion
- Risks factors: age >50 years, male, spinal cord trauma, syrinx
- Insidious onset of neck pain, upper limb sensory and motor deficit, gait and balance deficit, incontinence, reduced dexterity

- Natural course—highly variable. Periods of quiescence and stepwise progression
- Lhermitte's sign: <20% sensitive, >90% specific
- Hoffmann's sign: 50–80% sensitive, 78% specific
- Babinski's reflex: 10–70% sensitive, >90% specific
- Hyperreflexia: >65% sensitive
- Clonus: <50% sensitive
- MRI: for intramedullary hyperintensity. EMG: for spinal cord conduction deficits and anterior horn cell dysfunction
- Treatment:
  - Randomized trials found superior analgesia and mobility with steroid/LA epidurals, compared with the same solution given IM
  - Sometimes an indication for surgery; mixed outcomes for surgical and conservative management
  - Spondylotic myelopathy—substantial proportion of patients deteriorate, necessitating surgery. Consensus statement on conservative management: 20–60% will deteriorate at 3- to 6-year follow-up

Management

- Pharmacological:
  - NSAIDs: moderate evidence that topical NSAIDs are effective for acute and chronic neck pain. Weak evidence supports muscle relaxants for subacute neck pain associated with muscle spasm. Neither drug is superior to non-pharmacological alternative therapies
- Interventional (see 16.5 Cervical facet joint/medial branch blocks and radiofrequency denervation, p. 309; 20.5 Epidural injections (cervical, thoracic, lumbar), p. 377):
  - Blocks are usually 'diagnostic'
- Complementary and alternative therapies:
  - Strongest evidence is for exercise
  - Weaker evidence supports massage, acupuncture, yoga, and spinal manipulation
  - RCT showed spinal manipulation and exercise groups to have statistically significant improved outcomes with pharmacological treatment
- Surgery:
  - More effective than conservative management in short term, but not long term
  - Cervical radiculopathy: anterior cervical discectomy and fusion (ACDF) + physiotherapy versus physiotherapy alone showed surgical group to have less pain and disability at 5 and 8 years, but no difference in arm pain
  - Cervical spondylotic myelopathy: one study showed no difference in outcomes at 2 and 10 years between conservative management and surgery. Surgery associated with complication rates of 11–38%
  - Since only modest short-term benefits with surgery, conservative management and surveillance for neurological progression are reasonable
  - Cervical degenerative disc disease: ACDF and CDA. Scant research comparing with non-surgical outcomes

Conclusions

- Topical NSAIDs can be beneficial in non-specific neck pain

- Can use muscle relaxants for acute non-radicular pain
- Weak evidence to support ESI in cervical radiculopathy
- Weak evidence to support RF ablation in patients with a positive response to diagnostic block

Further reading

1. Cohen SP, Hooten WM. Advances in the diagnosis and management of neck pain. BMJ 2017;358:j3221
2. Tsui SL, Chen PP, Jacobus NG KF. Neck pain. In: Chin PH (ed). Pain Medicine: A Multidisciplinary Approach. 2010; pp. 199–205. Tin Wan: Hong Kong University Press

23.4 Whiplash injury

Definition

- Whiplash-associated disorders (WADs) are defined by the Quebec Task Force as: '*Whiplash is an acceleration–deceleration mechanism of energy transfer to the neck. It may result from rear-end or side-impact motor vehicle collisions, but can also occur during diving or other mishaps. The impact may result in bony or soft-tissue injuries (whiplash-injury), which in turn may lead to a variety of clinical manifestations called Whiplash-Associated Disorders*' (See Table 23.4.1 for classification of WADs)
- Common injury associated with vehicular collisions

Table 23.4.1 Classification of whiplash-associated disorders

Grade	Symptom	Radiography	Treatment
0	Asymptomatic	Not required	Not required
I	Neck pain/stiffness/ tenderness; no physical signs	Not required	Simple analgesics
II	Neck pain/stiffness/ tenderness on palpation, with decreased range of movement	X-ray of cervical spine usually NOT required unless: • Suspected bony injury • Impaired consciousness • High speed impact	• Non-opioid analgesics • NSAIDs
III	Neck pain/stiffness/ tenderness ± sensory deficits ± motor weakness ± decreased tendon reflexes	X-ray of cervical spine (AP, lateral, and open-mouth view) May need CT/MRI	• Non-opioid analgesics • NSAIDs • Opioids for a limited time
IV	Neck pain/stiffness/ tenderness + dislocation/ fracture ± spinal cord injury	CT, MRI, myelography, discography	• Non-opioid analgesics • NSAIDs • Opioids • Immediate referral to spinal surgeon

Source: Data from Spitzer, W., O., *et al.* (1995). Scientific monograph of the Quebec Task Force on Whiplash Associated Disorders: redefining 'whiplash' and its management. *Spine*. 20(8):8S–58S.

- Acute whiplash injury manifests with symptoms for up to 4 weeks; in subacute whiplash, symptoms persist until 12 weeks, beyond which the condition is termed chronic WAD

Mechanism of injury

(See Fig. 23.4.1.)

- WAD usually occurs in rear-end, low-impact collisions
- The vehicle occupant's trunk is forced back on the seat, with neck hyperextension, followed by forward recoil
- The risk is higher in people with thinner necks (women) or short necks, and if the collision is with a heavy vehicle
- Cervical facet joints (especially C2/3 and C5/6) have been implicated as the main source of whiplash pain

Treatment

- *Acute* whiplash—physiotherapy and manipulation improve neck pain and ROM. Hot and cold packs, hydrotherapy, traction, US, laser therapy, short-wave diathermy, TENS, and acupuncture may help. NSAIDs, amitriptyline, diazepam, epidural LAs, and steroids have variable benefits
- *Subacute* whiplash injury—postural training, eye fixation exercises, and psychological support help more than physical therapy alone. Multidisciplinary functional rehabilitation programmes may reduce pain and catastrophizing
- *Chronic* WAD—RF denervation of the cervical facet joints has shown reasonable benefit. Facet steroid injections, muscle Botox® injections, and traction may provide short-term benefit. Multimodal rehabilitation programmes combining physical and cognitive behavioural therapies result in better outcomes, compared to physical therapy alone

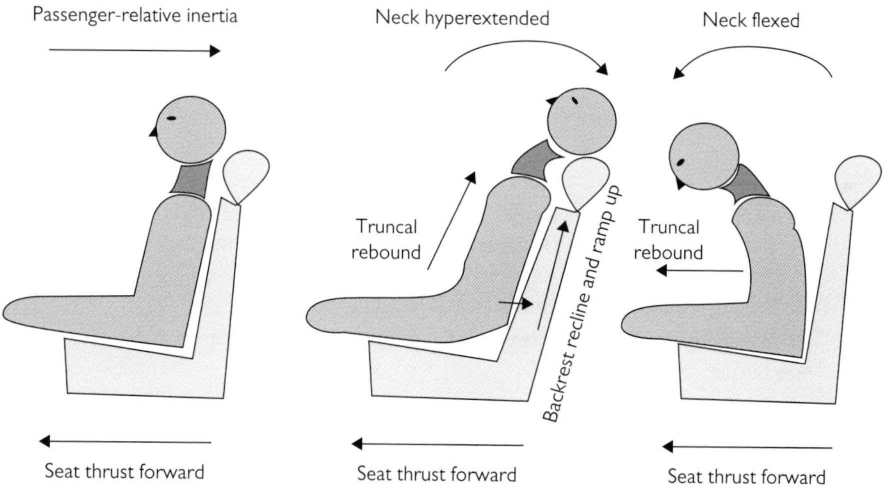

Figure 23.4.1 Mechanism of injury

Reproduced with permission from Tameem, A., Kapur, S., and Mutagi, H. (2014). Whiplash injury. *Continuing Education in Anaesthesia Critical Care & Pain*, 14(4);167–170. https://doi.org/10.1093/bjaceaccp/mkt052

- *Grade III or IV WAD*—may require surgical intervention, including cervical fusion or subacromial decompression

Medico-legal factors

- The UK has the highest incidence of WADs in Europe and make up three-quarters of all vehicle insurance claims
- Compensation-driven litigation culture has led to a rise in reported WADs
- Pain and disability can persist once chronic WAD has developed, even after receipt of compensation
- Around 40% of patients suffer from symptoms of WAD beyond 3 months (chronic whiplash) and up to 5% of patients develop persistent disability

Further reading

1. Spitzer WO, Skovron ML, Salmi LR, et al. Scientific monograph of the Quebec Task Force on Whiplash Associated Disorders: redefining 'whiplash' and its management. Spine 1995;20(8):8S–58S
2. Tameem A, Kapur S, Mutagi H. Whiplash injury. Contin Educ Anaesth Crit Care Pain 2014;14(4):167–70. https://doi.org/10.1093/bjaceaccp/mkt052

23.5 Shoulder pain

Introduction

- Pain arising from anatomical structures in the shoulder or described as such; also consider referred pain from nearby joints, the cervical plexus, and the cervical spine
- Very common—up to 66% lifetime prevalence, 60% incidence in women
- There is a correlation between atherosclerosis, diabetes, and shoulder pain

Anatomy

- Three bones:
  - Head of the humerus
  - Glenoid fossa (scapula)
  - Clavicle
- Three joints:
  - Glenohumeral joint between the humerus head and the glenoid fossa (scapula).The glenoid labrum (cartilage) increases the depth of the glenoid fossa to promote stability of the joint
  - The ACJ between the acromion (scapula) and the clavicle
  - Sternoclavicular joint (SCJ) between the sternum and the clavicle
- Three bursae:
  - Subacromial–subdeltoid bursa deep to the deltoid and coracoacromial arch, superficial to the supraspinatus tendon
  - Subcoracoid bursa located anterior to the subscapularis muscle and inferior to the coracoid process
  - Subscapular bursa between the subscapular tendon and the joint capsule

- Joint capsule:
  - From the anatomical neck of the humerus to the border of the glenoid fossa, lined by synovial membrane
- Five ligaments:
  - Glenohumeral ligaments (superior, middle, and inferior)
  - Coracohumeral ligament
  - Transverse humeral ligament
  - Coracoclavicular ligament
  - Coracoacromial ligament which forms the coracoacromial arc
- Muscles:
  - Deltoid muscle:
    - Innervated by the suprascapular nerve (C5)
    - Abducts the arm 30–90°
  - Four rotator cuff muscles:
    - Supraspinatus muscle
      - Innervated by the suprascapular nerve (C5)
      - Abducts the arm 0–30°
    - Infraspinatus muscle:
      - Innervated by the suprascapular nerve (C5)
      - Externally rotates the arm 90%
    - Teres minor muscle:
      - Innervated by the axillary nerve (C5)
      - Externally rotates the arm 10%
    - Subscapularis muscle:
      - Innervated by the subscapular nerve (C5–6)
      - Internally rotates the arm 90%
- Nerve supply from the suprascapular, axillary, subscapular, and lateral pectoral nerves
- Movements:
  - Shoulder joint is a ball-and-socket joint (synovial joint), covered with hyaline cartilage
  - Movements: extension, flexion, abduction, adduction, external and internal rotation
- Joint stability from rotator cuff muscles, the glenoid labrum, ligaments, and biceps tendons

Pathophysiology

- Tendon inflammation, tear, or degeneration (bursitis or tendinitis)
- Joint instability
- Arthritis (septic, OA, autoimmune)
- Trauma causing fracture, joint dislocation, and rupture of ligament

History

- Sudden versus chronic onset, history of trauma, previous dislocation, rheumatological symptoms, including joint swelling, morning stiffness, lethargy, weight loss, loss of appetite, fever, and malaise. Occupation, hobbies, and sports

Examination

- Inspection:
  - Posture, scar, asymmetry of shoulder girdle, swelling, wasting

    - Winging of the scapula when arms stretched against the wall (can be due to an injury of the long thoracic nerve)
    - Performance of a functional task (e.g. take off/put on shirt)
- Palpation:
    - Temperature, areas of tenderness, and allodynia (static mechanical, deep somatic, thermal)
    - Bones and joints:
        - Clavicle, humerus, scapula, SCJ, and ACJ
    - Muscle and tendons:
        - Rotator cuff, biceps, triceps, deltoid, pectorals, neck muscles
        - Tone (increased in UMN and decreased in LMN lesions)
- Movement active, passive, and against resistance:
    - Flexion (150°), extension (40°), abduction (180°), adduction (30°), external rotation (80°), internal rotation (reach T6 spinal level)
    - Power grade 0 (none) to 5 (normal)—Medical Research Council scale for muscle power
    - Palpate for joint crepitus and assess joint instability
    - Dynamic mechanical allodynia
- Sensation, reflexes, and coordination of upper limbs
- Rotator cuff muscles, tendons, and glenohumeral stability:
    - Rotator cuff muscles
        - Supraspinatus muscle (empty can test): arms at 90°, with elbows extended, full pronation, and internal rotation of the forearm. Thumbs are pointing down as if the patient were pouring liquid out of a can
        - Infraspinatus muscle and teres minor: externally rotate the arm against resistance
        - Subscapularis (belly off sign): patient rests hands on the abdomen and examiner tries to pull them away
    - Rotator cuff tendons—impingement tests:
        - Neer's test: the scapula is stabilized with the thumb pointing down and the arm is passively flexed
        - Hawkin's test: arms forward at 90°, elbows flexed, forceful internal rotation of the shoulder
    - Glenohumeral stability with the apprehension test:
        - Patient sitting or supine, with shoulder 90° abducted. Anterior pressure to the humerus, externally rotating the shoulder
- Cervical spine and elbow joint examination

Investigations

- Psychometric questionnaires (see 30.1 Psychometric assessments, p. 613). Shoulder Pain and Disability Index Questionnaire measures pain and disability in patients with shoulder pain
- Plain X-ray—fracture, dislocation, arthritis
- US—diagnostic for tendinitis and joint effusion
- MRI—soft tissue assessment, injury to ligaments and tendons
- EMG and NCS—can help identify the location of an injury (brachial plexus, peripheral nerve, or spinal cord)

Differential diagnosis

Primary shoulder pathology

- Shoulder joint/capsule—dislocation, trauma, arthritis degenerative, immune related or other cause, frozen shoulder, avascular necrosis
- Rotator cuff—tear, impingement
- Bursa—subacromial bursitis
- Shoulder instability—recurrent dislocation, trauma, collagen disorder

Referred pain

- Cervical origin—radicular and referred pain from cervical spondylosis, disc degeneration/prolapse, facet joint disease
- Pain from the diaphragm and of visceral origin such as angina and biliary colic
- Systemic disorders such as fibromyalgia and polymyalgia rheumatica

Treatment

- Vast majority of shoulder problems are treated conservatively initially, mainly with simple analgesics and physiotherapy
- Physical, pharmacological, and psychosocial interventions, as per chronic pain management principles, are used to preserve and promote shoulder function

Surgical interventions

- Shoulder arthroscopy
- Manipulation under anaesthesia for frozen shoulder
- Arthroscopic or open rotator cuff repair
- Shoulder joint replacement

Pain interventions

Further details about procedures are covered elsewhere in the book. Performed using either the landmark technique, X-rays, or US guidance:

- Nerve block and/or PRF treatment:
  - Suprascapular block—pathologies of the glenohumeral joint
  - Axillary nerve block—pain in the regimental badge area on the arm
- Subacromial bursa injection:
  - Subacromial impingement, rotator cuff disorder, adhesive capsulitis
- Glenohumeral joint injection:
  - Glenohumeral arthritis, adhesive capsulitis, labrum tears

Additional information

- 60% patients recover by 1 year from all causes of shoulder pain, but has a tendency to recur
- Adhesive capsulitis (most patients completely recover):
  - First phase (2–9 months): the pain is very prominent
  - Second phase (4–12 months): reduced range of motion is more prominent than pain
  - Third phase (5–24 months): gradual recovery

Further reading

1. Gray M, Wallace A, Aldridge S. Assessment of shoulder pain for non-specialists. BMJ 2016;355:i5783

23.6 Carpal tunnel syndrome

Introduction

- The carpal tunnel is a narrow canal on the volar aspect of the wrist, covered by the flexor retinaculum and bound on three sides by the carpal bones distally. It contains flexor tendons in their sheaths, the median nerve, blood vessels, and lymphatics
- Compression of the median nerve in the carpal tunnel results in carpal tunnel syndrome

Aetiology

- Idiopathic in >50% of patients
- Associated conditions: RA, diabetes, obesity, repetitive strain injury, pregnancy, CMT syndrome type 1, amyloidosis, hypothyroidism

History

- Pain, numbness, and paraesthesiae on the thumb, index, middle finger, and lateral half of the ring finger
- The pain may extend to the forearm
- Reduced grip and dropping items from the hand are common
- More frequent in women

Examination

- Sensory deficits of the thumb, index, middle finger, and lateral half of the ring finger
- Muscle weakness and atrophy of the thenar eminence in later stages
- Positive Tinel's sign and Phalen's test

Investigations

- Investigations to identify the underlying cause
- NCS
- EMG

Diagnosis

- Diagnosis mostly from clinical symptomatology. Other diagnoses to consider include cervical radiculopathy, arthritis, diabetic neuropathy, or other causes of peripheral neuropathy

Treatment

- NSAIDs, paracetamol, and physiotherapy
- Carpal tunnel decompression surgery—better outcomes than steroid injections
- Treatments with lower evidence:
  - Steroid injections
  - Neutral wrist splints, especially at night, but prolonged use may weaken the muscles
  - Others: acupuncture, US, yoga, and carpal bone mobilization

Further reading

1. Stevens JC, Beard CM, O'Fallon WM, et al. Conditions associated with carpal tunnel syndrome. Mayo Clin Proc 1992;67:541–8

23.7 Low back pain

Definition

- Low back pain is an imprecise term used to describe varying combinations of pain, muscle tension, and stiffness below the costal margins and above the inferior gluteal folds
- With or without radicular pain

Prevalence

- Low back pain is the most common chronic pain complaint
- Lifetime prevalence is 60–80% in industrialized countries, with 1-year prevalence of 15–45%
- Prevalence increases from age 30 to 60, then stabilizes
- Good prognosis of acute low back pain—90% of episodes resolve
- Prevalence of chronic low back pain in adults in a European survey: 18%
- In 2009, there were 1.6 million people with chronic back pain in the UK and the cost of back pain to the economy was £12.3 billion

Risk factors

- Obesity, smoking
- Sedentary lifestyle
- Heavy physical work (repetitive lifting, twisting)
- Prolonged standing in an awkward posture
- Lower socioeconomic status
- Depression

Pathophysiology

- The human spine accumulates degenerative ('wear and tear') changes from early adulthood onwards
- Facet joints and SIJs accumulate degenerative changes and can become osteoarthritic
- Discs with acute tears can leak nucleosus pulposus gel, which is inflammatory outside the disc
- Disc degeneration can lead to abnormal stress and inflammation in the adjacent vertebral endplates
- Pain from any cause in the spine promotes muscular tension and altered postural and movement patterns, which contribute to further pain

Aetiology

- Facet joint OA (arthropathy/degeneration)
- SIJ OA (arthropathy/degeneration)
- Discogenic back pain (from disc degeneration sequelae)
- 'Myofascial'—muscle motor pattern dysfunction with muscle tension and fatigue
- Spondylolisthesis—associated facet joint OA and myofascial pain
- Lumbar radicular pain—disc degeneration, stenosis, post-surgery
- Central sensitization—central amplification seen in chronic pain

- Less common causes of back pain that need to be kept in mind and excluded are:
  - Osteoporotic and traumatic fractures
  - Malignancy (e.g. myeloma, prostate cancer)
  - Infection: frank infection is rare, unless a complication of surgery, but discitis can occasionally occur through blood-borne spread of bacteria
  - There is some evidence that very low-grade infection of discs may be implicated in some cases of low back pain symptoms

Diagnosis

Exclusion of red and yellow flags

- Red flags trigger a more detailed history and examination ± investigations to avoid missing uncommon, but serious, underlying disease
- **Red flags:** severe pain, night pain, thoracic pain, fever, unexplained weight loss, history of carcinoma, immunocompromise, history of long-term corticosteroids, progressive neurological deficit, disturbed gait, bladder or bowel sphincter dysfunction, saddle anaesthesia, age of onset <20 years or >55 years
- **Yellow flags** (psychosocial factors indicating long-term chronicity and disability, interventions less likely effective, multidisciplinary treatment (MDT) approach needed):
  - Catastrophization—belief that back pain is harmful, progressive, and potentially severely disabling
  - Fear avoidance behaviour and reduced activity levels
  - Expectation that passive, rather than active, treatment will be beneficial
  - Tendency to depression, low morale, and social withdrawal
  - Social or financial problems

Distribution and pattern of pain

Axial pain versus radicular pain

- A useful way to look at low back pain is to determine if the pain has an axial or a radicular pattern

Axial pain

- Adjacent to the spine
- Usually associated with paraspinal muscle tension and tenderness, with any spread into limbs being proximal and limited
- Axial pain suggests spinal MSK drivers, including facet joint and SIJ arthropathy, lumbar disc degeneration with vertebral endplate inflammation, and muscle and ligament inflammation/injury

Radicular pain

- Travels down a limb or around the thorax in a band consistent with a nerve root distribution
- Result of nerve root inflammation/ischaemia/injury
- Usually with neuropathic features

Axial discogenic back pain

- Lumbar disc degeneration is normal as we age
- Discs do not have internal nerves and most degenerations are not painful
- Discogenic axial pain is worse with loading of the discs (flexion, sitting, and activities that increase disc pressure)
- Mechanisms whereby disc degeneration may produce axial pain:

- Leakage of nucleosus pulposus (rich in pro-inflammatory phospholipase A2) into adjacent structures
- Peripheral ingrowth of nociceptive nerves accompanying granulation tissue into damaged discs
- Possibly associated low-grade disc and vertebral endplate infection in some cases
- Altered mechanical loading on adjacent structures

Mixed presentations

- Elements of both axial and radicular pain present
- May be due to having both axial and radicular pathology
- Can also be due to severe 'axial' pathology pain being referred down a limb (e.g. in severe SIJ arthropathy)
- With primary radicular pain, secondary muscle tension and guarding of the spine can cause associated axial pain

Neurogenic claudication pain as a special case

- Usually seen in older patients
- Spinal nerve or cauda equina blood supply is limited by stenosis (spinal canal narrowing) or fibrosis following surgery, and flow cannot increase to meet the demands of activity
- A complaint of radicular symptoms in one lower limb with activity may be encountered with narrowing of one side of the spinal canal (lateral recess stenosis)
- In central lumbar spinal canal stenosis, the typical presentation is one of low back pain and bilateral lower limb heaviness and pain with walking—especially uphill
- Walking distance becomes limited and there is a tendency to stoop when walking
- Consider referral to spine surgery team

Examination

- Gait, posture, deformity, surgical scars, use of supportive braces, skin changes (e.g. from hot water bottle)
- Range of movement, muscle tone, tenderness
- Reduced straight leg raise, positive neural stretch tests (slump test)
- Neurological deficit (sensory, motor, reflex impairment), distribution of paraesthesiae or sensory loss, reduced ankle and great toe dorsiflexion, knee and ankle reflexes
- Test dermatomal (sensation) and myotomal (motor weakness) distribution of symptoms, which usually correlate with specific nerve roots for radicular pain (e.g. pain on top of the foot and foot drop - L5 nerve root) (see 1.4 Dermatomes and myotomes, p. 14)
- Pain behaviour (avoidance, guarding, inconsistencies)

Investigations (if appropriate)

- **X-ray—rarely indicated** (trauma, osteoporotic or malignant vertebral fractures, scoliosis, dynamic spondylolisthesis views)
- **CT and MRI—not** essential in non-specific low back pain, but indicated in radicular pain symptoms (disc degeneration, facet joint degeneration, foraminal narrowing, nerve root compromise, spinal canal stenosis, vertebral collapse/fracture) and other red flag presentations
- **DEXA scan** (to assess for osteoporosis)

Treatment

- Education, reassurance (the majority of acute low back pain exacerbations improve, and patients should be educated that back pain is common and degenerative spinal changes are normal, and reassured that their spine is stable and will benefit from remaining active)

- Patients should be considered holistically (biopsychosocial model)
- Emphasize and encourage positive lifestyle changes (e.g. maintenance of physical condition, avoidance of smoking, and weight control)
- Simple analgesics if they prove useful: paracetamol, NSAIDs (muscle relaxants for acute spasms should only be prescribed for a short and limited time)
- Physiotherapy may be offered (gentle and frequent exercising and stretching)

Axial low back pain

- When chronic axial low back pain is moderate to severe and refractory to the above conservative measures and red flag exclusion has been made, then interventional techniques may be considered
- Axial back pain should be regarded as 'back pain for investigation' as the contribution of any interventional target in driving axial pain is unclear until it is tested

Radicular pain

- Radicular pain is usually due to nerve root irritation
- If radiculopathy is present (numbness/weakness in addition to pain) or if the pain is persistent, then MRI of the lumbo-sacral spine is indicated prior to considering targeted nerve root (transforaminal epidural injection) or lumbar epidural injection
- Surgery in the case of refractory compressive radiculopathy

Axial discogenic back

- Education and reassurance (resume normal activities as soon as possible)
- Encourage return to work (manual handling and lifting may be needed), occupational health
- Interventional treatments for discogenic pain (none has strong evidence):
  - Injection of discs with steroids, sclerosants, methylene blue, or stem cells
  - Disc cauterization
  - Disc replacement surgery, spacer device surgery to offload the disc, spinal fusion surgery
  - Antibiotics in the presence of Modic type 1 vertebral endplate changes
  - SCS

Further reading

1. Albert HB, Sorensen JS, Christensen BS, Manniche C. Antibiotic treatment in patients with chronic low back pain and vertebral bone edema (Modic type 1 changes): a double-blind randomized clinical controlled trial of efficacy. Eur Spine J 2013;22(4):697–707
2. Donaldson L. Breaking through the barrier. Annual report of the chief medical officer 2009;17–18
2. Hoy D, Brooks P, Blyth F, Buchbinder R. The epidemiology of low back pain. Best Pract Res Clin Rheumatol 2010;24(6):769–81
3. Samanta J, Kendall J, Samanta A. Chronic low back pain. Primary care 10-minute consultation. BMJ 2003;326:535
4. Van Kleef M, Vanelderen P, Cohen SP, et al. Pain originating from the lumbar facet joints. Pain Pract 2010;10(5):459–69

23.8 Lumbo-sacral transitional vertebrae

Introduction

- Relatively common congenital spinal anomalies
- Refers to vertebrae with intermediate morphological features
- Could take the form of either an assimilation of the fifth lumbar vertebra to the first sacral vertebra *(sacralization)* or a transition of the first sacral vertebra to assimilate the lumbar vertebra morphology (*lumbarization*)
- An association with back pain was first described by Mario Bertolotti in 1917
- It alters the numerical labelling and counting of the vertebra; hence, in cases of lumbarization, it is *L6/S1* and in sacralization *L4/S1*

Incidence

- Generally reported to be 4–30%

Aetiology

- Not completely understood, but genetic factors are believed to be very important

Clinical significance

- Although the evidence is lacking, it is frequently associated with degenerative disc disease or herniation, spinal central canal or foraminal stenosis, and facet joint arthrosis
- Potential association with back pain
- Could lead to errors of identifying the correct level during surgery or pain interventions

Investigations

- Plain radiographs: AP and lateral of the lumbo-sacral spine. This can be combined with an AP and 30° cranial tilt film
- CT scan
- MRI scan

Castellvi diagnostic classification (1984)

- Type 1. Dysplastic TP—unilateral (1a) or bilateral (1b) TP (>19 mm wide)
- Type 2. Incomplete sacralization/lumbarization—unilateral (2a) or bilateral (2b) enlarged TP pseudarthrosis with the adjacent sacral ala
- Type 3. Unilateral (3a) or bilateral (3b) fused completely with the adjacent sacral ala
- Type 4. Mixed—type 3a and 2a on each side

Treatment

- Physical, pharmacological, psychological, and psychosocial interventions as per chronic pain management principles
- Surgical and interventional pain management treatments—unclear which of these treatments is more efficacious. Some of the available treatments include:
  - Injection of LA and steroids into the pseudarthrosis or contralateral facet joint
  - RF ablation of the nerve supply after a positive diagnostic block
  - Surgical resection of a partial TP or an anomalous articulation

Further reading

1. Konin GP, Walz DM. Lumbosacral transitional vertebrae: classification, imaging findings and clinical relevance. Am J Neuroradiol 2010;31:1778–86
2. Bron JL, Van Royen B, Wuisman P. The clinical significance of lumbosacral transitional anomalies. Acta Orthop Belg 2007;73:687–95

23.9 Failed back surgery syndrome

Introduction

- FBSS is usually diagnosed if pain recurs or gets worse 6 months after technically adequate spinal surgery, although variations exist in the description of this syndrome
- The aetiology is complex, with normally a mixture of nociceptive, neuropathic, and sympathetic contributors
- Around 30% of patients experience persistent or recurrent pain following technically adequate spinal surgery, which is a significant clinical and economic burden
- The role of certain surgeries such as spinal fusions is controversial, with a mixture of critical and supportive expert publications

Factors associated with positive pain outcomes in spinal surgery

- The patient has realistic expectations and understands the surgical risks
- Medically fit and motivated to get better
- Has had appropriate conservative management
- Surgery not delayed in cauda equina syndrome, potential unstable fractures, spinal malignancy (primary or metastatic), infections (discitis, osteomyelitis), significant spinal canal stenosis, and defects that worsen with time such as scoliosis in young patients

Factors associated with poorer pain outcomes in spinal surgery

- Unrealistic expectations by patient or clinician
- Surgery performed for pain relief in the absence of a clear pathology amenable to surgical correction
- Psychological factors:
  - Personality traits associated with anxiety, worry, agitation, and anger
  - Cognitive factors such as low self-efficacy, poor pain-coping skills, catastrophizing, sense of injustice
  - History of abuse (sexual, physical, verbal, neglect)
- Mental health conditions not optimized such as depression, anxiety, substance use disorders, and others
- Social factors: unemployment, ongoing litigation or disability benefit application, relationship difficulties, conflict with employer/insurance, poor working conditions, negative influence by significant others such as family
- Medical factors: physically deconditioned, smoking, poor nutrition, high BMI, older age, multiple medical comorbidities, opioid-tolerant

Causes of failed back surgery syndrome

- Surgical procedure was probably not indicated

- Other pathologies/pain generators that are contributing to the pain were not addressed during the surgical procedure
- Surgical complication such as epidural fibrosis at surgical site (common), trauma to nerve roots, or other complications
- Recurrence of pathology or development of a new pathology after the surgery such as disc herniation/herniation at adjacent level
- Pre-existing irreversible nerve damage caused by disc herniation/sequestered disc fragment/cauda equina syndrome

Treatments

- Treatment is controversial
- Exclude red flags
- Repeat surgery may not produce the expected improvement in pain relief
- Detailed biopsychosocial assessment with a multidisciplinary team approach, including patient education, exercise, physiotherapy, and psychological treatments are essential
- Trial of pharmacological agents for neuropathic pain (antidepressants, gabapentinoids, see Chapters 9 and 10.)
- Interventional pain medicine has limited evidence of efficacy. However, some specific patients benefit from specific interventions such as ESIs, sacroiliac or medial branch blocks ± RF denervations, epiduroscopy, and adhesiolysis
- There is evidence to support SCS for neuropathic pain in FBSS

Further reading

1. Chan C, Pang P. Failed back surgery syndrome. Pain Med 2011;12:577–606
2. Van Buyten JP, Linderoth B. The failed back surgery syndrome. Definition and therapeutic algorithms—an update. Eur J Pain Suppl 2010;4:273–86

23.10 Spondylolysis

Introduction

- Spondylolysis refers to an osseous defect of the pars interarticularis (isthmus) of the vertebral arch
- It is derived from the Greek words *spondylos* (vertebra) and *lysis* (defect)

Incidence

- Reports vary from 4–6% to 6–8% of the general population
- Could reach a staggering 63% in participants of certain sports
- With spondylolisthesis, it is the most common reported cause of low back pain in children and adolescents older than 10 years

Anatomy

- Unilateral or bilateral (more common)
- The pars interarticularis constitutes the junction between the laminae, articular facets, and the pedicles of the vertebra

- Bone formation/osteophytes (made of osseous, fibrous, and cartilaginous tissues) in vertebral discs, joints (facet and uncovertebral), and vertebral bodies, which can result in:
  - Foraminal neural narrowing, nerve root compression, and radicular symptoms from the bone growth at facet and uncovertebral joints
  - Compression of the spinal cord and myelopathy from changes in vertebral body margins and the posterior longitudinal ligament
- In bilateral cases, the upper vertebra can slide over the lower one (spondylolisthesis) or posterior neural arch displacement
- More commonly found in the cervical/lumbar spine than in the thoracic spine (most likely because the thoracic spine is more rigid)
- In lumbar cases, L5 is affected in 85–95%, followed by L4 in 5–15%

Pathophysiology

- Is not completely understood. Aetiology is multifactorial:
  - Genetic: high incidence amongst family members—up to 69% of cases
  - Ageing is a very important factor
  - Trauma, mechanical stress, fatigue fractures from repetitive mechanical loading
  - Repetitive spinal rotation/flexion/extension movements
  - Vertebral discs lose height and water content, with weakening of the annulus fibrosus
- It is hypothesized that a combination of the above factors results in increased mechanical stress in the vertebral endplates, facet joints, and uncovertebral joints. This leads to the development of osteophytes, hypertrophy of the ligaments, and osseous structures
- Strong association with spina bifida occulta

Clinical picture

- Red flags need to be excluded
- Most cases are asymptomatic, only accidentally discovered radiologically
- Can develop gradually over time, with flare-ups following particular events or movements, after an acute event, or with no precipitating factor/explanation
- Symptomatic cases tend to complain of focal mechanical low back pain radiating into the buttocks. This can particularly pose a problem in young athletes
- Normally aggravated by spinal hyperextension
- Patients sometimes complain of radicular pain:
  - Atypical radicular pain: position-dependent and not associated with neurological signs
  - Typical radicular pain: neurological symptoms and signs secondary to neural compression
- Physical examination may reveal:
  - Exaggerated lumbar lordosis, in addition to tightness of the hamstrings, although the exact explanation for this is unknown
  - Neurological signs of radiculopathy
  - Evidence of central sensitization

Investigations

- Plain radiographs: pars defect appears as an area of lucency in the pars interarticularis, resembling a break in the neck or 'collar' of the 'scottie dog'. However, detection of the defect may be difficult and require multiple views
- SPECT: more sensitive than plain X-rays in detecting the lesions
- CT scan: more sensitive than plain X-rays. It is considered by many to be the imaging modality of choice

- MRI
- Often >1 modality is used

Treatment

- Physical, pharmacological, psychological, and psychosocial interventions as per chronic pain management principles
- Development of active pain self-management strategies such as pacing, goal setting, thought resolution, exercise, management of flare-ups, etc.
- Some patients benefit from a spinal brace
- Surgery normally considered after failure of conservative management after 6 months in specific patients where surgery can correct anatomical deficits. Some of the procedures that can be done include:
  - Spinal fusion—sometimes an uninstrumented fusion of L5/S1 with an autogenous iliac crest bone graft is performed
  - Repair of the pars defect at L4 or above can be indicated in children and adolescents
  - Spinal decompression

Further reading

1. Standaert CG, Herring SA. Spondylolysis: a critical review. Br J Sports Med 2000;34:415–22
2. Leone A, Cianfone A, Cerase A, et al. Lumbar spondylolysis: a review. Skeletal Radiol 2011;40:683–700

23.11 Sacroiliac joint pain

Definition

- Pain localized in the region of the sacroiliac joint (SIJ), reproducible by stress and provocation tests, and reliably relieved by selective infiltration of the SIJ

Prevalence

- 16–30% amongst patients with axial low back pain (depending on the use of diagnostic criteria)

Anatomy—introduction

- SIJs are the largest joints in the body, and they join the sacral spine to the pelvis
- The upper part of the joint is fibro-cartilaginous, and the lower part is a synovial joint
- SIJs bear heavy loads when we are standing and walking
- SIJs normally have very limited movement
- Their function is to combine stability with a cushioning effect
- They may become painful due to degenerative change or injury
- Pain is felt at the lumbo-sacral level in the region of the joint and typically spreads into the buttock and thigh

Aetiology

- SIJ arthropathy is involved in around 5–10% of chronic low back pain
- SIJ arthropathy is usually due to degenerative/osteoarthritic processes
- Less common causes are inflammatory arthritis, including ankylosing spondylitis and gout

- Risk factors for SIJ instability: younger age, pregnancy, hypermobility, trauma
- Risk factors for SIJ arthropathy: leg length discrepancy, abnormal gait, trauma, scoliosis, lumbar fusion surgery with fixation of the sacrum (prevalence of 32–33% demonstrated with SIJ blocks), pregnancy, heavy physical exertion

History

- Pain in gluteal region (94%)
- Referred pain to lower lumbar area (72%), groin (14%), upper lumbar area (6%), abdomen (2%), lower limb (28%), and foot (12%)

Examination

- SIJ instability can present with severe lumbo-sacral pain and even with a sciatica type of pain
- Large forces are needed to stress the joint due to its size and immobility
- Tests: (1) stressing of the SIJ with distraction (antero-posterior pressure on ASIS in prone position); (2) thigh thrust; (3) Faber test; (4) compression (pressure on iliac crest in lateral position); and (5) Gaenslen's test. Three out of five positive tests indicates likely SIJ pathology (specificity of 79% and sensitivity of 85%). A single test is of little value

Imaging

- Indicated when red flags are present (X-ray, CT, MRI, bone scan)

Differential diagnosis

- Spondyloarthropathy (ankylosing spondylitis, reactive or psoriatic arthritis)
- Lumbar nerve root compression
- Lumbar facet joint arthropathy
- Hip pain
- Endometriosis
- Myofascial pain
- Piriformis syndrome

Treatment

Conservative

- Physiotherapy and manipulation (posture and gait disturbances)
- Immuno-modulators in rheumatological disorders (ankylosing spondylitis)

Pain interventions

- NICE Guideline 59 does not make specific reference to SIJ procedures
- IASP criteria support the confirmation of diagnosis by successful injection
- Injection of the SIJ with LA and steroid is supported by low to moderate evidence—can be carried out under X-ray or US control (see 18.2 Sacroiliac joint block and radiofrequency denervation, p. 340)
- *RF denervation of the SIJ:*
  - Supported by moderate evidence
  - Innervation of the SIJ is more complex and variable than that of the facet joint, and several different techniques are described
  - The anterior contribution to innervation of the joint cannot be lesioned
  - The majority of the nerve supply to SIJs is from the lateral branches originating from S1 and S2, but branches of L5, L4, S3, and S4 may contribute

- When instability is a major problem, SIJ injections and denervations do not produce lasting pain relief and prolotherapy (injections of fibrosing solutions into and along the joint ligaments) and surgical fixation may be considered

Further reading

1. Laslett M. Evidence based diagnosis and treatment of the painful sacroiliac joint. J Man Manip Ther 2008;16(3):142–52
2. Simopoulos T, Manchikanti L, Gupta S. Systematic review of the diagnostic accuracy and therapeutic effectiveness of sacroiliac joint interventions. Pain Physician 2015;18:E713–56
3. Vanelderen P, Szadek K, Cohen SP, et al. 13. Sacroiliac joint pain. In: Van Zundert J, Patijn J, Hartrick CT, et al. (eds). Evidence-Based Interventional Pain Medicine. 2012; pp. 96–102. Chichester: Wiley-Blackwell

23.12 Coccygodynia

Definition

- Inflammation or displacement of the coccyx (tailbone) presents with pain and tenderness at the tip of the tailbone

Incidence

- Female:male ratio = 5:1
- Female coccyx is longer and most posteriorly placed, and parturition predisposes to a high incidence
- 70% of traumatic births cause coccygeal joint injury
- Other risk factor: high BMI

Anatomical correlation

- Coccyx = final segment of the vertebral column
- 3–5 coccygeal vertebrae are present
- Attached to the sacrum at the sacro-coccygeal junction
- It is one leg of the weight-bearing tripod along with the ischial tuberosities in the sitting position
- Ligamentous attachments: sacro-coccygeal, sacro-spinal, sacro-tuberous, and anococcygeal ligaments
- Muscles: levator ani, gluteus maximus, gluteus medius, gluteus minimus, coccygeus muscle, and other deep gluteal muscles, such as obturator internus and piriformis, can refer pain to the coccyx region

Causes

- Acute trauma
- Traumatic parturition
- Repetitive stress injury such as cycling
- Incorrect sitting position
- Motor sports

Diagnosis

- Mostly history: history of trauma, dull and deep achy pain in coccygeal region
- Detailed history to exclude differential diagnoses listed below
- Chronic pelvic pain can be associated with coccygodynia; detailed psychosocial and sexual history is mandatory
- Manual examination (including per rectal examination)
- X-ray: plain X-ray, lateral view to exclude fracture and dislocation; dynamic radiology can be used in difficult cases
- MRI: mainly to rule out sinister pathology

Differential diagnosis

- Infection: shingles, osteomyelitis, local infection
- CNS tumours, cysts
- Malignancy: primary and secondary
- Referred pain: pelvic structures, such as rectum and lower part of the colon, urogenital structures, and lumbar disc herniation
- Nerve entrapments causing referred pain (cluneal nerves)

Treatments

- Multidisciplinary and multimodal approach is crucial for success of therapy as for other chronic pain conditions

Conservative management

- Up to 90% of cases get better with conservative treatment and simple analgesics
- Adapting sitting position
- Coccyx cushion
- Physiotherapy for pelvic floor structures and exercise
- Therapeutic US therapy
- Acupuncture
- Heat/cold application
- TENS
- CBT and other psychotherapies

(Some of these treatments have limited evidence.)

Pharmacological

- Simple analgesics, especially NSAIDs if there is no contraindication

Interventions

- LA and steroid injection under X-ray or US guidance (60–85% success rate)
- Caudal block
- Ganglion impar block
- RF or PRF denervation or pulsed RF of sacral nerve roots

Neuromodulation techniques

- Only in selected cases (currently limited evidence as it is an emerging treatment option and many are case series)
- TENS
- Peripheral field stimulation

- PNS
- SCS

Surgical

- Surgical removal (coccygectomy) is not recommended routinely due to high risk of post-surgical pain and fibrosis and only moderate long-term effect

Further reading

1. Howard PD, Dolan AN, Falco AN, et al. A comparison of conservative interventions and their effectiveness for coccydynia: a systematic review. J Man Manip Ther 2013;21(4):213–19
2. Lirette LS, Chaiban G, Tolba R, et al. Coccydynia: an overview of the anatomy, etiology, and treatment of coccyx pain. Ochsner J Spring 2014;14(1):84–7
3. Ravi P, Anoop A, Peter GW. Coccydynia. Curr Rev Musculoskelet Med 2008;1(3–4):223–6
4. Van Zundert J, Patijn J, Hartrick CT, et al. 14. Coccygodynia. In: Van Zundert J, Patijn J, Hartrick CT, et al. (eds). Evidence-based Interventional Pain Medicine. 2012; pp. 103–6. Chichester: Wiley-Blackwell

23.13 Piriformis syndrome

Definition

- '*Pain in the buttock and posterior thigh due to myofascial injury of the piriformis muscle itself or dysfunction of the sacroiliac joint or pain in the posterior leg and foot, groin and perineum due to entrapment of the sciatic or other nerves by the piriformis muscle within the greater sciatic foramen, or a combination of these causes*'(ISAP)

Incidence

- 5–8% of low back pain

Anatomy of piriformis muscle

- Origin: antero-lateral surface of the sacrum between the anterior sacral foramina, runs laterally and inferiorly through the greater sciatic foramen
- Insertion: upper margin of the greater trochanter of the femur

Function of muscle

- Adductor of flexed thigh and external rotator of extended hip

Adjacent structures

- Sciatic nerve, superior gluteal nerve, posterior femoral cutaneous nerve
- Nerves to superior and inferior gamelli, obturator internus, quadratus femoris, and gluteus maximus, medius, and minimus
- In 88% of the times, the sciatic nerve passes below the muscle. Sometimes it passes between a split muscle or is divided with one division passing above and the other below the muscle or through the muscle

Pathophysiology

- Pathology and dysfunction of the piriformis muscle can cause low back pain, buttock pain, and sciatica because of muscle spasm and compression of the sciatic nerve

Predisposing factors

- Trauma (50%):
  - Direct injury, prolonged sitting, sport injuries, e.g. cycling, dancing
- Obesity
- Pregnancy
- Cerebral palsy (increased muscle tone)
- Limb length discrepancy
- Abnormal posture

Diagnosis

- Symptoms and signs: ipsilateral (usually) pain in the buttock, lower back, and posterior thigh, occasionally radiating below the knee, dyspareunia and labial pain (females), scrotal pain (males), painful bowel movements
- Aggravating factors: walking, prolonged sitting
- Examination/tests:
  - Tenderness to palpation over the muscle
  - Lasegue's sign: pain and tenderness in the greater sciatic notch on voluntary flexion, adduction, and internal rotation of the hip
  - Pace's sign: pain and weakness on resisted abduction of the hip with the patient seated
  - Freiberg sign: pain on forced internal rotation of the extended thigh
  - Investigations: CT and MRI may show enlargement of the piriformis. EMG may show delay in the H reflex on flexion, adduction, and internal rotation (FAIR) of the hip

Treatment

- Conservative: physical therapy, in combination with analgesics, anti-inflammatory drugs, and muscle relaxants
- Treatment of a correctable cause such as posture, limb length discrepancy, weight reduction, and avoiding precipitating factors
- Injection treatment:
  - LA and steroid into the muscle
  - BTX-A (100 IU) into the muscle if there is a transient improvement of symptoms with steroid and LA
  - Injections performed under fluoroscopy guidance, but US- and CT-guided injections are more accurate
- Surgery:
  - Excision, thinning, or tendon release of the muscle may be considered for severe refractory cases

Further reading

1. Cohen SP, Benzon HT. Pain originating from the buttock: sacroiliac joint syndrome and piriformis syndrome. In: Benzon HT, Raja S, Liu AA et al. (eds). Essentials of Pain Medicine. 2011; pp. 337–8. Philadelphia, PA: Elsevier Saunders
2. Foreman W, Mahajan G, Fishman SM. Piriformis syndrome. In: Wallace MS, Staats PS (eds). Pain Medicine and Management. 2005; pp. 331–5. New York: McGraw-Hill

23.14 Greater trochanteric pain syndrome

Introduction

- Regional pain syndrome with chronic intermittent pain around the bony prominence over the lateral aspect of the hip (greater trochanter region)
- Previously known as trochanteric bursitis—now thought that the bursa perhaps has a smaller role and inflammation is not always present

Pathophysiology

- Greater trochanter provides lubrication and cushioning to tendons, allowing muscles to flex and extend. Inflammation or trauma (acute or recurrent) in muscles, tendons, fascia, or bursae is associated with this condition
- More common in women aged 40–60 years
- Common associations:
  - Gait disturbances and postural abnormalities secondary to sacroiliac, spinal, and muscular disorders
  - Low back pain, knee pain, RA, and fibromyalgia
  - Previous hip surgery
- Risk factors for a poorer outcome: older age, poorly controlled acute pain, long duration of pain, greater movement restriction or functional impairment

History and examination

- Lateral hip pain, possible radiation of pain to the infero-lateral aspect of the thigh
- Pain aggravated on hip movement
- Spasticity in the muscles and tendons attached to the greater trochanter
- Pain on palpation of the greater trochanter (point tenderness)
- Positive Trendelenburg test
- Rule out an infected bursitis: tender palpable mass, warmth, redness, or oedema

Investigations

- It is a clinical diagnosis. Imaging and/or blood tests are warranted if suspicion of fracture, hip arthritis, avascular necrosis of the head of the femur, malignancy, tendon tears, or tendinopathies (e.g. gluteus medius tendinopathy)

Differential diagnosis

- Sports hernia
- Infection of the bursa or surrounding structures
- Pain referred from the hip and lumbar area (e.g. lumbar nerve root compression), abdomen, or other surrounding structures

Treatment

- Reassure: 90% recover with conservative measures
- In the acute phase, avoid repetitive hip movements or lying on the affected hip, ice packs (apply for 10–20 minutes several times a day), simple analgesics (paracetamol or NSAIDs), and weight reduction (if appropriate)
- Physiotherapy and correction of underlying gait disturbances

- If pain persists, consider:
  - Intra-bursa injections of LA and steroid (landmark technique or under X-ray or US guidance)
  - Other options: TENS, shockwave therapy, surgical bursectomy (very rarely performed)
  - Refer to rheumatologist or orthopaedic surgeon if in doubt with diagnosis, persistent pain despite maximal medical treatment, suspected infection, previous hip problems (hip surgery or fracture femur)

Further reading

1. Canoso J, Isaac Z, Curtis MR. Greater trochanteric pain syndrome. 2018. https://www.uptodate.com
2. Reid, D. The management of greater trochanteric pain syndrome: A systematic literature review. J Orthop 2016;13(1):15–28.

23.15 Plantar fasciitis

Definition

- Persistent heel pain resulting from chronic overuse, or degenerative and reparative process affecting the origin of the plantar fascia at the distal calcaneum

Incidence

- 11–15% of foot symptoms, and 80% of heel pain
- Lifetime prevalence 10%

Pathophysiology

- Chronic degeneration resulting from repetitive stretching and tearing, rather than from inflammation

Anatomy

- Triangular thickened fibrous aponeurosis
- Five digital bands providing investing sheaths for plantar flexor tendons and small plantar nerves
- Shock absorber
- Provides tension and support to the arch of the foot

Innervation of heel skin

- The medial calcaneal nerve, a branch of the tibial nerve, can be involved proximally in tarsal tunnel syndrome
- First branch of the lateral plantar nerve (Boxter's nerve), distal to medial of the calcaneal tuberosity. This nerve is at risk of entrapment between the adductor hallucis muscle and the medial belly of the quadratus plantae muscle

Risk factors

- Chronic axial overload:
  - Physical exercise, e.g. long-distance running, ballet
  - Obesity

- Occupational—teachers, factory workers, policemen
- Anatomical—flat feet, high-arched feet, shortened Achilles tendon
- Biomechanical—overinversion, limited ankle dorsiflexion, weak plantar flexors, weak intrinsic muscles of the foot
- Environmental—deconditioning, walking barefoot or on hard surfaces, poor footwear

Symptoms and signs

- Common in those aged 40–60, who are on their feet for extended periods of time
- Under-surface of the heel is very painful on weight-bearing, worse after a period of immobility
- Gradual onset of pain on the medial side of the heel, intense in the morning and radiating to the arch of the foot
- Tenderness over the medial calcaneum
- Windlass test: pain reproduced on passive dorsiflexion of the toes

Investigations

- Imaging—not necessarily useful:
  - USS—swelling of plantar fascia
  - X-ray—calcaneal spur

Differential diagnosis

- Achilles tendinitis:
  - Tenderness over posterior aspect of the heal and along Achilles tendon
  - Pain radiates up to calf muscles
  - Pain can be reproduced by foot extension or standing on tiptoes
- Calcaneal stress fracture:
  - Presents with diffuse, warm swelling, characterized by resting pain and reproduced by squeezing the calcaneum
- Subcalcaneal bursitis:
  - Posterior heel pain under the calcaneal fat pad
  - Not reproduced by foot or toe dorsiflexion
- Tarsal tunnel syndrome:
  - Poorly localized pain
  - Numbness and burning on medial foot and ankle and sometimes over calf muscles
  - Reproduced by Tinel's test: tapping with fingers or tendon hammer posterior to the medial malleolus

Management

- Early plantar fasciitis—conservative treatment; majority will completely recover within 6 months; heat, cold
- Patient education and intensive rehabilitation
- Correct reversible causes
- Insoles and heel pads to correct foot pronation
- Physical therapies:
  - Stretching of plantar fascia—towel looped around foot which is pulled with extended knees, causing active dorsiflexion
  - Calf stretches with slightly flexed soleus and fully extended knee
  - Night splints or Strasbourg socks, hold foot in dorsiflexion, facilitating passive plantar fascia stretch
  - Massage with golf ball beneath painful arch

- Pharmacological management, as per NICE recommendations:
  - Paracetamol ± codeine
  - NSAIDs
- Interventional management:
  - Steroid injection, preferably US-guided, from the side of the fascia as there is a risk of rupture of the plantar fascia in 10% of cases if direct injection into the plantar fascia
  - RF ablation of the sensory branch of the medial calcaneal nerve and the first branch of the lateral plantar nerve
  - Localized injection of autologous PRP—promising early result; however, lack of long-term evidence
  - Plantar fascia release surgery may be tried when conservative management has been tried for 6–12 months without success
  - Extracorporeal shockwave therapy (ECSWT): NICE-approved for intractable plantar fasciitis

Further reading

1. Cutts S, Obi N, Pasapula C, Chan W. Plantar fasciitis. Ann R Coll Surg Engl 2012;94(8):539–42
2. Goff JD, Crawford R. Diagnosis and treatment of plantar fasciitis. Am Fam Physician 2011;84(6):676–82
3. Liden B, Simmons M, Landsman AS. A retrospective analysis of 22 patients treated with percutaneous radiofrequency nerve ablation for prolonged moderate to severe heel pain associated with plantar fasciitis. J Foot Ankle Surg 2009;48:642–7

CHAPTER 24

Neuropathic Pain Conditions

Sabina Bachtold, Owen Bodycombe, Sumit Gulati, Rajesh Gupta, Rahul Guru, Nofil Mulla, Ashok Puttapa, Erlick Pereira, Jan Rudiger, Thomas E Smith, Kantharuby Tambirajoo, Alifia Tameem, and Athmaja Thottungal

CONTENTS

24.1 Post-stroke pain

Definition

- Pain caused by a primary lesion or dysfunction in CNS or peripheral nervous system associated with abnormal sensitivity to temperature and noxious stimulation
- Arises within weeks to months after stroke
- Associated with the presence of depression, cognitive dysfunction, and impaired QoL
- Chronic pain syndromes are present in up to half of the patients

Types and incidence

- Post-stroke pain—30–40% initially, decreasing to 20% after 1 year
- MSK pain (including shoulder pain and subluxation)—70%
- Central post-stroke pain—8–30%
- CRPS type 1—10–30%
- Painful spasticity

Pathophysiology

- Interplay between peripheral nociceptive pain generators and central neuropathic generators, in concert with altered CNS pain signal processing and neuromodulation
- Any lesion of the CNS can be implicated
- Central post-stroke pain occurs due to a lesion in the spino-thalamo-cortical pathway and arises more often from non-thalamic than from thalamic lesions. Common after lateral medullary infarct or lesions in the ventro-posterior thalamus

- Central and peripheral sensitization plays a significant role
- No patterns of symptoms pertaining to any particular lesion
- Can occur after haemorrhagic or ischaemic cerebral events
- Loss of afferent input causes neuronal hyperpolarization. Hyperpolarization of neurons with disinhibition of the CNS descending pathway

Clinical features

- Nociceptive pain is associated with tissue damage and is mediated by an intact nervous system
- Neuropathic pain is caused by injury to, or dysfunction of, the peripheral and/or central nervous system
- Central post-stroke pain—spontaneous and continuous pain and sensory changes in the area corresponding to the stroke lesion; may present as burning, lancinating pain, with allodynia and hyperpathia

Management

- Central post-stroke pain—challenging to treat, with mixed results; principles include reducing peripheral and central sensitization, decreasing DRG activity, and increasing central inhibition
    - Pharmacological—trial of antidepressants, anticonvulsants, antiarrhythmic drugs (mexiletine), ketamine, cannabinoids, topical lidocaine/capsaicin, opioids. Evidence suggests cannabinoids and TCAs > pregabalin/lamotrigine
    - Neurostimulation—TENS, cervical spinal cord stimulator, epidural motor cortex stimulation (MCS), thalamic DBS, motor cortex repetitive transcranial magnetic stimulation (rTMS)
- Spasticity—baclofen, local neuromuscular blockade (botulinum toxin). LA blocks may provide short-term relief of pain and spasm, and allow active and passive movement of the joints
- Pain related to posture and immobility—specific mobilization procedures, alterations to nursing
- Shoulder pain—could result from glenohumeral subluxation, and strategies designed to improve the ROM and function of the glenohumeral joint (surface electrical stimulation, passive mobilization) should be used
- Rehabilitation: experienced physiotherapists teaching desensitization techniques, biofeedback, relaxation, family education, and involvement in rehabilitation

Other/additional information

- Dejerine–Roussy syndrome is the best-characterized central post-stroke pain syndrome. This thalamic pain syndrome is due to infarction of the ventroposterolateral thalamus, accounts for approximately one-third of the cases of central post-stroke pain, and is characterized by severe and paroxysmal pain, accompanied by allodynia and hyperalgesia

Further reading

1. Boivie J. Central pain. In: Wall P, Melzack R (eds). Textbook of Pain. 4th edition, 1999; pp. 879–914. London: Churchill Livingstone
2. Klit H, Finnerup NB, Jensen TS. Central post-stroke pain: clinical characteristics pathophysiology, and management. Lancet Neurol 2009; 8: pp. 857–68.

24.2 Chronic inflammatory demyelinating polyneuropathy

Introduction

- Immune-mediated disorder of the peripheral nervous system
- Rare condition—30% of patients are cured or in long-term remission, and 18% have unstable active disease (progressive/relapsing) which may lead to substantial disability
- The pathogenesis is incompletely understood and includes several humoral and cell-mediated mechanisms
- Similar to Guillain–Barré syndrome but produces chronic weakness, which is either progressive or relapsing and remitting

Clinical features

- Most patients have a slowly progressive symmetrical polyneuropathy
- In some patients, the course can be relapsing or progressive for >2 months
- Prominent proximal and distal muscle weakness
- Sensory loss in distal limbs—loss of vibration sense and joint position is more pronounced than loss of pain and temperature sensation
- Poor balance, pain, and impaired ambulation
- Generalized hyporeflexia or areflexia
- Different presentations of this condition:
  - Sensory-predominant: dysfunction of large sensory fibres
  - Distal and sensory demyelinating symmetric neuropathy
  - Proximal variant affecting the dorsal sensory nerve roots (large-fibre sensory dysfunction). Presents with symmetrical sensory ataxia and decreased vibration and proprioception
  - Lewis–Sumner syndrome: asymmetrical, multifocal sensory and motor neuropathy

Investigations

- Lumbar puncture: raised protein without pleocytosis in the CSF
- MRI: gadolinium enhancement and/or hypertrophy of brachial or lumbo-sacral plexuses, lumbo-sacral or cervical nerve roots, or cauda equina
- NCS: evidence of demyelinating neuropathy
- Nerve biopsy: segmental demyelination (without or with inflammation)

Treatments

Disease-specific treatments—immune-modulating therapy

- First line: corticosteroids, plasma exchange, or IV immunoglobulin (Ig) on their own or used in combination in severe cases
- Second line: azathioprine, methotrexate, ciclosporin, cyclophosphamide, tacrolimus, mycophenolate, etanercept
- Other: stem cell transplant

Multidisciplinary treatments

- Multimodal addressing biological (disease-specific, surgical, analgesic), physical, psychological (psychiatric or psychological), and social (work, litigation, social support network) contributors to pain, disability, and distress
- Regular exercise, nutrition, and healthy lifestyle

Additional information

- Accurate diagnosis can be improved using the European Federation of Neurological Societies and Peripheral Nerve Society diagnostic criteria
- Other neuropathies can have a similar presentation:
  - Infections: diphtheria, *Borrelia burgdorferi* infection (Lyme disease), drugs, or toxins
  - Hereditary demyelinating neuropathy
  - Multifocal motor neuropathy
  - IgM monoclonal gammopathy
  - Other demyelinating neuropathies: osteosclerotic myeloma, diabetic and non-diabetic lumbo-sacral radiculopathic neuropathy, peripheral nervous system lymphoma, amyloidosis

Further reading

1. Lewis AR, Shefner JM, Dashne JF. Chronic inflammatory demyelinating polyneuropathy. 2020. https://www.uptodate.com

24.3 Multiple sclerosis

Definition

- An immune-mediated disorder of the CNS characterized by demyelination at multiple times over multiple sites

Incidence

- In 2010, the prevalence was 285.8 and 113.1 per 100 000 women and men, respectively
- Peak incidence occurs between the ages of 40 and 50
- Female:male ratio—close to 3:1
- A total of 203 people per 100 000 were living with MS, and 6003 new cases were diagnosed in that years

Pathophysiology

- MS involves a two-stage degenerative process
- Acute phase (inflammatory stage)—inflammatory cells enter the CNS and, via several mechanisms, damage endothelial cells, while also attracting macrophages which create further demyelination
- Chronic phase—involves ongoing loss of axonal support, causing chronic degeneration. Loss of oligodendrocytes, astrogliosis, and demyelination occur. Loss of myelin sheath is responsible for cross-excitation and can eventually cause peripheral and central (deafferentation) neuropathic pain

Aetiology/risk factors

- Genetic factors play a significant role, with first-degree relatives having a 20- to 40-fold increased risk
- Geographic factors also contribute, with incidence increasing away from the equator to the poles

Diagnosis

- The McDonald criteria (revised in 2010) provide a framework on which a diagnosis of MS can be made; it stipulates a combination of clinical and radiological (MRI) findings to demonstrate damage to the CNS in both space and time (see Table 24.3.1)
- Clinical presentations can include: loss or reduction of, or double, vision; ascending sensory or motor symptoms; cerebellar disturbance; or Lhermitte's syndrome (sensory changes on neck flexion)
- Exclusion of any other diagnosis
- The differential diagnosis can be extensive and can be approached by looking for suggestions that another presentation is more likely. These may be rare symptoms in the presentation of MS, such as peripheral neuropathy or hearing loss, or patient factors such as age (presentation before the age of 20 or after 50) or a strong family history of other diseases

Treatment

Education

- Lifestyle advice, such as stopping smoking and taking exercise, helps reduce relapse rates

Physical and psychological therapy

- Can help with fatigue, spasticity, and mobility issues, as well as with mood disturbances

Pharmacological management

- **Management of relapses**—confirm relapse by ruling out infection and disease fluctuation. The mainstay of treatment of a relapse is methylprednisolone 0.5 g/day for 5 days
- **Disease-modifying therapy** (DMT), e.g. alemtuzumab, β-interferon and glatiramer acetate, cladribine
- **Symptomatic treatment** for pain, incontinence, mobility, fatigue, memory, and spasticity

Table 24.3.1 McDonald criteria for MS

Number of clinical attacks	Objective evidence of lesions on MRI	Additional criteria
≥2	≥2	None needed
≥2	1	DIS (or wait for another clinical attack at another site)
1	2	DIT (or wait for another clinical attack at another site)
1	1	DIS and DIT (or wait for another clinical attack at another site)
0		Disease progression in 1 year and at least two or three points mentioned below: 1. DIS in brain 2. DIS in spinal cord 3. CSF positive

DIS, dissemination in space; DIT, dissemination in time.

Adapted with permission from McDonald W., Compston, A., Edan, G. et al. (2001). Recommended Diagnostic Criteria for Multiple Sclerosis: Guidelines from the International Panel on the Diagnosis of Multiple Sclerosis. *Ann Neurol.* 50(1):121-7. doi:10.1002/ana.1032

- Neuropathic pain is best treated using NICE neuropathic pain guidance, while baclofen can be used for spasticity and amantadine for fatigue
- Botulinum toxin and IT baclofen have both been used in people with resistant spasticity. Sativex® (THC:CBD spray) is no longer recommended for treatment of spasticity in MS patients

Other/additional information

- NICE recommends that all patients with MS have an annual comprehensive review covering all aspects of their care by people expert in the field

Further reading

1. Polman CH, Reingold SC, Banwell B, et al. Diagnostic criteria for multiple sclerosis: 2010 Revisions to the McDonald criteria. Ann Neurol 2011;69(2):292–302
2. National Institute for Health and Care Excellence. Multiple sclerosis in adults: management. 2014; updated 2019. https://www.nice.org.uk/guidance/cg186

24.4 Spinal cord injury

Introduction

- Trauma is the most common cause of SCI. More common in males
- Incidence in the UK is 12–16 per million of the population
- Chronic pain is common (70%) and normally associated with significant impact on mood, functioning, QoL, and productivity
- Most common types of pain are nociceptive (MSK or visceral) and neuropathic

Pathophysiology

- Nociceptive pain from activation of MSK and/or visceral nociceptors
- Neuropathic pain:
  - Peripheral pain generators from the peripheral somato-sensory nervous system can be involved
  - Spinal cord mechanisms:
    - Hyperexcitable neurons
    - Autonomic, inflammatory, and immunological changes (e.g. glial activation)
    - Structural neuroplasticity (e.g. dendritic sprouting)
    - Functional changes in ion channels (e.g. Na^+ and Ca^{2+}) and receptors (e.g. NMDA)
    - Spinal cord deafferentation (partial or complete) leads to white matter loss and hypersensitivity in the spinal cord
  - Supra-spinal mechanisms (may develop as a consequence of the SCI):
  - Cortical reorganization (functional and structural)
  - Changes in anterior cingulate cortex and prefrontal cortex
  - Changes in thalamus (abnormal bursting, thalamo-cortical dysrhythmia)
  - Below-level neuropathic pain is mostly centrally mediated (neuronal hyperexcitability), but the mechanism is not clear. The mechanism of evoked and spontaneous pain is different in complete and incomplete injuries. Functioning peripheral nerve fibres (polysynaptic, A-delta, C-fibres, or other) in incomplete SCI patients transmit peripheral

thresholds to the spinal cord from the injury site and periphery. Some patients have subclinical preservation of some spinal cord pathways on neurophysiological testing (QST) despite having a 'complete' SCI

Clinical features

Neuropathic pain

- SCI commonly presents with several types of neuropathic pain outlined in the IASP taxonomy of pain after an SCI. Criteria for SCI-related neuropathic pain include:
  - History and diagnostic test confirming SCI
  - Pain distribution is at or below the neurological level
  - Negative or positive sensory symptoms and clinical signs of neuropathic pain
  - Other causes of pain excluded or unlikely
- Neuropathic pain is common and classified as follows:
  - Above-level neuropathic pain originates from pathologies above the level of the SCI such as CRPS or peripheral nerve injury
  - At-level neuropathic pain arises from the spinal cord and/or nerve roots. Presents in two dermatomes above or below the level of the injury
  - Below-level neuropathic pain is localized below the level of the injury
  - Other causes of neuropathic pain such as diabetic neuropathy, PHN or other causes

Musculoskeletal pain

- Acute MSK pain from inflamed or damaged MSK structures (tendons, muscles, bones, ligaments, joints)
- Chronic MSK pain commonly caused by MSK overuse or strain. Chronic wheelchair use can cause carpal tunnel syndrome, nerve entrapments, and thoracic outlet syndrome. Back and neck MSK pain is common, especially in patients with paraplegia and spinal fusion surgery. Pain from muscle spasms is also common

Visceral pain

- From nociceptors located in the pelvis, abdomen, or thorax. Some examples include constipation, peptic ulcer, appendicitis, cholecystitis, and MI

Other causes of pain

- Nociceptive causes such as surgical scar incision, autonomic dysreflexia headache, etc.
- Other causes of pain such as fibromyalgia, interstitial cystitis, etc.
- Sometimes the cause of the pain is unknown

Assessment

- Pain-orientated detailed history, questionnaires, system based examination (neurological and musculoskeletal systems are normally very important)
- Important to assess psychosocial factors and associated pain-related disabilities
- Neurological examination to determine the sensory and motor level, whether injury is complete or incomplete (incomplete injuries have sensory and/or motor function in S4–5), and score on the American Spinal Injury Association Impairment scale
- Investigations:
  - Blood tests such as folate, metabolic profile, vitamin B12, and vitamin D which can contribute to neuronal dysfunction

- X-ray, CT, and MRI if suspected spinal segmental instability, compression, peripheral nerve compression, syringomyelia, hardware instability, or structural pathology
- Endoscopy, barium studies, cystoscopy, and urodynamic studies may be indicated for visceral pain in the pelvis, abdomen, or thorax
- NCS for neuropathies
- Bone scans for inflammatory processes in bone such as infections, fractures, and CRPS
- QST and contact pain-evoked potentials not available in clinical practice routinely

Treatment

- Whenever possible, treat the underlying pathology. Most treatments for pain management are aimed at providing symptomatic relief and have limited evidence of efficacy
- Gold standard is multidisciplinary treatments with input from a psychologist, physiotherapist, OT, nursing, pharmacy, dietician, and doctor, targeting function, productivity, rest, leisure, vocation, relationships, motivation, and mood
- CBT improves pain behaviour, mood, and coping mechanisms
- OT and physiotherapy improve overuse syndrome, fitness, abnormal postures, and gait. Treatments can include education, exercise, hydrotherapy, training with day-to-day activities (transferring, using the wheelchair, changing lifestyle), and environmental modifications
- Pharmacological treatments:
  - Long-term use of analgesics should be minimized due to associated S/Es and adverse effects (particularly opioids and benzodiazepines)
  - MSK pain: paracetamol, NSAIDs, and opioids as per WHO ladder. Baclofen, botulinum toxin, and BZDs can be considered for pain from muscle spasms
  - Neuropathic pain can be treated with antidepressants (amitriptyline, duloxetine, dosulepin), anticonvulsants (pregabalin, gabapentin), and opioids (e.g, tramadol, tapentadol) ketamine and lidocaine can be effective in acute neuropathic pain
  - Severe vasomotor changes with regional pain: sympathomimetics, Ca^{2+} channel blockers, interventional blocks
  - Regional trophic changes and osteopenia: bisphosphonates, calcitonin
  - Depression, insomnia, anxiety: antidepressants that have analgesic properties ideally, anxiolytics, psychotherapy
- Surgery may be required to reverse structural problems that are contributing to pain (e.g. surgical decompression for peripheral nerve compression, drainage of syringomyelia, dorsal root entry zone lesioning)
- Neuromodulation can be considered for refractory pain:
  - IT pumps can be used to treat neuropathic pain or muscle spasticity. Combination therapies are successful, involving baclofen, clonidine, morphine, and ziconotide
  - SCS efficacy is controversial probably due to impaired DH function. Patients with incomplete injuries get more pain relief with SCS than the complete lesion
  - Other neurostimulation techniques that can be considered include TENS, transcranial magnetic stimulation, PNS, and MCS

Further reading

1. Bryce TN, Biering-sorenson F, Finnerup NB, et al. International spinal cord injury pain classification: Part I. Background and description. Spinal Cord 2012;50:413–17
2. Finnerup NB. Pain in patients with spinal cord injury. Pain 2013;154(1):S71–6

3. Kirshblum SC, Burns SP, Biering-Sorensen Fin, et al. International standards for neurological classification of spinal cord injury. J Spinal Cord Med 2011;34(6):535–46
4. Siddall PJ, Yezierski RP, Loeser JD. Taxonomy and epidemiology of spinal cord injury pain. In: Burchiel KJ, Yezierski RP (eds). Spinal Cord Injury Pain: Assessment, Mechanisms, Management. Progress in Pain Research and Management. 2002; pp. 9–24. Seattle, WA: IASP Press

24.5 Cauda equina syndrome

Introduction

- Presents commonly with acute-onset urinary retention or incontinence or faecal incontinence accompanied by altered perineal sensation secondary to a large central lumbar disc prolapse compressing the cauda equina nerves in the spinal canal

Incidence

- 4/10 000 adults with back pain
- 1–2% of surgically treated lumbar disc prolapses
- Can be either sudden onset without previous problems or can occur in patients with chronic non-cancer low back pain radiating down the leg

Anatomy

- Sacral nerve roots pass centrally in the theca in the spinal canal. S2–4 supply sphincter function. Central lumbar spinal canal compression can compromise innervation of the sphincters and perineum

Pathophysiology

- Rupture of the annulus fibrosus, causing the nucleus pulposus to herniate posteriorly
- More common in young adults <60 years old as discs degenerate and desiccate with age
- More common in obese patients due to greater axial loading of the spine and relatively weaker paraspinal musculature limiting load distribution

Diagnosis

- Diagnosis is mostly made from the history
- Loss of sensation of micturition or defecation
- Acute-onset urinary dysfunction, progressing to painless urinary retention and overflow incontinence
- Faecal incontinence
- Perineal paraesthesiae/anaesthesia
- Sexual dysfunction (impotence)
- Leg pain and weakness (often bilateral)

Examination and investigations

- Saddle anaesthesia
- Reduced or absent anal tone in two-thirds of patients
- Reduced or absent anal wink reflex
- Reduced or absent bulbocavernosus reflex
- Absent ankle jerk reflexes
- MRI scan of the lumbo-sacral spine is mandatory to make diagnosis

Aetiology

- Usually massive herniated lumbar disc
- Sometimes tumour (metastatic spinal cord compression or intradural lesion)
- Occasionally trauma (burst fracture with retropulsed fragment)
- Seldom spondylodiscitis
- Rarely spinal epidural haematoma or abscess
- Non-surgical causes include septic thrombophlebitis, ischaemia, inflammation, and paraneoplastic or metastatic tumour seeding

Treatment

- Surgical emergency: urgent decompression by discectomy within 48 hours of symptom onset provides the best chance of recovery of sphincter function
- Generous bilateral laminectomy before discectomy is often preferred to a limited microdiscectomy approach. Occasionally, an intradural approach is needed
- If >1-week history of double incontinence, then expedient surgery desirable, but less urgent as sphincters usually irreversibly impaired
- Post-operative bladder function assessment by catheter clamping before removal; post-voiding residual measurement is important and prompt urology referral should be made for residual sphincter impairment
- Recovery of sensory and motor function may continue for up to 2 years. Recurrent disc prolapse is a small, but important, risk
- Medical management: steroids and radiotherapy

Further reading

1. Gleave JR, Macfarlane R. Cauda equina syndrome: what is the relationship between timing of surgery and outcome? Br J Neurosurg 2002;16(4):325–8
2. Todd NV. Neurological deterioration in cauda equina syndrome is probably progressive and continuous. Implications for clinical management. Br J Neurosurg 2015;29(5):630–4

24.6 Trigeminal neuralgia

Introduction

Trigeminal neuralgia is:

- A rare condition, characterized by recurrent paroxysmal, unilateral, brief electric shock-like pains, abrupt in onset and termination
- Limited to the distribution of one or more divisions of the trigeminal nerve
- Triggered by innocuous stimuli
- Idiopathic or secondary to other disorders
- Persistent background facial pain may be present

Epidemiology

- Incidence of approximately 12/100 000 people/year
- More common in women

- Commonly in people over the age of 50 but can occur at any age
- MS may be a possible secondary cause in young adults

Anatomy

(See 16.2 Anatomy of the trigeminal nerve and trigeminal ganglion block, p. 301.)

- The trigeminal nerve exits the brainstem laterally at the mid-pons level and has two roots—a larger sensory root and a smaller motor root
- The motor root also contains sensory nerve fibres that mainly mediate pain sensation
- The Gasserian ganglion, located in Meckel's cave in the middle cranial fossa, is the ganglion of the trigeminal nerve and contains first-order general somatic sensory fibres that carry pain, temperature, and touch sensation
- The peripheral processes of neurons in the ganglion form the three divisions—ophthalmic, maxillary, and mandibular
- The sensory trigeminal nerve nuclei are the largest of the cranial nerve nuclei and extend from the midbrain to the high cervical cord

Pathophysiology

- Vascular compression from either an artery or a vein of the trigeminal nerve root occurs, with morphological changes in the nerve in about 95% of patients
- The exact pathophysiology of compression causing pain is unknown
- A combination of central demyelination of the nerve root entry zone and reinforcing electrical excitability may be a hypothesis. This demyelination leads to impairment of the nociceptive system
- In patients with more background facial pain, there seems to be loss of central inhibition of the nociceptive system, which persists even after successful surgery, manifesting as some form of abnormality of somato-sensory function
- There are also trigeminal neuralgia cases associated with MS plaques or infarcts within the brainstem or cerebellopontine mass lesions

Diagnosis

Classical trigeminal neuralgia

- Pain usually occurs in the V2 or V3 distributions
- Evidence of neurovascular compression of the trigeminal root with morphological changes on MRI or during surgery
- The hallmarks include memorable onset, initial long remission periods that become shorter with time, and longer attacks of pain
- 65% of newly diagnosed patients with classical trigeminal neuralgia have a second episode within 5 years, and 77% within 10 years
- 50% may have remission periods of at least 6 months' duration
- Attack frequency can vary throughout the day
- Two subcategories exist: classical trigeminal neuralgia, purely paroxysmal, and classical trigeminal neuralgia with concomitant persistent facial pain (atypical trigeminal neuralgia)
- Autonomic features are rare
- Diagnostic criteria for the two forms of classical trigeminal neuralgia (see table 24.6.1)

Table 24.6.1 Diagnostic criteria for the two forms of classical trigeminal neuralgia

	Classical trigeminal neuralgia, purely paroxysmal	Classical trigeminal neuralgia with concomitant persistent facial pain
Features	Recurrent paroxysmal attacks lasting seconds to minutes Severe intensity Electric shock-like shooting, stabbing or sharp in quality Precipitated by innocuous stimuli to affected side of the face Occurs in one or more divisions of the trigeminal nerve No radiation beyond the trigeminal distribution No clinically evident neurological deficit	
Facial pain	No persistent facial pain between attacks	Persistent facial pain of moderate intensity in the affected area
Response to treatment	Responds well initially to medical treatment; good response to microvascular decompression	Responds poorly to conservative treatment and surgical intervention
Other features	Never crosses to opposite side, rarely may be bilateral	

Source: Data from *The International Classification of Headache Disorders*, Third Edition. London, United Kingdom: International Headache Society.

Secondary trigeminal neuralgia

- Other causes of pain include MS plaques, tumours in the cerebellopontine angle, and arterio-venous malformation
- Patients with MS present at a much younger age, with atypical pain, without the trigger zones and the lancinating brief paroxysmal period. It can be bilateral and can be challenging to manage
- Imaging is mandatory for diagnosis

Treatment

Medical treatment

- First-line treatment of trigeminal neuralgia
- Carbamazepine is the drug of choice, which provides excellent initial pain relief in the majority of patients. It should be started at a low dose and gradually increased every 3–7 days to achieve best pain control with minimal S/Es
- Common S/Es include tiredness and poor concentration. At higher doses, balance impairment and hyponatraemia are common, especially in the elderly. Occurrence of a rash requires discontinuation of the drug
- The second drug of choice is oxcarbazepine, a keto derivative of carbamazepine, with similar efficacy, but with increased tolerability and fewer drug interactions
- If patients are intolerant of the above drugs, then lamotrigine, baclofen, pregabalin, or phenytoin can be tried
- Patients should be referred onwards to a specialist in managing trigeminal neuralgia, as S/Es with combination therapy are high and best managed in a specialized setting

Surgical treatment

- Indicated for patients in whom medical treatment has failed or S/Es associated with medical treatment are unacceptable

- Surgical options fall into two categories: microvascular decompression or destructive procedures

Microvascular decompression

- Has the highest success rate in maintaining long-term pain relief
- Offers an 80% chance of being pain-free without the need for any further treatment, with a recurrence rate of about 10% over 20 years
- It consists of a small craniotomy in the mastoid region, gently separating the nerve from the offending blood vessel and holding it in place with a small piece of Teflon. In cases where vascular compression is not evident, a partial neurectomy of the nerve near the root entry zone may be performed. A neurectomy causes numbness in the face, with the risk of causing anaesthesia dolorosa
- Risks of surgery include hearing loss, damage to the trigeminal nerve causing permanent facial numbness, CSF leak, and meningitis

Destructive procedures

These procedures involve partial controlled damage to the trigeminal nerve root with the aim to relieve pain. It can be used for all causes of trigeminal neuralgia and is performed with either sedation or light general anaesthesia, ideal in the elderly or medically unfit patients. Some options include:

- Balloon compression: a soft catheter with a balloon is inserted into the foramen ovale through the cheek under radiological guidance and inflated to compress the nerve. Pain relief usually lasts 1–2 years and can be repeated. A common S/E is numbness of the face, including that of the cornea
- Glycerol injection: glycerol is injected via a needle inserted through the cheek into the foramen ovale, with the patient in the sitting position (glycerol is heavier than spinal fluid). The glycerol bathes the ganglion and damages the nerve fibres. Recurrence within a year or two is frequent and the procedure can be repeated. Facial sensation loss is a common S/E
- RF ablation: via a needle inserted into the foramen ovale to target the area of pain, the nerve area is gradually heated with an electrode, injuring the nerve fibres. Symptoms recur in 50% of patients 3–4 years following lesioning. Production of more numbness can extend the pain relief even longer but increases the risks of anaesthesia dolorosa
- Stereotactic radiosurgery: highly focused radiation beams are delivered to the nerve root exit zone at the brainstem. Radiation causes the formation of a lesion on the nerve that disrupts sensory signal transmission to the brain. Pain relief is usually evident weeks to months later and appears to be as effective as with other percutaneous procedures. Recurrence rates are around 25% between 1 and 3 years

Emergency treatment

- Severe acute pain can stop the patient eating and drinking and can lead to severe dehydration and possible hyponatraemia caused by oral medications
- Opioids use has no effect
- Admission to hospital for pain management, correction of biochemical abnormalities, and IV hydration is required
- In many cases, a single dose of IV phenytoin with cardiac monitoring helps to break the pain cycle and can be instituted together with an increase in oral medications
- Good oral hygiene required to prevent any additional dental pain
- Percutaneous procedures (e.g. balloon compression) can be utilized to manage the acute pain

- Stereotactic radiosurgery is not recommended as an emergency treatment, given the lag time before results are noted

Further reading

1. Headache Classification Committee of the International Headache Society (IHS): The International Classification of Headache Disorders, 3rd edition. Cephalalgia 2018;38(1):1–211. doi: 10.1177/0333102417738202
2. Burchiel KJ. A new classification of facial pain. Neurosurgery 2003;53(5):1164–7. doi:10.1227/01.neu.0000088806.11659.d8
3. Nurmikko TJ, Eldridge PR. Trigeminal neuralgia—pathophysiology, diagnosis and current treatment. Br J Anaesth 2001;87(1):117–32. doi:10.1093/bja/87.1.117

24.7 Glossopharyngeal neuralgia

Introduction

- Glossopharyngeal neuralgia presents with pain in the sensory distribution of CN IX
- First described by Weissenberg in 1910 in a patient with a cerebellopontine angle tumour
- Clinically resembles trigeminal neuralgia but occurs 100 times less often
- Incidence rate is 0.7 cases per 10 000 population

Clinical features

- Usually affects patients in the fifth decade of life but may occur at any age
- Patients present with otalgia (most common), tonsillar pain, laryngeal pain, and glossal pain—in that order
- Paroxysmal pain lasting seconds to minutes
- Common triggers are swallowing, chewing, talking, and coughing
- 'Overflow pain'—20% of patients have pain in the sensory areas supplied by CN V, CN X, and upper cervical segments. This is due to spillover of nociceptive impulses from CN IX through the nucleus tractus solitarius of the medulla to CN V or convergence with the descending portion of CN V
- Several hypotheses describe a synapse between CN IX and CN X that results in pain associated with bradycardia and syncope

Investigations

- Baseline blood tests and MRI to rule out a cerebellopontine angle tumour and demyelinating diseases

Management

- Multidisciplinary and multimodal treatments
- Pharmacotherapy:
  - First line: carbamazepine
    - Start with 200 mg nocte, and increase in 200 mg increments up to a maximum dose of 1200 mg daily
    - Common S/Es: dizziness, sedation, confusion, and rash

    - Monitor FBC, serum chemistry, and urinalysis
    - Monitor actively for life-threatening blood dyscrasias
  - Second line: oxcarbazepine, gabapentinoids, antidepressants, baclofen
- Glossopharyngeal nerve block:
  - Transoral, transnasal, and lateral infratemporal approaches
  - Potential complications: haematoma formation (injury to internal jugular vein or carotid artery), CSF leak, LA toxicity
  - A successful diagnostic block may be followed by RF procedures
  - Neuro-destruction with phenol, alcohol, and glycerol is reserved for selective patients in whom drug therapy has failed
- Microvascular decompression (Jannetta technique): a neurosurgical procedure that identifies the nerve root close to the brainstem and decompresses the offending blood vessel, with positioning of the sponge in between the vessel and the glossopharyngeal nerve

Further reading

1. Bajwa Z, Ho CC, Khan SA, Garza I. Overview of craniofacial pain. 2018. https://www.uptodate.com

24.8 Occipital neuralgia

Definition

- Stabbing and shooting paroxysmal pain, along the dermatome of the GON (90%) and LON (10%)
- Damage and/or irritation of the nerves causes neuralgia
- Pain elicited by pressure over the nerves, along the nuchal ridge or on rotation and lateral flexion of cervical spine, with constant pain in between episodes

Course of the nerve

- The GON is formed by the dorsal ramus of C2, has a medial course under the IO muscle, bending cranially, and finally turns laterally, piercing the semispinalis muscle and the aponeurosis of the trapezius muscle, after which it divides and lies SC

Causes

- Vascular—irritation of C1/C2 nerve roots by aberrant branch of the posterior inferior cerebellar artery, giant cell arteritis, arterio-venous fistula at the cervical dural level
- Neurogenic—MS, C2 myelitis, schwannoma of the occipital nerve
- Muscular/tendon involvement
- Bone—C1/C2 arthritis, dysfunction of the atlas bone, osteolytic lesions of the cranium
- Post-vitrectomy surgery

Clinical features

- Pain in the neck radiating to the posterior cranium to the top of the head, over the ear, and parotid gland
- Attacks lasts for seconds to minutes

- Sharp pain and electric shock-like sensation, and may be triggered by brushing hair, neck movements, or resting the head on a pillow
- Pain may be referred in the retro-orbital and frontal head regions, and felt usually unilaterally and occasionally bilaterally

Examination

- Sensory changes and tenderness in the dermatome
- Positive Tinel's sign—pain on percussion of the nerve

Investigations

- Baseline blood tests, CT, and MRI are needed to rule out tumours, cervicalgia, and other causes of secondary headaches
- Open-mouth X-ray—arthritis of the C2 facet joint
- Diagnostic blocks of GON and LON are helpful

Differential diagnosis

- Tension-type headache, migraine, cervicogenic headache
- Occult tumour, congenital anomalies (Arnold–Chiari malformation)
- Cervical disc disease, OA
- Gout, diabetes
- Infection, vasculitis

Treatment

Conservative

- Physical therapy, massage, improving posture, and reducing secondary muscle tension
- Pharmacological therapy:
  - Anti-inflammatories
  - Antidepressants (especially TCAs)
  - Antiepileptics (gabapentinoids, carbamazepine)
  - Muscle relaxants (baclofen, tizanidine)

Interventions

- Occipital nerve blocks (GON and LON, and occasionally TON) with LA and steroid mixtures
- BTX-A injection
- PRF of the occipital nerve may help
- PRF of the C2 DRG—very limited evidence
- PENS and ONS can be helpful. Electrical impulses are delivered via insulated lead wires tunnelled under the skin. It is relatively minimally invasive and can offer long-term benefit
- Microvascular decompression of C2 nerve root, DRG, or post-ganglionic nerve is practised in some specialist centres

Further reading

1. Gradient PM, Smith JH. The neuralgias: 'diagnosis and management'. Curr Neurosci Rep 2014;14(7):459

2. Vanelderen P, Lataster A, Levy R et al. Occipital Neuralgia. In: Zundert JV, Patjin J, Hartrick C, et al. il, Maarten Van Kleef. Evidence-Based Interventional Pain Medicine; According to Clinical Diagnosis, 2012; pp. 49–54. Wiley-Blackwell

24.9 Post-herpetic neuralgia

Definition/introduction

- Post-herpetic neuralgia (PHN) is neuropathic pain in a dermatome due to damage to a peripheral nerve during an outbreak of shingles (pain that continues for >3 months)
- PHN is the most common complication of shingles (sensory nerve fibres and skin are affected; motor fibres are rarely affected)
- Chickenpox (varicella) is caused by initial infection with the varicella zoster virus (VZV) (skin rash, small itchy blisters ± fever, tiredness, headaches)
- VZV is one of the herpesviruses
- Shingles (herpes zoster) are caused by reactivation of the herpes zoster virus (approximately 20% lifetime prevalence)

Incidence

- For herpes zoster: 0.34%, but almost tripled in the elderly population above the age of 80
- Even higher in individuals with low cell-mediated immunity
- Incidence in the elderly will become even higher with universal immunization of children with varicella, as the boosting effect on cell-mediated immunity due to exposure to varicella will be lost
- For PHN: 10–18% of patients with herpes zoster (under 60 <10%, over 60 up to 30–40%)

Pathophysiology/anatomy

- After initial infection (chickenpox, varicella), the VZV remains dormant in the DRG
- All individuals once infected with varicella undergo seroconversion. They remain at risk of developing shingles and its complications, including PHN
- VZV is reactivated whenever there is a decline in immunity, causing shingles
- During reactivation, the VZV travels down the axons from DRGs to the skin in the periphery to cause a rash or blisters
- VZV can also end up travelling centrally to affect the meninges and spinal cord, resulting in their inflammation
- The course of the disease is usually mild, with pain in most cases subsiding, with scabbing of the rash or even before that
- Shingles can also result in other complications, including visceral, neurological, and ophthalmic disorders
- Mostly affected areas: thoracic dermatomes, ophthalmic division of the trigeminal nerve (ophthalmic shingles)

Risk factors to develop post-herpetic neuralgia after shingles

- Age: older than 50
- Severity of shingles: extensive/severe rash and severe pain and associated sensory abnormality in the early phase
- Other illness: chronic disease (diabetes), immunosuppression
- Shingles location: on the face or torso
- Delay in shingles antiviral treatment for >72 hours after the rash appeared

Diagnosis

- Mainly clinical diagnosis, with signs and symptoms limited to the skin area where the shingles outbreak first occurred (usually unilateral in a band around the trunk)
- Pain lasting >3 months after the shingles rash has healed; presentation of burning, sharp, and stabbing or deep and aching pain (usually T4–6 dermatomes but can also affect cervical and trigeminal nerves)
- Frequently with allodynia (even touching clothes can cause pain)
- Less commonly with itching and areas of numbness/reduced sensation
- Although it presents as a continuum of pain after the rash, it can also present years after the initial rash; in these patients, polymerase chain reaction (PCR) test detecting VZV in the CSF may help the diagnosis
- Antibodies to herpes zoster (4-fold increase) to support subclinical herpes zoster
- Viral culture or immunofluorescence to differentiate between herpes simplex and herpes zoster

Possible complications

- Depending on the duration of PHN and the severity of pain, patients can develop depression, fatigue, difficulty sleeping, lack of appetite, and concentration problems

Treatment

- Biopsychosocial approach
- Pain can persist for years and can be difficult to treat

Pharmacological options (tricyclic antidepressants, anticonvulsants, topical agents, opioids)

Tricyclic antidepressants

- These are found to be effective for PHN treatment as their action is multimodal, i.e. by potentiation of the effects of neurotransmitters in the descending pain modulatory pathways, blockade of Na^+ channels, and blockade of α-adrenoceptors
- Amitriptyline, nortriptyline (NNT = 3.7)

Anticonvulsants

- Gabapentin and pregabalin are effective
- Pregabalin with superior bioavailability and less associated adverse effects. Also improved stage 4 sleep, resulting in improved QoL in patients

Topical agents

- Lidocaine patch:
  - Several studies and systemic reviews support the use of lidocaine patches (5%) in the treatment of PHN (NNT = 4.4 for pain)
- Topical capsaicin:
  - Vanilloid receptor agonist with multiple modes of action, including inactivation of receptive terminal of nociceptors, depletion of SP, and as a C-fibre nerve toxin
  - Effective in low concentration of 0.025% or 0.075% (cream), applied 4–5 times per day, as well as in high concentration of 8% (patch), applied for 30–60 minutes (higher concentration more effective in a double-blind RCT)

Opioids (e.g. codeine, tramadol, morphine)

- Opioids can be quite effective for PHN, with morphine having an NNT value of 2.79 against an NNT of 3.73 for nortriptyline in a double-blind crossover study
- Considered as second or third choice due to S/Es and tolerance, and dependence with prolonged use

Non-pharmacological options

- Wear comfortable clothes, ice packs
- TENS or acupuncture (lack of evidence)
- SCS in the PHN (lack of trials)
- Self-management strategies for chronic pain

Prevention

- Varicella vaccine to prevent chickenpox which reduces overall incidence and reduces severity of the disease (Zostavax® from Merck seems to reduce the incidence of PHN)
- Vaccination above the age of 60 (with live attenuated VZV vaccine) causes a boosting of immunity against VZV
- In a double-blind RCT, vaccination of adults aged over 60: reduction of shingles by 61.1% over 3.12 years' surveillance period
- Vaccination is recommended to all adults aged over 60 who have had chickenpox or not

Further reading

1. Jung BF, Johnson RW, Griffin DRJ, Dworkin RH. Risk factors for postherpetic neuralgia in patients with herpes zoster. Neurology 2004;62:1545–51
2. Sindrup SH, Otto M, Finnerup NB, Jensen TS. Antidepressants in the treatment of neuropathic pain. Basic Clin Pharmacol Toxicol 2005;96:399–409
3. Backonja M, Wallace MS, Blonsky ER, et al. NGX-4010, a high concentration capsaicin patch, for the treatment of postherpetic neuralgia: a randomised, double-blind study. Lancet Neurol 2008;7(12):1106–12
4. Mayo Foundation for Medical Education and Research. Postherpetic neuralgia. November 2020. https://www.mayoclinic.org/diseases-conditions/postherpetic-neuralgia/symptoms-causes/syc-20376588

24.10 Meralgia paraesthetica

Definition

- Pain, tingling, and numbness felt in the distribution of the lateral cutaneous nerve of the thigh (antero-lateral thigh)

Incidence

- In the general population: 4.3 in 10 000 person-years
- In people with diabetes: 24.7 per 10 000 person-years

Anatomy

- The lateral cutaneous nerve of the thigh arises from the lumbar plexus from contributions from L2 and L3 nerve roots
- It runs along the lateral border of the psoas muscle before entering the thigh by passing through the lateral part of the inguinal ligament adjacent to the ASIS (although the course can vary)
- The most common cause of meralgia paraesthetica is focal entrapment of the nerve as it passes through the inguinal ligament

Risk factors

- Obesity, pregnancy
- Wearing heavy tool belts or body armour
- Traumatic injury (e.g. seat belt injury, prone surgery)
- Rarely, masses within the pelvis can injure the nerve more proximally
- The higher incidence in diabetics may indicate that the nerve is more vulnerable due to added metabolic injury

Diagnosis

- Diagnosis is made on clinical grounds
- Pain, dysaesthesia, and/or paraesthesiae in the nerve distribution (lateral thigh)
- Sensory changes are found on examination—hypoaesthesia and/or dysaesthesia are common
- Deep palpation just below and medial to the ASIS often elicits the symptoms
- The nerve is pure sensory, so motor function is not affected

Treatment

- Address risk factors (tight clothing/belts, obesity, diabetes)
- Neuropathic pain medications
- Focal LA and steroid nerve blocks—with or without US
- Surgical decompression—has been described but is rarely performed

Prognosis

- Pain and paraesthesiae usually resolve with time, but numbness may remain

Further reading

1. Carai A, Fenu G, Sechi E, et al. Anatomical variability of the lateral femoral cutaneous nerve: findings from a surgical series. Clin Anat 2009;22(3):365–70
2. Hara K, Sakura S, Shido A. Ultrasound-guided lateral femoral cutaneous nerve block: comparison of two techniques. Anaesth Intensive Care 2011;39(1):69–72
3. Parisi TJ, Mandrekar J, Dyck PJ, Klein CJ. Meralgia paresthetica: relation to obesity, advanced age, and diabetes mellitus. Neurology 2011;77(16):1538–42
4. Patijn J, Mekhail N, Hayek S, et al. Meralgia paresthetica. Pain Pract 2011;11(3):302–8
5. Simpson G, Krol A, Silver D, Nicholls B. 5.7 Lateral femoral cutaneous nerve. In: Simpson G, Krol A, Silver D, Nicholls B. (eds). Ultrasound-guided Interventions in Chronic Pain Management. 2019; pp. 201–204. UK: European Society of Regional Anaesthsia & Pain Therapy (ESRA)
6. Van Slobbe AM, Bohnen AM, Bernsen RM, et al. Incidence rates and determinants in meralgia paresthetica in general practice. J Neurol 2004;251(3):294–7

24.11 Complex regional pain syndrome

Definition

- As per IASP, CRPS is a syndrome characterized by continuing (spontaneous and/or evoked) regional pain that is seemingly disproportionate in time or degree to the usual course of pain after trauma or other lesion

Types

- Type 1: minor injuries or fracture of a limb precede the onset of symptoms (fractures, sprains, surgery, immobilization)—90% of cases
- Type 2: develops after injury to a major peripheral nerve—10% of cases
- NOS: not otherwise specified (recent addition to the classification)

Impact

- Associated with significant disability and reduced QoL
- Variable progress
- Increased health care costs and societal costs

Pathophysiology

- Peripheral sensitization
- Sympathetically mediated pain (red/warm, cold/blue)
- Central sensitization (intense and repeated stimulus leads to hypersensitivity), NMDA receptor-mediated (treatment with ketamine and IV Mg^{2+})
- Autoimmune processes (treatment with IV Ig)
- Motor and sensory dysfunction
- Protective disuse—cortical reorganization sustains CRPS (the limb can feel strange, disfigured, out of place → treatment: graded motor imagery)
- Aberrant healing and exaggerated inflammation
- CRPS due to nerve damage

Epidemiology

- Women are 3–4 times more likely to be affected
- Peak incidence between 37 and 50 years
- Prevalence: 12–60/100 000 population
- 85% of patients improve within the first year
- 2% recurrence rate
- Association with female sex, asthma, migraine, osteoporosis, and intake of ACEIs

Diagnosis (Budapest criteria: signs and symptoms)

1. Continuous pain (which is disproportionate to the inciting event)
2. At least one symptom in three categories of (i) to (iv):
   i. Sensory (allodynia = touch is painful; hyperalgesia = hypersensitivity to painful stimulus; hypoaesthesia = reduced sensation)
   ii. Vasomotor (temperature, colour changes)
   iii. Sudomotor (oedema = swelling; sweating abnormalities)
   iv. Motor/trophic changes (weakness, tremor, hair/nail growth changes, skin changes)

3. At least one sign (at evaluation) in two or more categories of (i) to (iv):
   i. Sensory (hyperalgesia to pinprick; allodynia = light touch and temperature are painful; deep somatic pressure; joint movement)
   ii. Vasomotor (temperature asymmetry >1°C, skin colour changes)
   iii. Sudomotor changes/oedema (sweating changes)
   iv. Motor/trophic changes:
      a. Motor: reduced ROM ± motor dysfunction, weakness, tremor, dystonia
      b. Trophic: skin changes, hair and nail growth changes
4. No other diagnosis can better explain the signs and symptoms

CRPS severity score

Self-reported symptoms

- Allodynia, hyperpathia (1)
- Temperature asymmetry (1)
- Skin colour (1)
- Sweating (1)
- Oedema (1)
- Trophic changes (hair, nail, skin) (1)
- Motor changes (weakness, tremor, dysfunction) (1)
- Reduced ROM (1)

Signs on examination

- Hyperpathia to pinprick (1)
- Allodynia (touch, brush, cold, warm, vibration, pressure) (1)
- Temperature asymmetry (1)
- Skin colour (1)
- Sweating asymmetry (1)
- Oedema asymmetry (1)
- Trophic changes (1)
- Motor changes (1)
- Reduced active ROM (1)

Tests

- Thermography (temperature)
- Sweat testing
- Imaging (X-ray, bone densitometry to check for osteoporosis)
- Electrophysiology (EMG)

Treatment

- Need a multidisciplinary and multimodal approach
- Education (self-management) → stroke gently and frequently

Specialized physiotherapy/occupational therapy

- Desensitization (rubbing limb), weight-bearing
- Stretching, fine motor exercises
- Tactile discrimination therapy
- Mirror therapy, graded motor imagery (imagined hand movements)

Medication

- Anti-neuropathics (nortriptyline/amitriptyline, pregabalin/gabapentin)
- Corticosteroids in early CRPS (if onset <6 months), e.g. prednisolone
- Bisphosphonates if onset <6 months (to increase bone strength)
- Calcitonin
- Nifedipine (vasodilator) in cold extremity CRPS
- Spasmolytics (in dystonia, tremor, myoclonus): baclofen, BZDs
- N-acetylcysteine 600 mg: trial of 3 months (three times per day) blue/white/cold limb
- Dimethylsulfoxide (DMSO) cream: trial of 3 months (five times per day)—hot/warm/ swollen limb
- Ketamine (low dose)

Injections

- Stellate ganglion block (injection in the neck for arm symptoms)
- T2–3 sympathetic block for upper limb CRPS resistant to stellate ganglion block
- Lumbar sympathetic block (injection in the lower back for leg symptoms)
- Peripheral nerve blocks (for arm and leg symptoms)
- Epidural and IT therapy
- SCS (spinal cord stimulators are recommended by NICE and their long-term effect is under evaluation)

Defer elective operations in early CRPS until symptoms subside.

For ongoing pain

- Physiotherapy, psychological support, and doctor appointments
- Self-support groups
- Leisure and social activities

Other supportive therapies

- CBT (specialized centres)
- Education of health care professionals about CRPS (e.g. GPs)
- Patient-centred approach and facilities in place to request top-up support
- EEG biofeedback
- Psychotherapy
- Relaxation techniques, hypnosis

Further reading

1. Dworkin RH, O'Connor AB, Kent J, et al. Interventional management of neuropathic pain: NeuPSIG recommendations. Pain 2013;154(11):2249–61
2. Grieve S, Perez RSGM, Birklein F, et al. Recommendations for a first Core Outcome Measurement set for complex regional pain syndrome. Clinical studies (COMPACT). Pain 2017;158(6):1083–90
3. Marinus J, Moseley GL, Birklein F, et al. Clinical features and pathophysiology of complex regional pain syndrome. Lancet Neurol 2011;10(7):637–48
4. Pons T, Shipton EA, Williman J, Mulder RT. Potential risk factors for the onset of complex regional pain syndrome type 1: a systematic literature review. Anesthesiol Res Pract 2015;2015:956539

5. Van Eijs F, Stanton-Hicks M, Van Zundert J, et al. 16 Complex regional pain syndrome. In: Van Zundert J, Patijn J, Hartrick CT, et al. (eds). Evidence-based Interventional Pain Medicine. 2012; pp. 123–36. Chichester, UK: Wiley-Blackwell

24.12 Phantom limb and stump pain

Definition

- Removal or amputation of a part of the body such as a limb, breast, or other, usually resulting in an awareness of phantom sensations in the amputated part—can range from a feeling of the part being present to severe pain

Types

- Phantom awareness: a feeling of the missing part being present
- Phantom sensation: any specific sensation of the missing limb, except pain, e.g. paraesthesiae, specific position or shape
- Phantom pain: painful, unpleasant sensations in the distribution of the missing limb—can be cramping, burning, shock-like, sharp, or dull pain
- Stump pain: pain referred to the residual stump, unlike phantom pain
- Stump contractions: spontaneous movement of the stump, ranging from small jerks to visible contractions
- Telescoping: this is retraction of the phantom part sensation towards the residual stump

Incidence

- 85% of amputees experience phantom sensations in the initial weeks after amputation
- 60–80% of amputees experience phantom pain. However, substantially fewer patients (5–10%) experience severe pain
- Lower in young children
- More frequent in upper limb amputees
- Lasts from a few weeks to many years. In many of the cases, it gradually reduces in severity

Risk factors

- Uncontrolled pre-amputation pain and persistent perioperative/stump pain
- Psychological factors, such as anxiety, depression, and lack of social support, play a role
- Genetic predisposition

Diagnosis

- Mainly history

Phantom pain

- Onset: within the first few weeks of an amputation, but in a small number of cases, it may develop months to years after an amputation
- Site: usually experienced in the distal parts of the limbs in limb amputees. Amputation of another part (e.g. breast) results in pain in that region
- Timing: usually intermittent, rather than constant. Frequency can vary from every day to weekly
- Quality: shooting, burning, aching, pins and needles, cramping

Stump pain

- Onset: common in the early post-amputation period but can persist beyond the surgical healing stage
- Site: on the residual stump
- Quality: throbbing, burning, stabbing, spontaneous movements
- Examination findings: areas of hypoaesthesia, hyperalgesia, or allodynia
- 60% of amputees with phantom pain have coexisting stump pain

Examination/investigations

- Skin for erythema, temperature, allodynia, neuroma, and infection
- X-ray, US, and MRI to look for pathology
- Wound swabs for infection
- Heterotropic ossification in >60% of trauma amputations where there is a deposit of Ca^{2+} in the stump. Can be see on X-ray

Pathophysiology

- Not completely understood
- Changes occur at the peripheral, spinal, and supra-spinal levels

Peripheral mechanisms

- Peripheral sensitization occurs
- *Neuromas* after amputation can show spontaneous abnormal activity and sensitivity that can cause phantom and stump pain
- Cell bodies in the *DRGs* also show similar abnormal activity
- Cross-talk of the sympathetic and sensory nervous systems at the level of the DRGs contributes to the increased pain response following a change in sympathetic activity

Spinal mechanisms

- Central sensitization occurs because of an increase in sensitivity and abnormal activity in DH neurons, expansion of the receptive field, and increased activity in the NMDA receptor complex

Supra-spinal mechanisms

- *Cortical reorganization* plays an important role in the development of phantom pain
- The somato-sensory cortex of the amputated part starts receiving sensory input from the adjacent areas
- This abnormal input may result in amplification of sensation and pain
- Normally dormant thalamic neurons also start to respond to stimuli

Management

- High-quality evidence for treatment of phantom and stump pain is lacking
- General guidelines for treatment of neuropathic and nociceptive pain should be followed
- Management of phantom and stump pain is not very effective and is challenging

Prevention

- Epidural infusion ideally instituted before amputation (good result, but may not be practical)
- Prolonged perineural infusion of LA (very good analgesia and may prevent phantom pain)

- Ketamine perioperative bolus and infusion
- Memantine PO at 5 mg, maximum 20 mg/day
- Gabapentinoids perioperatively reduces opioid consumption but may not prevent phantom pain
- Multimodal, multidisciplinary, pragmatic perioperative pain management pathway involving the inpatient pain team (see Fig. 24.12.1)

PREOPERATIVE REGIME:

- Once decision for amputation, contact Acute Pain Team (Bleep ....) during office hours to optimize preoperative analgesia
- Commence Gabapentinoids (after discussion with the surgeons and acute pain team) – Refer to Box 1
    - Gabapentin
        - If already prescribed, optimize dose – If previous treatment failed with Gabapentin, consider Pregabalin
    - Pregabalin
        - Start at dose of 75mg BD, first dose in the immediate preoperative period (2 hours prior to surgery)

INTRAOPERATIVE REGIME:

- Anaesthesia (GA/RA) – as per the anaesthetist choice
- Insertion of a perineural sciatic nerve catheter with an epidural catheter kit by surgeons +/- insertion of femoral nerve catheter with an epidural catheter kit or single shot femoral nerve block by the anaesthetist
- Initial intraoperative bolus of 10ml of 0.25% bupivacaine through both catheters irrespective of mode of anaesthesia
- Continuous infusion – 0.2% Ropivacaine using an Ambit pump
    - Basal rate – 10ml/hr (10ml/hr even if femoral + sciatic nerve catheters)
    - Bolus – 10ml of 0.2% Ropivacaine, 2 hour lockout
- PCA morphine if appropriate

POSTOPERATIVE REGIME:

- Gabapentinoids titrated to effect/side effects
- POD4 – Trial cessation of sciatic nerve catheter infusion. If pain recurs, restart 0.2% Ropivacaine infusion after a bolus of 10ml of 0.2% Ropivacaine via the pump
- POD6 - Repeat trial cessation

Figure 24.12.1 Sample of a multimodal perioperative pain management guideline

Reproduced from Aladin, H., Jennings, A., Hodges, M., and Tameem, A. (2018). Major lower limb amputation audit – introduction and implementation of a multimodal perioperative pain management guideline. *British Journal of Pain*, 12(4):230–237. http://doi.org/10.1177/2049463718769339

Early stump pain

- Should be treated with paracetamol, NSAIDs, and opioids with neural blockade if appropriate
- If neuropathic features are present, then TCAs and gabapentinoids should be instituted
- TENS—some evidence of its use in acute cases
- Baclofen, especially if stump contractions present

Acute phantom pain

- Salmon calcitonin:
  - Neuropeptide hormone
  - Alters β-endorphin, inhibits PG and cytokine production, and modulates central serotonergic pathways
  - SC for 5–7 days (100 IU/day)

Chronic stump and phantom pain

- Pharmacological treatment:
  - Anti-neuropathic agents—amitriptyline, gabapentin (moderate-quality evidence)
  - Anticonvulsants—carbamazepine, lamotrigine (for lancinating pain)
  - Opioids—morphine, tramadol (both have been shown to be beneficial)
  - NMDA antagonists—IV ketamine over 1 hour reduces phantom pain
  - Other drugs—calcitonin, capsaicin, lidocaine plasters, IT opioids (no good-quality evidence for these drugs)
  - Capsaicin 8% patches (Qutenzas®)—reduction in pain and stump hypersensitivity, enabling wearing stump prosthesis

Interventions

- Stump revision can be performed if there is stump pathology
- Neuroma excision
- Excision of Ca^{2+} deposits in heterotropic ossification
- SCS and dorsal root entry zone lesioning have had disappointing results
- Botulinum toxin injections have improved phantom pain

Psychological interventions

- Education, CBT, biofeedback, and hypnosis reduce severity of pain (low-quality evidence)

Other treatments

- Graded motor imagery (laterality, imagery, mirror therapy)
- TENS
- Physiotherapy, OT, and desensitization
- Prosthetics

Sample of a checklist used for major lower limb amputations in vascular surgery (see fig 24.12.2)

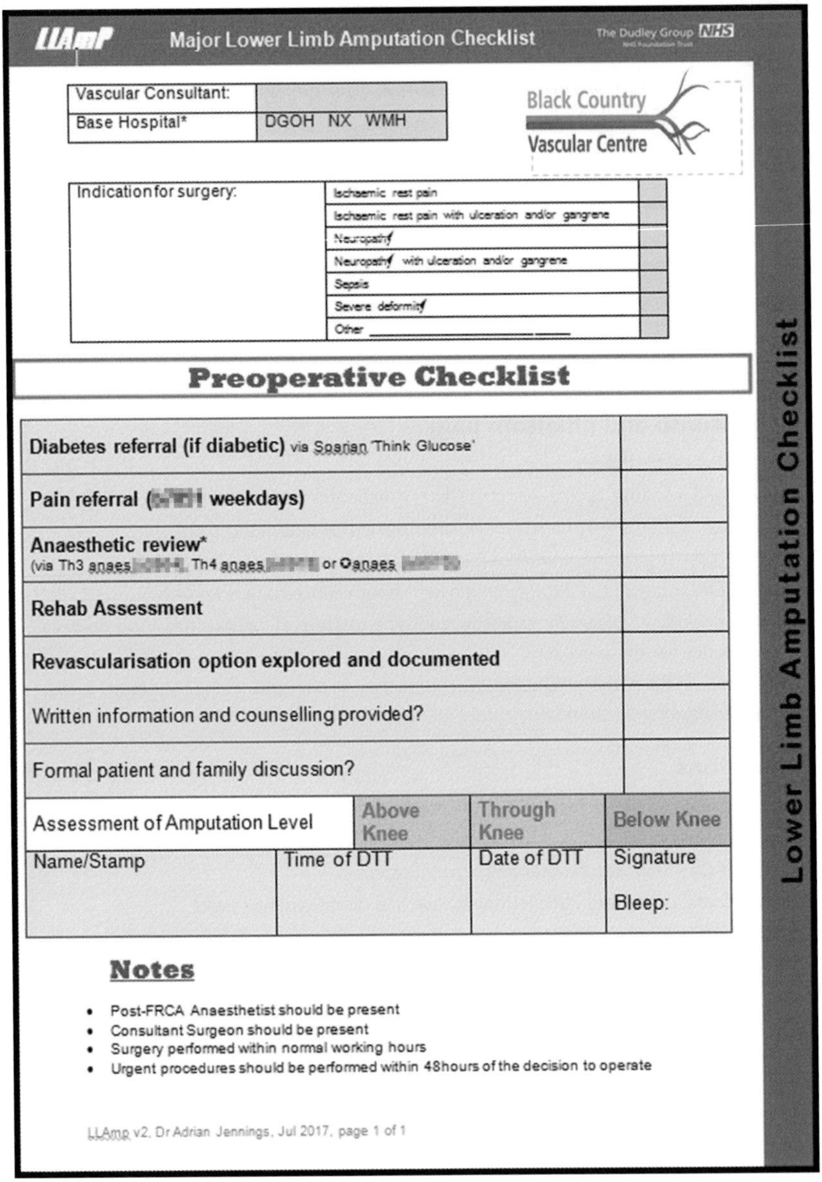

LLAmP Major Lower Limb Amputation Checklist The Dudley Group NHS

Vascular Consultant:	
Base Hospital*	DGOH NX WMH

Black Country Vascular Centre

Indication for surgery:		
	Ischaemic rest pain	
	Ischaemic rest pain with ulceration and/or gangrene	
	Neuropathy	
	Neuropathy with ulceration and/or gangrene	
	Sepsis	
	Severe deformity	
	Other ______________	

Preoperative Checklist

Diabetes referral (if diabetic) via Sparian 'Think Glucose'			
Pain referral ([redacted] **weekdays)**			
Anaesthetic review* (via Th3 anaes [redacted], Th4 anaes [redacted] or Oanaes [redacted])			
Rehab Assessment			
Revascularisation option explored and documented			
Written information and counselling provided?			
Formal patient and family discussion?			
Assessment of Amputation Level	Above Knee	Through Knee	Below Knee
Name/Stamp	Time of DTT	Date of DTT	Signature Bleep:

Notes

- Post-FRCA Anaesthetist should be present
- Consultant Surgeon should be present
- Surgery performed within normal working hours
- Urgent procedures should be performed within 48hours of the decision to operate

LLAmp v2. Dr Adrian Jennings, Jul 2017, page 1 of 1

Lower Limb Amputation Checklist

Figure 24.12.2 Sample of a checklist used for major lower limb amputations (vascular)

Reproduced from Aladin, H., Jennings, A., Hodges, M., and Tameem, A. (2018). Major lower limb amputation audit – introduction and implementation of a multimodal perioperative pain management guideline. *British Journal of Pain*, 12(4):230–237. http://doi.org/10.1177/2049463718769339

Further reading

1. Nikolajsen L. Phantom limb. In: Koltzenburg M, Tracey I, Turk D, McMahon SB (eds). Wall and Melzack's Textbook of Pain. 2013; pp. 915–25. Philadelphia, PA: Saunders.
2. Alviar MJM, Hale T, Dungca M. Pharmacologic interventions for treating phantom limb pain. Cochrane Database Syst Rev 2016;10:CD006380. doi: 10.1002/14651858.CD006380.pub3

24.13 Diabetic polyneuropathy

Definition

- Diabetic neuropathy is a type of nerve damage in diabetic patients without any other demonstrable causes of peripheral neuropathy
- High blood sugar levels can cause injury in nerves throughout the body, but most frequently in the legs and feet
- It is a common complication of diabetes but can often be prevented or slowed with tight blood sugar control and a healthy lifestyle
- It may or may not be painful

Types of diabetic neuropathy

- Several classifications—based on anatomical distribution (two main types)

Diffuse or generalized symmetrical neuropathy (most common)

- Chronic distal sensorimotor polyneuropathy (in feet/legs, then hands/arms)—most common cause of painful diabetic neuropathy. Pain affects QoL in 56% of these patients
- Acute sensory neuropathy
- Autonomic neuropathy—cardiovascular, GI, and genitourinary systems

Focal mononeuropathy (damage to a specific nerve) or multifocal neuropathy

- Cranial—face
- Truncal
- Focal limb neuropathy (usually in legs)
- Proximal neuropathy (diabetic amyotrophy) in thighs, hips, buttocks, and legs (sensory and motor systems can be affected)
- Chronic inflammatory demyelinating polyneuropathy—infiltration of inflammatory cells causes damage to myelin sheaths and vasa nervosum

Epidemiology and incidence

- Incidence and prevalence are difficult to verify (no consistent diagnostic criteria in studies)
- One-third of diabetic patients suffered from painful neuropathy (large community study in England)
- >50% of patients with chronic distal sensorimotor polyneuropathy complain of pain affecting their QoL
- Prevalence of chronic distal sensorimotor neuropathic polyneuropathy in type 1 diabetes is 5%, while in type 2 diabetes, it is 15–20%
- Incidence: men = women
- The incidence of non-painful versus painful diabetic polyneuropathy is higher

Pathophysiology (three theories)

Polyol pathway

- Conversion of excessive intraneural glucose to sorbitol and fructose via polyol pathway
- This causes reduced Na-K-ATPase activity, thus reduced production of NO and glutathione (vasodilators and buffer against oxidative injury), leading to chronic ischaemia

Microvascular damage theory

- Neural ischaemia due to endothelial hyperplasia and thickening of the basal membrane

Glycosylation end-product theory

- Reduced axonal transport in chronic hyperglycaemia, leading to accumulation of oxidative end-products around peripheral nerves, resulting in oxidative stress and damage

Other contributors to nerve injury

- Abnormal Ca^{2+} channel function and Na^{+} channel activity (role in painful neuropathy)

Risk factors

- Poor diabetic control (most important factor)
- Duration of diabetes
- Old age
- Overweight
- Dyslipidaemia (increased low-density lipoprotein or triglycerides)
- Hypertension
- Coexisting: kidney damage, smoking/alcohol
- Genetic predisposition

Symptoms

- Some with mild symptoms
- Can be quite painful and disabling

Distal symmetrical painful neuropathy

- Gradual onset, normally starts with sensory symptoms
- At the beginning, patients commonly have distal symmetrical burning or aching pain, which spreads proximally over time
- Length-dependent diabetic neuropathy (affects longer nerves first), involving the feet and legs in a stocking distribution
- Upper limb (hands/arms—glove distribution) may be involved in more severe cases
- Often worse at night
- Numbness (reduced pain/temperature sensation), tingling, burning, sharp, cramps, allodynia (pain on walking/standing/touching clothes), muscle weakness, loss of reflexes (ankle), loss of balance, foot ulcers/infections, bone and joint pain

Autonomic neuropathy

- Hypoglycaemia unawareness
- Bladder problems (infections, retention, incontinence)
- Constipation/diarrhoea or both
- Gastroparesis (nausea, vomiting, bloating, loss of appetite)

- Swallowing, sweating, and body temperature may be affected
- Accommodation of eyes affected
- Tachycardia at rest, postural hypotension
- Erectile dysfunction, vaginal dryness, reduced libido

Proximal neuropathy (diabetic amyotrophy)

- More common with type 2 diabetes and older adults
- Usually one-sided, but can spread to the other side of the body
- Severe pain in hip, thigh, and buttock area
- Weak, shrinking thigh muscles
- Difficulty rising from sitting position
- Weight loss
- Abdominal swelling is possible

Focal neuropathy (mono-neuropathy)

- Damage to a single nerve in the face, trunk, and legs
- More common in the elderly
- Can cause sudden, severe pain which usually goes away after weeks/months without treatment
- Pain in the shin/foot, anterior thigh, lower back, pelvis, chest, and abdomen
- Bell's palsy (one-sided facial paralysis)
- Eye (double vision, difficulty focusing, ache behind the eye)
- Carpal tunnel syndrome due to nerve compression

Diagnosis (exclusion of other factors)

Clinical history (symptoms)

- Burning pain, allodynia
- Sharp electric, current-like sensations
- Paraesthesiae, hyperaesthesia, and deep aching pain
- Pain usually worst at night, lower limbs more affected than upper limbs
- ANS involvement, particularly in long-standing diabetes (tachycardia, orthostatic hypotension, sexual dysfunction, altered gut motility, and loss of gastro-oesophageal function)

Neurological examination

- Loss of touch and pin prick pain sensation (early), filament test
- Loss of proprioception
- Loss of vibration sense
- Absent ankle reflex
- Gait ataxia
- Signs of peripheral autonomic dysfunctions in peripheries (e.g. cold feet, engorged veins)

Neuropathic pain questionnaires

- DN4, NPS, LANSS, NPSI, NPQ

Specific investigations

- NCS/EMG—detect large myelinated nerve dysfunction (α, β); cannot detect small fibre polyneuropathies (A-delta, C)

- Blood tests: sugar levels, HbA1c (glycosylated haemoglobin, e.g. twice per year)
- QST (vibration, temperature)—an increased sensory threshold correlates with sensory loss, and lowered thresholds with allodynia/hyperalgesia
- Autonomic function testing (supine and postural BP, sweating tests)
- Skin testing for epidermal nerve fibre density and morphology

Differential diagnoses

- Peripheral vascular disease
- Morton's neuroma
- Vitamin B12 deficiency
- Malnutrition
- Hypothyroidism
- Uraemia
- Restless legs syndrome
- Neuropathy from toxins, e.g. alcohol

Management/treatment

- Education—lifestyle modification (healthy diet, exercise, stopping smoking/drinking alcohol)
- Optimal glycaemic control (between 4.4 and 7.2 mmol/L before meals, below 10 mmol/L 2 hours after meals
- Care of diabetic ulcers
- Management of cardiovascular risk factors
- Pain management (symptomatic)

Pharmacological pain management

Tricyclic antidepressants

- Amitriptyline (NNT = 3.5)—increased risk of sudden cardiac death if >100 mg/day

Serotonin–noradrenaline reuptake inhibitors

- Good for coexisting depression
- First line is duloxetine—no significant difference between 60 mg once daily and 60 mg twice daily (both doses better than placebo)
- Venlafaxine NNT 4.5 for 150–225 mg of extended-release formulations

Antiepileptics

- Also useful in generalized anxiety disorder
- Gabapentinoids (pregabalin, gabapentin) bind to α-2 delta-1 subunit of Ca^{2+} channels, resulting in reduced release of excitatory neurotransmitters
- Evidence is weak for lamotrigine, topiramate, and carbamazepine
- Note: pregabalin facilitates sleep; duloxetine increases sleep fragmentation and reduces the rapid eye movement phase of sleep

Intravenous lidocaine infusion

- For further information, see 6.2 Lidocaine, p. 104

Topical capsaicin

- Focal treatment with capsaicin 0.025 or 0.075%, Qutenza® (8% capsaicin patches) 2–3 times per year (see 13.6 Capsaicin, p. 240)

Non-pharmacological pain management

- CBT, ACT, multidisciplinary pain management
- TENS, acupuncture (limited evidence)
- SCS (RCT showed reduced pain and improved QoL with refractory painful diabetic neuropathy in the lower extremities)

Management of complications

- Loss of toe, foot, or leg (infections, ulcers) → check feet daily; dry, clean, trimmed toenails
- Joint damage (Charcot joint)—surgical and non-surgical management
- Recurrent urinary infections and urinary incontinence (medication, strict schedule, self-catheterization)
- Hypoglycaemia (reduced awareness due to autonomic changes)—check blood sugar levels regularly
- Orthostatic hypotension (drink plenty of water, get up slowly, medication, sleep with head up, compression stockings)
- Digestive problems (eat smaller, more frequent meals; reduce fibre and fat; eat soups/pureed food; change diet for constipation, diarrhoea, and nausea)
- Sexual dysfunction (some medications, vacuum devices in men, lubricants in women)
- Increased or decreased sweating

Further reading

1. Daouisi C, Nurmikko TJ. Painful diabetic neuropathy. In: Stannard C, Kalso E, Ballantyne J (eds). Evidence-based Chronic Pain Management. 2010: pp. 204–221. Chichester, UK: Wiley-Blackwell
2. Haanpää M, Hietaharju A. Halting the march of painful diabetic neuropathy. International Association for the Study of Pain. Pain: Clinical Updates 2015;Vol. XXIII (No. 2)
3. Mayo Foundation for Medical Education and Research. Diabetic neuropathy. March 2020. https://www.mayoclinic.org/diseases-conditions/diabetic-neuropathy/symptoms-causes/syc-20371580
4. Rajan RS, de Gray L, George E. Painful diabetic neuropathy. Contin Educ Anaesth Crit Care Pain 2014;14:230–5

24.14 Charcot–Marie–Tooth syndrome

Introduction

- Charcot-Marie-Tooth syndrome (CMT) syndrome is a spectrum of inherited disorders caused by mutations of genes that are expressed in peripheral nerves (axons and/or myelin)
- Includes over 30 different disorders, the most common being types 1 and 2 and the primary X-linked form
- Autosomal dominant condition
- Rate of disability generally increases with age, with considerable variability, depending on the CMT subtype, age of onset, and clinical severity

Clinical features

CMT disease type I

- Demyelinating sensorimotor neuropathy
- Several types—CMT1A and CMT1B are the most common
- CMT1A, the most common mutation, is a duplication of the peripheral myelin protein gene on chromosome 22
- Onset typically in the first two decades of life
- Presents normally with walking difficulties and ankle sprains from:
  - Muscle weakness initially in leg calves. Distal wasting may produce the classical inverted champagne bottle deformity
  - Sensory loss: gradual, normally involves proprioception and vibration sense
  - Later changes: atrophied intrinsic muscles of the hands and feet
  - Pes cavus foot and kyphoscoliosis are normally associated
  - Sometimes there are palpable thickening of peripheral nerves
  - Life expectancy not affected

CMT disease type 2

- Axonal sensorimotor neuropathy—demyelination does not normally occur
- Onset in the second decade or later
- Sensory symptoms (decreased proprioception and vibration sense) are more marked than motor symptoms
- Usually there is areflexia in the legs only
- Structural deformities are not common
- Nerve conduction is slow, but always >38 m/s
- There is no palpable thickening of peripheral nerves

Management

- Specific treatment for CMT is currently unavailable
- Exclude other neuropathies (e.g. diabetes, immune-mediated, nutritional, etc.)
- Multidisciplinary interventions as per chronic pain management principles to improve function and well-being:
  - Physical treatments: strengthening, stretching, endurance, orthotics
  - Psychological treatments: CBT, ACT, cognitive restructuring, distraction, relaxation, mindfulness
  - Pharmacotherapy can be considered: TCAs, gabapentinoids, or SNRIs
- Avoid drugs that exacerbate the weakness and/or may harm the patient:
  - Definite risk: vinca alkaloids (vincristine), taxols (paclitaxel, docetaxel, cabazitaxel)
  - Moderate/significant risk: amiodarone, cisplatin, colchicine, fluoroquinolones
  - Minor risk: 5-fluorouracil, adriamycin, chloroquine, griseofulvin, hydralazine
  - Negligible risk: allopurinol, amitriptyline, chloramphenicol, clofibrate
- Alcohol is not a neurotoxic drug but affects balance and coordination, and overconsumption of alcohol is generally not recommended
- Surgery may be indicated to improve pain, function, and significant deformities associated with CMT such as:
  - Osteotomy—severe flat feet
  - Arthrodesis—severe flat feet and correcting heel deformities

    - Plantar fascia release—persistent heel pain from inflamed tendons
    - Spinal surgery—scoliosis causing severe functional impairment
- Research of new treatments:
    - Stem cells (cells at an early stage of development) to repair nerve damage
    - Hormonal and gene therapy to slow progression of CMT
    - Ascorbic acid has been used in some trials

Further reading

1. Kang PB. Charcot–Marie–Tooth disease: genetics, clinical features and diagnosis. 2020. https://uptodate.com
2. Kang PB. Charcot–Marie–Tooth disease: management and prognosis. 2020. https://uptodate.com.

Rheumatological Conditions

Sian Griffith

CONTENTS

25.1 Biomarkers and investigations in rheumatology

Inflammatory markers (ESR and CRP)

- ESR is an indirect measure of inflammatory response
- CRP is produced by the liver during an inflammatory response
- ESR and CRP can be increased in infection, inflammation, malignancy, and tissue injury
- ESR and CRP discrepancy can be due to difference in kinetics, with CRP rising and decreasing more rapidly than ESR
- ESR and/or CRP are usually elevated in patients with polymyalgia rheumatica, giant cell arteritis, vasculitides, and acute crystal arthropathy (vasculitides are a heterogenous group of autoimmune diseases, characterized by inflammation of blood vessels (vasculitis) and subsequent ischaemia and organ damage)
- ESR and/or CRP may, or may not, be increased in patients with RA and seronegative spondyloarthritis
- ESR and CRP are not increased in patients with OA or joint hypermobility syndrome
- Patients with SLE can have isolated elevation of ESR without an increase in CRP

Serum uric acid

- It is possible to have elevated serum uric acid without having gout
- Uric acid crystals should be present in synovial fluid to confirm diagnosis

Immunological tests

- Both rheumatoid factor and anti-cyclic citrullinated peptide (CCP) antibody should be tested in patients with suspected RA
- Patients with RA can test positive for anti-CCP antibody, rheumatoid factor, both antibodies, or neither antibody
- Anti-CCP is more specific, but rheumatoid factor is more sensitive

- High titre of rheumatoid factor is a better predictor for severe disease with extra-articular manifestations
- Anti-nuclear antibodies (ANA) are present in 3–15% of the healthy population
- ANA are present with varying frequency in patients with SLE, scleroderma, Sjögren's syndrome, polymyositis/dermatomyositis, mixed connective tissue disease, drug-induced lupus, juvenile inflammatory arthritis, and autoimmune hepatitis
- Patients with suspected connective tissue diseases are further characterized according to clinical features and the presence of other autoantibodies (anti-double-stranded DNA (dsDNA), anti-Ro, anti-La, anti-Sm, anti-RNP, anti-phospholipid, anti-centromere antibodies, anti-Scl-70)
- Creatine kinase (CK) should be measured if myositis suspected
- Measurement of complement activation (C3 and C4) can be useful in patients with SLE
- Anti-neutrophil cytoplasmic antibodies (ANCA) are frequently found in patients with granulomatosis with polyangitis, microscopic polyangitis, and eosinophilic granulomatosis with polyangitis, which are collectively known as the ANCA-associated vasculitides
- Any patient with suspected connective tissue disease or vasculitis must have urinalysis to look for haematuria and proteinuria

Imaging

- X-rays show characteristic changes in patients with long-standing rheumatic diseases (ankylosing spondylitis, gout, RA, and OA)
- US with power Doppler is used to detect synovitis in early inflammatory arthritis
- MRI with gadolinium enhancement, or MRI (T1 and STIR) is also used to detect early inflammatory arthritis in peripheral joints and the spine, respectively

Further reading

1. Bijlsma JWJ, Hachulla E. EULAR Textbook on Rheumatic Diseases. 2nd edition, 2015. London: BMJ Publishing Group Ltd
2. American College of Rheumatology. https://www.rheumatology.org
3. UpToDate. https://www.uptodate.com

25.2 Ankylosing spondylitis

Definition

- The term **ankylosing spondylitis (radiographic axial spondyloarthritis)** is reserved for patients with spinal symptoms and X-ray changes of sacroiliitis
- Patients often have other manifestations (enthesitis 40–60%) and/or acute anterior uveitis (30–50%)
- The term **non-radiographic axial spondyloarthritis** (nr-ax SpA) is used for patients with symptoms of inflammatory back pain (insidious onset, pain at night, age at onset <40 years, improvement with exercise but not with rest) without sacroiliitis on X-rays, although 70% have visible inflammation in the SIJs and/or the spine when MRI of the whole spine and SIJ (T1 and STIR) is done
- Axial spondyloarthritis (radiographic and non-radiographic) is also found in patients with psoriatic arthritis, inflammatory bowel disease (ulcerative colitis and Crohn's disease), reactive arthritis, and juvenile spondyloarthritis.

Prevalence

- 0.2–0.5% (this varies according to the prevalence of the HLA-B27 gene in different ethnic groups)
- The chance of developing ankylosing spondylitis in HLA-B27-positive patients is 1–5%; it increases to 15–20% in the case of an affected first-degree relative

Pathophysiology

- Aetiology is unknown
- Thought to reflect a complex interplay of genetic and environmental factors
- Inflammation affecting SIJs, entheses, vertebral bodies, peripheral joints, GI tract, and the eyes

Diagnosis

- It is suspected in patients with symptoms of inflammatory back pain and confirmed by X-ray (ankylosing spondylitis), or alternatively by specialized MRI (patients with nr-ax SpA)
- Usually diagnosed by a rheumatologist, or referred to rheumatology services shortly after diagnosis

Treatment of early disease

1. **Education** about diagnosis and prognosis
2. Importance of **exercise** to help symptoms and maintain posture, ROM, and aerobic fitness. Referral to physiotherapists and patient support groups (National Ankylosing Spondylitis Society (NASS))
3. Strongly advised to **stop smoking**
4. NSAIDs and **simple analgesics**
5. **Injection** of SIJs with corticosteroid (image-guided)
6. Injection of costochondral joints, peripheral joints, entheses, and plantar fascia if required
7. **Ongoing assessment** of patients using standard scores such as BASDAI (Bath Ankylosing Spondylitis Disease Activity Index) and BASFI (Bath Ankylosing Spondylitis Functional Index), measuring ROM
8. Identification of patients not responding to NSAIDs and exercise—for treatment with **biologic medication (TNF alpha inhibitor or other agent)**
9. Biologic medication prescribed by a rheumatologist (national guidance)
10. **Conventional disease-modifying anti-rheumatic medication** (cDMARD) such as sulfasalazine, methotrexate, or leflunomide if there is peripheral arthritis
11. **Advice** with regard to workplace, conception, and pregnancy
12. **Ongoing monitoring** for complications of disease or treatment

Treatment of long-standing disease

1. Assessment to distinguish mechanical problems (fixed rigid spine, osteoarthritic hips and shoulders) from **ongoing inflammatory problems**
2. **Further investigations** if spinal fracture (this can occur after minor trauma in patients with rigid osteoporotic spines), spinal instability, or spinal stenosis suspected
3. **Management of inflammatory disease**, as for early disease
4. **Surgical referral**, if required, for shoulder and hip disease
5. Diagnosis and treatment of **coexisting osteoporosis**
6. **Ongoing surveillance** for aortic regurgitation, risk factors for IHD and apical pulmonary fibrosis
7. Appropriate **exercise** regimes for established disease
8. **Environmental modifications** to help with physical limitations due to loss of spinal mobility (prism spectacles, large driving mirrors, domestic aids and appliances)

9. Adequate **pain relief** (paracetamol, occasionally opioids and anti-neuropathics)
10. Occasionally facet joint injection (if thought to be source of pain)

Further reading

1. Bijlsma JWJ, Hachulla E. EULAR Textbook on Rheumatic Diseases. 2nd edition, 2015. London: BMJ Publishing Group Ltd
2. National Axial Spondyloarthritis Society. http://nass.co.uk/

25.3 Gout

Definition

- Gout is a monosodium urate (MSU) crystal deposition disease

Prevalence

- 3% of the population
- Male:female ratio 20:1
- Increasing prevalence linked to increased longevity, age-associated cardiovascular, metabolic, and renal disease, medications, and increased consumption of foods that contribute to obesity and diabetes mellitus

Pathophysiology

- Serum uric acid (SUA) levels are influenced by the total amount of SUA produced, renal clearance of urate, and intestinal excretion of urate
- Release of MSU crystals results in an intense inflammatory response involving neutrophils, monocytes/macrophages, and lymphocytes
- Joints most often affected are the feet, ankles, and knees, although Achilles tendons, olecranon bursae, wrists, and metacarpophalangeal (MCP) and proximal interphalangeal joints can also be involved

Diagnosis

- Usually presents as episodes of acute monoarthritis (podagra = gouty arthritis in the metatarsophalangeal joint of the big toe has high specificity >97% and sensitivity >96%)
- Tophi occur in long-standing undertreated gout and represent deposits of MSU crystals
- Identification of MSU crystals in synovial fluid from joints (needle aspiration) during an acute attack (specificity: 100%, sensitivity: 84%), asymptomatic joints during inter-critical periods, or tophi allows a definitive diagnosis
- Blood test: elevated serum uric acid > 6mg/dL (normal range: 3-8 mg/dL or 0.18-0.48 mmol/L, but age and gender differences) low sensitivity: 67% and specificity: 78%)
- 'Punched-out' erosions with sclerotic margins and overhanging edges in a marginal and juxta-articular distribution on X-rays
- US to identify the characteristic 'double contour sign' in articular cartilage, erosions, and tophaceous deposits

Treatment

1. Management of gout is often suboptimal, leading to undertreated patients with ongoing symptoms

2. Acute attacks managed with low-dose **colchicine** (0.5 mg three times daily), NSAIDs, intra-articular steroid, or PO steroids
3. **Allopurinol** is started at a low dose (100 mg daily), and titrated upwards in 100 mg increments, every few weeks, until SUA <300 micromoles/L (allopurinol dose reduced in patients with renal dysfunction)
4. Patients often need treatment with low-dose colchicine, **NSAIDs, or low-dose steroids** for the first 3–6 months of treatment with any urate-lowering medication
5. **Febuxostat** can be used in patients with renal insufficiency or intolerance of allopurinol, but it is avoided in patients with IHD or heart failure
6. **Benzbromarone** is an effective uricosuric drug, which can be used in patients with mild to moderate renal impairment or who are refractory to allopurinol. Specialist use on a named-patient basis only in many countries
7. **Losartan and fenofibrate** have modest SUA-lowering effect and can be used as co-adjuvants in patients also requiring treatment for hypertension and hyperlipidaemia
8. Patients should be given **lifestyle advice** (maintaining healthy BMI, avoiding large quantities of shellfish, offal, and sugar-sweetened soft drinks, and reducing alcohol intake in line with national guidance)
9. Cardiovascular risk factors should be addressed, as gout is independently associated with risk of MI

Further reading

1. Bijlsma JWJ, Hachulla E. EULAR Textbook on Rheumatic Diseases. 2nd edition, 2015. London: BMJ Publishing Group Ltd
2. Hui M, Carr A, Cameron S, et al. for the British Society for Rheumatology Standards, Audit and Guidelines Working Group, The British Society for Rheumatology Guideline for the Management of Gout. Rheumatology, Volume 56, Issue 7, July 2017, p. e1–e20. http://academic.oup.com/rheumatology/article/56/7/e1/3855179
3. Gaffo AL, Dalbeth N, Romain PL. Clinical manifestations and diagnosis of gout. UpToDate. 2019 https://www.uptodate.com/contents/clinical-manifestations-and-diagnosis-of-gout
4. Zhang W, Doherty M, Pascual E et al. EULAR evidence based recommendations for gout. Part I: Diagnosis. Report of a task force of the Standing Committee for International Clinical Studies Including Therapeutics (ESCISIT). Ann Rheum Dis. 2006;65:1301–11

25.4 Joint hypermobility syndrome

Prevalence

- 10–20% of the population have joint hypermobility
- 10–20% of those with joint hypermobility report additional symptoms of fibromyalgia, GI disturbance, bladder symptoms, and autonomic dysfunction
- This is sometimes referred to as joint hypermobility syndrome (JHS), although there is debate about whether this is a discreet entity from fibromyalgia/chronic widespread pain

Pathophysiology

- Lack of well-defined biologic marker contrasts with other hereditary conditions of connective tissue (Marfan's syndrome, osteogenesis imperfecta, Ehlers–Danlos syndrome (EDS)—classic type or vascular type)

Diagnosis

- Joint hypermobility is ascertained if a patient scores ≥4 points using the Beighton score for hypermobility:
  - Passive apposition of thumb to forearm (2 points)
  - Passive dorsiflexion of fifth MCP joint (2 points)
  - Hyperextension of the elbow (2 points)
  - Hyperextension of the knee (2 points)
  - Flexion of lumbar spine with the hands flat on the floor (1 point)
- The Brighton criteria (1998) can be used to screen patients for JHS
- Diagnosis is usually based on clinical features without additional testing. Thought to be indistinguishable from EDS-hypermobility type (previously referred to as EDS type III)
- Occasional need for cardiovascular investigations, ophthalmology review, skin biopsy, or genetic testing if features of Marfan's syndrome, EDS-classic type, or EDS-vascular type

Treatment

1. **Physiotherapy** with emphasis on self-management, specific advice as required, for localized issues (joint subluxation, soft tissue problems)
2. **Holistic care** with advice on symptom management to avoid referral to multiple specialties
3. **Reassurance and psychological support** as association with anxiety and depression
4. Input from **OT** with regard to workplace or ADL
5. Pain managed with **simple analgesics** and short courses of NSAIDs
6. **Multidisciplinary approach** if features of chronic widespread pain/fibromyalgia
7. **Referral to specialist services** if symptomatic orthostatic hypotension or postural tachycardia syndrome
8. Urological or gastroenterology advice if bladder symptoms (dysuria, frequency) or bowel symptoms (reflux, irritable bowel symptoms) not controlled with usual measures
9. Reports of reduced response to LAs in some patients with JHS

Further reading

1. Hakim AJ, Grahame R, Norris P, et al. Local anaesthetic failure in joint hypermobility syndrome. J R Soc Med 2005;98(2):84–5
2. UpToDate. https://www.uptodate.com

25.5 Osteoporosis

Definition

- Osteoporosis is a generalized bone disease, characterized by decreased bone mass and deterioration of bone microarchitecture, resulting in increased fracture risk
- Osteoporosis does not cause pain. Pain occurs acutely with fragility fractures. Vertebral fractures can be associated with chronic spinal pain, reduced QoL, and reduced life expectancy

Prevalence

- In Caucasian populations, 50% of women and 20% of men over the age of 50 will experience a fragility fracture in their remaining lifetime

Pathophysiology

- Increased risk of fracture is associated with low peak bone mass, old age, sex steroid deficiency, lipid oxidation, decreased physical activity, use of steroids, and a propensity to fall
- Low bone mass may be secondary to underlying disease
- The following investigations may be required: FBC, ESR, urea and electrolytes, LFTs, bone profile, 25-hydroxyvitamin D, thyroid-stimulating hormone (TSH), coeliac screen, testosterone, serum and urine immunoelectrophoresis, 24-hour urinary Ca^{2+}, 24-hour urinary cortisol

Diagnosis

- Diagnosis can be made clinically (patients with vertebral fragility fracture or patients >75 years with low trauma impact fracture) without the need for bone mineral density (BMD) measurement
- In other patients, BMD measurement is combined with validated risk factors for fracture to give a treatment intervention threshold (e.g. FRAX® = Fracture Risk Assessment Tool)
- For epidemiological purposes, osteoporosis has been defined as a BMD of >2.5 SDs below the mean peak BMD in healthy adults of the same gender, which is expressed as T-score <−2.5 (see Bone density scan (DEXA scan = Dual-Energy X-ray Absorptiometry) in 1.7 Investigations in pain medicine, p. 22)
- Any patient with a vertebral fragility fracture as an incidental finding should be investigated for underlying disease and offered treatment

Management of acute vertebral fracture

1. Can be asymptomatic or painful (6–12 weeks)
2. Pain usually treated with **paracetamol, ibuprofen, naproxen, or co-codamol**
3. **Tramadol and opioids** may be needed
4. **Calcitonin** daily or on alternate days can be given for 2–4 weeks
5. **Vertebroplasty or kyphoplasty** can be used if pain, due to recent unhealed fracture, not controlled by analgesics (see 22.9 Vertebroplasty, p. 438)
6. **Malignancy needs to be excluded** as a cause of acute vertebral collapse
7. All patients with osteoporotic vertebral collapse need to commence appropriate **long-term treatment** in accordance with local pathways (PO and IV bisphosphonates: alendronic acid, risedronate sodium, IV zoledronic acid; human monoclonal antibodies: denosumab; parathyroid hormone analogue: teriparatide)
8. **All treatments are given in conjunction with calcium and vitamin D supplementation**
9. **Education** about the need for long-term medication, and follow-up to check adherence
10. **Physiotherapy and OT** to restore functional status

Management of chronic vertebral fracture

1. Some patients suffer chronic pain as a result of spinal deformity
2. May need regular oral analgesia such as **paracetamol, opioids, and/or anti-neuropathics**
3. **Change osteoporosis** medication if evidence of progressive vertebral collapse
4. **Psychological support** to help with problems associated with spinal deformity
5. **Environmental and workplace modifications** to help with physical limitations
6. **Occasional use of facet joint injection** if secondary OA thought to be source of pain (systemic absorption is low, with minor impact on osteoporosis; consider LA alone or LA with low-dose steroid, particularly in frail/elderly patients)

Prevention of osteoporosis

- Healthy balanced diet (high in calcium)
- Increased exposure to sunlight (to help increase vitamin D levels) and/or vitamin D supplementation
- Regular weight-bearing exercises (e.g. walking, running)

Further reading

1. Bijlsma JWJ, Hachulla E. EULAR Textbook on Rheumatic Diseases. 2nd edition, 2015. London: BMJ Publishing Group Ltd
2. Fracture Risk Assessment Tool (FRAX®). http://www.shef.ac.uk/FRAX/
3. UpToDate. https://www.uptodate.com

25.6 Rheumatoid arthritis

Definition

- Rheumatoid arthritis is a chronic inflammatory disorder that typically affects small and medium-sized joints in a symmetrical fashion
- Heterogenous disease with variable mode of disease onset and disease course

Prevalence

- 0.5–1% of European and North American adults
- Female:male ratio 3:1

Pathophysiology

- Generally accepted to be an autoimmune disease despite failure to identify a dominant arthritogenic antigen
- Aetiology thought to be an interplay of genetic (in particular, HLA-DRB1 alleles) and environmental factors (most importantly smoking)
- Many important cell types and cytokines (T cells, B cells, mast cells, monocytes, and inflammatory cytokines), which are now therapeutic targets

Diagnosis

- Clinical diagnosis based on signs and symptoms
- Swelling of MCP, proximal interphalangeal, wrists, and metatarsophalangeal (MTP) joints is typical of disease at onset
- ESR/CRP not always elevated
- Anti-CCP antibodies (or ACPA) is found in 60–70% of RA patients and is more specific than rheumatoid factor for the disease
- US can detect synovitis and erosions in early disease
- MRI can detect early erosions and bone marrow oedema (non-specific). Synovitis can be seen with gadolinium enhancement
- X-ray of hands and feet: joint space loss and erosions in established disease

Treatment of early disease

1. Early introduction of **cDMARDs** as priority (methotrexate is the anchor drug, in both monotherapy and combination therapy, due to favourable efficacy:toxicity ratio)

2. **Alternative cDMARDs** (leflunomide, sulfasalazine, and hydroxychloroquine) can be used in combination with methotrexate or as an alternative to methotrexate
3. **Steroids** in low to moderate doses can be used in early disease, although long-term use should be avoided
4. Patients who do not respond to maximum-dose methotrexate, or an alternative cDMARD (sequentially or in combination), are considered for **biologic therapy (T cell co-stimulation inhibitor, TNF alpha inhibitor, B cell inhibitor, IL6 inhibitor, JAK inhibitor)**
5. Patients on biologic therapy are usually continued on methotrexate, or an alternative cDMARD
6. Flare-ups can be helped by short-term **NSAIDs or intra-articular steroid**, with upward titration of cDMARD/biologic therapy to avoid further disease flare
7. **Education and emotional support** to include pregnancy and work issues
8. Access to **physiotherapists, podiatrists, and occupational therapists**

Treatment of long-standing disease

1. **Ongoing assessment** to distinguish mechanical from inflammatory problems
2. **Surgical referral** for carpal tunnel decompression, tendon repairs, and arthroplasty
3. Cervical spine assessment prior to anaesthesia because of risk of atlanto-axial subluxation
4. **Detection of systemic complications** such as vasculitis, neuropathies, secondary Sjögren's syndrome, and pulmonary fibrosis
5. Detection and management of **risk factors for cardiovascular disease**
6. Treatment for **osteoporosis**
7. **Adequate analgesia** (paracetamol, **NSAIDs**, occasionally opioids and anti-neuropathics)
8. Encouragement to **exercise**
9. Help with **mobility aids and home adaptations** if required
10. Occasional use of blocks (e.g. occipital nerve block, suprascapular nerve block)

Further reading

1. Bijlsma JWJ, Hachulla E. EULAR Textbook on Rheumatic Diseases. 2nd edition, 2015. London: BMJ Publishing Group Ltd

25.7 Systemic lupus erythematosus

Definition

- Systemic lupus erythematosus (SLE) is a multisystem autoimmune disease with a broad spectrum of clinical presentation encompassing almost all organs and tissues

Incidence

- 20–150 per 100 000 (depending on ethnicity)
- Female:male ratio 9:1

Pathophysiology

- Interaction between hormonal status, genes, and environment changing immune tolerance to endogenous nuclear antigens

Diagnosis

- Requires integration of symptoms, physical examination findings, and results of diagnostic tests
- 65% of patients have disease onset aged between 16 and 55 years
- Most common symptoms are arthralgia, constitutional symptoms, rashes, and arthritis
- Clinical manifestations also include: renal disease, Raynaud's, cognitive and psychiatric symptoms, fits, vasculitis, mouth ulcers, pancreatitis, inflammatory bowel disease, lymphadenopathy, pleurisy, pericarditis, interstitial lung disease, and thrombotic disease
- Patients with suspected SLE should be specifically asked about rashes, photosensitivity, Raynaud's phenomenon, oral ulcers, arthritis, hair loss, shortness of breath, pleuritic chest pain, fever, and fatigue
- Physical examination to look for rashes, alopecia, oral ulceration, lymphadenopathy, splenomegaly, pericardial or pleural effusion, and peripheral oedema. Fundoscopy to look for cotton wool spots
- **BP and urinalysis at every clinical encounter because of risk of occult renal involvement**
- Haematological findings include anaemia, leucopenia, or thrombocytopenia
- ANA is 95% sensitive but has a low specificity
- 70% of patients have antibodies to dsDNA, with 95% specificity
- Anti-Sm antibody in 10–30%
- Patients may have positive anti-phospholipid antibodies, anti-Ro, anti-La, and anti-ribonucleoprotein (RNP)
- Complement (C3 and C4) can be reduced in active disease
- Further investigations: neuropsychiatric symptoms (MRI, EEG, NCS), cardiorespiratory symptoms (ECG, CXR, cardiac echocardiography, high-resolution CT chest), musculoskeletal symptoms (X-ray, US, MRI, CK, EMG), suspected renal involvement (renal biopsy), GI (amylase, CT)

Treatment

1. **Hydroxychloroquine**, alone for mild joint and skin disease, and in combination with other medications for more severe disease
2. **Corticosteroid** (high dose for severe disease)
3. **Azathioprine, ciclosporin A, methotrexate, mycophenolate mofetil, cyclophosphamide**, depending on organ involvement and severity
4. **B cell-targeted therapies** (rituximab and belimumab for refractory disease)
5. Detection and management of **risk factors** for cardiovascular disease
6. **Prevention of steroid-induced osteoporosis**
7. **Detailed advice** on fertility, pregnancy, and breastfeeding
8. **Simple analgesics/NSAIDs** if required to manage joint pain
9. Advice on **pacing and graded exercise** to help with fatigue

Further reading

1. Bijlsma JWJ, Hachulla E. EULAR Textbook on Rheumatic Diseases. 2nd edition, 2015. London: BMJ Publishing Group Ltd

Visceral Pain Conditions

Enrique Collantes, Paolo Pais, Jan Rudiger, and Athmaja Thottungal

CONTENTS

26.1 Overview of visceral pain

Introduction—classification of visceral pain

- True visceral pain (tissue insult): nociception arising from neural sources in deep organs of the body
- Visceral hyperalgesia (visceral allodynia): stimuli which are not noxious are interpreted as pain due to alterations in nerves carrying sensations from the viscera, causing changes in visceral sensitivity at either the peripheral or the central level
- Referred pain:
  - Viscero-visceral referral: one sensitized organ causes sensitization of another visceral organ
  - Viscero-somatic referral: visceral pain causes referred somatic pain
  - Somatic-visceral referral: somatic pain causes referred visceral pain

Overview

- Common and high prevalence, e.g. renal colic, dysmenorrhoea, IBS, MI
- Pain arising from internal organs of the body, including cardiac, airway structures, GI tract, and upper abdominal, renal, and reproductive organs
- Prompt assessment is important as can be part of a life-threatening presentation such as MI, acute pancreatitis, bowel obstruction, and peritonitis. Due to its diffuse nature, poor localization, and changing nature over time, it is difficult to distinguish life-threatening from non-life-threatening visceral pain syndromes such as IBS
- Concurrence of visceral and somatic pain syndromes is common
- Multiple factors cause and/or modify visceral pain such as psychosocial stress, mental health disorders, genetic factors, life events (e.g. abuse, life-threatening event, trauma), and biomedical factors

True visceral pain/visceral nociception

- Vague, diffuse, poorly defined sensation felt in the midline, regardless of the internal organ of origin
- There are various causes such as infection, inflammation, mechanical stretch/distension/obstruction, neoplasm, ischaemia, e.g. myocardial ischaemia, and renal stones
- Pain from the pancreas, gall bladder, duodenum, heart, stomach, and oesophagus is normally felt in the upper abdomen and lower sternum. Palpation in this area does not normally worsen the pain
- Can be described as a compression or pressure
- Poor correlation between the intensity of pain and the magnitude of internal organ damage, e.g. patients with angina can have severe pain, compared with silent MI which is painless
- Can be associated with strong emotional (anxiety, fear, angry) and autonomic (pallor, sweating, discomfort, nausea, vomiting, bradycardia, low BP, diarrhoea) responses

Visceral hyperalgesia/visceral allodynia

- Slow and poorly localized, and may not even feel like pain, e.g. colic, abdominal distension/bloating
- Pain from normal physiological visceral stimulus due to increased sensitivity of that organ when there is no tissue insult, e.g. eating food in functional dyspepsia or passing urine in painful bladder syndrome
- Visceral hyperalgesia can be associated with a nociceptive, neuropathic and/or an inflammatory process
- It can also be associated with a traumatic event such as abuse, maternal separation, war, and torture
- Some causes of visceral hyperalgesia:
  - Thorax: non-cardiac chest pain, functional dyspepsia
  - Abdomen: idiopathic dyspepsia, IBS, functional abdominal pain
  - Pelvis: painful bladder syndrome, urethral pain syndrome, persistent interstitial cystitis, chronic non-bacterial prostatitis, pudendal neuralgia, vaginal pain syndrome, vulvar pain syndrome, anorectal pain syndrome

Viscero-visceral referral

- One sensitized organ causes sensitization of another organ when the two internal organs share a common sensory afferent nerve or from afferent 'cross-talk' in the DH
- Some causes of viscero-visceral referral:
  - The heart and gall bladder have overlapping (T5) afferent pathways: in patients with IHD and gall bladder disease, treatment of gall bladder calculi can reduce the number of angina attacks and coronary revascularization can reduce the number of biliary colics
  - The renal system and the uterus have overlapping afferent nerve pathways (T10–L1 afferents)—patients treated with hormonal therapy for dysmenorrhoea can decrease the frequency of renal colics

Viscero-somatic referral

- Visceral pain causes referred somatic pain. Thorough history, examination, and investigations must be done to determine if pain is somatic or referred
- Somatic referred pain is better localized, sharper, and less likely to be associated with emotional and neurovegetative signs. It can have a similar presentation to deep somatic nociceptive pain

- Somatic referred pain can be associated with hyperalgesia, resulting in increased sensitivity in muscles, skin, and SC tissue innervated by the somatic spinal nerve. For example, patients with dysmenorrhoea can have tenderness on deep palpation of the suprapubic area between painful periods
- Example of pain syndromes with viscero-somatic referral:
  - Renal colic: hypersensitive lumbar muscles (quadratus lumborum, obliques) and pain in flank and groin, even after the calculi have been passed
  - Acute myocardial ischaemia: pain in the chest radiating down the arm (C8–T1 dermatomes)

Somatic-viscero referral

- Similar mechanisms to those of viscero-somatic referral
- Deep palpation of muscle can reproduce visceral pain in people with profound muscle hyperalgesia. For example, deep palpation in flank and groin can elicit visceral pain from the genitourinary system even after a renal calculi has been passed
- Treatment of somatic referred pain can improve visceral pain.

Management

- Good patient/doctor relationship
- Address the underlying pathology
- Ensure that there are no red flags/pathologies amenable to treatment. Sometimes the cause of the pain is not identified
- Patient education, realistic goal setting, healthy lifestyle, and weight control
- Multidisciplinary and multimodal approaches
- Important to address the psychosocial components of the presentations
- Psychology: CBT, hypnotherapy, ACT, or other psychological treatments
- Physiotherapy: pacing, regular exercise/stretching, or other treatments that improve function and prevent deconditioning
- Interventional pain medicine can be highly effective in some visceral presentations:
  - SCS can be effective in selective patients with chest pain from angina (improved myocardial oxygen delivery and reduction of frequency of angina attacks), IBS (sacral SCS), functional dyspepsia (may work by improving gastroparesis), and refractory pelvic pain
  - Neurolytic blocks are highly effective for cancer pain, e.g. coeliac block in pain from pancreatic cancer (its use in pain from chronic pancreatitis is controversial)
- Pharmacotherapy:
  - Anti-neuropathic agents: TCAs, SNRIs, gabapentinoids (more information on antidepressants and gabapentinoids can be found in Chapters 9 and 10)
  - Spasmolytics: antispastics (e.g., baclofen), benzodiazepines (e.g., diazepam, clonazepam, temazepam), non-benzodiazepine antispasmodics (carisoprodol, cyclobenzaprine, metaxalone, methocarbamol, thiocolchicoside, tizanidine, tolperisone, orphenadrine) and miscellaneous (botulinum toxin, eszopiclone). The choice of muscle relaxant and evidence supporting different muscle relaxants is very variable and long-term use of some of these medications are associated with patient harm. Some of these spasmolytics are discussed in more detail in Chapter 13 (13.1 baclofen, 13.3 botulinum toxin, 13.7 clonazepam, 13.15 orphenadrine)
  - Anxiolytics: atypical antipsychotics such as quetiapine, α-2 agonists, antidepressants, BZDs in highly selected patient groups in the short term
  - Avoid reliance on opioids

Visceral pain in the elderly

- Visceral pain is more common in the elderly
- Visceral pathologies have more atypical presentations in the elderly:
  - Cardiovascular—some studies quote up to 30% of MIs in the elderly are silent MIs
  - Respiratory—pneumothorax
  - Abdominal complaints—up to 45% of the elderly with appendicitis do not have right lower quadrant abdominal pain

Visceral pain and gender

- Gender-specific conditions: menstrual pain, labour pain, post-partum visceral pain
- Anatomical differences in different genders: women are more likely to develop genitourinary tract infections due to having a shorter urethra
- Some conditions are more common in one gender, with no clear organic explanation, likely due to genetic factors. For example:
  - Females—higher prevalence of IBS and gall bladder disease
  - Males—higher prevalence of IHD

Further reading

1. IASP Global Year against visceral pain 2012 available on: https://www.iasp-pain.org/advocacy/global-year/visceral-pain/
2. Giamberardino MA. Visceral Pain. IASP Pain Clinical Updates. Volume XIII, No.6. Dec 2005. IASP Press.

26.2 Chronic abdominal pain

Definition

- Chronic abdominal pain is continuous or intermittent abdominal pain or discomfort lasting for at least 6 months

Incidence

- The incidence of chronic abdominal pain and the aetiology in paediatric, adolescent, and adult populations vary and treatment modalities differ
- The aetiology is multifactorial and variable in each age group
- Unspecified abdominal pain is reported in 22.9 per 1000 person-years
- Epidemiological studies describe 25% of the population reporting abdominal pain
- Differences in reporting, depending on ethnicity and geographical regions

Anatomical correlation

- Pain may arise from any structures inside the abdomen, or it could be referred pain
- It may originate from visceral organs, MSK parts, or neural tissue

Common causes

- Broadly classified as:
  - Gastrointestinal
  - Genitourinary

- Gynaecological
- Neurological
- Metabolic
- Psychological
- Functional

Pathophysiology

- Induced by stimulation of visceral nociceptors
- This can lead to both peripheral and central sensitization, which explains the amplification of pain perception and referred pain to other parts of the body
- The interaction between visceral pathology and altered central pain processing causes discrepancy between objective signs peripherally and increased central pain perception
- Central sensitization and psychological causes have a poor prognostic outcome

Common underlying pathologies

Inflammatory causes

- Inflammatory bowel disease
- Chronic pancreatitis
- Chronic appendicitis
- Coeliac disease
- Pelvic inflammatory disease
- Primary sclerosing cholangitis
- Fibrosing mesenteritis
- Eosinophilic gastroenteritis

Infection

- Parasites
- TB
- Viral infections
- Other bacterial infections (*Helicobacter pylori*)

Vascular

- Mesenteric ischaemia
- Coeliac artery syndrome
- Superior mesenteric artery syndrome

Metabolic

- Diabetic neuropathy
- Hereditary angio-oedema
- Familial Mediterranean fever
- Porphyria

Neuromuscular causes

- Anterior cutaneous entrapment syndrome
- Myofascial pain syndromes, e.g. rectus abdominis syndrome
- Twelfth rib syndrome
- Thoracic neuropathy

- Radiculopathy secondary to back problems
- Hernias
- Levator ani syndrome

Functional

- Constipation
- IBS
- Sphincter of Oddi dysfunction
- Functional abdominal pain syndrome
- Dyspepsia
- Gastroparesis

Other

- Peptic ulcer
- Gallstones
- Endometriosis
- Adhesions
- Neoplasms
- Intestinal obstruction
- Lactose intolerance
- Food allergies
- Intestinal malrotation

Diagnosis

History

- Detailed history is paramount, including history of origin, duration, character, radiation, relationship to food, medications (opioid-induced constipation and OIH), changes with body position, previous abdominopelvic surgeries, and positioning, especially prolonged lithotomy positioning if pelvic pain is present with abdominal pain
- Type of pain—visceral, somatic, or referred
- In chronic abdominal pain associated with pelvic pain ± depression, detailed psychosocial and sexual history is mandatory
- Menstrual and obstetric history for females
- History suggestive of any red and yellow flags

Examination/tests

- General examination (a quadrant-based examination will help to identify potential pain generators, followed by inspection, palpation, percussion, and auscultation)
- Manual examination of the abdomen, including per vaginal and per rectal examination
- Routine blood tests—FBC, LFTs, amylase, lipase, Hb electrophoresis, porphyrin levels, lead, inflammatory markers (CRP, ESR)
- Stool examination—parasites, occult blood
- Urine examination—infection
- Endoscopy—gastroscopy, colonoscopy, cystoscopy, sigmoidoscopy
- Barium studies
- Laparoscopic examination
- USS/MRI/CT—mainly to rule out sinister pathologies

Differential diagnosis

- Differential diagnosis is difficult as multifactorial aetiology in chronic abdominal pain. Depending on the clinical picture, a possible differential diagnosis is made based on the primary organ involved and neighbouring structures

Treatment

- A multidisciplinary and multimodal approach is crucial for success of therapy as for other chronic pain conditions

Conservative (some with limited evidence)

- Lifestyle change—to avoid constipation and food if intolerance, weight reduction, to stop smoking, and to avoid excessive alcohol consumption
- Adapting sitting position
- Physiotherapy for MSK structures
- Acupuncture
- Heat/cold application
- TENS
- CBT and other psychotherapies
- Biofeedback techniques
- Nutritional therapy

Pharmacological

- Simple analgesics
- Anti-neuropathic medications—anticonvulsants, antidepressants
- Avoid chronic use of opioids as can cause constipation and OIH
- Proton pump inhibitors if indicated
- Treat infections
- Nutritional supplements

Interventions (under X-ray, CT, or US guidance as indicated)

- Nerve blocks—peripheral, DRG, nerve root block, and neuraxial block
- LA and steroid injection (TPIs or facial plane blocks)
- Epidural—thoracic/lumbar/caudal
- Sympathetic block—coeliac ganglion, aorto-renal ganglion, superior mesenteric ganglion, mesenteric ganglion, and hypogastric plexus

Neuromodulation techniques

- RF denervation or pulsed RF of DRG, nerve roots, peripheral nerves, or sympathetic chain
- SCS/DRG stimulator or peripheral nerve stimulator—only in selected cases (currently limited evidence as it is an emerging treatment option—many are case series)

Further reading

1. Eccleston C, Palermo TM, Williams AC, et al. Psychological therapies for the management of chronic and recurrent pain in children and adolescents. Cochrane Database Syst Rev 2014;5:CD003968 [Review]

2. Farmer AD, Aziz Q. Mechanisms and management of functional abdominal pain. J R Soc Med 2014;107(9):347–54 [Review]
3. Koop H, Koprdova S, Schürmann C. Chronic abdominal wall pain. Dtsch Arztebl Int 2016;113(4):51–7 [Review]
4. Korterink J, Devanarayana NM, Rajindrajith S, et al. Childhood functional abdominal pain: mechanisms and management. Nat Rev Gastroenterol Hepatol 2015;12(3):159–71 [Review]
5. Rana MV, Candido KD, Raja O, Knezevic NN. Celiac plexus block in the management of chronic abdominal pain. Curr Pain Headache Rep 2014;18(2):394 [Review]
6. Spee LA, Lisman-van Leeuwen Y, Benninga MA, et al. Predictors of chronic abdominal pain affecting the well-being of children in primary care. Ann Fam Med 2015;13(2):158–63

26.3 Chronic pancreatitis

Definition

- Chronic pancreatitis is defined as progressive inflammatory response of the pancreas, leading to irreversible morphological changes of the parenchyma
- It is characterized by mononuclear infiltration and fibrosis

Incidence

- More common in men (3:1)
- Black population has 2–3 times increased incidence
- Developed world: 10/100 000; tropical countries: 20–125/100 000
- 50% mortality within 20–25 years of diagnosis
- 33-fold increase in pancreatic cancer

Anatomical correlation

- Pain may arise from any structures inside the abdomen or it could be referred pain
- It could originate from visceral organs or MSK parts, or it could be neuropathic pain

Aetiology

- Alcohol
- Smoking
- Genetic/hereditary
- Obstructive anomalies
- Autoimmune
- Metabolic
- Idiopathic

Pathophysiology of chronic pancreatic pain

- There are different mechanisms:
    - Neuropathic pain
    - Nociceptive pain
    - Neurogenic inflammation
- There is also a central sensitization process which contributes to hyperalgesia that is common in chronic pancreatitis

Diagnosis

- Early diagnosis is difficult due to lack of sensitive imaging or functional markers
- Clinical diagnosis is made based on:
  - History—pain could be intermittent. Normally in epigastric region radiating to the back. History of diarrhoea and steatorrhoea
  - Examination—no specific examination findings. Pain area can be confirmed and might reveal a pseudocyst
  - Presence of risk factors
  - Pancreatic function test—limited use
  - Imaging—CT/MRI/US
  - Endoscopy

Differential diagnosis

- Pain originating from the pancreas or neighbouring structures such as the stomach, spleen, gall bladder (e.g. stones), and IBS

Treatment

- A multidisciplinary and multimodal approach is crucial for success of therapy as for other chronic pain conditions

Conservative (some with limited evidence)

- Lifestyle change—stopping smoking and alcohol consumption
- Nutritional therapy

Pharmacological

- Simple analgesics
- Anti-neuropathic medications: antidepressants (e.g. TCAs, SNRIs), antiepileptics
- Avoid chronic use of opioids as this will cause increased pressure at the sphincter of Oddi and can cause deterioration of pain. It can also cause OIH
- Pancreatic enzyme replacement therapy
- Antioxidant therapy

Interventions

- Sympathetic block: splanchnic plexus block/coeliac plexus block, followed by PRF/RF/chemical neurolysis—CT-, US-, endoscopy-, or X-ray-guided
- SCS (limited evidence)

Neuromodulation techniques

- RF denervation or pulsed RF of DRG, nerve roots, peripheral nerves, or sympathetic chain
- Spinal cord stimulator/DRG stimulator or peripheral nerve stimulator—only in very selected cases (currently limited evidence as it is an emerging treatment option—many are case series)

Surgical

- Endoscopy
- Pseudocyst removal
- Pancreatectomy with auto-transplant

Further reading

1. Anderson MA, Akshintala V, Albers KM, et al. Mechanism, assessment and management of pain in chronic pancreatitis: recommendations of a multidisciplinary study group. Pancreatology 2015;16(1):83–94
2. Bouwense SAW, de Vries M, Schreuder LTW, et al. Systematic mechanism-orientated approach to chronic pancreatitis pain. World J Gastroenterol 2015;21(1):47–59
3. Conwell DL, Lee LS, Yadav D, et al. American Pancreatic Association Practice Guidelines in Chronic Pancreatitis: evidence-based report on diagnostic guidelines. Pancreas 2014;43(8):1143–62
4. D'Haese JG, Ceyhan GO, Demir IE, et al. Treatment options in painful chronic pancreatitis: a systematic review. HPB (Oxford) 2014;16(6):512–21
5. Puylaert M, Kapural L, Van Zundert J, et al. Pain in chronic pancreatitis. In: Van Zundert J, Patijn J, Hartrick CT, et al. (eds). Evidence-based Interventional Pain Medicine. 2012; pp. 202–11. Chicester, UK: Wiley-Blackwell

26.4 Chronic pelvic pain

Definition

- Pelvic pain is abdominal pain located below the level of the umbilicus, including frequently lower back pain with or without radiation into the thighs
- Such pain may be acute, chronic, or intermittent and may be simulated by GI disease, such as diverticulitis, or by lumbo-sacral arthritis
- In females: chronic pelvic pain can be defined as intermittent or constant pain in the lower abdomen or pelvis of a woman of at least 6 months' duration, not occurring exclusively with menstruation or intercourse and not associated with pregnancy

Incidence

- More prevalent in females: 14–40% in the reproductive age group
- Prevalence comparable to that of asthma and low back pain
- 20–70% have improper/wrong diagnosis
- Time period from presentation to diagnosis varies between 6.7 ± 6.2 years

Anatomical correlation of pain generators

- Most of the time, there can be one or more anatomical structures as pain generators

Female pelvic pain

- Urethra
- Bladder
- Vulva
- Vagina
- Uterus
- Ovaries
- Pelvic floor
- Peritoneum/endometriosis
- Bowel
- Post-surgical/neuropathic

- MSK
- Psychosocial

Male pelvic pain

- Urethra
- Bladder
- Penis
- Scrotum
- Prostate
- Pelvic floor
- Peritoneum
- Bowel
- Post-surgical/neuropathic
- MSK
- Systemic
- Psychosocial

Causes

Gynaecological conditions

- Endometriosis
- Adhesions
- Chronic pelvic inflammatory disease
- Pelvic congestion syndrome
- Ovarian remnant syndrome
- Recurrent haemorrhagic ovarian cysts
- Myomata uteri (degenerating)
- Adenomyosis
- Uterine retroversion
- Pelvic floor and hip muscle pain
- Visceral hyperalgesia
- Neoplasms

Urological conditions

- Urinary retention
- Urethral syndrome
- Interstitial cystitis
- Pyelonephritis
- Neoplasms

Abdominal conditions

- Neuropathies
- Porphyrias
- IBS
- Bowel obstruction
- Diverticulitis
- Hernia
- Neoplasms

Neurological conditions

- Nerve entrapment syndromes
- Generalized myofascial pain syndrome
- Fibromyalgia

Musculoskeletal conditions

- SIJ pain
- Hip pain
- Pubic dysfunction
- Spine pathology

Psychological conditions

- Depression
- PTSD (history of abuse/trauma)
- Anxiety disorders
- Personality disorder

Diagnosis

- History—a detailed history is paramount. Take a detailed history of origin, duration, character, radiation, previous abdominopelvic surgeries, and positioning during surgery, especially prolonged lithotomy positioning
- In chronic pelvic pain associated with depression, a detailed psychosocial and sexual history is mandatory
- Menstrual and obstetric history for females
- History suggestive of any red and yellow flags
- General examination
- Manual examination, including vaginal and rectal examination
- Laparoscopic examination
- USS/MRI/CT—mainly to rule out sinister pathologies
- Colonoscopy, cystoscopy, and sigmoidoscopy

Differential diagnosis

- Differential diagnosis is very difficult as multifactorial causes found in chronic pelvic pain
- Depending upon the clinical picture, a possible differential diagnosis is made, based on the primary organ involved and neighbouring structures

Treatments

- A multidisciplinary and multimodal approach is crucial for success of therapy as for other chronic pain conditions

Conservative (some with limited evidence)

- Lifestyle changes
- Adapting sitting position
- Coccyx cushion if appropriate
- Physiotherapy for pelvic floor structures and manipulation
- Therapeutic US therapy
- Acupuncture

- Heat/cold application
- TENS
- CBT, other psychotherapies
- Biofeedback techniques
- Nutritional therapy

Pharmacological

- Simple analgesics, especially NSAIDs if there is no contraindication
- Anti-neuropathic medications—TCAs (e.g. amitriptyline), anticonvulsants (e.g. pregabalin, gabapentin), SNRIs (e.g. duloxetine)
- Opioids—may be used only for acute flare-ups. Opioids used as long-term treatment is associated with worse outcome

Interventions

- LA and steroid injection under X-ray or US guidance (60–85% success rate)
- Caudal block
- Ganglion impar block
- Sacral nerve root block
- RF denervation or pulsed RF of nerve roots

Neuromodulation techniques—only in selected cases

(Currently limited evidence as it is an emerging treatment option—mostly case series)

- TENS
- Peripheral field stimulation
- PNS, depending on pathology
- Pudendal nerve stimulation
- Sacral stimulation
- DRG stimulation
- SCS

Surgical

- Depending on the cause of pelvic pain, appropriate surgery may be indicated

Additional information

- Most of the time, chronic pelvic pain is associated with chronic abdominal pain and presents as chronic abdominopelvic pain
- Treatment depends upon the pain generator and also the pathophysiology
- There may be a need to treat both conditions together (see 26.2 Chronic abdominal pain, p. 530)

Further reading

1. Close C, Sinclair M, Liddle SD, et al. A systematic review investigating the effectiveness of complementary and alternative medicine (CAM) for the management of low back and/or pelvic pain (LBPP) in pregnancy. J Adv Nurs 2014;70(8):1702–16 [Review]

2. Engeler DS, Baranowski AP, Dinis-Oliveira P, et al. The 2013 EAU guidelines on chronic pelvic pain: is management of chronic pelvic pain a habit, a philosophy, or a science? 10 years of development. European Association of Urology. Eur Urol 2013;64(3):431–9 [Review]
3. Hunter CW, Stovall B, Chen G, et al. Anatomy, pathophysiology and interventional therapies for chronic pelvic pain: a review. Pain Physician 2018;21(2):147–67
4. Nelson P, Apte G, Justiz R, et al. Chronic female pelvic pain—part 2: differential diagnosis and management. Pain Pract 2012;12(2):111–41 [Review]

26.5 Vulvodynia

Definition

- The International Society for the Study of Vulvovaginal Disease (ISSVD) definition of vulvodynia is vulvar pain of at least 3 months' duration without a clear identifiable cause which may have potential associated factors
- It is a diagnosis of exclusion and is an idiopathic pain disorder

Incidence

- 3–7% of reproductive age group
- Only 1.4% of women seeking medical advice are correctly diagnosed

Aetiology

- Cause is unknown

Contributing factors

- Neuropathy (increased nerve fibres in the region or spinal nerve injury)
- Chronic vaginal dryness
- Sjögren's syndrome
- Genetic predisposition to inflammation
- Allergy or sensitivities
- Pelvic floor dysfunction

Anatomical correlation and pathophysiology

- It is very complex due to variation in the innervation
- The vulva is innervated by:
  - Anterior labial branch of the IIN
  - GFN
  - Branches of pudendal nerve
- Pelvic floor muscles are divided into three groups:
  - Superficial (urogenital diaphragm)
  - Middle
  - Deep pelvic floor muscles (anal triangle muscles and associated pelvic and hip muscles)
- The pudendal artery, vein, and nerve passing through Alcock's canal provide neurovascular function of the pelvic floor

Classification

- Generalized or localized
- Primary or secondary

- Provoked or unprovoked
- Intermittent, persistent or constant
- Immediate or delayed

Differential diagnoses to rule out

Infection

- Candidiasis
- Trichomoniasis
- Herpes
- Human papillomavirus

Inflammation

- Lichen planus
- Lichen sclerosus
- Lichen simplex
- Contact dermatitis

Neurologic disorders

- Pudendal nerve, IIN, or GFN injury, entrapment, or neuropathy
- Tarlov cysts

Trauma

- Straddle injury
- Female genital mutilation
- Accidents
- Sexual abuse

Neoplastic conditions

- Squamous cell carcinoma

Oestrogen deficiencies

Iatrogenic

- Persistent post-surgical pain
- Nerve injury
- Surgical positioning: lithotomy, laparoscopic trocar injury

History and physical examination

- Detailed pain history, including psychosocial and sexual history, should be taken
- Complete gynaecological examination, including external genitalia, per vaginal, and per rectal examination

Examination

- Cotton sensory test
- Neurosensory check—cotton vs pin prick
- Pelvic floor muscle examination

Pain comorbidities

- Interstitial cystitis
- Endometriosis
- Chronic headache
- Hypermobility syndrome
- Temporomandibular dysfunction

Contributing factors

- Emotional well-being
- Sleep interference
- Relationship problems
- Physical functioning
- Sexual functioning

Treatment

- A multidisciplinary and multimodal approach is crucial for success of therapy as for other chronic pain conditions

Conservative/self-management

- Exercise and physical therapy—pelvic floor muscle exercises, yoga, massage, soft tissue work, dilators, and biofeedback
- Healthy diet—especially low-oxalate diet
- Stress management
- Psychotherapy, including mindfulness and CBT
- Sexual therapy
- Acupuncture

Medications

- Simple analgesics
- TCAs—commonly amitriptyline and nortriptyline
- SNRIs—commonly duloxetine and venlafaxine
- Anticonvulsants—commonly gabapentin, pregabalin, topiramate, lamotrigine, and carbamazepine
- Topical—antifungal, corticosteroids, lidocaine, oestrogen, testosterone, ketamine, and gabapentin

Interventions

- Mainly targeting nerves supplying the vulvar region
- Nerve blocks—GFN, IIN, or pudendal nerve block
- Pulsed RF of nerves
- *Neuromodulation:*
    - TENS
    - Peripheral nerve neuromodulation
    - SCS

Surgery

- Reserved for provoked vestibular vulvodynia

Further reading

1. Corsini-Munt S, Rancourt KM, Dubé JP, et al. Vulvodynia: a consideration of clinical and methodological research challenges and recommended solutions. J Pain Res 2017;10:2425–36
2. De Andres J, Sanchis-Lopez N, Asensio-Samper JM, et al. Vulvodynia—an evidence-based literature review and proposed treatment algorithm. Pain Pract 2016;16(2):204–36
3. Falsetta ML, Foster DC, Bonham AD, Phipps RP. A review of the available clinical therapies for vulvodynia management and new data implicating pro-inflammatory mediators in pain elicitation. BJOG 2016;124(2):210–18
4. Sadownik LA. Etiology, diagnosis, and clinical management of vulvodynia. Int J Womens Health 2014;6:437–49

26.6 Refractory angina pectoris

Definition

- Severe chest pain, heavy retrosternal pain, referred pain (arm, neck, jaw)
- It is refractory if conservative treatments fail

Pathophysiology

- Due to coronary obstruction or spasms (insufficient blood and oxygen supply to the heart, increased oxygen consumption)

Risk factors

- Smoking, obesity, hypertension, diabetes, high cholesterol

Diagnosis

History

- Retrosternal pain often radiating to the arms, neck, throat, jaw and teeth (especially on the left side)
- Sweating, nausea, vomiting
- Symptoms provoked by exertion and disappear at rest
- Triggered by emotional stress, exposure to cold, meals, and smoking
- Refractory if repeated reversible myocardial ischaemia occurs despite optimal treatment with severe coronary stenosis (>75%)

Examination/tests

- Cardiological workup needed
- 12-lead ECG at rest or exercise stress test on ergometer (ischaemic signs)
- Stress echocardiography
- Angiography, CT angiography

Differential diagnosis

- Respiratory (pulmonary hypertension, pulmonary embolism, pleuritis, pneumothorax, pneumonia)
- Cardiac valve disease (mitral prolapse, cardiac syndrome X)
- GI: peptic ulcer, pancreatitis, oesophageal spasms, reflux, cholecystitis
- MSK: costochondritis, Tietze's syndrome, thoracic trauma, cervical arthritis, myositis, cancer
- Spinal cord injury, thoracic radiculopathy
- Aortic dissection, post-herpetic neuralgia, panic disorder

Treatment

Conservative (under cardiology)

- Reduce oxygen demand (β-blockers, Ca^{2+} channel blocker)
- Increase oxygen supply (nitrates, angioplasty, coronary artery bypass grafting (CABG))
- Anti-cholesterol and antiplatelet drugs
- Good progress has been made with anti-cholesterol and anti-anginal drugs, and better quality of percutaneous angioplasty

Spinal cord stimulator

- Patients with substantial limitation due to angina despite all conservative and surgical therapies (must have been investigated by a cardiologist)
- Indications are controversial
- Evidence: 2B+ (recommended in specialized centres)
- *Effects:*
  - Less pain (↑ GABA, ↑ dopamine, ↑ glycine)
  - Anti-anginal (normalization of the cardiac nerve system)
  - Less medication use, higher exercise tolerance
  - Anti-ischaemic effects, fewer attacks (increased angina pectoris threshold, redistribution of coronary blood flow?)
  - Angiogenesis (collaterals)
  - SCS does not mask acute myocardial infarcts
- *Efficacy:*
  - Better exercise tolerance, improved QoL after 12 months
  - Improved symptoms after 12 months
  - Reduced mortality, reduced cerebrovascular accidents (versus CABG patients)
  - SCS may be an alternative to surgery in selected patients
- *Complications:*
  - Lead migration, electrode fracture (7%)
  - Battery failure, SC infection
  - No major complications described
- *Absolute contraindications:*
  - Defibrillating pacemaker
  - Bleeding diathesis
  - Neuraxial malignancies
  - Severe cognitive disorders
- *Technique:*
  - Asepsis, prophylactic antibiotics
  - Tuohy needle insertion at T8/T9

- Electrode tip at T2/T3 (four or eight contacts)
- Mapping of painful area
- Stimulator (implantable pulse generator) in buttock or upper abdomen

Further reading

1. Van Kleef M, Staats P, Mekhail N, Huygen F. Chronic refractory angina pectoris. In: Van Zundert J, Patijn J, Hartrick CT, et al. (eds). Evidence-based Interventional Pain Medicine. 2012; pp. 191–5. Chichester, UK: Wiley-Blackwell

CHAPTER 27

Widespread Chronic Pain

Enrique Collantes, Nofil Mulla, and Kavita Poply

CONTENTS

27.1 Chronic fatigue syndrome

Introduction

- Chronic fatigue syndrome, or myalgic encephalitis or systemic exertion intolerance disease, is characterized by a wide range of symptoms, the most common being extreme fatigue
- More common in women and between second and fourth decades

Pathophysiology

Pathophysiology is not well understood and some of the mechanisms involved include:

- Altered pain processing—descending inhibitory serotonergic pathways
- Genetic factors—familial, methylenetetrahydrofolate reductase gene
- Infections—many patients describe the onset after an infection:
    - Viral infections such as Epstein–Barr virus, retroviruses, enteroviruses, and others
    - Bacterial infections such as pneumonia
- Immune system changes—higher levels of cytokines and active $CD8^{+}$ T cells
- Endocrine–metabolic imbalance—hypometabolic state, high levels of insulin-like growth factor, low cortisol, low corticotropic hormone secretion, abnormalities in metabolism of lipids, amino acids, and sugars to make energy
- Mental health problems—depression, PTSD
- Sleep disorders
- Environmental stressors
- Psychosocial contributors

Investigations

- Investigations are not needed for diagnosis
- Investigations are performed to exclude other causes such as FBC, inflammatory markers (CRP, ESR), CK, thyroid studies, and other tests assessing for other causes

Diagnostic criteria

- Chronic fatigue lasting >6 months
- Plus at least one of the following clinical features of moderate to high severity at least half of the time: post-exertional malaise (>24 hours), subjective memory impairment, tender lymph nodes, MSK pain, headache, unrefreshing sleep, and orthostatic-related symptoms
- Major interference with productivity, leisure, rest, and daily activities

Differential diagnosis

- Fibromyalgia
- Somatoform disorder, conversion disorder, illness anxiety disorder
- Hypothyroidism/hyperparathyroidism
- Autoimmune disorders—RA, SLE, Sjögren's syndrome, polymyalgia rheumatica, myositis
- HIV, Lyme disease, hepatitis C
- Drug-related—statins, aromatase inhibitors, bisphosphonates
- Sleep apnoea
- Malignancy—multiple myeloma, metastatic cancer

Treatments

- Validate, use an empathic approach, and develop trust with the patient
- Patient education on chronic fatigue syndrome:
  - It is not life-threatening but can cause significant disability
  - The cause is not completely understood, but multiple mechanisms are involved—genetic, endocrinological, neurological, metabolic, immunological, environmental, psychosocial, and mental health factors
  - Address the patient's concerns, beliefs, and expectations
  - Treatment focuses on reducing symptoms, impairment, and disability
- Treating modifiable perpetuating factors—depression, cognitive impairment, sleep, unhelpful thoughts/behaviours, disconnection from the community
- Healthy lifestyle (weight control, balanced diet, improving general fitness, not smoking or drinking alcohol, exercise)
- CBT
- Graded exercise therapies with pacing
- Short drug trials addressing specific presentations—pain, mood, anxiety, etc.
- Workplace and non-work-related ergonomic changes

Additional information

- Conditions that can coexist:
  - Regional pain syndromes: IBS, temporomandibular joint dysfunction, tension headaches, idiopathic low back pain, vulvodynia
  - Depression, panic attacks, generalized anxiety disorder, PTSD

Further reading

1. Committee on the Diagnostic Criteria for Myalgic Encephalomyelitis/Chronic Fatigue Syndrome; Board on the Health of Select Populations; Institute of Medicine. https://www.nap.edu/initiative/committee-on-the-diagnostic-criteria-for-myalgic-encephalomyelitischronic-fatigue-syndrome

2. Larun L, Brurberg KG, Odgaard-Jensen J, Price JR. Exercise therapy for chronic fatigue syndrome. Cochrane Database Syst Rev 2015;2:CD003200
3. Meeus M, Nijs J, Meirleir KD. Chronic musculoskeletal pain in patients with the chronic fatigue syndrome: a systematic review. Eur J Pain 2007;11(4):377–86

27.2 Fibromyalgia

Introduction

- Widespread chronic pain syndrome, with a prevalence of 2% in the general population
- Heterogenous condition affecting all four quadrants of body. It presents with pain being a dominant symptom, but it can also be associated with fatigue, mood swings, and cognitive impairment as part of a spectrum

Pathophysiology

- There are several proposed mechanisms, but no clear pathophysiological mechanism exists:
  - CNS pain processing abnormalities resulting in hyperexcitability of pain-transmitting neurons
  - Dysfunction of descending inhibitory pathways
  - Abnormal function of HPA axis
  - Disturbances in the balance between serotonergic and dopaminergic mechanisms
  - Strong familial component—first-degree relatives of patients with fibromyalgia are 8.5 times more likely to have the disorder than the general population

Investigations

- Not needed for diagnosing fibromyalgia
- Investigations are performed to exclude other causes. Investigations routinely performed include FBC, inflammatory markers (CRP, ESR), CK, thyroid studies, and other tests assessing for other causes

Differential diagnosis

- Chronic fatigue syndrome
- Somatoform disorder, conversion disorder, illness anxiety disorder
- Hypothyroidism/hyperparathyroidism
- Autoimmune disorders—RA, SLE, Sjögren's syndrome, polymyalgia rheumatica, myositis
- HIV, Lyme disease, hepatitis C
- Drug-related—statins, aromatase inhibitors, bisphosphonates
- Sleep apnoea
- Malignancy—multiple myeloma, metastatic cancer

Diagnosis—American College of Rheumatology diagnostic criteria

- 1990 diagnostic criteria: traditionally diagnosed as specific tender points on palpation (>11/18)
- 2010 diagnostic criteria: physician-based criteria valid for individual patient diagnosis. It accounted for both peripheral and somatic symptoms, simplifying the diagnosis of fibromyalgia. Suitable for use in primary care without requiring a tender point examination
- 2011 diagnostic criteria: revised criteria more patient-reported and suitable for research purposes. It led to misclassification when applied to regional pain syndromes
- Median sensitivity and specificity of the 2010 and 2011 criteria were 86% and 90%, respectively, providing an improved diagnostic accuracy to the previous 1990 criteria

Table 27.2.1 American College of Rheumatology 2016 diagnostic criteria for fibromyalgia

1. Generalized pain, defined as pain in at least four of five regions (axial plus upper and lower segments plus left- and right-sided pain), is present
2. Symptoms have been present at a similar level for at least 3 months
3. Widespread pain index (WPI) ≥7 and symptom severity scale (SSS) score ≥5 or WPI of 4–6 and SSS score ≥9
4. A diagnosis of fibromyalgia is valid, irrespective of other diagnoses. A diagnosis of fibromyalgia does not exclude the presence of other clinically important illnesses. Now a more recent 2016 revision has been proposed adding a widespread pain criterion

WPI:
Note the number of areas in which the patient has had pain over the past week (score will be between 0 and 19): left shoulder girdle, right shoulder girdle, left hip (buttock, trochanter), right hip (buttock, trochanter), left jaw, right jaw, upper back, lower back, left upper arm, right upper are, left lower arm, right lower arm, left upper leg, right upper leg, left lower leg, right lower leg, neck, chest, abdomen

SSS score:
A. Fatigue, waking unrefreshed, cognitive symptoms. For each of these three symptoms, indicate the severity over the past week, using the following scale:
 a. Score 0: no problem
 b. Score 1: generally mild or intermittent
 c. Score 2: often present at a moderate level
 d. Score 3: severe, pervasive, continuous, life-disturbing problems
B. Somatic symptoms: indicate whether the patient has 0, no symptoms; 1, few symptoms; 2, a moderate number of symptoms; or 3, many symptoms. Somatic symptoms that might be considered: muscle pain, irritable bowel syndrome, fatigue/tiredness, thinking or remembering problem, muscle weakness, headache, pain/cramps in the abdomen, numbness/tingling, dizziness, insomnia, depression, constipation, pain in the upper abdomen, nausea, nervousness, chest pain, blurred vision, fever, diarrhoea, dry mouth, itching, wheezing, Raynaud's phenomenon, hives/welts, ringing in ears, vomiting, heartburn, oral ulcers, loss of/change in taste, seizures, dry eyes, shortness of breath, loss of appetite, rash, sun sensitivity, hearing difficulties, easy bruising, hair loss, frequent urination, painful urination, and bladder spasms

 The SSS score is the sum of the severity of the three symptoms (fatigue, waking unrefreshed, cognitive symptoms) plus the extent of the somatic symptoms in general. The final SSS score is between 0 and 12

Reproduced from Wolfe, F., et al. (2010). The American College of Rheumatology Prelimininary Diagnostic Criteria for Fibromyalgia and Measurement of Symptom Severity. *Arthiritis Care and Research*. 62(5): 600–610. DOI 10.1002/acr.20140.

- 2016 diagnostic criteria: provides a better diagnostic accuracy by combining physician and questionnaire criteria, minimizing misclassification of regional pain disorders, and eliminating the previously confusing recommendation regarding diagnostic exclusions (see Table 27.2.1)

Management

- Early diagnosis and patient education form the key components of a multidisciplinary management approach recommended by the European League against Rheumatism (EULAR)
- At the outset, patients need to be offered individual graded exercise therapy that can be combined with non-pharmacological. If symptoms are predominantly associated with depression, anxiety, and poor coping skills, psychological therapies such as CBT should be considered. On the other hand, pharmacotherapy may be helpful in managing the pain component with sleep disturbance and anxiety

Non-pharmacological management

- Should be considered as the first step in the management of fibromyalgia—a key component of multimodal pain management, avoiding pharmacological-related S/Es:

- Exercise: strongly recommended early in treatment pathway. Both aerobic and strengthening exercise programmes are recommended
- CBT: effective at producing modest long-term reductions in pain and disability, and improving mood
- Acupuncture: can be offered early in management as added to standard therapy—resulted in 30% (21%, 39%) improvement in pain and fatigue
- Mindfulness/mind–body therapy: results in short-term improvements in pain and QoL
- Meditative movement therapies: t'ai chi, yoga, qigong, or body awareness therapy have demonstrated improvements in sleep, fatigue, and QoL. Regular use of these therapies may result in improvement, some of which is maintained longer term

Pharmacological management

- Should be considered in relation to individual symptoms in association with pain such as fatigue and disability
- Amitriptyline (TCA):
  - 30% pain reduction, risk reduction (RR) 1.60, 95% CI 1.15–2.24
  - NNT 3.54, 95% CI 2.74–5.01
  - Moderate effect on sleep and fatigue
  - 25 mg daily has been shown to improve pain intensity, with no additional benefit demonstrated at 50 mg dose
- Pregabalin (gabapentinoids):
  - 75–300 mg twice daily
  - NNT 9, 95% CI 7–13
  - RR 1.37, 95% CI 1.22–1.53
  - Very small effect on fatigue and sleep. Minimal effect on disability. Evidence on gabapentin is limited to a single moderate-quality study, with, however, a significant effect of 30% pain reduction (RR 1.65, 95% CI 1.10–2.48) and a similar small effect on sleep and a larger effect on improvement in disability
- Duloxetine (SNRI):
  - 60 mg/day has been effective at reducing >30% pain (RR 1.38, 95% CI 1.22–1.56), with NNT 6 and 95% CI 3–12, with small effects on sleep and disability, but no effect on fatigue
- Milnacipran has been reported to have 30% pain reduction (RR 1.38, 95% CI 1.25–1.51), a small benefit on fatigue and disability, and no effect on sleep
- Opioids, NSAIDs, and SSRIs have poor evidence. Furthermore, opioids should be avoided because of the risk of addiction, dependence, and other adverse effects (see Chapter 7)

Further reading

1. Wolfe F, Clauw DJ, Fitzcharles MA, et al. The American College of Rheumatology preliminary diagnostic criteria for fibromyalgia and measurement of symptom severity. Arthritis Care Res (Hoboken) 2010;62(5):600–10
2. MacFarlane GJ, Kronisch C, Dean LE, et al. EULAR revised recommendations for the management of fibromyalgia. Ann Rheumatol Dis 2017;76(2):318–28
3. Mease P. Fibromyalgia syndrome: review of clinical presentation, pathogenesis, outcome measures, and treatment. J Rheumatol 2005;32:2063
4. Wolfe F, Clauw DJ, Fitzcharles MA, et al. Fibromyalgia criteria and severity scales for clinical and epidemiological studies: a modification of the ACR preliminary diagnostic criteria for fibromyalgia. J Rheumatol 2011;38:1113–22

Other Pain Conditions

Enrique Collantes, Anthony Gubbay, Sumit Gulati, Sarah Harper, Tommy Lwin, Nofil Mulla, Paolo Pais, David Pang, Shankar Ramaswamy, Jan Rudiger, Kantaruby Tambirajoo, Victoria Winter, and Ivan Wong

CONTENTS

28.1 Acute pain

Introduction

- Acute pain is pain of recent onset and limited duration (<3 months)
- Chronic pain usually persists for longer than 3 months or beyond the usual duration of an acute injury or disease
- There are differences between acute and chronic pain and require different approaches to treatment
- Poorly controlled acute pain may contribute to the development of chronic pain which has wider ramifications for the patient and society
- More attention is needed for patients who are pregnant, elderly, opioid-tolerant, or disabled (physical, cognitive, visual/hearing impairments), those with substance abuse disorder, sleep apnoea, or renal or liver disease, and those who do not speak English and from ethnic minorities

Pathophysiology

- Normally nociceptive (somatic and/or visceral) and/or neuropathic
- Tissue injury in the peripheral and/or central nervous system causes an inflammatory response
- Peripheral and/or central sensitization can develop, which results in increased sensitivity of the somato-sensory nervous system to noxious and non-noxious stimuli. Complex interplay of mechanisms that go beyond the sensory/discriminative aspects can result in long-term reorganization of the nervous system (see Chapter 2 for further information)

Characteristics of acute pain

- Short-lived
- Types of pain

    - Nociceptive pain (somatic pain ± visceral pain)
    - Neuropathic pain
- Leads to adaptive behaviours
- Appropriate biological responses
- Normal baseline neuronal sensitivity
- Does not usually lead to disability

Advantages of effective acute pain management

- Improved patient and staff satisfaction
- Improved quality of care, patient safety, and cost-effectiveness
- Earlier mobilization
- Reduced patient complications
- Reduced duration of stay and re-admissions to hospital for pain management problems
- Less use of health care resources
- Well-controlled acute pain may reduce the incidence of persistent pain

Assessment

- Biopsychosocial approach
- Consider if the pain is neuropathic ± nociceptive (somatic ± visceral)
- Detailed pain-orientated history
- Relevant medical and surgical history
- Identify perpetuating factors: expectations, beliefs, mood disorders, psychosocial stressors, litigation, coping skills
- Current and previous treatments
- Pain assessment tools:
    - For initial assessment, ongoing evaluation and response to treatments
    - Unidimensional tools commonly used are the NRS, VRS, and VAS. Pain scores should never be used alone to determine pain intensity
    - Functional assessment is crucial, e.g. functional activity score
    - Observational pain assessment tools should be used if patients cannot respond verbally or cannot self-report
    - Pain-orientated physical examination and exclude red flags

Management

General overview

- Address the underlying organic cause
- Address patient expectations and beliefs, and develop a good therapeutic relationship with the patient. Patients need to understand that being completely pain free is usually not achievable and the key goal of analgesia is to facilitate recovery, mobilization and physiotherapy
- Patient and staff education, and multidisciplinary and multimodal approaches positively influence outcomes
- Frequent assessment and reassessment of the effect of all interventions are essential. Slow analgesic titration and avoidance of a rapid increase in opioid analgesia or other analgesics with sedating properties is important

- Unexpected onset of pain or poorly controlled pain may be from an established or new surgical, medical, and psychiatric diagnosis
- Acute neuropathic pain is normally under-recognized and undertreated. Treatments which can work more quickly and may be appropriate include opioids (tramadol and tapentadol), gabapentinoids, and ketamine
- Preventative analgesia—level 1 evidence for ketamine, LAs, and certain regional techniques (refer to other sections of the book)
- PROSPECT (PROcedure-SPECific post-operative pain managemenT) provides evidence-based treatments of pain for specific operations

Multimodal pain management

- Multimodal pain management combining pharmacological and non-pharmacological techniques provide more effective analgesia reducing S/Es and adverse effects
- Non-pharmacological treatments
  - Input from physiotherapy, OT, and psychology
  - Pain management strategies can include activity pacing, problem-solving, attention diversion (book, music, videos, or others), thought management, goal setting, acupuncture, TENS, biofeedback, hypnosis, and relaxation/meditation techniques
- Pharmacological treatment
  - Multimodal Analgesia: paracetamol ± NSAIDs ± opioids ± adjuvants
  - PCA is indicated in the early post-operative setting and when patients cannot have oral intake
  - Due to patient factors, environmental factors, and individual opioid characteristics (e.g. in renal failure, avoiding opioids that have active metabolites, etc.), some opioids may be more appropriate in some circumstances (see Chapter 7 for further reading). Patients on sedating agents and/or opioids need to be adequately assessed and monitored for ventilatory impairment
  - Adjuvants are opioid-sparing and decrease opioid-related S/Es
  - Adjuvants include ketamine, lidocaine, gabapentinoids, α-2 receptor agonists (clonidine, dexmedetomidine), steroids (dexamethasone), and antidepressants
  - Consider drugs, such as Entonox® and methoxyflurane, for analgesia during procedures
- Regional analgesia and continuous peripheral nerve blocks
  - Neuraxial analgesia: good evidence in abdominal and thoracic surgery
  - Epidural analgesia is underutilized due to potential serious S/Es
  - Continuous peripheral nerve blocks provide better analgesia than single-injection peripheral nerve blocks. Peripheral nerve blocks generally have a better safety profile than neuroaxial blocks

Further reading

1. Prospect (PROcedure-SPECfic post-operative pain managemenT). https://esraeurope.org/prospect/
2. Schug SA, Palmer GM, Scott DA, Halliwell R, Trinca J. Acute Pain Management: Scientific Evidence. 4th edition, 2015. Melbourne: Australian and New Zealand College of Anaesthetists and Faculty of Pain Medicine

28.2 Chronic post-surgical pain

Definition (IASP)—multiple definitions exist

- Chronic post-surgical pain is pain that develops or worsens in intensity after a surgical procedure and persisting beyond the healing process
- Pain lasting for at least 3 months after surgery, significantly affecting QoL
- The pain can be a continuation of acute post-surgical pain or develop after an asymptomatic period (after several months or even years)
- Pain is localized to the surgical field or projected to the innervation territory of a nerve or referred to a dermatome
- Other causes for pain excluded (e.g. malignancy, infection, pain from pre-existing pain problem)
- It is one of the most common complications after surgery

Incidence

- On average, CPSP occurs in 1–2 of ten surgical patients, but it varies with the type of surgery (see Table 28.2.1)
- The incidence of severe CPSP is between 2% and 25%
- 2% of post-operative patients reported severe CPSP one year after surgery
- Intolerable CPSP occurs in about one of every 100 operations
- Neuropathic pain is present in up to 80% of patients with CPSP

Pathophysiology

- Damage to major nerves during surgery (however, CPSP can develop in the absence of nerve damage)
- Persistent peripheral noxious stimulation

Table 28.2.1 Incidence of chronic post-surgical pain (CPSP)

Type of surgery	Incidence of CPSP
Amputation	30–85%
Caesarean section	6–55%
Cholecystectomy	3–50%
Coronary bypass	30–50%
Craniotomy	7–30%
Dental surgery	5–13%
Hip arthroplasty	27%
Inguinal herniotomy	5–63%
Knee arthroplasty	13–44%
Melanoma resection	9%
Mastectomy	11–57%
Sternotomy	7–17%
Thoracotomy	5–65%
Vasectomy	0–37%

- Enduring maladaptive neuroplastic changes at the spinal DH and/or higher CNS structures
- Compromised inhibitory modulators of noxious stimulation in medullary-spinal pathways
- Impaired descending facilitatory modulation
- Maladaptive brain remodelling in structure, function, and connectivity

Risk factors

- Demographic factors:
  - Young age (but not very young age)
  - Female sex
  - Sociodemographic (educational, socioeconomic, compensatory, employment-related factors)
- Genetic predisposition:
  - Heritability of chronic pain is estimated between 30% and 70%
  - Genetic variations exist in drug metabolism and neurological pain pathways
  - Some genetic polymorphisms are associated with CPSP (e.g. COMT on pain inhibition or *OPRM1* encoding the mu receptor)
  - Monozygous twins manifest partial concordance in the development of pain and inflammation; therefore, epigenetics may also play a role in the development of CPSP
- Psychosocial factors:
  - Depression, psychological vulnerability, stress, late return to work
  - Anxiety, catastrophizing, fear avoidance
  - Comorbid stress symptoms (e.g. sleep disturbance, PTSD)
  - In children, parental catastrophizing can contribute to CPSP
- Pain as risk factor:
  - Strongest predictor of CPSP is poorly controlled pain with severe pain in the preoperative and post-operative period
  - Severe post-operative pain could be an early manifestation of subsequent CPSP
  - Acute post-operative pain and the duration of severe post-operative pain on day 1 post-surgery. For every 10% increase in time spent in severe pain, the risk of developing CPSP increased by 30%
- Surgical factors:
  - Surgical procedure influences the incidence (see Table 28.2.1)
  - CPSP is procedure-specific (influence of nerve injury, increased risk of CPSP with longer duration of surgery, more traumatic and extensive approaches, repeated revisions, and when surgical complications occur; role of nerve sparing/handling surgical techniques is inconclusive)
  - Even minor procedures can lead to CPSP
- Medical factors:
  - CPSP risk is higher with multiple comorbidities and preoperative disability (e.g. IBS, RA, Raynaud syndrome)
  - The addition of chemotherapy/radiotherapy as an additional therapeutic modality
  - Preoperative opioid use. Chronic opioid users may require 3–4 times the amount of opioids, compared to opioid-naïve patients

Preventative and pre-emptive measures

- Surgical:
  - Modification of surgical technique to minimize the impact of tissue trauma and intraoperative nerve injury
  - Surgery duration also plays a role, although this may be a reflection on complex pathology and related to the degree of intraoperative tissue damage

- Anaesthetic:
  - Regional anaesthesia has the potential to reduce the severity of acute and chronic pain after surgery
  - Pre-emptive epidural analgesia has a significant benefit on post-operative pain
- Pharmacological:
  - IV lidocaine, anti-neuropathic agents, gabapentinoids, antidepressants—efficacy increases with duration of treatment
  - These therapies appear promising as part of a multimodal analgesic strategy (the exact dosage and duration are yet to be determined)
  - Perioperative ketamine infusion appears ineffective in reducing CPSP
- Psychological:
  - Psychological support (including preoperative counselling)

Treatment (physical, medical, surgical, pain interventions, alternatives)

- Transitional pain services aim to prevent the transition from acute to chronic pain (concept of a fully integrated peri-operative pain service)
- Preoperative:
  - Risk stratification
  - Discussion with surgeon (surgical approach), and anaesthetic and analgesic planning
  - Transitional pain service (for perioperative management of pain)
- Intraoperative:
  - Surgical technique
  - Anaesthetic and analgesic technique (regional anaesthesia, multimodal analgesia)
- Post-operative:
  - Effective analgesia
  - Early management of potentially developing chronic pain
- Physical therapies:
  - Massage, physiotherapy, and acupuncture
- Pharmacological treatment—in neuropathic pain:
  - Treatment recommendations are generally extrapolated from data for other types of chronic pain, especially in neuropathic pain:
    - Anticonvulsants, TCAs, and SNRIs for neuropathic pain (first line)
    - Paracetamol and NSAIDs can also be used in accordance with symptom severity
    - Strong opioids should be used with caution after considering the risks and benefits
- Pain interventions:
  - Consider various other interventions such as nerve blocks, nerve ablation, and neuromodulation for patients in whom pharmacological intervention has not worked
- Psychological interventions:
  - CBT may be useful

Further reading

1. Fletcher D, Stamer UM, Pogatzki-Zahn E, et al. Chronic postsurgical pain in Europe: an observational study. Eur J Anaesthesiol 2015;32(10):725–34
2. Humble SR, Varela N, Jayaweera A, Bhaskar A. Chronic postsurgical pain and cancer: the catch of surviving the unsurvivable. Curr Opin Support Palliat Care 2018;12(2):118–23

3. International Association for the Study of Pain. Factsheet 4: Chronic postsurgical pain: definition and impact. https://www.iasp-pain.org/GlobalYear/AfterSurgery
4. Parineeta T, Pramote E. Chronic postsurgical pain: current evidence for prevention and management. Korean J Pain 2018;31(3):155–73
5. Richebe P, Capdevila X, Rivat C. Persistent postsurgical pain: pathophysiology and preventative pharmacologic considerations. Anaesthesiology 2018;129:590–607
6. Schug, SA, Bruce J. Risk stratification for the development of chronic postsurgical pain, PAIN clinical updates. Pain Rep 2017;2(6):e627

28.3 Erythromelalgia

Introduction

- Rare neurovascular disorder of unknown aetiology, with an incidence rate of approximately 1 in 50 000 people per year, with a higher incidence in women
- Can be inherited or acquired

Clinical features

- Intermittent intense burning sensations, redness, and increased temperature in the periphery, primarily affecting the feet, but can affect hands

Aggravating factors

- Exposure to heat
- Lowering the affected limb, i.e. feet/hands
- Exercise
- Pressure

Relieving factors

- Cooling of the affected limbs
- Lowering the affected limbs

Types

- Various subtypes, but two main classes:
  - Idiopathic
  - Secondary

Pathophysiology—primary or idiopathic form

- Usually early-onset type presenting in childhood
- It is caused by gain in function as a result of mutations in the *SCN9A* gene, which is responsible for coding Nav 1.7 channels, mainly localized in the DRG and sympathetic ganglia
- Functional characterization of mutant Na^+ channels has been done by patch clamp technique and suggests slowed deactivation and increased firing frequency following stimulation
- Nav 1.8 channels, which are more resistant to inactivation following depolarization, are also present in the DRG, and gain in function or hyperexcitation is the outcome manifesting as neuropathic pain
- Nav 1.8 channels are not present in the sympathetic ganglion; mutation in the *SCN9A* gene results in hypoexcitation and dysfunction of sympathetic regulation, which, in turn, results in vasomotor manifestations seen in the periphery

- The mechanism is thought to be similar to diabetic neuropathy, i.e. due to microvascular derangement leading to peripheral arterio-venous shunting, causing hypoxia despite increased skin blood flow, pain, and swelling, along with increased temperature (the increased temperature, in turn, can alter Na^+ channels, resulting in a potential vicious cycle)

Secondary form

- Usually secondary to thrombocytosis in myeloproliferative syndromes, as a result of altered platelet functions, which, in turn, affect the microvasculature
- Erythromelalgia may present years before the onset of myeloproliferative disorders (therefore, patients with erythromelalgia should be tested regularly for any abnormality of blood cells and Hb; any such abnormality should warrant full evaluation for myeloproliferative disorders, as about 10% of cases of erythromelalgia are associated with these disorders)

Diagnosis

- It is an exclusion diagnosis
- Based on history and clinical examination during the symptomatic period
- Skin biopsy not useful in diagnosing erythromelalgia, although it can be used to exclude other conditions

Management

- The aim should be to identify the disease early to achieve the best prognosis in terms of remissions and a better QoL; as such, there is no cure for the condition
- Avoiding precipitating factors
- Treatment of secondary causes (e.g. myeloproliferative disorders):
  - Non-pharmacological measures:
    - Cooling the affected extremities (patients may end up having frostbite after using ice too frequently)
    - CBT, pain rehabilitation programme, patient support group (Erythromelalgia Association)
  - Pharmacological treatment:
    - Aspirin has been found to be very effective in treatment of pain, particularly in patients with myeloproliferative disorders
    - Lidocaine patches
    - Other anti-neuropathic agents are used when the above-mentioned non-pharmacological and topical measures have failed to treat the symptoms. The ones considered to be useful from case reports and case series include gabapentinoids, venlafaxine, and TCAs
    - Other treatments with possible beneficial effects are IV lidocaine, Na^+ channel blockers, vasodilators, and IV Ig
    - Systemic steroids may also be helpful if used at early stages before central sensitization takes place

Further reading

1. Davis MDP, Callen J, Ofori AO. Erythromelalgia. UpToDate. 2021. https://www.uptodate.com/contents/erythromelalgia

2. Farrar MA, Lee M-J, Howells J, Andrews P, Lin, C S-Y. Burning pain: axonal dysfunction in erythromelalgia. Pain 2017;158(5):900–11
3. Pagani-Estévez GL, Sandroni P, Davis MD, Watson JC. Erythromelalgia: identification of a corticosteroid-responsive subset. J Am Acad Dermatol 2017;76(3):506–11

28.4 Headaches

Introduction

- Prevalence of current headache disorder (symptomatic at least once within the year) amongst adults is estimated globally to be about 50%
- Impose a significant burden on personal suffering, financial cost, QoL, and employment
- The long-term effort of coping with headaches may also predispose the individual to other illnesses

Diagnosis of headache

- No specific diagnostic tests, relies on accurate history
- A headache diary kept over a few weeks is helpful as the pattern of attacks is a critical pointer in the diagnosis
- Conditions requiring more urgent interventions must first be ruled out

Warning features in the history

- New or unexpected headache
- A thunderclap (abrupt or 'explosive' onset) headache
- Headache with atypical aura (duration >1 hour or including motor weakness)
- Aura occurring for the first time in a patient during use of combined oral contraceptives
- New-onset headache in a patient older than 50 years or younger than 10 years
- Persistent morning headache with nausea
- Progressive headache, worsening over weeks or longer
- Associated with postural change
- New-onset headache in a patient with a history of cancer or a history of HIV infection

Types of headache disorders

- Headaches are broadly classified as either primary or secondary
- Primary headaches are benign, recurrent headaches not caused by any underlying disease or structural problems
- Secondary headaches are caused by an underlying disease process which, in some cases, may be life-threatening

Primary headaches

- Encompasses 90% of headaches
- Include migraines, tension-type headaches, trigeminal autonomic cephalgia (TAC), and other primary headache disorders
- Improved recognition of common headache disorders and better targeting of available treatments should reduce the headache burden
- Specialist advice from a neurologist or a headache specialist should be sought in refractory or complex cases

Migraines

- A common disabling primary headache disorder, usually begins at puberty, and mostly affects those aged between 35 and 45 years
- 2:1 times more common in women, because of hormonal influences
- Moderate or severe in intensity, unilateral and pulsating, can last from 4 to 72 hours
- Associated with GI symptoms that limit activity
- Dark and quiet environments are preferred during an attack
- Migraines can occur with or without an aura
- Auras are focal neurological symptoms that can precede or accompany a headache, usually visual (transient hemianopic disturbances or spreading scotoma) and lasting 5–60 minutes
- Other reversible focal deficits include unilateral paraesthesiae of the hand, arm, or face, or dysphasia
- Some patients also experience a premonitory phase (hours or days before a headache) and a headache resolution phase
- Premonitory and resolution symptoms include hyperactivity, hypoactivity, depression, cravings for particular foods, repetitive yawning, fatigue, and neck stiffness or pain
- Acute treatment options:
  - Combination therapy with an oral triptan and an NSAID or a triptan and paracetamol
  - Oral triptan, NSAID, aspirin, or paracetamol as monotherapy
  - Antiemetic, even in the absence of nausea or vomiting
  - If one triptan is ineffective, others may work as lack of effectiveness is not a class effect
  - If oral therapy not effective or not tolerated, then non-oral metoclopramide or prochlorperazine can be used, in addition to a non-oral NSAID or triptan if these have not been tried
  - No ergots or opioids to be offered
- Prophylactic treatment options:
  - Recommended if >4 attacks of migraine per month, headaches lasting longer than 12 hours or very disabling
  - Some patients need long-term prophylaxis, but review the need at 6 months after starting prophylactic treatment
  - Topiramate is a recommended first-line option but has a teratogenic risk in women of childbearing age
  - Propranolol and amitriptyline are also recommended as first-line agents
  - Do not offer gabapentin as prophylaxis
  - A course of acupuncture can be considered in those patients for whom topiramate and propranolol are unsuitable or ineffective
- Special considerations:
  - Combined hormonal contraception should not be used if a woman has migraine with aura because of a possible increased risk of ischaemic stroke
  - Migraine without aura often improves during pregnancy. Paracetamol is suggested as first choice in pregnancy. Triptan or an NSAID can be considered after weighing the risk–benefit ratio for use in pregnancy. If prophylaxis is necessary during pregnancy, discussion with, or referral to, a specialist is recommended

Tension-type headaches

- Lifetime prevalence in the general population between 30% and 78%
- Begins during the teenage years, affecting more women than men
- Stress-related or associated with MSK problems in the neck

- The episodic form is described as typically bilateral, pressing or tightening in quality, of mild to moderate intensity, lasting minutes to days, with no nausea or vomiting
- The infrequent subtype occurs <12 days per year, and the frequent subtype occurs 1–14 days per month, on average for 12–180 days per year
- The chronic form evolves over time and occurs >15 days per month, on average for >180 days per year
- Acute treatment with aspirin, paracetamol, or NSAID is recommended
- No pharmacological prophylaxis is indicated, but acupuncture can be considered

Trigeminal autonomic cephalgias

- TACs share the clinical feature of lateralizing headaches with prominent ipsilateral cranial parasympathetic features. Different subtypes exist with characteristic features

Cluster headache

- Age 20–40 years; male:female 3:1
- At least five attacks which are unilateral orbital, supraorbital, or temporal
- Severe intensity and variable quality, associated with restlessness or agitation, lasting for 15–180 minutes
- Frequency can vary from one every other day to 8/day; episodic: 7 days to 1 year, with remission lasting at least 1 month; chronic: attacks occur for >1 year, without remission or with remission periods <1 month
- Other symptoms include ipsilateral conjunctival injection or lacrimation, nasal congestion or rhinorrhoea, forehead and facial sweating or flushing, eyelid oedema, miosis, and/or ptosis
- Treatment: acute—oxygen therapy, nasal or SC triptan; prophylactic—verapamil during cluster bout

Paroxysmal hemicrania

- Onset in adulthood
- At least 20 attacks which can be unilateral orbital, supraorbital, or temporal, lasting for 2–30 minutes
- Severe intensity and variable quality
- Frequency is about 5/day for more than half of the time; *episodic:* at least two bouts lasting 7 days to 1 year, separated by remission periods of ≥1 month; *chronic:* attacks without remission or with remission of <1 month for at least 1 year
- Other symptoms include ipsilateral conjunctival injection or lacrimation, nasal congestion or rhinorrhoea, forehead and facial sweating or flushing, eyelid oedema, miosis, and/or ptosis
- Responds absolutely to indomethacin

Short-acting unilateral neuralgiform headaches

- Onset in adulthood
- At least 20 attacks which can be unilateral orbital, supraorbital, temporal, and/or other trigeminal distribution, lasting for 1–600 seconds
- Moderate to severe in intensity and can be single stab, series of stabs, or saw-tooth pattern
- Frequency is 1/day for more than half of the time; *episodic:* 7 days to 1 year, with remission lasting at least 1 month; *chronic:* attacks occur for >1 year, without remission or with remission periods <1 month
- Symptoms include ipsilateral conjunctival injection or lacrimation, nasal congestion or rhinorrhoea, forehead and facial sweating or flushing, eyelid oedema, miosis, and/or ptosis
- SUNCT (short-lasting unilateral neuralgiform headache attacks with conjunctival injection and tearing): both conjunctival injection and lacrimation

- SUNA (short-lasting unilateral neuralgiform headache attacks with cranial autonomic symptoms): only one or neither of conjunctival injection and lacrimation
- Treatment is difficult. First line: lamotrigine; second line: topiramate, gabapentin

Hemicrania continua

- Onset in adulthood
- Attacks should be present for >3 months and are unilateral
- Moderate to severe in intensity and of variable quality
- Present for >3 months with exacerbations; *remitting subtype:* not continuous pain but has remission of at least 1 day; *unremitting subtype:* daily and continuous for at least 1 year without remission of ≥1 day
- Other symptoms include ipsilateral conjunctival injection or lacrimation, nasal congestion or rhinorrhoea, forehead and facial sweating or flushing, eyelid oedema, miosis, and/or ptosis
- Responds absolutely to indomethacin

Medication overuse headache

- Headache occurring on 15 or more days per month, developing as a consequence of regular overuse of acute or symptomatic headache medication (on 10 or more, or 15 or more days per month, depending on the medication) for >3 months
- It usually, but not invariably, resolves after overuse is stopped
- A public health problem, with a worldwide prevalence of 1–2%
- Aims of treatment are withdrawal of overused drugs, to provide the patient with pharmacological and non-pharmacological support, and to prevent relapse
- The Severity of Dependence Scale (SDS) score is a significant predictor of medication overuse amongst headache patients
- Withdrawal symptoms lasts for 2–10 days after detoxification
- The most common symptom is initial worsening of the headache, accompanied by various degrees of nausea, vomiting, hypotension, tachycardia, sleep disturbances, restlessness, anxiety, and nervousness
- The duration of withdrawal headaches has been found to vary with different drugs, being shorter in patients overusing triptans (approximately 4 days) than in those overusing ergotamine (approximately 7 days) or analgesics (approximately 10 days)
- Improvements are seen in two out of three patients after detoxification treatment

Further reading

1. Headache Classification Committee of the International Headache Society (IHS). The International Classification of Headache Disorders, 3rd edition. Cephalgia 2018;38(1):1–211
2. National Institute for Health and Care Excellence. Headaches in over 12s: diagnosis and management. NICE Clinical Guideline [CG150]. 2021. https://www.nice.org.uk/guidance/cg150
3. Matharu MS, Goadsby PJ. Trigeminal autonomic cephalgias. J Neurol Neurosurg Psychiatry 2002;72(2):19–26

28.5 Orofacial pain

Definition

- Pain localized to the region above the neck, in front of the ears, and below the orbitomeatal line, as well as pain within the oral cavity

- Comprises a large group of disorders, including temporomandibular disorders (TMDs), headaches, neuralgia, pain arising from dental or mucosal origins, and idiopathic pain

Of specific note

- There is an inherent complexity in shared care, including diagnosis, between dental and medical professionals
- An acute dental problem can masquerade as any of the other diagnostic groups, and vice versa, as dental pain can be referred, poorly localized, or misdiagnosed and can become chronic
- Common dental conditions may well coexist with other chronic pains

Incidence

- 12–26% of British adults report >1 day of orofacial pain within the past month
- Up to 50% of this is chronic

Classification

Dental

- Pulpitis
- Cracked tooth
- Dentine sensitivity
- Abscess

Non-dental

(See Table 28.5.1.)

Table 28.5.1 Types of non-dental pain

Oral non-dental pain	Neurovascular and tension	Cranial neuralgia	Persistent idiopathic
1. Oral malignancy 2. Mucosal lesions 3. Salivary gland pathology (lithiasis or tumour) 4. Atypical odontalgia	1. Tension-type headache 2. *Migraine:* i. Neurovascular orofacial pain (NVOP) ii. A subset of migraine usually in the distribution of the trigeminal nerve 3. *Trigeminal autonomic cephalgias:* i. Cluster headache ii. Paroxysmal hemicranias iii. Short-lasting unilateral neuralgiform headaches with conjunctival tearing (SUNCT) iv. Short-lasting unilateral neuralgiform headaches with cranial autonomic features (SUNA) d. Hemicrania continua	*Primary:* 1. Trigeminal neuralgia 2. Glossopharyngeal neuralgia *Secondary:* 1. Post-herpetic neuralgia 2. Diabetes mellitus 3. Multiple sclerosis 4. HIV 5. Post-traumatic neuropathy = anaesthesia dolorosa	1. Temporomandibular joint dysfunction (TMD) = facial arthromyalgia 2. Stomatodynia = burning mouth syndrome 3. Persistent idiopathic facial pain (PIFP) = atypical facial pain (AFP) = atypical odontalgia 4. Giant cell arteritis (GCA)

Diagnosis and triage to appropriate clinician

- Based on history, examination, and investigation

Investigation and treatment

Dental

- Specific treatment by a dental surgeon

Non-dental oral

- Specific investigation, including biopsy for histological diagnosis, followed by multidisciplinary discussion to determine the optimum treatment pathway which may include surgery/chemotherapy and/or radiotherapy

Atypical odontalgia

- Continuous dull ache or burning pain in teeth (normal or treated teeth), sometimes felt in extracted teeth site, worse on chewing
- May spread to neighbouring teeth
- Absent radiological findings
- Links with psychological issues, somatization, and other chronic pain conditions
- Treatment—reassurance, anti-neuropathics

Neurovascular and tension

(See 28.4 Headaches, p. 561.)

- Multidisciplinary pain management input for chronic pain

Tension-type headache

- Conservative multidisciplinary treatment

Migraine/neurovascular orofacial pain

- Simple analgesics/NSAIDs and antiemetics
- Triptans
- Prophylactic β-blockers, TCAs, topiramate, valproate, gabapentin
- Botulinum toxin

Cluster headache

- Oxygen
- Triptans
- Prophylactic prednisolone, verapamil, lithium, methysergide

Paroxysmal hemicrania

- Indomethacin

SUNCT/SUNA

- Lamotrigine, oxcarbazepine, topiramate, gabapentin

Hemicrania continua

- Indomethacin

Cranial neuralgias

Trigeminal neuralgia

(See 24.6 Trigeminal neuralgia, p. 490.)

- Multidisciplinary pain management input
- Carbamazepine/oxcarbazepine, lamotrigine, pregabalin
- Microvascular decompression, RF, or thermal ablative techniques

Glossopharyngeal neuralgia

(See 24.7 Glossopharyngeal neuralgia, p. 494.)

- Pain in the soft palate, ear and mastoid, base of tongue, and posterior pharynx, may be triggered by yawning, swallowing, talking, or coughing
- Multidisciplinary pain management input
- As for trigeminal neuralgia

Post-herpetic neuralgia

(See 24.9 Post-herpetic neuralgia, p. 497.)

- One or more dermatomal distributions of the trigeminal nerve can be affected—second most commonly affected nerve after thoracic nerves
- Ramsay Hunt syndrome—herpes zoster infection of the geniculate ganglion, causing facial palsy with earache
- Vaccination against VZV/herpes zoster
- Early systemic antiviral medication
- Multidisciplinary pain management
- TCAs, antiepileptics, opioids, NMDA receptor antagonists, topical lidocaine, capsaicin

Diabetic polyneuropathy

(See 24.13 Diabetic polyneuropathy, p. 509.)

- Optimization of underlying diabetes
- Multidisciplinary pain management input
- Anti-neuropathic medication

Multiple sclerosis-related neuropathy

- Optimization of underlying neurological condition
- Multidisciplinary pain management

HIV-related neuropathy

- Optimization of the underlying condition
- Multidisciplinary pain management

Post-traumatic neuropathy = anaesthesia dolorosa

Pathophysiology of anaesthesia dolorosa

- Rare deafferentation pain that occurs after traumatic (including radiotherapy) or surgical injury to the trigeminal nerve.
- Risk of 1.6% after glycerol rhizotomy, 0.8–2% after RF rhizotomy, and 2% after percutaneous controlled thermocoagulation
- Numbness associated with severe disabling pain

Treatment of anaesthesia dolorosa

- TCAs
- Anticonvulsants
- Multidisciplinary pain management

Persistent idiopathic

Temporomandibular disorders

Clinical features

- The most common causes of orofacial pain
- Affect 10–15% of the population over a lifetime, more in females
- Pain localized to pre- and post-auricular areas and the mandible
- Unilateral or bilateral, can radiate to the head and neck
- Associated clicking or crepitus and locking of temporomandibular joints, with tightness felt around the face
- Intermittent or continuous pain, sharp, dull, or shooting in nature
- Typically exacerbated by yawning and mastication, can be associated with bruxism
- Dysregulation of the adrenergic system with decreased COMT activity may be seen

Risk factors for TMDs

- **Degenerative TMDs rare but should be excluded, e.g. RA**
- Higher levels of distress, catastrophizing, and hypervigilance than controls
- Linked with anxiety/depression and other chronic painful conditions, including fibromyalgia and back pain

Management of TMDs

- Rule out red flags (dysfunction of the cranial nerve, sudden onset in >50-year-old patients, extremely limited mouth opening, lymphadenopathy, discharge/bleeding from the nose)
- Primarily a self-limiting disorder which should be treated conservatively
- Simple analgesics, TCAs, anticonvulsants
- Occlusal splints or mouth guards
- Multidisciplinary pain management input (education, acupuncture, psychological support, and self-management strategies)
- Surgery rarely, e.g. after failure of conservative management, degenerative joint disease, or disc dysfunction

Persistent idiopathic stomatodynia = burning mouth syndrome (BMS)

- A benign condition presenting as a burning sensation/pain in the absence of any abnormal clinical findings in the mouth or abnormal blood tests
- Primarily located in the anterior two-thirds of the tongue but can involve the lips, gingivae, and hard palate ± altered sensation of taste
- Pathophysiology largely unexplained, but some evidence of small-fibre sensory neuropathy ± central changes on fMRI scanning
- Commonly presents around/after the menopause and can be associated with anxiety/depression and other benign painful conditions, e.g. fibromyalgia, interstitial cystitis, IBS
- Affects 2% of the population
- Female:male 7:1

Treatment of BMS

- Clonazepam (PO or topical)
- TCAs
- Anticonvulsants
- Multidisciplinary pain management

Atypical facial pain (AFP) = persistent idiopathic facial pain (PIFP)

- A persistent idiopathic orofacial pain, which does not fit the clinical pattern for any other diagnosis, present for 6 months or more
- Affects the middle-aged female population, often unilateral
- Not restricted by neurological anatomical boundaries
- Pain can be deep, vague, wandering, and constant and can extend into the neck
- Examination may reveal some areas of decreased sensations in the painful area
- Often associated with psychological comorbidity and other chronic benign painful conditions, needing a thorough psychological workup
- Treatment outcome is usually unsatisfactory; along similar lines to trigeminal neuralgia, but evidence base weak as heterogeneity of patients and rarity of the condition limit research opportunities. TCAs and anticonvulsants may help and invasive interventional procedures should be avoided

Giant cell arteritis

- Important differential diagnosis in patients over 50 years
- Daily headaches, sensitivity in the scalp, generalized fatigue ± pain in the tongue
- Throbbing, continuous temporal, or pre-auricular pain
- Usually unilateral
- Reduced pulse in a dilate, tortuous temporal artery on examination suspicious
- Blood ESR can be markedly elevated, and CRP and temporal artery biopsy diagnostic
- Potentially vision-threatening, so requires urgent diagnosis and treatment with high-dose steroids (if necessary before test results back)
- Biopsy can be positive within 7–10 days of starting steroids
- Urgent referral to ophthalmology
- May be associated with jaw claudication, systemic illness, and polymyalgia rheumatica
- Giant cell arteritis can be active for up to 2 years; hence, steroids should be continued to prevent vision complications

Further reading

1. Romero-Reyes M, Uyanik JM. Orofacial pain management: current perspectives. J Pain Res 2014;7:99–115
2. Woda A, Tubert-Jeannin S, Bouhassira D, et al. Towards a new taxonomy of idiopathic orofacial pain. Pain 2005;116(3):396–406
3. Shephard MK, MacGregor EA, Zakrzewska JM. Orofacial pain—a guide for the headache physician. Headache 2014;54(1):22–39

28.6 Paediatric chronic pain

Introduction

- Paediatric chronic pain is increasingly recognized
- However, chronic pain in children has been less extensively studied and the evidence base is smaller than in adults
- Pain in neonates was only recently recognized and many procedures were done without any analgesia or anaesthesia in the past

Pain pathways and mechanisms in children

- Pain pathways in children differ functionally from those in adults due to a maturing nervous system:
  - Little descending inhibition from higher CNS centres in the first week
  - Dendritic spine density 2–3 times of that of adults
  - Highest dendritic spine density in the prefrontal cortex at 2.5–7 years
  - The RVM switches from a facilitator of nociception to an inhibitor with age
  - Animal studies show that the PAG area does not produce analgesia at early ages
- Prolonged neonatal intensive care is associated with increased nociceptive sensitivity, and fMRI studies show increased central sensitivity of brain pain pathways

Epidemiology of paediatric pain

(See Table 28.6.1.)

- A cross-sectional Dutch study of 5425 children showed that 54% experienced pain within the last 3 months and 25% suffered from chronic pain of >3 months' duration (8% of this pain was described as severe). Girls were more likely to suffer from chronic pain than boys

Pain assessment

(See Table 28.6.2.)

- Assessment of pain is age-dependent, and both self-reporting and physiological measures are commonly used
- Assessment must be age-appropriate and younger children may not easily verbalize or self-report their pain

Table 28.6.1 Epidemiology of paediatric pain

Pain type	Prevalence (%)	Age
Headache	8–82	Older
Abdominal	3.8–53.4	Younger
Back	13.5–24	Older
Musculoskeletal	3.9–40	Older
Multiple	3.5–48.8	Unknown
Other	5–88	Unknown

Table 28.6.2 Pain assessment in children

Pain	Pain intensity Pain description Temporal aspects
Associated symptoms	Fatigue Sleep
Emotional	Anxiety Depression
Cognitive	Coping Catastrophizing Avoidance
Social	School attendance Family function Parental anxiety and depression

Therapeutic basis of management

- Paediatric chronic pain requires a multidisciplinary approach and a biopsychosocial model is the current model of care
- Evidence for the use of adult management strategies is limited in the paediatric population
- Strategies must be age-appropriate and the impact of pain on the family is a significant consideration in long-term management

Specific pain presentations

- Although many chronic pain syndromes are present in both the paediatric and adult populations, there are important differences in their presentation, aetiology, and prognosis

Complex regional pain syndrome

- Peak incidence is in early adolescence, with a female predominance
- Compared with adults, there is a greater incidence in the lower limb, but prognosis is better
- Fewer physical signs are present
- Diagnostic criteria are similar to those for adult CRPS using the Budapest criteria (see 24.11 Complex regional pain syndrome, p. 501)
- Initial management is with physiotherapy, and this is associated with a good outcome in 90% of patients
- Refractory cases benefit from an interdisciplinary approach
- The role of interventions (nerve blocks, neuromodulation) is unknown and its use must be combined with a multidisciplinary pain management strategy

Neuropathic pain

- Due to the immaturity and capacity for plasticity of the nervous system, neuropathic pain has a number of significant differences in childhood
- Many medical conditions seen in adults are uncommon in children such as diabetic neuropathy and PHN
- Obstetric brachial plexus palsy is rarely associated with neuropathic pain

- The incidence of neuropathic pain after never injury is lower in children and approaches adult levels after adolescence
- Post-surgical neuropathic pain is increasingly recognized in children (after inguinal hernia repair, 13.5% of children reported chronic pain and 2% described it as severe in intensity)
- The proportion of SCI patients who are paediatric is 3–5%
- Neuropathic pain is less common in children, compared with adults
- Injury in under 20-year olds have a 26% risk of developing persistent pain, whereas the risk is 45% in those above 20 years of age
- Anti-neuropathic analgesia (e.g. TCAs and gabapentinoids) are useful adjuncts in children and doses must be age-appropriate
  - Gabapentin (5–10 mg/kg three times daily)
  - Amitriptyline (0.5 mg/kg at night)
- S/Es must be balanced with analgesic benefit, as CNS S/Es can have significant effects on school and exam performance
- Topical therapies such as lidocaine plasters or 8% capsiacin are especially useful due to their lack of systemic effects

Abdominal pain

- A high proportion of abdominal pain in children is associated with a functional cause
- The diagnosis is made on the basis of:
  - Episodic or continuous pain
  - Insufficient criteria for other functional GI disorders
  - No evidence of inflammatory, anatomic, metabolic, or neoplastic processes that can explain the symptoms
- Functional abdominal pain includes IBS, functional dyspepsia, and abdominal migraine
- Apart from abdominal migraine, symptoms must be present for at least 8 weeks
- Despite a lack of organic pathology, affected children have frequent school absences, functional impairment, and psychological distress with depression and anxiety
- Although pharmacological approaches are common, there is a lack of evidence of their long-term efficacy
- CBT has been associated with beneficial outcomes

Headache

- Headache in children is among the most common causes for medical consultations in children
- The diagnostic criteria for migraine are modified

Ages affected

- All ages are affected by headache:
  - 3–8% by 3 years of age
  - 20% by 5 years
  - 37–51% by 7 years
  - 57–82% by 15 years

Important causes

- Although there are a large number of diagnoses, the important causes are:
  - Migraine (most common cause of chronic daily headache)
  - Medication overuse headache (second most common cause)

- ■ Tension-type headache and new daily persistent headache
- ■ TAC

Features that indicate imaging

- Recent onset of severe headache
- Change in severity or frequency
- Fixed or unusual location
- Early morning or waking from sleep
- Postural headache
- Abnormal neurological examination
- Abnormal growth or puberty
- Deterioration in school function

Management principles

- Although medication is the most common approach, it is important to balance the risk and benefits
- Excessive use of analgesia can result in analgesic overuse headache, and opioids must be avoided
- Lifestyle management, education, and behavioural therapies are important in long-term management
- The use of occipital nerve blocks can be a useful and low-risk adjunct

Musculoskeletal pain

- Most MSK pains in children are benign, but a full assessment is crucial to rule out inflammatory arthritis, infection, and malignancy
- About 7–15% of all schoolchildren suffer from MSK pain
- Back pain is an increasingly recognized problem in children
- By the age of 18 years, at least half will have reported episodes of back pain, but few of these will present themselves to health professionals
- It is important to rule out serious pathology, and a careful clinical assessment is required to make a diagnosis and to identify red flags that may constitute serious underlying pathology
- Radiological imaging often starts with plain radiographs to look for infections, structural abnormalities, and tumours
- Further imaging (CT or MRI) can then be used if appropriate
- Most mechanical low back pain responds to physiotherapy, but refractory cases will benefit from a multidisciplinary approach
- The role of interventions is limited and their use is less than that seen in adults

Important causes of back pain in children

Intervertebral disc pathology

- Disc degeneration is seen in 6–19% between 10 and 18 years of age
- It is possible that many cases of adult back pain start in childhood

Scheuermann's disease

- Presents with thoracic and thoracolumbar kyphosis
- Symptoms improve with skeletal maturity
- Refractory cases may benefit from spinal bracing

Juvenile idiopathic arthritis

- Commonly affects the cervical spine
- In older children, SIJ pain may be present

Osteomyelitis and discitis

- Infants and children differ from adults in that the disc has widespread anastomotic channels
- This allows for pyogenic osteomyelitis and TB to occur in the spine, but also decreases the risk of infarction and increases the chance of bacterial clearance
- Unlike in adults, discitis in children is often self-limiting and an infectious cause is uncommon

Neoplasia

- Nocturnal pain and progressive increase in symptoms should alert the clinician

Conclusions

- Chronic non-cancer pain is increasingly recognized as a significant cause of functional impairment and disability in children
- It has an impact on the child's QoL, school performance, and peer networks
- Therapy must be aimed at recognizing the differences in the aetiology and natural history of pain in children, with an understanding of the complex relationships involving their family, school, and social networks
- A multidisciplinary biopsychosocial approach should be applied, as single interventions are often insufficient

Further reading

1. Hechler T, Kanstrup M, Lewandowski HA, et al. Systematic review on intensive interdisciplinary pain treatment of children with chronic pain. Pediatrics 2015;138(1):115–27
2. King S, Chambers CT, Huguet A, et al. The epidemiology of chronic pain in children and adolescents revisited: a systematic review. Pain 2011;152:2729e38
3. Perquin CW, Hazebroek-Kampschreur AA, Hunfeld JA, et al. Pain in children and adolescents: a common experience. Pain 2000;87:51–8
4. Rajapakse D, Liossi C, Howard R. Presentation and management of chronic pain. Arch Dis Child 2014;99:474–80

28.7 Pain in the elderly

Introduction

- Chronic pain prevalence increases with age—chronic pain affects 63% of patients over 75 years of age
- There is an increased prevalence of chronic pain in care home residents (>80% compared with >50% in the community)
- Chronic pain in older adults tends to be constant, of moderate to severe intensity, and lasting for several years (multifocal and multifactorial)
- Persistent pain or its inadequate treatment is associated with a number of adverse outcomes in older people, including functional impairment, falls, slow rehabilitation, mood changes

(depression and anxiety), decreased socialization, sleep and appetite disturbance, and greater health care use and costs

Aetiology

- The most common sites of chronic pain in the elderly are the hips, knees, and back
- Pain conditions which are more common in older adults include:
  - MSK—myofascial pain syndrome, OA
  - Cancer-related—due to cancer itself and/or cancer treatments
  - Neuropathic—peripheral neuropathies, PHN, post-stroke pain
  - Other—fibromyalgia

Physiology/psychology

- A meta-analysis showed that while pain threshold increases with age, pain tolerance thresholds do not show age-related changes. Therefore, ageing reduces pain sensitivity for lower pain intensities
- Some studies suggest an increased vulnerability amongst older adults to severe and persistent pain
- Psychological factors may affect pain reporting in older adults, including altered pain beliefs and attitudes, fear of addiction, misattribution of symptoms, and stoicism

Risk factors

- Loneliness and social isolation
- There is a strong link between pain in the elderly and low mood—each being a risk factor for the other
- Increased risk of mood disorder, cognitive decline, and falls in elderly patients with chronic pain

History

- Assessment of pain in older adults may be more difficult due to communication issues (visual/hearing loss), concurrent illness, cognitive ability, and socio-cultural factors
- Patient self-reporting of pain is the most valid and reliable indicator of pain, even in the presence of mild to moderate dementia—the NRS or verbal descriptors should be used to establish pain intensity
- A self-report measure of function should also be used such as the Pain Disability Index
- For patients with severe cognitive impairment (e.g., scoring <18 on Mini-Mental Status Examination), the PAINAD, Abbey or Doloplus-2 scales are recommended. Also gain a history from carers/family members to determine the patient's function, rest, leisure, and productivity
- The PAINAD scale involves observation of the patient for 3–5 minutes during an activity to note breathing, negative vocalizations, facial expressions, body language, and consolability. Each domain is scored 0–2, with a total possible score of 10
- Comorbidities may contribute to pain or influence the treatment of pain
- Drug history essential to anticipate potential drug–drug interactions

Examination

- In addition to a general examination, including cardiorespiratory, consider the following specific examinations:
  - Neurological—central, peripheral, and autonomic nervous systems
  - MSK and rheumatological—look, feel, move joints and muscles

- Assessment of mobility/balance—impacts on falls risk
- Assessment of mental state especially the cognitive function

Investigations

- Imaging only indicated for patients in whom there is suspicion of a disease which requires specialist intervention, e.g. hip OA, neurogenic claudication, etc.
- Consider imaging in the presence of 'red flags', e.g. worsening pain with a history of cancer, risk factors for infection (e.g. immunosuppressive therapy), constitutional signs/symptoms, recent trauma or risk of fractures

Treatment

General principles

- Stepped approach—the least potentially toxic interventions should be used initially, followed by therapies with greater risks
- Systemic medications are used as a later step due to the risk of S/Es, toxicity, and interactions with other medications used for chronic illness
- Local treatments/topical treatments may be preferable due to lack of systemic S/Es
- High risk of drug–drug and drug–disease interactions in patients on multiple medications for other comorbidities
- Altered pharmacokinetics with ageing include:
  - Absorption: altered from the gut due to slowing of GI transit time (may increase absorption of continuous-release enteral drugs)
  - Distribution: altered due to increased fat:lean body weight ratios
  - Metabolism: altered due to altered function of the hepatic system and CYP450 enzymes
  - Excretion: due to reduced glomerular filtration and renal clearance

Pharmacological treatments

Paracetamol

- Well tolerated
- Caution in dosing for low-weight elderly adults

NSAIDs

- Should be used with great caution in elderly adults—risk of adverse effects significantly higher in older adults, especially those with chronic kidney disease, gastropathy, and cardiovascular disease, or those who may be intravascularly deplete, e.g. heart failure.
- If used, use at the lowest dose for the shortest period of time, co-prescribed with a proton pump inhibitor
- Naproxen and celecoxib have been shown to be the most appropriate of NSAIDs for patients with cardiovascular risk factors
- COX-2 selective inhibitors have a lower risk of GI S/Es, but cardiovascular risk factors are higher

Opioids

- Effective in the short term (<12 weeks), but long-term data are lacking
- May be appropriate in moderate to severe pain in highly selected patients with functional impairment or impaired QoL

- Modified-release or transdermal preparations aim to provide relatively constant plasma concentrations for continuous pain, although short-acting opioids are preferred to reduce opioid induced ventilatory impairment and other opiod related adverse effects
- Risk of S/Es will necessitate antiemetic and laxative co-prescription. May also affect level of consciousness/thinking processes and increase the risk of falls
- Caution in renal failure with renally cleared drugs, e.g. hydromorphone/morphine/oxycodone

Adjuvant medications

- Primarily used for neuropathic pain
- Use at the lowest dose and titrate upwards slowly to the lowest effective dose
- Caution with tramadol and TCAs which have anticholinergic S/Es (sedation, cognitive dysfunction, orthostatic hypotension)
- Caution with pregabalin and gabapentin especially in renal impairment—risk of S/Es: dizziness, somnolence, fatigue, cognitive impairment, falls, peripheral oedema, depression
- Carbamazepine/oxcarbazepine may be used for trigeminal neuralgia—risk of hyponatraemia/SIADH
- Duloxetine—evidence effective for treatment of neuropathic pain and some studies suggest use for non-neuropathic pain, e.g. OA/lower back pain

Topical treatments

- Lidocaine/capsaicin/menthol—limited efficacy for management of localized neuropathic pain but have a good safety profile with minimal adverse effects
- Topical NSAIDs for localized MSK pain

Pain interventions

- Use in older population—evidence is weak/mixed/lacking
- Procedures most commonly performed:
  - Intra-articular injections of corticosteroids/hyaluronic acid, e.g. knee OA
  - Spinal nerve blocks for degenerative lumbar disease/spinal stenosis
- Other procedures:
  - Condition-specific neural blocks
  - Percutaneous procedures for trigeminal neuralgia in elderly patients with comorbidities
  - Epidural corticosteroid injections, e.g. spinal stenosis—limited evidence (less evidence in radicular pain/sciatica)
  - Facet joint injections/RF denervation of medial branch nerves
  - Sympathectomy—weak evidence in older population for neuropathic pain

Physical treatments

- Must be tailored and individual-specific to optimize function and independence
- Aim to strengthen the core, improve flexibility and endurance for physical activity, improve function, and reduce falls risk
- Use of assist devices to enable engagement in ADLs may enable the patient to remain more independent and reduce functional decline

Psychological treatments

- Aim to influence how people respond and cope with pain
- CBT improves chronic pain, disability, and mood

- Limited evidence for biofeedback training, relaxation, mindfulness, meditation, and enhancing emotion regulation in elderly patients with chronic pain

Complementary therapies

- Limited research for effectiveness of TENS/massage/reflexology/acupuncture in elderly with chronic pain
- However, anecdotal evidence suggests some benefit

Interventional/surgical treatments

- Vertebroplasty/kyphoplasty for the treatment of acute painful vertebral fractures
- Joint replacement for OA

Further reading

1. Fayaz A, Croft P, Langford RM, et al. Prevalence of chronic pain in the UK: a systematic review and meta-analysis of population studies. BMJ Open 2016;6:e010364
2. Reid MC, Eccleston C, Pillemer K. Management of chronic pain in older adults. BMJ 2015;350:h532
3. Abdulla A, Adams N, Bone M, et al. Guidance on the management of pain in older people. Age Ageing 2013;42(1):1–57

28.8 Human immunodeficiency virus

Introduction

- The HIV targets the immune system and weakens people's defence systems against infections and some types of cancer
- Undertreatment of pain in HIV patients is common, particularly in patients with less education and a history of IV drug use, and in females

Incidence

- Globally, 36.7 million people were living with HIV at the end of 2016, with 1.8 million people becoming newly infected. An estimated 0.8% of adults aged 15–49 years are living with HIV worldwide; 54% of adults and 43% of children living with HIV worldwide are currently receiving lifelong antiretroviral therapy
- Approximately 30–60% of patients have severe pain associated with a profound negative impact on psychological and physical functioning, as well as on overall QoL. Prevalence of poorly controlled pain has been reported in up to 97% of terminally ill HIV patients
- Patients are more likely to be unemployed and disabled and to have less social support
- Patients with HIV who experience pain are more likely to be distressed, depressed, and hopeless and to have suicidal thoughts (40%), compared to those without pain (20%)

Aetiology of pain

- Direct damage caused by HIV
- Immunosuppression
- Therapies for HIV/acquired immunodeficiency syndrome (AIDS)

- Associated disorders with HIV/AIDS
- Causes unrelated to HIV/AIDS
- A review found the mechanisms of HIV-related pain were 45% somatic, 15% visceral, 19% neuropathic, and 4% unknown

Pain syndromes in HIV patients

Nervous system

Neuropathies

- Distal symmetrical polyneuropathy and antiretroviral toxic neuropathy are the most common
- Acute herpes zoster, acute varicella zoster, and post-herpetic neuropathy are also common
- Others: autonomic neuropathy, acute zoster pain, post-herpetic neuropathy, mononeuritis multiplex, mononeuropathies, diffuse inflammatory lymphocytosis syndrome, lumbo-sacral polyradiculopathy, demyelinating polyradiculoneuropathy, HIV-associated neuromuscular weakness syndrome

Brain disorders

- HIV encephalopathy: aseptic/bacterial/viral (cytomegalovirus (CMV) or HIV)/fungal (*Cryptococcus*)
- Toxoplasmosis
- Malignancies: lymphoma, sarcomas such as Kaposi's or others
- Other conditions such as migraines, tension headaches, and sinusitis

Gastrointestinal system

- Oral cavity: oral lesions, infections (*Candida*), mouth ulcers
- Oesophagitis related to infections or HIV therapies
- Infections: gastroenteritis, hepatobiliary, etc.
- S/Es of medications
- Peptic ulcer disease
- Pancreatitis
- Neoplasms: Kaposi's sarcoma, non-Hodgkin's lymphoma, and others
- Anorectal pain

Cardiothoracic system

- Pneumonia (commonly *Pneumocystis carinii*), lung malignancy
- Endocarditis, pericarditis, myocarditis, especially in patients who use IV drugs

Rheumatic system

- Reiter's syndrome, septic arthritis, psoriatic arthritis
- Polymyositis from HIV itself or from medications (e.g. azathioprine)

HIV-associated sensory neuropathy

- Most common cause of peripheral nerve dysfunction in HIV (between 30% and 60% of individuals affected)
- Two clinically almost indistinguishable entities, with different causes, often coexisting:
  - Distal sensory polyneuropathy (HIV-related)
  - Antiretroviral toxic neuropathy (antiretroviral treatment-related)

Clinical presentation

- Distal symmetrical small-fibre neuropathy in a 'stocking and glove' distribution, with the feet being affected first. Progressive onset of symmetrical paraesthesiae, numbness, and painful dysaesthesia of the lower extremities. Hyperalgesia and allodynia are common
- Descriptors used by patients are commonly 'burning', 'numb', and 'tingling'
- Wearing shoes can become problematic, although some patients report the most pain when they are barefoot in bed (allodynia provoked by contact with linen)
- As the course of the disease progresses, the symptoms can ascend to the legs
- When the pain reaches the knees, the upper limbs may become involved (fingertips)
- Hyporeflexia of the lower extremities is common (reduced/absent Achilles reflex)
- Weakness is rare (if it occurs, explore alternative diagnoses)
- Insidious onset for distal sensory polyneuropathy; sudden and rapidly progressive onset for antiretroviral toxic neuropathy, temporally associated with exposure to antiretroviral therapy (as early as 1 week from the start, and usually within the first year of use). These are the only true differentiating elements

Pathophysiology

- Distal sensory polyneuropathy: neuronal apoptosis induced directly by the Gp120 HIV protein, and exposure of Schwann cells and macrophages to Gp120 results in the release of neurotoxins
- Antiretroviral toxic neuropathy: exposure to nucleoside reverse transcriptase inhibitors (NRTIs), in particular stavudine, didanosine, and zalcitabine, can lead to mitochondrial toxicity and resulting nerve damage
- In both of these neuropathies, there is distal axonal degeneration and dying-back axonopathy of long axons affecting both myelinated and unmyelinated fibres

Risk factors

- Advanced HIV disease: low CD4 T cell count, high viral load
- Exposure to NRTIs and neurotoxic medications (antibiotics, chemotherapy)
- Diabetes, hypothyroidism, hypovitaminosis (especially B12)
- Increasing age and height (longer nerve fibres)
- Alcohol and recreational drug use
- Concurrent infections (hepatitis C, syphilis)

Diagnosis

- Mainly based on history, clinical picture, and physical examination
- Investigations:
  - To screen for other causes
  - Electrodiagnostic studies warranted in cases of weakness or asymmetry (may point to other types of neuropathy)
  - Biopsy (tissue, sural nerve)—not routine clinical practice and commonly in research

Management

- Prompt initiation of HIV treatment in antiretroviral-naïve patients
- Change to non-neurotoxic agents in patients on treatment
- Mitigation of other sources of nerve insult (see Risk factors, p. 580)
- Physical, pharmacological, and psychosocial interventions as per general pain management principles

- Pharmacotherapy that can be used:
  - Anticonvulsants: gabapentin, pregabalin, lamotrigine
  - Antidepressants: amitriptyline, nortriptyline, duloxetine, venlafaxine
  - Topical: lidocaine 5% patch, capsaicin 8% patch or topical 0.0075% or 0.0125%
  - Cannabis (evidence is controversial and is unlicensed in many countries for chronic non-cancer pain management)
  - Opiates to be used with great caution as:
    - There is little evidence for efficacy of opioids in HIV neuropathic pain
    - There is a high risk of opioid misuse or abuse in HIV patients
    - Opioids may have pro-nociceptive effects (activation of glia, secretion of pro-nociceptive mediators such as cytokines, ILs, TNF) and may promote HIV infectivity from opioid-related immunosuppressive effects

Further reading

1. Hewitt DJ, McDonald M, Portenoy RK, et al. Pain syndromes and etiologies in ambulatory AIDS patients. Pain 1997;70:117–23
2. Phillips TJC, Cherry CL, Moss PJ, Rice ASC. Painful HIV-associated sensory neuropathy—IASP clinical updates. 2010;18(3):1–8
3. Nardin RA, Freeman M. Epidemiology, clinical manifestations, diagnosis, and treatment of HIV-associated peripheral neuropathy. UpToDate. 2018. https://www.uptodate.com

28.9 Sickle cell disease

Definition of sickle cell disease

- Inherited autosomal recessive disorder of the Hb molecule
- The normal glutamic acid is replaced by valine on the β-globin gene, producing a variant Hb called HbS
- Homozygotes have sickle cell disease, and heterozygotes have sickle cell trait
- HbS in combination with other variants produces Hb-thalassaemia
- The major sequelae are haemolysis, anaemia, and pain

Incidence

- Incidence 1/5000—the most common severe genetic disease in the UK
- More common in African, Afro-Caribbean, Asian, Mediterranean, and Middle Eastern people
- Carriers exhibit partial resistance to all forms of *Plasmodium falciparum* malaria

Physiology

- HbS causes the red cell to become sickle-shaped and inflexible under certain physiological conditions
- 'Sickle cells' cause microvascular occlusion and increased haemolysis

Pain in sickle cell disease

- Acute painful crises:
  - Vaso-occlusion leads to a combination of hypoxia–reperfusion injury, ischaemic tissue damage, and chronic vascular inflammation

- Inflammatory mediators, especially ATP, H^+, and glutamate, activate receptors on A-delta and C-fibres within the nociceptive system
- Chronic pain:
    - Inflammatory response secondary to repeated episodes of microvascular occlusion and resultant tissue damage
    - Central sensitization and 'wind-up' of the nervous system in response to recurrent acute painful crises, causing long-term amplification and maintenance of the pain signal
- Neuropathic pain:
    - Putative mechanism is via microvascular occlusion of the vasa vasorum
    - Common presentations include mental neuralgia, trigeminal neuralgia, and more rarely orbital or spinal cord infarction

Risk factors for acute painful crises

- Acidosis, hypoxia, exposure to cold, exercise, stress
- Frequent, severe acute painful crises with inadequate analgesia increase the risk of chronic pain

Diagnosis

- Hb electrophoresis
- Screening of at-risk pregnant women and their partners in early pregnancy to detect carriers
- Heel-prick blood spot test in newborns in the UK
- Perioperative screening of high-risk patients for sickle cell trait

Treatment

- Supportive treatment:
    - Balanced diet, sleep, hydration, folic acid, regular surveillance. Multidisciplinary input to address the sequelae of chronic pain and illness
- Symptomatic management:
    - Blood transfusion for anaemia, analgesic plan for acute painful crises, as well as for chronic pain, antibiotics for infection
- Preventative management:
    - Prophylactic daily penicillin V until age of 5, pneumococcal vaccination, stress management, HbF induction with hydroxyurea, avoidance of precipitating conditions
- Abortive management:
    - Prompt, aggressive treatment of acute painful crises
    - Blood parameters can support the diagnosis of acute painful crises (decreased red blood cell (RBC) deformability, increased number of dense cells, reticulocytes, leucocytes, and relative thrombocytopenia) in complex cases, e.g. to exclude opioid-seeking behaviours
    - Provide a pain management plan for patients to institute at home (commonly short-acting opioids and paracetamol)
    - Treat preferably in a rapid access medical day case admission unit rather than via the emergency department
    - Future avenues include anti-adhesion molecules and inhaled NO
- Curative therapy:
    - Stem cell transplantation, future gene therapy

Further reading

1. Mousa SA, Qari MH. Diagnosis and management of sickle cell disorders. Methods Mol Biol 2010;663:291–307
2. Brousse V, Makani J, Rees DC. Management of sickle cell disease in the community. BMJ 2014;348:g1765

28.10 Vascular insufficiency pain

Introduction

- A number of terms describe a spectrum of peripheral vascular disorders:
  - Peripheral arterial disease—a disease of the peripheral arterial system characterized by insufficient blood flow to the limbs to support normal function
  - Intermittent claudication—a clinical syndrome that consists of leg pain induced by walking; the pain improves with rest
  - Critical limb ischaemia—persistent pain at rest due to insufficient blood supply to a limb, leading to poor tissue perfusion, tissue loss, skin ulceration, and loss of limb function
  - Acute limb ischaemia—an acute emergency caused by sudden loss of blood supply to a limb, leading to rapid tissue loss and limb function

Incidence

- Age-related increase in prevalence of up to 15% of the population aged above 50 years
- Important modifiable risk factors include poor nutrition, smoking, diabetes, hypertension, obesity, high alcohol use, and hyperlipidaemia

Pathophysiology

- Reduction of blood flow causing a mismatch between the supply of nutrients and the removal of toxic metabolites from tissues by:
  - Atherosclerotic plaque causing arterial stenosis or occlusion (most common mechanism)
  - Embolization of an artery from a thrombus or arterial dissection perioperatively
- Nociceptive and/or neuropathic pain plus autonomic dysfunction

History

- Assess the psychological, physical, and social impact of the pain on the person and the functional limitations as a result of the pain. Characteristics of vascular insufficiency pain:
  - Nature of the pain:
    - Ischaemic pain is normally worse on elevation and relieved by dependency. In critical limb ischaemia, there is rest pain and/or claudication pain (exacerbated by exercise and immediately relieved by rest)
    - Neuropathic pain can present as burning, altered sensation, shooting, or allodynia, and may be worse at rest and relieved by exercise
    - Nociplastic pain: mixed presentation of nociceptive and neuropathic pain
  - Time frame can be acute, subacute, or chronic
  - Can affect sensory (small or large fibres), motor, autonomic, or multiple nerve fibres
  - Distribution most commonly:
    - Aorto-iliac disease manifesting with pain in the thigh and buttock
    - Femoral–popliteal disease presenting as pain in the calf

Examination

- Cardiorespiratory examination focusing on the peripheral vascular system
- Relevant examination for other causes as infections, ulcers, haematomas, compartment syndrome, deep vein thrombosis, etc.
- Assess for signs of:
  - Ischaemic limb—hair loss, shiny skin, skin ulcer, pale skin colour, brittle nails, weakness, weak/absent peripheral pulses, sensory loss, and muscle wasting
  - Neuropathy—large, small, motor, autonomic fibre involvement with sensory gain or loss and pattern (polyneuropathy, mononeuropathy, symmetrical)

Investigations

- Psychometric questionnaires—e.g. BPI, Depression Anxiety Stress Scales (DAAS), the Leeds Assessment of Neuropathic Symptoms and Signs (LANNS) Pain Detect, Neuropathic Pain Questionnaire (NPQ), Identification Pain Questionnaire (ID Pain)
- Blood tests—FBC, lipid profile, metabolic and diabetic screen
- Ankle–brachial pressure index <0.8 indicates significant peripheral artery disease
- US Doppler study
- CT angiogram or MRI
- Angiogram and interventional radiology

Differential diagnosis

- Lumbar spinal canal stenosis—this produces neurogenic claudication
- CRPS
- Phantom limb pain
- Spinal cord, lumbar plexus, and peripheral nerve palsy
- Idiopathic
- Other causes of peripheral neuropathies such as metabolic (e.g. diabetes), toxic (e.g. alcohol, antineoplastic agents, antiretrovirals), autoimmune (e.g. lupus, vasculitic neuropathy), infective (e.g. HIV), and inherited (e.g. hereditary sensory neuropathy, Fabry's disease)

Treatment

Disease-specific treatments

- Healthy diet, smoking cessation, BP, exercise, and weight optimization
- Statins and antiplatelet agents
- If conservative treatments fail to improve QoL and function, consider:
  - Minimally invasive endovascular revascularization—angioplasty, stenting
  - Open bypass operations
  - Amputation

Multidisciplinary treatments

- Address physical, psychological (psychiatric or psychological), and social (work, litigation, social support network) contributors to pain, disability, and distress:
  - Patient education is one of the primary goals to empower patients to adapt and achieve QoL that is as optimal as possible
  - Development of pain management strategies (e.g. activity pacing, exercises, desensitizing, goal setting, thought challenging, and others)

- CBT, ACT, cognitive restructuring, distraction, relaxation, mindfulness, and other psychological strategies individually or in a pain programme according to the patient's needs

Pharmacological treatment

- Several agents can be considered, including:
  - Anticonvulsants (e.g. gabapentin, pregabalin)
  - Antidepressants (e.g. TCAs, SNRIs, SSRIs)
  - Opioids (e.g. tramadol, tapentadol, morphine)—no long-term studies showing efficacy
  - Other medications with lower evidence include ketamine, lidocaine, topical capsaicin, and IV PG

Pain intervention

- Subarachnoid, epidural, or peripheral nerve blocks—effective in acute limb ischaemia
- Sympathetic block for critical limb ischaemia:
  - Lumbar sympathetic block has inconsistent results for lower limb pain
  - Stellate ganglion block for upper limb ischaemic pain has variable success
- SCS—RCT has shown benefit for peripheral vascular disease and refractory angina. The British Pain Society guidelines recommend these as good clinical indications for SCS. SCS could not be recommended by NICE due to inadequate RCT data and insufficient economic evaluation

Further reading

1. Laoire ÁN, Murtagh FEM. Systematic review of pharmacological therapies for the management of ischaemic pain in patients with non-reconstructable critical limb ischaemia. Br Med J Support Palliat Care 2018;8(4):400–10
2. Morley RL, Sharma A, Horsch AD, et al. Peripheral artery disease. BMJ 2018;360:j5842

SECTION 6

CANCER AND PAIN

Cancer and Pain

Kasia Chmiel, Mahesh Choudhari, Alix Dumitrescu, Yehia Kamel, Ashok Puttapa, and Alifia Tameem

CONTENTS

29.1 Cancer pain mechanisms

Introduction

- Cancer pain is a complex syndrome involving inflammatory, neuropathic, and ischaemic mechanisms, and most patients experience mixed pain (80%)
- 30% of patients at an early stage of cancer suffer from pain, increasing to 75–90% in advanced stages

Types of pain

Neuropathic pain

- Due to damage to neurons, either peripheral or central, via mechanical compression, ischaemia, haemorrhage, chemical changes, and oedema, further impeding oxygen supply, and transection
- There is peripheral and central sensitization, leading to spontaneous and ectopic discharges and activation of NMDA receptors

Inflammatory pain

- Peripheral and central mediators of inflammation, such as bradykinins and cytokines, establish a feed-forward loop that results in sensitization of primary afferents, recruitment of silent nociceptors, and peripheral hyperalgesia

Nociceptive/visceral pain

- Diffuse, poorly localized pain with symptoms of spasm and heavy feeling. It can be secondary to bowel obstruction or ischaemic bowel

Pain due to direct effect of malignant tumours (70%)

- Deposits of abnormal cancer cells are very active metabolically and divide rapidly, which causes an imbalance between oxygen supply and demand, causing necrosis. These cells secrete a large amount of pain chemical mediators such as TNF alpha, NGF, and ILs, leading to an inflammatory response attracting lymphocytes and macrophages
- Tumour expansion and fascia and capsular stretching, causing mechanical pressure locally
- Direct mechanical compression, infiltration, or entrapment of nerves and plexuses, causing neuropathic pain and direct infiltration of tissues, bone, and viscera
- Obstruction of hollow viscus and blood vessels results in inflammation and ischaemia. This causes diffuse pain due to peritoneal stretching

Bone metastasis

- Metastatic disease of bone is a very common cause of severe pain and occurs in nearly 90% of patients, mainly arising from cancers affecting the prostate, breast, lung, kidney, and thyroid gland, and spreads to the axial skeleton, ribs, arms, and long bones of the leg
- Increased osteoblastic activity in the bone leads to enhanced structure of the bony matrix, causing periosteal stretch pain. Increased osteolytic or bone destruction activity of the bone marrow affects and destroys the sensory nerve endings and causes neurochemical reorganization of the spinal cord
- Increased bone loss due to resorption of bone by osteoclasts causes painful pathological fractures in patients with advanced disease:
    - Paraneoplastic phenomenon causing the production of antibodies against neurons, leading to peripheral neuropathy or neuritis
    - Secondary infection and open ulcer formation

Pain related to cancer therapy (20%)

Chemotherapy

- Chemotherapeutic drugs can be neurotoxic, especially vinca alkaloids (vincristine, vinblastine); alkylating agents containing platinum (cisplatin, carboplatin, oxaliplatin); and paclitaxel, docetaxel, and bortezomib causing peripheral neuropathy and mucositis
- Steroids can cause osteonecrosis; immunocompromised individuals can have infections (herpes zoster)
- Neurotoxicity is dose-dependent and worse when used in combination

Radiotherapy

- Radiation causes inflammation, fibrosis, and necrosis, as well as injury to the peripheral and central nervous systems, causing severe neuropathic pain, plexopathies, myelopathy, osteonecrosis, mucositis, and cystitis

Surgical

- Pain due to neuroma formation, post-thoracotomy pain syndrome, post-mastectomy pain syndrome, phantom pain

Pain due to other factors (10%)

- Impaired mobility resulting in decubitus ulcer and bedsores
- Constipation, dehydration, and OIH
- Psychological stress
- Cancer-associated symptoms, such as malaise, cachexia, anxiety, and myofascial dystrophy, aggravate pain symptoms
- Pre-existing medical conditions such as arthritis, low back pain, migraine, and fibromyalgia

Characteristics of cancer pain

- Cancer and its metastatic disease are progressive and dynamic, in comparison to CNCP which is static. This may lead to requirement of escalated and higher doses of potent opioids
- Cancer pain can occur from diagnosis till the end and can range from procedural/surgical pain initially to treatment-related pains, pain due to metastasis, and finally pain at the end of life. Another entity seen is pain in long-term survivors affecting their QoL
- People with cancer pain suffer from depression and psychological stress, in addition to physical discomfort—hence, psychological elements, such as depression, anxiety, and stress, pose more challenges in pain management
- Cancer patients suffer from other disabilities such as insomnia, cachexia, nausea and vomiting, dysphagia, constipation, anorexia, skin conditions, and complications of treatment
- Identifying specific pain associated with specific neoplasm helps in offering effective therapy at an early stage and preventing pain and suffering later, e.g. brachial plexopathy secondary to Pancoast tumour extension, lumbo-sacral plexopathy secondary to colorectal or prostate tumour extension or metastases from the breast
- Breakthrough pain is any transient and clinically significant pain that rises over adequately controlled baseline pain. It affects roughly about two-thirds of patients with cancer pain and is associated with more severe pain, reduced response to opioid medications, increased psychological distress, and worsening functional impairment
- Incidental pain which occurs due to movement, e.g. unstable pathological fractures

Further reading

1. Scott-Warren J, Bhaskar A. Cancer pain management—Part I: general principles. Contin Educ Anaesth Crit Care Pain 2014;14(6):278–84
2. Schwei MJ, Honore P, Rogers SD, et al. Neurochemical and cellular reorganization of the spinal cord in a murine model of bone cancer pain. J Neurosci 1999;19(24):10886–97

29.2 Overview of cancer pain management

Assessment of cancer pain

- Adequate and regular reassessment of cancer pain, with accurate documentation, should be carried out in order to provide optimal treatment
- Comprehensive assessment of this pain using a multi-dimensional model, with assessment of the underlying disease
- History and examination to confirm the presence of background, incident, or breakthrough pain should be obtained
- Include the type of pain and its intensity and localization, along with aggravating and relieving factors, the presence of neuropathic pain, and current management of pain relief
- A thorough psychological, social, and spiritual assessment using assessment tools prior to initiating a management plan. Assessment of other cancer-related symptoms, especially anxiety, depression, and sleep disturbances, which can affect the patient's family relationships and QoL
- Knowledge about the patient's coping strategies, economic impact, and spiritual beliefs can influence the treatment plan
- Newer-onset pain or change in pain should be addressed immediately and investigated, as it may highlight worsening in the patient's condition or worsening of existing pain needing analgesic modification

Management of cancer pain

- A biopsychosocial approach, rather than simply following the WHO ladder, should be used. Care of a patient suffering from cancer pain requires a holistic approach, combining psychological support, social support, rehabilitation, and pain management, in order to provide the best possible QoL or quality of death.

Principles of cancer pain management

Education

- Explaining to patients the cause of pain and the treatment options available, as well as their adverse effects, to help the patient manage their condition in a better and more satisfactory way

Modification of pain threshold

- Improving activity, mood, sleep, and social support can work positively towards raising the pain threshold in these patients
- Situations which increase pain may need to be avoided
- Patients need to plan ahead and may need aids to change their lifestyle to reduce pain
- Physiotherapy and OT play a very important role in recognizing and minimizing the impact of the disease on the day-to-day functioning of the patient

Lifestyle modification

- Situations which increase pain may need to be avoided
- Patients need to plan ahead and may need aids to change their lifestyle to reduce pain
- Physiotherapy and occupational therapy play a very important role in recognising and minimising the impact of the disease on the day to day functioning of the patient

Oncological management

- Anti-cancer treatment significantly helps in relieving pain either by treating the cancer or by palliation
- *The main approaches to shrink the size of the tumour and metastasis are:*
  - **Surgery** may be indicated for various procedures, e.g. stabilization of pathological fractures, resection of necrotic tumours, drains and shunt surgery for ascites and obstructive hydrocephalus
  - **Hormone therapy** has been shown to have good results in patients who have hormone-sensitive tumours such as prostate and breast cancers
  - **Chemotherapy**—patients with widespread metastases respond well to chemotherapy if the tumours are chemosensitive. Multiple myeloma and bronchus and breast cancers respond well to this modality of treatment
  - **Radiotherapy**—radiation produces free electrons and free radicals which destroy tumour cells and decrease pain; it can be delivered either systemically with radionuclides or as external local-field or wide-field radiotherapy. Osteoblastic lesions respond very well to radiotherapy

Modification of pain perception

- Perception of pain can be modified through pharmacological, as well as non-pharmacological, methods
- **Non-pharmacological methods**—heat and cold therapy, acupuncture, TENS
- **Complementary therapies**—improve well-being: aromatherapy, homeopathy, herbal medicines, hypnotherapy, massages, reflexology relaxation, and music therapy

Pharmacological management

- Systemic analgesics are considered the first-line treatment modality for cancer pain, with opioids being the ideal systemic medication
- It should be via an oral route, unless not tolerated or inadequate, and customized to the patient's requirement, ranging from simple non-opioid analgesics for mild pain to weak opioids, such as codeine, for moderate pain and strong opioids, such as morphine, for moderate to severe pain, and should provide background analgesia, as well as rescue analgesia
- It is important to monitor both short- and long-term S/Es of the drugs and treat aggressively

Interruption of pain pathways by interventional therapies

- Neuroablation can be carried out by longer-lasting nerve-blocking procedures—either physical (heat, cold, mechanical pressure, surgery) or chemical (alcohol, phenol, glycerol)
- This works well for localized pain along the distribution of a nerve or nerve plexus

Psychological interventions

- Some patients benefit from psychological interventions such as coping skills training, attention diversion strategies, and cognitive coping strategies
- The WHO ladder has significantly helped in cancer pain management but is not without limitations. We need to embrace a new model of management, which uses multimodal combination therapies, is mechanism-based, and includes interventions to optimize pain relief and limit adverse effects
- The Sheffield model of care encompasses the above and recommends pain therapies throughout the illness by using: (1) disease-directed therapy; (2) patient-directed therapy; and (3) family-directed therapy (see Figs. 29.2.1 and 29.2.2)

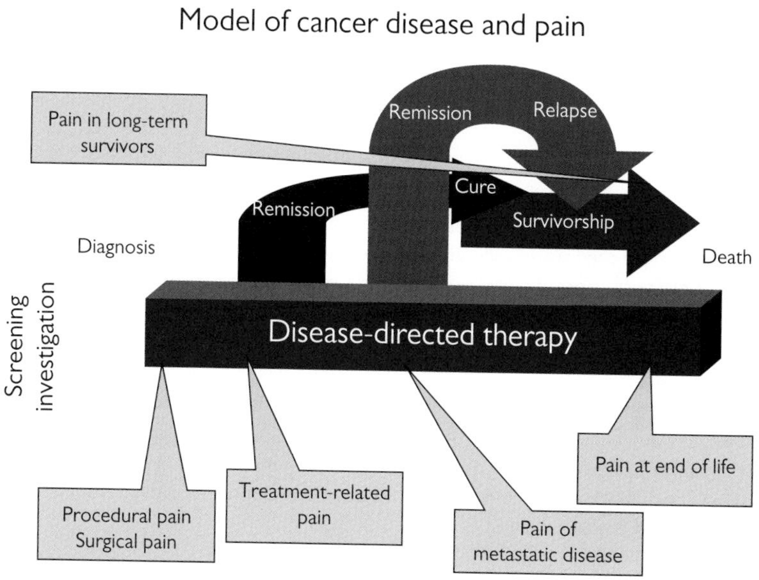

Figure 29.2.1 Cancer disease and pain

Adapted with permission from Ahmedazai, S., H. and Walsh, D. (2000). Palliative medicine and modern cancer care. *Seminars in Oncology*, 27(1):1–6

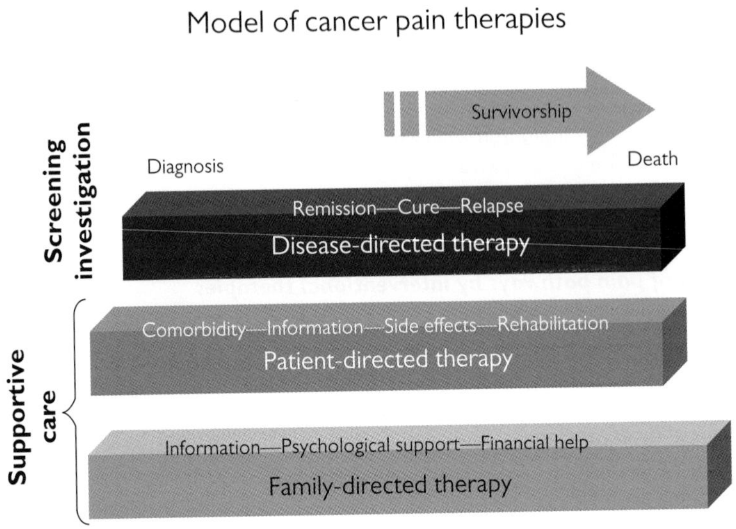

Figure 29.2.2 Pain therapies for cancer
Adapted with permission from Ahmedazai, S., H. and Walsh, D. (2000). Palliative medicine and modern cancer care. *Seminars in Oncology*, 27(1):1–6

Further reading

1. The British Pain Society. Cancer pain management. 2010. https://www.britishpainsociety.org/static/uploads/resources/files/book_cancer_pain.pdf
2. Bennett MI, Bagnall AM, Jose Closs S. How effective are patient-based educational interventions in the management of cancer pain? Systematic review and meta-analysis. Pain 2009;143:192–9

29.3 Cancer pain and psychology

- The diagnosis of cancer can have a massive psychological impact on both the patient and the family
- They suffer from grief, anxiety, depression, and psychological stress, in addition to physical discomfort, which can cause significant challenges in management, especially at certain points such as at diagnosis, start of treatment, relapse or recurrence, and treatment failure, and at the thought of dying
- **Psychological distress**, such as worries about death, pain, family issues, and financial strain, exacerbates the pain and, in turn, further worsens the psychological disturbances
- **Fear** can generate high anxiety, resulting in poor coping strategy, and reduces the threshold for pain
- 25% of cancer patients suffer from **depression**, which results in feeling of worthlessness, impaired concentration, and disinterest in daily activities. Depressed patients may develop hopelessness and helplessness

Management

- Assessment of psychosocial factors influencing the experience of pain will include the patient's understanding of their condition, what the pain means to the individual and their family, how the pain may impact upon relationships within the patient's family, whether the pain influences the patient's mood, coping strategies adopted by the patient, and the patient's sleep pattern

- Proper assessment of emotional and psychological status of cancer pain patients is an essential step in management
- The HADS is very helpful in quantifying the impact. Counselling, relaxation, and education reduce anxiety in cancer patients
- Psychological approaches in pain management include coping skills training, attention diversion strategies, and cognitive coping strategies. They teach the patients various behavioural and cognitive skills to cope with their pain and reduce their physical and psychological distress
- Pain management programmes aim to help the patient improve their QoL and achieve optimal functioning despite their medical conditions. CBT has been shown to produce promising results for cancer pain management in the acute period

Palliative care in managing other symptoms associated with cancer

- Palliative care is defined as active total care of patients whose disease is not responsive to curative treatment. The goal is to achieve the best QoL for patients and their families
- Management of other symptoms causing distress in cancer patients, which include constipation, general weakness, cachexia, dry mouth, oral ulceration, disabilities related to malignant infiltration such as paraplegia and bowel obstruction, anorexia, and dyspnoea, as well as familial and social distress
- A multidisciplinary team with different specialists and allied health professionals is essential to palliative care
- The Sheffield model of supportive care is a good multimodal, comprehensive model of cancer pain management

Further reading

1. Ahmedzai SH, Walsh TD. Palliative medicine and modern cancer care. Semin Oncol 2001;27:1–6
2. The British Pain Society. Cancer pain management. 2010. https://www.britishpainsociety.org/static/uploads/resources/files/book_cancer_pain.pdf
3. Anderson KO, Cohen MZ, Mendoza TR, et al. Brief cognitive-behavioural audiotape interventions for cancer-related pain: immediate but not long-term effectiveness. Cancer 2006;107(1):207–14

29.4 Opioids and adjuvants in cancer pain management

- Since 1986, the WHO's 3-step analgesic ladder has been widely adopted as a simple guideline for cancer pain management, based on the recommendations of an international group of experts. It relied on a simple, stepwise escalation of treatment, resulting in adequate pain relief in 70–80% of patients

Opioids

- Opioids are the most important option in cancer pain management and all patients with pain should be offered a trial
- Highly effective in somatic and visceral pain in the short and medium term
- Helps with neuropathic pain relief at sufficiently high doses, although not recommended
- Regulatory barriers still prevent access to opioids due to potential misuse and addiction in many countries

Principles of opioid administration

- The goal—a balance between clinically significant, sustained pain relief and S/Es with improved QoL
- Traditionally, pure mu agonist opioids were used in cancer pain management, whether weak (codeine) or strong (morphine)
- Partial mu agonist drugs, such as buprenorphine, have a limited role due to their analgesic ceiling effect and potential precipitation of withdrawal effects in patients already on strong opioids
- Drugs with a mixed action acting centrally through the noradrenergic pathway, such as tramadol and tapentadol, may play a role

Drug selection

- Opioids are selected according to intensity of pain—codeine or low-dose morphine for moderate pain, and morphine, oxycodone, fentanyl, oxymorphone, and hydromorphone for severe pain
- Opioids with short t1/2 are used first due to ease of titration
- Increasingly, methadone is being used for cancer pain management due to high oral bioavailability, longer dosing intervals, absence of active metabolites, long t1/2, cheap costs, and dual mechanism of action as a mu receptor agonist and NMDA antagonist
- The equianalgesic dose conversion relationship between morphine and methadone is curvilinear (methadone: morphine)
    - Low-dose oral morphine (30–300 mg) → 1:4–1:6
    - High-dose oral morphine(>300 mg) → 1:10–1:12

Opioid rotation

- Some patients may not respond to a particular type(s) of opioids, suffer from adverse effects, or become opioid-tolerant → successive trials of different types until one with a favourable response is identified is known as *opioid rotation*
- Due to incomplete cross-tolerance between different opioids and receptor polymorphism
- Automatically cause a 25–50% reduction in the equianalgesic dose of the chosen opioid
- Increase or decrease by 15–30% and prescribe 5–15% of the total daily dose for breakthrough pain

Routes of administration

- Ideally the least invasive and painful, most reliable, and safest route. Oral route whenever possible
- If vomiting or pathology involving the bowel, other routes could be chosen
- Transdermal route: fentanyl patches are an important advancement in cancer pain management and cause less constipation
- Rectal route: almost equianalgesic to the oral route. Oxycodone, oxymorphone, hydromorphone, and morphine suppository formulations exist
- Invasive routes: if need for rapid control of pain, more suitable regimen, and very high opioid requirements → oral route not practical
    - Intermittent or continuous infusions via IV or SC routes are most commonly used. The IM route is painful with no pharmacological advantage

- SC infusion ± *PCA*: through a 25–27G device such as a 'butterfly'. Could infuse opioids + other drugs such as ketamine and antiemetics. Oxymorphone, hydromorphone, morphine, diamorphine, and fentanyl are suitable as they are absorbable, and soluble methadone is not recommended due to its irritating effect
- Neuraxial infusion

Scheduled administration

- 'Around the clock': regular, preferably with controlled-release preparations → continuous sustained pain relief with provision of as needed (PRN) or 'rescue doses' → 50–100% of 4-hourly dose or 5–15% of total dose/24 hours
- PRN dosing: as sole regimen, useful during initiation of opioid therapy until stabilized on opioid therapy

Dose titration

- Doses increased by 30–100% of fixed dose or by an increment equal to the total consumed as 'rescue doses' in the previous 24 hours divided over the fixed dose
- Assess effect of each increment: 2–3 days for modified-release preparations, 3–6 for patches, and 5–6 for methadone

Breakthrough pain

- Short-acting drug on a PRN basis, opioid, or opioid–non-opioid drug combination
- *Transmucosal fentanyl*—specifically indicated due to rapid absorption → faster pain relief

Opioid side effects

- Nausea, vomiting, and constipation: worse in this cohort due to immobility, poor diet, abdominal pathology, polypharmacy
- Respiratory depression: tolerance develops over time
- Somnolence and mental clouding, due to high doses used, could be compounded by other factors related to disease, e.g. metabolic derangement or cerebral tumour. Patients may benefit from a psychostimulant such as dexamfetamine or methylphenidate 2.5–10 mg once or twice daily
- Delirium and confusion: compounded by other factors, such as somnolence, and can be managed by a small dose of a neuroleptic drug, e.g. haloperidol
- Multifocal myoclonus: can cause breakthrough pain; could benefit from opioid rotation, BZD, or an anticonvulsant
- Other S/Es include urinary retention, hypogonadism, dry mouth, pruritus, disorientated sleep, tolerance, and OIH. OIH is treated with gradual dose reduction, opioid rotation, or an alternative strategy other than opioids

Adjuvant analgesics

Adjuvants for neuropathic pain

- *Antidepressants:* such as TCAs, e.g. amitriptyline and imipramine. Secondary amine TCAs, such as nortriptyline and desipramine, have fewer S/Es. Starting dose 10–25 mg; aim for 75–125 mg/day. Also used are selective serotonin–noradrenaline reuptake inhibitors (SSNRIs), e.g. duloxetine

- *Anticonvulsants:* gabapentinoids especially useful. Some clinicians use carbamazepine, based on favourable experience with trigeminal neuralgia
- *LAs:* topical lidocaine such as 5% patches, oral mexiletine

Adjuvants for bone pain

- Usually treated by a combination of GCs and bisphosphonates. Bisphosphonates: inorganic analogues of pyrophosphate → inhibition of osteoclast activity. Pamidronate at a dose of 15–30 mg/2 weeks or 60 mg/4 weeks (more effective)

Adjuvants for visceral pain

- Oxybutynin: useful in bladder spasm pain due to anticholinergic and papaverine-like antispasmodic effect
- Octreotide: a somatostatin analogue useful in inoperable bowel obstruction
- Anticholinergics (hyoscine): useful for inoperable bowel obstruction

Multipurpose adjuvants: breakthrough pain

- GCs, such as dexamethasone and prednisolone, have been shown to result in analgesic benefit and improved QoL. Their effects include reduction of oedema, inflammation, and stabilizing electrical activity in affected nerves
- Useful in conditions such as headache caused by raised ICP, acute spinal cord compression, and hepatic capsular distension

Further reading

1. Raphael J, Ahmedzai S, Hester J, et al. Cancer pain: Part 1: pathophysiology; oncological, pharmacological, and psychological treatments: a perspective from the British Pain Society endorsed by the UK Association of Palliative Medicine and the Royal College of General Practitioners. Pain Med 2010;11:742–64
2. Cherny NI. The management of cancer pain. In: Melzack R, Wall P (eds). Handbook of Pain Management: A Clinical Companion to Wall and Melzack's Textbook of Pain. 2nd edition, 2008; pp. 641–66. London: Elsevier
3. Vargas-Schaffer G. Is the WHO analgesic ladder still valid? Twenty-four years of experience. Can Fam Physician 2010;56:514–17
4. Portenoy RK. Treatment of cancer pain. Lancet 2011;377:2236–47

29.5 Neurolytic procedures for cancer pain management

Introduction

- The WHO analgesic ladder forms a useful framework for initial cancer pain management
- 10–15% of patients with pain that is poorly responsive to opioids, or where S/Es are particularly problematic, may greatly benefit from invasive procedures designed to interrupt pain signals along neural pathways
- Such procedures should not be seen as the 'fourth step' on the WHO analgesic ladder but can, and should, be considered at each step, depending on patient preference and need
- Various methods are used for neurolysis (see Table 29.5.1)

Table 29.5.1 Methods used for neurolysis

Pharmacological	Physical	Surgery
Alcohol (50–100%) Phenol (3–12%) Glycerol Ammonium sulfate	Heat—alternating current of 50–100 kHz, producing lesions causing neuroablation; thermocoagulation Cold—cold saline, cryoprobe Mechanical—balloon compression for Trigeminal nerualgia	Rare, e.g. midline myelotomy, presacral neurotomy

Intrathecal neurolytic or neuro- destructive lesions

- Corning in 1884 reported the use of IT cocaine; however, it was Dogliotti who first described the use of IT alcohol for chronic pain management in 1931
- Since then, many authors have described IT injection of various neurolytic substances for treatment of oncologic pain
- Maher in 1955 suggested the use of phenol in glycerine
- Other chemical agents, such as chlorocresol, ethyl ether, ammonium salts, silver nitrates, and hypertonic saline, have been used
- By the mid- twentieth century, central neuraxial techniques were associated with significant incidences of infection due to poor aseptic practices, which led to poor acceptance of central neuraxial procedures for pain relief
- In recent years, alcohol and phenol have been the substances most commonly used for this purpose
- There are no controlled studies, so the literature consists of observations, reports, and book chapters reflecting the opinions of experienced clinicians
- Use of neurolytic blocks is particularly relevant if pain does not respond to analgesics, S/Es of analgesics are intolerable, or the IT catheter technique for cancer pain relief is not an option

Intrathecal thoracic/cervical neurolytic block

- IT thoracic/cervical neurolysis can be used to relieve unilateral intractable malignant pain in upper thoracic and/or lower cervical dermatome
- At lower thoracic dermatomal levels, the spinal cord level does not correspond quite well to the vertebral level, and therefore, deciding about the level at which injection is required to be performed, to address pain, is quite challenging
- The presence of the denticulate ligament, a fibrous structure separating the sensory (dorsal) and motor (ventral) fibres of the spinal nerves as they emerge from the spinal cord, and the baricity of the injected neurolytic solution allow to target selective sensory nerve fibres by positioning the patient appropriately
- The patient is placed in a lateral position at a 45° semi-prone angle if a hypobaric drug is used or in a lateral position at a 45° semi-supine angle if a hyperbaric neurolytic solution is injected intrathecally
- The procedure is performed with aseptic precautions and under fluoroscopy guidance
- A 22G, or narrower-gauge, spinal needle is used
- Usually 0.2 mL of neurolytic solution for each dermatome is used and no more than 0.8–1 mL should be injected at a single level, to minimize the risk of inadvertent spread to motor nerve roots

- Dehydrated alcohol (50–100%) is generally used for IT thoracic/cervical neurolysis as it is hypobaric and floats in the CSF, blocking only sensory fibres in the painful (upper) side
- It is also less uncomfortable for the patient to lie on the non-painful side while in a lateral position at a semi-prone angle
- The patient should be warned about a burning sensation in the painful area which occurs immediately on injection of alcohol intrathecally, which settles down gradually over a few minutes
- After injecting alcohol and prior to withdrawal, the spinal needle should be flushed with about 0.3 mL of plain bupivacaine to avoid alcohol tracking back in its path
- The patient is then kept in same position for at least 30 minutes, so that alcohol fixes to sensory fibres only

Intrathecal saddle block

- IT saddle neurolytic block is effective in managing pain in the perineum related to pelvic organ malignancy
- Phenol with glycerol is hyperbaric, as compared to the CSF, and available in various concentrations ranging from 5% to 10%
- Being a saddle block, it affects both sensory and motor components of the sacral nerves and therefore can affect bowel and bladder sphincters, causing incontinence
- However, often due to the nature of malignancy, patients usually have either a stoma and/or a urinary catheter *in situ*, and incontinence as a complication of the procedure is not always a significant issue in most patients
- Phenol with glycerol is a highly viscous solution, hence the need of a wider-gauge spinal needle (22G or 20G)
- Injection is performed at the lowest possible (L5/S1 or L4/L5) vertebral level in the sitting position, tilted at 45° backwards, which is maintained for at least 30 minutes after injection of phenol, so that only the lower sacral nerves are blocked
- Dose 0.1–0.3 mL aliquots up to a volume of 1 mL to be injected. If patient has urinary and faecal incontinence, then a higher dose could be used. Motor function should be monitored at all times when injecting the drug

Mechanism of action of intrathecal neurolytic block

- Experimental animal post-mortem studies suggest that neurolytic solutions cause demyelination and degeneration of nerve fibres
- Although they affect all types of nerve fibres indiscriminately, the degree of destruction depends on the concentration of the agent used
- Affected nerve fibres do eventually regenerate, and therefore, the effect of the neurolytic agent usually lasts for 10–12 weeks only

Informed consent

- For any neurolytic procedure, it is mandatory that realistic success rates, common S/Es, and complications are discussed with the patient/family members
- The patient also should be provided with written information leaflets, as most patients requiring these blocks are often on high doses of opiates and neuropathic agents and therefore may not completely understand only verbal explanation of the procedure/its complications

- The patient should be made aware of failure of the procedure, loss of touch/temperature sensation in the blocked area, undesirable adjacent/motor nerve blockade, deafferentation pain, and infection
- It is also important to inform the patient that these blocks may not relieve all the pain and may not be effective beyond a few months, requiring a repeat of the procedure, if appropriate

Post-procedure

- Haemodynamic changes are minimal following the above-mentioned IT neurolytic blocks
- Transient weakness may occur which usually improves in a few days
- Once pain reduction is achieved, patients on high-dose strong opiates and neuropathic agents may become stuporous with respiratory depression
- Careful close observations for the first 24 hours at least (hospice/hospital) and changes to the usual doses of strong opiates may be warranted

Epidural or intrathecal drug delivery systems

(See 20.5 Epidural injections, p. 377; 29.6 Intrathecal drug delivery treatment for cancer pain, p. 602.)

- Used when patients are opioid-responsive but struggle with S/Es at higher opioid doses
- Can be externalized systems or implanted systems which deliver pharmacological agents such as background infusions ± intermittent boluses

Cordotomy

(see 20.7 Percutaneous cordotomy, p. 382.)

- Creation of RF lesion in the lateral spinothalamic tract at the C1/2 level on the opposite side of pain, eliminating pain and temperature sensations from half of the body

Midline myelotomy

- A surgical technique, which involves sagittal division of the spinal cord in the lumbar region for severe pelvic pain as it disrupts the spinothalamic tracts
- Rarely done as causes paralysis and incontinence

Vertebroplasty and kyphoplasty

(See 22.9 Vertebroplasty, p. 438.)

- Performed for vertebral body disease where cement is injected into the vertebral body under fluoroscopy

Neurolytic/neuroablative procedures of peripheral nerves/plexus and visceral blocks

- Can be performed with pharmacological and RF lesioning
- Nerve root blocks, brachial/lumbar plexopathy, e.g. tumour infiltration
- Intercostal nerve block, e.g. phenol for rib metastasis
- Paravertebral blocks
- Coeliac and splanchnic plexus blocks, e.g. chemical neuroablation for pancreatic cancer
- Hypogastric blocks, e.g. abdominopelvic malignancies
- Ganglion impar blocks, e.g. perineal pain

Further reading

1. Scott-Warren J, Bhaskar A. Cancer pain management: Part II: interventional techniques. Contin Educ Anaesth Crit Care Pain 2015;15(2):68–72.
2. McGarvey ML, Ferrante FM, Patel RS, et al. Irreversible spinal cord injury as a complication of subarachnoid ethanol neurolysis. Neurology 2000;54:1522
3. Lauretti GR, Trevelin WR, Frade LCP, et al. Spinal alcohol neurolysis for intractable thoracic postherpetic neuralgia after test bupivacaine spinal analgesia. Anaesthesiology 2004;101(7):244–7

29.6 Intrathecal drug delivery treatment for cancer pain

- Analgesia is achieved by direct deposition of the drug into the CSF through continuous infusion
- It avoids the BBB, hence allowing the use of small doses
- This affords a reduction in S/Es and possibly a quicker and more efficacious response
- ITTD allows the use of LA infusions in the management of cancer pain
- Various receptors, such as opioid receptors (MOP, KOP, and DOP), NMDA, GABA, Na+, Ca^{2+}, dopaminergic, and α-2, can be targeted within the DH of the spinal cord
- It could be achieved through either an external device or a fully implantable pump
- Although a subject of debate, the common practice is to perform a trial infusion before proceeding to full implantation
- (See also 20.8 Intrathecal drug delivery systems, p. 384)

External ITDD

- There are two external methods of delivery:
  - One connected to a percutaneous catheter that may or may not be tunnelled. This is more suitable in patients with limited life expectancy
  - The other is a completely implanted catheter that has an SC port connected to an external pump. This is more suitable in patients with a short life expectancy
- Usually performed percutaneously under fluoroscopy guidance
- The medication could be either infused continuously or administered intermittently

Drugs commonly used

- Morphine, ziconotide, LAs, and others such as ketamine, adenosine, octreotide, neostigmine, midazolam, baclofen, and clonidine, have been tried
- Various combinations have been used

NICE and National Health Service England (NHSE) guidance on ITDD

- NHSE will routinely commission this service for patients with severe cancer pain that is refractory to conventional pain management techniques, after an appropriate selection process
- Evidence suggests that ITDD is a cost-effective analgesic management strategy, compared to standard opioid treatment, in these patients after 6 months of therapy
- Patients will need a comprehensive multidisciplinary team assessment with pain management, oncology, and palliative care
- It is an option for patients who have exhausted other options and/or are intolerant of the systemic S/Es of systemic analgesics and after a successful IT opioid trial, if appropriate
- Class 1 evidence for clinical efficacy in cancer pain

Management of a patient with an ITDD system

- Based upon the dosing regimen, a plan should be made about the refill intervals, documented, and handed over to the team looking after the patient
- A plan should be in place to manage common S/Es of the drugs used in the pump, with adequate provision of drugs that might be needed
- It is highly recommended that all clinicians inserting the ITDD system and involved in managing the patient should familiarize themselves with the particular pump being used, its make and model, and its manual

Pump-related failures

- **Pump:** a well-known, preventable cause of pump failure is corrosion, most likely resulting from infusing off-label drug preparations that could result in stalling. This has led Medtronics to issue a notice against the use of unapproved drug combinations. This could result in either withdrawal symptoms or uncontrolled pain, or overdosing
    - Pump–catheter misconnection: more common soon after implantations, yet could manifest late
    - Loss of pump propellant: resulting in either reduced delivery, manifesting as withdrawal and aggravated pain, or overdosing
    - Motor stalling due to gear shaft wear: resulting in slowing of infusion
- **Catheter:** by far more common as they are more vulnerable:
    - Migration: resulting in CSF leakage which could result in a hygroma
    - Kinking: which could take place anywhere between the pump and the catheter-receiving device. It is evidenced by inability to aspirate or inject
    - Drug leakage: which may occur at the pump–catheter connection. It could be immediately post-insertion or delayed
    - Microfractures, breakages, occlusion, and inflammatory mass
- Symptoms of ITDD failure due to the catheter are usually subtle and primarily noticed and reported by the patient in the form of inadequate analgesia or possibly withdrawal
- Workup to identify the cause should start with the history and complaint and then work its way logically
- First start by identifying the position of the catheter spread and the flow rates
- To explore possible catheter dislodgement or migration, proceed with AP and lateral X-rays
- If the catheter is accessible (such as through a port or in the case of external devices), then an attempt should be made at aspirating and injecting under strict aseptic precautions to prevent introducing infection
- A minimum of 1.5 mL should be aspirated to remove any drug
- Ease of aspiration: 2–3 mL of CSF is easily aspirated, such that it is unlikely that the tip is obstructed
- Holes in the catheter: interrupted flow on CSF aspiration
- A total of 2–4 mL of contrast is used to identify the catheter tip location after aspirating the active drug
- Radioactive indium: this is the most informative test of catheter integrity. This is reserved for stable patients where catheter withdrawal is not planned in the next 24–48 hours
- (See Figs. 29.6.1 and 29.6.2 for management of patients who report increased pain)

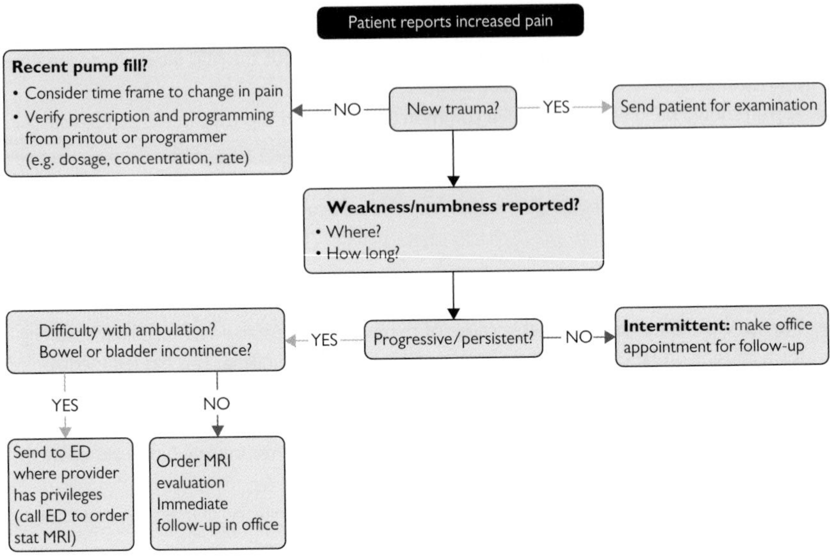

B. Office visit

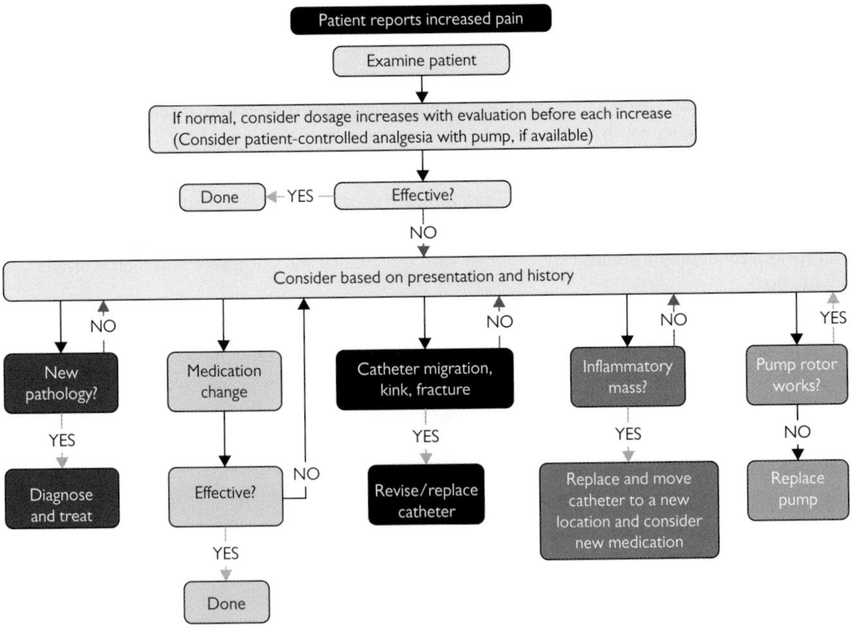

Figure 29.6.1 Flow chart for the management of patients who report increased pain

Reproduced courtesy of Medtronic. https://www.medtronic.com/uk-en/index.html

Conceptual framework for diagnosing and managing inadequate analgesia office visit considerations

C. Office visit

History:
- If original presenting pain condition has worsened: neurological changes?
- If new pain: what is quality, intensity, location?
- Do medication adjustments improve or not improve pain?
- In what dermatome is catheter tip located?
- History of pump regarding accuracy of medication remaining?

Physical:
- Neurological exam at presumed catheter tip location and at pain location: evaluate gait, balance, and sensory changes
- Mental status - is patient sedated? Cognitively intact? Agitated? Having hallucinations?

Pump:
- Can CSF be withdrawn through the catheter access port?
- Is a bolus dose effective?
- Is bolus painful?
- Are there any volume discrepancies?

Drug:
- Is the medication in the pump?
- Is refill medication as ordered?
- Have medications been administered within the stability specifications?
- Consider possibility of diversion of pump medication?

Radiologic workup:
- Catheter tip location: has location shifted? Catheter location to be used to determine location for thin slice study; see below
- Catheter access port contrast study: can CSF be easily aspirated? Can contrast be injected and visualized? Is there pain with the contrast injection?
- Imaging study in reservoir versus catheter?
- T1 MRI with gadolinium (thin slice) or CT myelogram to rule out inflammatory mass
- Consider MRI/CT to evaluate new pain location and dermatome level if granuloma workup is negative
- Does pump rotor work (movement can be visualized with CT)?

Figure 29.6.2 Flow chart for the management of patients who report increased pain

Reproduced courtesy of Medtronic. https://www.medtronic.com/uk-en/index.html

Further reading

1. Bhatia G, Lau ME, Koury KM, et al. Intrathecal drug delivery (ITDD) systems for cancer pain. F1000Res 2013;2:96
2. Xing F, Yong RJ, Kaye AD, et al. Intrathecal drug delivery and spinal cord stimulation for the treatment of cancer pain. Curr Pain Headache Rep 2018;22:11
3. The British Pain Society. Intrathecal drug delivery for the management of pain and spasticity in adults: recommendations for best clinical practice. 2008. https://www.britishpainsociety.org
4. Prager J, Deer T, Levy R, et al. Best practices for intrathecal drug delivery for pain. Neuromodulation 2014;17:354–72
5. Clinical Commissioning Policy: Intrathecal Pumps for Treatment of Severe Cancer Pain. Specialised Commissioning Team, NHS England. July 2015. Local Team A. https://www.england.nhs.uk/commissioning/wp-content/uploads/sites/12/2015/10/d08pb-intra-pumps-trtmnt.pdf

29.7 Chemotherapy for cancer pain

Introduction

- Chemotherapy is treatment of disease by use of chemical substances, especially treatment of cancer with cytotoxic and other drugs. The aim of chemotherapy is based on one of the following three therapeutical effects:
  1. Cure: to destroy cancer to the point of being undetectable, with the hope of no recurrence in the future
  2. Control: to keep cancer from spreading to other parts of the body or to slow progression
  3. Palliate: to ease symptoms related to malignancy, shrink/downsize tumours that cause pain or pressure on critical structures, or improve QoL
- Chemotherapy can have one of the following three intents:
  1. Neoadjuvant: to reduce the size before definitive surgery or radiotherapy
  2. Adjuvant: to destroy any residual microscopic cells following surgery or radiotherapy, increasing the chance of cure
  3. Palliative: to relieve symptoms of cancer or potentially extend life without the intention to cure the disease
- There are many agents used for a variety of cancers, which may include chemotherapy, hormonal therapy, tyrosine kinase inhibitors, immunological/biological agents, and bone-modifying drugs. Some of these agents result in predictable S/Es that can cause pain, especially painful neuropathies

The role of chemotherapy for pain management

- Malignancy does not always cause pain, but it can be painful, especially if critical structures are involved, or infiltrated or compressed by a lesion, or there is metastatic deposit. Chemotherapy itself rarely causes pain and treatment can often be the best option for pain related to progressive cancer. Chemotherapy can provide effective analgesia when the cancer burden/volume is high and the tumour is chemo-, immune-, or hormone-sensitive, e.g. extensive small cell lung cancer, neuroendocrine tumours, multiple myeloma, metastatic melanoma, hormone-sensitive breast cancer, or bony lesions from prostate cancer
- If cancer responds to chemotherapy, it is important to sequentially reduce analgesia as the cause of pain is removed. Risk of addiction in cancer pain is low, but opioid safety and a weaning plan should be part of regular management, especially in patients with the potential for cure or long-term survival, e.g. localized sarcoma. Opioid minimization strategies are associated with fewer S/Es and there are increasing concerns about opioids stimulating cancer growth (in animal studies)
- Pain is not always a sign of cancer being poorly controlled—it should be addressed as an issue of its own, separate from cancer progression (this must be excluded) or treatment. Widespread pain may be a manifestation of existential distress, for example.
- Patients who receive support from well-resourced and multidisciplinary palliative care teams experience less pain at their end of life, so advocating for early referrals to the palliative care team is an important strategy in pain management in advanced disease. This allows for not only good symptom management, but also management of psychological, social, carer, and spiritual needs, as well as advance care planning and planning for bereavement support

Chemotherapy causing pain

- Chemotherapy infusions are usually painless. Some chemotherapy agents can cause a stinging/burning sensation in the arm during infusion, but this should be mild and subside with infusion. If any pain, check for extravasation, which can be a severely painful event. Acute chemotherapy S/Es can include nausea and vomiting, diarrhoea, mucositis, and very rarely enteritis and typhlitis (if severe toxicity, often accompanied by severe neutropenia). These can lead to issues with absorption of regular analgesics and medications, requiring conversion to SC or IV administration
- Myalgias, arthralgias, and headaches can also occur, e.g. with taxol and many hormone-blocking agents. In the medium term, especially if the tumour is particularly responsive to treatment, pain crisis or pain flare-up post-treatment can occur (acute swelling with tumour death). Tumour lysis syndrome (renal failure post-extensive tumour lysis) is of particular concern, especially in haematological malignancies. Immune therapies can cause a cytokine storm, requiring significant support in the intensive care unit (ICU) setting
- Cancers can cause bone complications, causing significant disability and movement-related pain. Cancers causing lytic lesions can cause pathological fractures and crush fractures of vertebral bodies. Long-term use of aromatase inhibitors for hormone-sensitive breast cancer can lead to osteopenia and later to osteoporotic (non-malignant) fractures, arthralgia, and myalgia. Management of cancer bone pain includes paracetamol, NSAIDs, opioids, and adjuvants. Current medical management also includes bisphosphonates (pamidronate, zoledronic acid), denosumab, and rarely calcitonin (usually for resistant malignant hypercalcaemia). Vertebral deposits can lead to malignant spinal cord compression (not always painful). It is essential to order full-spine MRI, rather than single-level MRI (i.e. lumbo-sacral MRI) if malignant spinal cord compression is a clinical concern as it can often be multi-level. A review of patients with malignant spinal cord compression identified cancer at thoracic (77%), lumbar (29%), cervical (12%), and sacral (7%) levels, as well as at multilevel (25%). Some patients need surgery which can have a curative or symptom control intent (see 24.5 Cauda equina syndrome, p. 489)
- In the long term, some chemotherapies can lead to painful peripheral neuropathy and paraesthesiae (numbness), and altered taste, smell, and hearing. Platinum drugs (cisplatin > carboplatin), taxanes (paclitaxel > docetaxel), and vincristine are commonly prescribed chemotherapies that can cause neuropathy. Treatment options include pregabalin, gabapentin, duloxetine, amitriptyline, opioids such as tapentadol, and methadone. Most patients get better with time, over many months in most cases (requiring weaning of medications as symptoms settle)

Further reading

1. Cassidy J, Bissett D, Spence RPM. Oxford Handbook of Medical Oncology. 3rd edition, 2010. Oxford: Oxford University Press
2. University of Wollongong Australia. Palliative Care Outcomes Collaboration. https://ahsri.uow.edu.au/pcoc/index.html
3. McLinton A, Hutchison C. Malignant spinal cord compression: a retrospective audit of clinical practice at a UK regional cancer centre. Br J Cancer 2006;94(4):486–91
4. Watson M, Lucas C, Hoy A, et al. Oxford Handbook of Palliative Care. 2nd edition, 2009. Oxford: Oxford University Press

29.8 Radiotherapy for cancer pain

Introduction

- Ever since its discovery in around 1895, the analgesic effect of ionizing radiation has been well documented
- Hence, radiotherapy is used for the dual purpose of oncological treatment, whether to achieve cure or palliation, and subsequently for its analgesic effect
- It offers a quick, effective, and relatively cheap method of managing the *focal* symptoms of advanced malignancy whether due to primary disease or metastases
- In advanced malignancy, up to 70% of cases have shown bone metastases on post-mortem studies
- The analgesic effect is achieved through a reduction in tumour mass size, hence decreasing its infiltration and pressure
- This may be due to decompression of nerves and nerve plexuses, such as the brachial plexus in Pancoast tumour, or decreased irritation and stretching of periosteal nociceptors in osseous tumours

Mechanism of action and delivery methods

- Methods of delivery include percutaneous radiotherapy, radionuclide therapy, stereotactical thalamotomy, and radiodissection of the pituitary gland

Percutaneous radiotherapy—the most common method

- High-energy X-rays targeted at the tumour result in cellular DNA damage and eventually death
- Linear accelerators are used for its delivery in specialized centres
- It could be either:
  - Curative: delivered daily in multiple small doses called 'fractions', with the aim of avoiding as much as possible damage to adjacent normal tissues
  - Palliative: using lower doses with the primary aim of symptom control
- 60% of patients treated with palliative radiotherapy gain an element of pain reduction within 2–3 weeks on average

Common indications

- Bone metastases
- Locally advanced thoracic cancer
- Malignant spinal cord compression resulting in pain and neurological symptoms
- Brain metastases
- Head and neck cancers
- Advanced pelvic cancers

Side effects and complications

- Dependent on tissues receiving the treatment and on adjacent normal tissues
- Common examples:
  - Bone: up to 35% may experience a flare-up in the first week
  - Oral cavity and oropharynx: mucositis and pharyngitis (63%), with dysphagia and risk of aspiration pneumonia
  - Brain: fatigue and headache (32%) are the most common. The patient may also suffer from nausea, vomiting, and otitis externa in a minority of cases
  - Lung: coughing

    - Mediastinum: oesophagitis with resulting dysphagia in up to 22% of lung cancer patients and 28% of oesophageal cancer patients
    - Stomach and bowel: nausea, diarrhoea, and discomfort
    - Bladder: frequency, nocturia, and dysuria
    - Skin: erythema and hair loss
- Fatigue: common—up to two-thirds of patients may complain of it
- Long-term S/Es are rare, with acute ones resolving within 4–6 weeks of treatment
- They are managed by supportive measures to treat symptomatically, with opioids and antiemetics forming the mainstay of treatment

Further reading

1. Kuttig H. Radiotherapy of cancer pain. In: Zimmermann M, Drings P, Wagner G (eds). Pain in the Cancer Patient. Recent Results in Cancer Research. Vol. 89, 1984. Berlin, Springer Heidelberg
2. Spencer K, Parish R, Henry A. Palliative radiotherapy. BMJ 2018;360:k821

29.9 Palliative Surgical Procedures

Introduction

- Palliative care is defined by the WHO as an approach that improves the QoL of patients and their families facing problems associated with a life-threatening illness, through the prevention and relief of suffering by means of early identification and appropriate assessment and treatment of pain and other physical, psychosocial, and spiritual problems
- There are several surgical procedures that may be helpful in improving QoL or prolonging life in patients receiving palliative care input. These procedures should be carefully discussed with the patient and the person responsible, as well as health care professionals involved in their care
- For information on procedures performed for palliative patients, including spinal decompression and/or fusion, ITDD systems, cordotomy, vertebroplasty/kyphoplasty, and neurolytic blocks, see Chapter 4, and previous sections of this chapter.

Commonly performed surgeries in patients receiving palliative care

Surgical fixation of a pathological fracture

- A pathological fracture is a fracture that develops through an area of bone pathology, typically either spontaneously or following minimal trauma
- The goal of treatment is to minimize pain and maximize function. The nature of the surgical procedure is best determined by an experienced orthopaedic surgeon and may include arthroplasty or internal fixation with intramedullary nailing or plate/screw fixation devices
- An impending fracture is where the extent of bone pathology is such that a fracture is expected but has not yet occurred. Prophylactic surgical fixation may be considered for impending fractures
- Radiotherapy should be considered following surgical fixation of a pathological or impending pathological fracture or may occasionally be considered as primary treatment for an impending pathological fracture
- Patients with pathological fractures may benefit from perioperative LA blocks or catheters as part of their multimodal analgesia, i.e. a fascia iliaca block/catheter for a neck of femur fracture or an interscalene block/catheter for a pathological fracture of the proximal humerus

Venting gastrostomy, defunctioning ileostomy, or colostomy formation

- When a patient with metastatic cancer has an unresectable lesion or lesions causing multi-level bowel obstruction, a stoma may be created from the most proximal unobstructed segment of the GI tract to relieve the obstruction and associated nausea and vomiting. This may be an ileostomy or a colostomy
- A venting gastrostomy allows a patient to drink and have a soft diet and then contents of the stomach are drained out via a gastrostomy tube. The person does not absorb nutrients but can retain the pleasure and social aspect of eating, with reduced nausea or vomiting
- A person with a defunctioning ileostomy or colostomy may still effectively absorb nutrients, depending on the length of the residual small bowel

Oesophageal, duodenal, colonic, or rectal stent

- It may be possible to relieve a single-level obstruction due to malignancy with endoscopic stent insertion by a gastroenterologist or an upper GI or colorectal surgeon

Biliary stent

- A biliary tree stent may be placed via endoscopic retrograde pancreaticocholangiography (ERCP) for malignant pancreaticobiliary obstruction
- The most common complications are stent occlusion and stent migration
- If it is not possible to relieve biliary obstruction via ERCP and stent insertion, it may be possible to relieve biliary obstruction with an external drain via percutaneous transhepatic cholangiography
- Biliary decompression can relieve jaundice and pruritus and minimize the likelihood of cholangitis

Ureteric stent, percutaneous nephrostomy, or suprapubic catheter

- Malignant obstruction to urine flow may occur at any level of the urinary tract
- Ureteric obstruction may be relieved by insertion of a ureteric stent via cystoscopy or by surgical or interventional radiology placement of percutaneous nephrostomy
- Ureteric stents and percutaneous nephrostomies may be performed unilaterally or bilaterally
- Obstruction below the level of the bladder may be relieved by insertion of an indwelling urinary catheter or a suprapubic catheter
- Post-procedure, one needs to diligently monitor and manage any post-obstructive diuresis

Airway stent

- Airway stents are devices with a hollow lumen that are inserted into an airway bronchoscopically to relieve central airway obstruction

Further reading

1. Moss AC, Morris E, Leyden J, et al. Malignant distal biliary obstruction: a systematic review and meta-analysis of endoscopic and surgical bypass results. Cancer Treat Rev 2007;33:213
2. Zucchi E, Fornasarig M, Martella L, et al. Decompressive percutaneous endoscopic gastrostomy in advanced cancer patients with small-bowel obstruction is feasible and effective: a large prospective study. Support Care Cancer 2016;24:2877.

SECTION 7

PSYCHOLOGY OF PAIN MEDICINE

Psychology and Pain

Sabina Bachtold, Caroline Burrow, Rahul Guru, and Karen LeMarchand

CONTENTS

30.1 Psychometric assessments

Definition

- Chronic pain is often accompanied by symptoms of psychological distress and psychiatric disorders, including depression, anxiety, and anger
- Psychometrics permit the quantification of cognition, affect, and behaviour, thus enabling the identification of both the pathology and the degree of deviation from normality

Psychometric assessment tools

Diagnostic and Statistical Manual of Mental Disorders, fifth edition (DSM-5)

- A significant portion of patients presenting with chronic pain also have a history of primary psychiatric comorbidity
- It is important to distinguish patients with an underlying psychiatric illness from those whose psychological symptoms (anxiety, depression, or other expressions of psychopathology) arise secondary to their pain

Beck Depression Inventory (BDI)

- A brief, 21-item questionnaire that assesses the degree to which depressive symptomatology is present

Hospital Anxiety and Depression Scale (HADS)

- A highly validated scale which consists of 14 items—seven for anxiety and seven for depression. Each item scores from 0 to 3 points
- A total score of >8 out of 21 for anxiety and/or depression represents a clinically significant risk of these entities

General Health Questionnaire (GHQ)

- A psychometric screening tool to identify common psychiatric conditions
- There are versions with 12, 28, 30, and 60 questions, valid for use in adults and adolescents, but not in children; available free

Minnesota Multiphasic Personality Inventory-2 (MMPI-2)

- An extensive true/false questionnaire consisting of >500 items factored across ten clinical scales, as well as a variety of validity, secondary, and experimental scales
- The MMPI-2 has been used to verify clinical impressions about the psychological aspects of a patient's chronic pain and to predict responses to medical and surgical pain treatments

Profile of Mood States (POMS)

- A relatively new psychological rating scale used to assess transient, distinct mood states
- Advantages of using this assessment include simplicity of administration and ease of participant's understanding
- The POMS measures six different dimensions of mood swing, i.e. tension or anxiety, anger or hostility, vigor or activity, fatigue or inertia, depression or dejection, and confusion or bewilderment over a period of time

Patient Health Questionnaire-9 (PHQ-9)

- Multipurpose instrument for screening, diagnosing, and monitoring of depression
- It is brief, completed by the patient in minutes, and rapidly scored by the clinician

Generalized Anxiety Disorder-7 (GAD-7)

- A questionnaire with seven items, which measure the severity of various signs of generalized anxiety disorder according to reported response categories with assigned points
- The BDI, HADS, and GHQ can be used as self-report measures and all have standardized cut-off points that can be used to indicate a possible psychiatric state

Additional information

- Given the multiple measurement scales used in clinical practice, the IMMPACT recommended **BDI** and **POMS** to be used as core outcome measures of emotional functioning in chronic pain clinical trials
- They have well-established reliability and validity in the assessment of symptoms of depression and emotional distress, and they have been used in numerous clinical trials in psychiatry and chronic pain

Further reading

1. Bendinger T, Plunkett N. Measurement in pain medicine. BJA Educ 2016;16(9);310–15
2. Holdcroft A, Jaggar S. Core Topics in Pain. 2010. Cambridge: Cambridge University Press

30.2 Affective component of pain

Introduction

- Two components to pain:
    - Sensory/discriminative
    - Affective/emotional

- The affective component of pain is the emotional reaction and perceived sense of experience and is usually associated with some emotional distress
- It varies in individuals, depending on certain factors, including:
  - Situational context
  - Pain characteristics and previous pain experiences
  - Patient's understanding, family, and cultural background
  - Coping responses

Stages

- Immediate stage—unpleasantness/distress associated with intensity/arousal in the moment
- Secondary stage—memories, imagination, prediction of long-term consequences
- Common emotional reactions include anxiety, fear, frustration, anger, sadness, irritability, and depression

Assessment

- Assessment of symptoms, such as fatigue, activity level, and sleep disturbance, may be difficult in chronic pain patients due to the impact of the affective component
- Such symptoms may be as a result of the pain, emotional distress, or medication/treatments
- Multidimensional assessment necessary

Psychosocial evaluation

Comprehensive psychosocial evaluation should include:

- Impact (physical, emotional, psychological, spiritual)
  - Be aware of patients who may find it difficult to label/communicate their affective/emotional experience
- Response to pain/coping skills (adaptive and maladaptive)
- Avoidance (pain, stressors)
- Meaning of the pain to the patient and previous experience of pain/treatment and expectations (of the patient, of others)
- Medication and other health conditions (physical, psychological/psychiatric)
- History of trauma/PTSD
- Current support, contextual issues (additional stressors, family, social, work-related, benefits, legal)
- Assess for suicidal thoughts and intentions (follow local risk protocol/procedures)

Questionnaires

- Self-reporting scales proposed to measure the affective component:
  - Pain Discomfort Scale
  - VRS
- Self-reporting measures, which capture aspects of the affective component:
  - *Anxiety and depression:*
    - HADS
    - BDI
    - Beck Anxiety Inventory (BAI)
  - *Stress and anxiety symptoms:*
    - Stress Symptoms Checklist (SSCL)
  - *Cognition/beliefs:*
    - Pain Cognition Questionnaire

- *Coping:*
  - Coping Strategies Questionnaire (CSQ)
- *Acceptance:*
  - Chronic Pain Acceptance Questionnaire (CPAQ)
- *Mood and emotional functioning:*
  - POMS
- *Psychological functioning:*
  - Symptom Checklist-90 Revised (SCL-90R)

- Examples of self-report multi-dimensional measures, which include some measure of the affective component:
  - McGill Pain Questionnaire (MPQ) (short-form MPQ-SF)—most widely used measure
  - Brief Pain Inventory (BPI)
  - Multi-dimensional Pain Inventory
- Questionnaires recommended by IMMPACT in the United States:
  - Multi-dimensional Pain Inventory
  - BDI and/or POMS

Special points

- Questionnaire scores should be interpreted with caution
- Measures should be validated for chronic pain patients or criteria may require modification to avoid false positives
- Should be relevant to the intervention
- Specific scales may be available for special populations, e.g. pain assessment checklist for seniors with severe dementia (PACSLAC)

Further reading

1. Breivik H, Borchgrevink C, Allen SM, et al. Assessment of pain. Br J Anaesth 2008;101(11):17–24
2. British Pain Society/Royal College of Anaesthetists. Core standards for pain management services in the UK. First edition. 2015. https://fpm.ac.uk/sites/fpm/files/documents/2019-07/Core%20Standards%20for%20Pain%20Management%20Services.pdf
3. Dansie RJ, Turk DC. Assessment of patients with chronic pain. Br J Anaesth 2013;111(1):19–25
4. Dworkin RH, Turk DC, Wyrwich KW, et al. Interpreting the clinical importance of treatment outcomes in chronic pain clinical trials IMMPACT recommendations. J Pain 2008;9:105–21

30.3 Opioid risk assessment tools

Introduction

- All patients who are to be commenced on opioids need to be assessed for characteristics that increase the likelihood of opioid abuse
- Opioid risk assessment tools help in making this assessment

Tools

CAGE-AID (adapted to include drugs)

- This screening tool has four questions. This is not specific for opioids

Prescription Drug Use Questionnaire—patient version (PDUQp)

- A validated, 31-item questionnaire for assessing and predicting problematic opioid medication use in chronic pain patients
- Data are obtained regarding the patient's pain condition, opioid use, social and family history, and any psychiatric issues

Screening Instrument for Substance Abuse Potential (SISAP)

- The SISAP is a 5-item screening tool that assesses the risk of opioid abuse, based on a patient's alcohol consumption, marijuana use, tobacco use, and age (non-validated)

Screener and Opioid Assessment for Patients with Pain-Revised (SOAPP-R)

- A revised and validated version of the original self-report SOAPP to predict aberrant medication-related behaviours amongst chronic pain patients considered for long-term opioid therapy
- It helps determine the level of monitoring required. This version contains 24 items and psychometric values

Opioid Risk Tool (ORT)

- A validated 5-question tool to assess the risk of opioid abuse or aberrant behaviour
- It helps determine the level of monitoring required by stratifying patients as low, medium, and high risk

Current Opioid Misuse Measure (COMM)

- A highly sensitive and specific, validated 17-question tool designed to identify aberrant drug-related behaviour (ADRB) during chronic opioid therapy

Severity of Opioid Dependence Questionnaire (SODQ)

- This is a tool used as an indicator of opioid dependence
- Three items are especially important in identifying opioid dependency: the tendency to increase the analgesic dose or frequency, the tendency to have a preferred route of administration, and the tendency to consider oneself addicted

Patient Medication Questionnaire (PMQ)

- This is a validated 26-item questionnaire to assess ADRB in patients already on opioids (score <25: low risk of opioid abuse; 25–30: problematic use; >30: patient requires close monitoring and titration off opioids should be considered)

Additional points

- None of the opioid risk assessment tools are perfect in predicting the risk of opioid abuse. They have to be used in conjunction with other methods of assessment, which include a thorough history, physical examination, and tests such as urine toxicology
- SOAPP-R and ORT are the most accurate in predicting the risk of opioid abuse before starting therapy
- PMQ and COMM are better at predicting ADRB once opioid therapy has been initiated
- Risk assessment should be done before commencing opioid therapy and at regular intervals during therapy

Further reading

1. Smith HS, McCleane G. Identifying patients at risk for analgesic misuse. In: Smith HS (ed). Current Therapy in Pain. 2009. Philadelphia, PA: Saunders
2. Ducharme J, Moore S. Opioid use disorder assessment tools and drug screening. Mo Med 2019;116(4):318–24

30.4 Depression, anxiety, and suicidal ideation

Introduction

- Mood disorders can be commonly associated with chronic pain
- The most common symptoms are anxiety and depression
- Changes in mood are as a result of the impact of chronic pain
- Some patients may also have a premorbid psychological or psychiatric history

Depression—criteria

- Psychological symptoms that have persisted for >2 weeks
- Continuous low mood, irritability, intolerance (subjective report: feels sad/empty; observation: angry/tearful)
- Feeling hopeless and helpless
- Feeling guilty/worthless (guilt is usually inappropriate or excessive)
- No motivation or interest in things
- Difficulty in decision-making (inability to concentrate/indecisiveness)
- No enjoyment in life
- Suicidality (having suicidal thoughts or thoughts of self-harm)

Anxiety—criteria

- Fear and worry are normal emotions and can be appropriate emotions for those suffering from chronic pain
- Clinical anxiety presents with the following symptoms:
  - Excessive worry and feelings of apprehension (persistent for at least 6 months)
  - Physical symptoms such as palpitations, sweating, and tension
  - Symptoms cause significant distress or impairment in social, occupational, and other areas of functioning
  - Symptoms are not related to physiological substances, such as medications and drug abuse, or a medical condition such as heart problems and hyperthyroidism

Suicidality

- Substantially increased risk of suicide in those living with chronic pain
- Main predictors are negative pain-coping strategies and the degree of pain-related catastrophizing
- Suicidal ideation may be active or passive:
  - Passive: involves a desire to die, but without a specific plan of how the patient might end their life
  - Active: involves a wish to die accompanied by a plan of how they intend to end their life
- **Parasuicide** is an attempt at suicide where the aim is to deliberately fail and the person puts in plans to be discovered

- Co-occurring disorders should also be noted, as sometimes suicidal ideation could be a symptom of diagnosed or undiagnosed mental health
- Patients may use catastrophic terms, 'I would be better off dead'—this may not mean they intend to end their life but nonetheless should be followed up with questions about intent

Assessment

- Clinical interview to include risk assessment of suicidal intent

Questionnaires

- GAD-7—this may be used as a screening tool to measure levels of anxiety
- Patient Health Questionnaire-2 (PHQ-2) may be used in screening for depression, and PHQ-9 for monitoring depression
- Refer to DSM-IV, which can be found online

Treatment/referral

- Give an explanation to the patient of how mood impacts on pain, and vice versa, causing a circular effect
- Mood disorders related to psychosocial symptoms—referral for **counselling**
- Mild anxiety and depression—referral for Improving Access to Psychological Therapies (**IAPT**)
- Moderate anxiety and depression—referral for **CBT**
- Severe anxiety and depression affective of pain symptoms—referral to specialist pain/ **physical health psychology** services
- Severe anxiety and depression not related to pain symptoms—referral to adult mental health team (**AMHT**)
- Passive suicidal ideation—mood must be monitored
- Active suicidal ideation—referral to **mental health crisis team** and psychiatry

Further reading

1. American Psychiatric Association. Diagnostic and Statistical Manual of Mental Disorders. 4th edition, 1994. Washington, DC: American Psychiatric Association
2. Edwards RR, Smith MT, Kudel I, et al. Pain-related catastrophising as a risk factor for suicidal ideation in chronic pain. Pain 2006;126(1–3):272–9
3. Kroenke K, Spitzer RL, Williams JB. The Patient Health Questionnaire-2: validity of a two-item depression screener. Med Care 2003;41:1284–94
4. McWilliams LA, Cox BJ, Enns M. Mood and anxiety disorders associated with chronic pain: an examination of a nationally representative sample. Pain 2003;106:127–33
5. Spitzer RL, Kroenke K, Williams JB. A brief measure for assessing generalized anxiety disorder: the GAD-7. Arch Intern Med 2006;166(10):1092–7

30.5 Fear avoidance behaviour, catastrophizing, and pain behaviours

Fear avoidance behaviour

- The fear avoidance model uses a cognitive behavioural model
- Components include pain experience, catastrophizing, fear of pain, avoidance/escape, disuse, and disability/depression
- Chronic MSK pain is developed as a result of avoidant behaviour
- Pain is initially experienced; the patient then engages in avoidant behaviour (e.g. restricting movement, not bending/carrying) as a result of fear of pain
- Resulting lack of pain reinforces the avoidant behaviours, which leads to deconditioning/further pain
- Hypervigilance to pain/discomfort and avoidant behaviours lead to a vicious cycle
- Experience/anticipation of further pain reinforces avoidant behaviours and fears, exacerbating hypervigilance to pain/discomfort
- Misdirected problem-solving—pain is perceived to cause damage, leading to behavioural priority of escape/avoidance and increased vigilance for pain
- Influenced by characteristics of the pain (bottom–up processing) and cognitive and emotional appraisals/experiences/memories/expectations (top–down processing)
- Associated with poorer outcomes for employment, inactivity, greater disability/impaired physical performance, increased pain, catastrophizing, anxiety, and depression
- **Fear Avoidance Beliefs Questionnaire (FABQ)** is helpful in understanding the patient's beliefs

To address fear avoidance

- Reinstate normal activity levels
- Fear hierarchy—graded exposure
- Pacing activity
- Change perceptions of pain (i.e. non-threatening/temporary)

Catastrophizing

- Cognitive process characterized by:
  - Interpretation of negative events as being more negative than they really are
  - Perceiving events/sensations as 'out of proportion'
  - Overestimating the probability of negative events occurring
  - Excessive/exaggerated negative self-statements
- Pain is perceived as being 'extremely threatening'

Associated with

- Fear avoidance behaviour
- Low frustration tolerance and high levels of psychological/emotional distress
- Activity intolerance/lower levels of activity
- Intensified experience of pain
- Pain disability and related fear
- Negative control beliefs and coping outcomes

- Perceptions of poor self-efficacy
- Depression
- Higher rates of analgesic use
- The **Pain Catastrophizing Scale (PCS)** measures pain-related catastrophic thoughts.

Pain behaviours

- Expression of distress—verbalizing, crying, groaning, grimacing
- Changes to movement—guarding, limping, bracing, rubbing body parts
- Changes to posture—tense, rigid, slouching, bending
- Avoidance of activity
- Other pain behaviours—medication/alcohol/drug use, treatment seeking

Pain behaviours may be

- Learnt responses to pain/habit in an attempt to reduce pain and distress and seek help and support
- Indication of exaggeration/faking
- Associated with excessive concern from others (particularly partners)

Managing pain behaviours

- Make conscious, if unaware, and explore reinforcers
- Assertiveness skills
- Set clear goals
- Teach adaptive behaviours
- Explore others' responses to pain (family, professionals)

Treatment

- Fear avoidance behaviour, catastrophizing, and pain behaviours are ameliorable to CBT and ACT
- Behavioural aspects of the therapies focus upon fear exposure and building skills in more helpful behavioural strategies for pain management and expression of distress
- Cognitive aspects of the therapies focus upon reducing the belief that the pain requires medical intervention, shifting focus from cure to management of the pain by the individual

Further reading

1. Eccleston C. Psychology of chronic pain and evidence-based psychological interventions. In: Stannard CF, Kalso E, Ballantyne J (eds). Evidence-based Chronic Pain Management. 2010; pp. 59–67. Oxford: BMJ Books
2. Eccleston C, Palermo TM, Williams ACDC, et al. Psychological therapies for the management of chronic and recurrent pain in children and adolescents. Cochrane Database Syst Rev 2014;5:CD003968
3. Williams AC, Eccleston C, Morley S. Psychological therapies for the management of chronic pain (excluding headache) in adults. Cochrane Database Syst Rev 2012;11:CD007407

30.6 Personality disorders

Introduction

- A person with a PD may have limited ways of feeling, behaving, or thinking
- Impacts upon relationships, interactions with others, and coping and life skills
- People with a PD generally feel isolated and have a higher risk of suicide and higher levels of self-harm and addictive tendencies
- PDs can typically coexist with other mental health conditions (depression, bipolar disorder, substance abuse, eating disorder, anxiety disorders)
- No clear definition of why people develop PD
- Research suggests several causal factors that tend to be grouped into internal, genetic, and external factors (victims of abuse, childhood neglect, childhood trauma, chaotic family life, parental alcohol/drug abuse, parental mental health)
- Research carried out in 2006 suggests that approximately one in 20 people will have a PD at any given time

Definition

- Ten specific PDs, placed into three clusters, as identified in DSM-5 (see Table 30.6.1)

Table 30.6.1 Personality disorders

Clusters1	Key attributes
Cluster A—suspicious	• Paranoid (distrust others, suspicious and guarded, very sensitive, have difficulty maintaining close relationships) • Schizoid (behave introvertedly, emotionally cold, indifferent, little pleasure in life) • Schizotypal (odd/eccentric behaviour, believe they can read minds and have special power, prone to developing schizophrenia)
Cluster B—emotional and impulsive	• Antisocial (disregard for others, impulsive, aggressive, prioritize their needs) • Borderline (lack sense of self, fear of being abandoned, difficulty in controlling anger/maintaining relationships, increased suicidal thoughts, prone to developing paranoia) • Histrionic (lack self-worth, attention-seeking behaviour, influenced by others) • Narcissistic (entitled, self-absorbed behaviour, controlling, lack empathy, constant need to be admired)
Cluster C—anxious	• Avoidant (feel socially inept and inferior, isolated and lonely, avoid interactions with others and relationships, fear of rejection) • Dependent (feel helpless and lack self-confidence, cannot make independent decisions, passive and submissive, fear of being abandoned) • Obsessive–compulsive* (perfectionism, inflexible, set unrealistic high standards for all and self, preoccupied with orderliness and control, fear of making mistakes)

* Obsessive–compulsive personality disorder (OCPD) is separate from obsessive–compulsive disorder (OCD). OCD is an anxiety disorder, not a type of personality disorder.

Source: Data from American Psychiatric Association. (2013). *Diagnostic and statistical manual of mental disorders: DSM-5*. Arlington, VA: American Psychiatric Association.

Treatment

- Complex nature of PD makes treatment very challenging
- Previously thought to be 'untreatable' and a 'diagnosis of exclusion' from services
- People with PD tend to find it difficult to engage in therapy and often drop out of therapy due to:
    - Self-damaging behaviours
    - Inability to form relationships (including therapeutic relationships)
- Specialist treatment is required:
    - Dialectical behaviour therapy (DBT) is a cognitive behavioural treatment developed to specifically treat people who experience intense emotions
    - Therapeutic communities (TCs) are structured environments for people with complex psychological conditions

Referral (useful websites for NHS referral)

- http://www.nhs.uk/Conditions/Borderline-personality-disorder/Pages/Treatment.aspx

Further reading

1. American Psychiatric Association. Diagnostic and Statistical Manual of Mental Disorders (DSM-5). 5th edition, 2013. Washington, DC: American Psychiatric Association
2. Coid, J, Yang M, Tyrer P, et al. Prevalence and correlates of personality disorder in Great Britain. Br J Psychiatry 2006;188:423–31
3. Krysinska K, Heller TS. Suicide and deliberate self-harm in personality disorders. Curr Opin Psychiatry 2006;19(1):95–101
4. Linehan MM. Cognitive-Behavioural Treatment of Borderline Personality Disorder. 1993. New York: Guilford Press
5. National Institute for Mental Health in England. Personality disorder: no longer a diagnosis of exclusion. Policy implementation guidance for the development of services for people with personality disorder. Department of Health. 2003. http://personalitydisorder.org.uk/wp-content/uploads/2015/04/PD-No-longer-a-diagnosis-of-exclusion.pdf

30.7 Somatic symptom disorder

Introduction

- Somatic symptom disorder (SSD), previously referred to as somatization disorder
- The diagnostic class for SSD emphasizes distressing somatic symptoms with extreme reactions and behaviour and distress towards the symptoms, rather than the absence of a medical explanation for somatic symptoms
- Prevalence of SSD is 5–7% in the general population, and higher in neurology settings (25%)

Criteria

- The patient presents with extreme anxiety about physical symptoms
- The diagnostic criteria for SSD are summarized from DSM-5:
    - One or more somatic symptoms that cause major distress and result in significant disruption of daily life

- Excessive thoughts, feelings, or behaviours related to symptoms or associated health concerns, as evident by at least one of the following:
    1. Disproportionate and persistent thoughts about the seriousness of one's symptoms
    2. Persistently high level of anxiety about health or symptoms
    3. Excessive time and energy devoted to these symptoms or health concerns[1]
- Although any one somatic symptom may not be continuously present, the state of being symptomatic is generally persistent for >6 months
- Severity:
    - Mild—only one of symptoms (1) to (3) are specified
    - Moderate—two or more of symptoms (1) to (3) are specified
    - Severe—two or more of symptoms (1) to (3) are specified plus there are multiple somatic complaints or one very severe somatic symptom
- Generally dominant symptoms are somatic complaints, health anxiety, and pain
- Sexual abuse has also been associated with an increased risk of SSD
- Associated comorbidities include depression, IBS, and PTSD

Treatment—psychological therapy

- CBT
- Mindfulness
- The main aim is to empower and help the patient cope with the symptoms

Special notes

- After appropriate diagnostic tests are performed, a consultation explaining and describing the condition must be carried out with caution and without implication of a psychosomatic illness
- A patient with SSD is not purposely faking their symptoms—the pain they feel is real
- Patients will benefit from support within a trusting relationship, as this will help avoid unnecessary future investigations, while enabling observation of symptoms that may require investigation

Referral

- A psychiatric referral may be beneficial
- However, CBT has been shown to be more effective than psychiatric intervention

Further reading

1. Allen L, Woolfolk R, Escobar J, et al. Cognitive-behavioral therapy for somatization disorder: a randomized controlled trial. Arch Intern Med 2006;166(14):1512–18
2. American Psychiatric Association. Diagnostic and Statistical Manual of Mental Disorders (DSM-5). 5th edition, 2013. Washington, DC: American Psychiatric Association

1. Source: Data from American Psychiatric Association. (2013). *Diagnostic and statistical manual of mental disorders: DSM-5*. Arlington, VA: American Psychiatric Association.

3. Ghanizadeh A, Firoozabadi A. A review of somatoform disorders in DSM-IV and somatic symptom disorders in proposed DSM-V. Psychiatr Danub 2012;24(4):353–8
4. Kallivayalil RA, Punnoose VP. Understanding and managing somatoform disorders: making sense of non-sense. Indian J Psychiatry 2010;52(1):240–5
5. Shaw RJ, Bernard RS, DeMaso DR. Somatoform disorders. In: Steiner H (ed). Handbook of Developmental Psychiatry. 2011; pp. 397–429. Singapore: World Scientific Publishing

30.8 Post-traumatic stress disorder

Introduction

- PTSD is a chronic and debilitating condition that can develop in response to a traumatic life event or events
- Symptoms of PTSD are divided into three clusters:
  - Re-experiencing
  - Avoidance
  - Hyperarousal
- Other symptoms include feelings of guilt, dissociation, alterations in personality, difficulty with affect regulation, and marked impairment in ability for intimacy and attachment
- Comorbid disorders include severe anxiety, depression, dissociative disorder, substance abuse, suicidal feelings, and a range of physical complaints

Definition

- Trauma is defined when:
  - A person experiences, witnesses, or has been confronted with an event or events that involved actual or threatened death or serious injury or a threat to the physical integrity of self or others
  - The person's response involves intense fear, helplessness, or horror
- Can occur following a single traumatic incident or can be related to a series of events/prolonged event (complex PTSD)

Assessment

- Referral to a mental health professional for assessment if symptoms have persisted for longer than 4 weeks

Questionnaires

- Clinician-Administered PTSD Scale (CAPS)
- The Impact of Event Scale–Revised (IES-R)

Treatment

- Watchful waiting—monitoring in initial stages (symptoms for <4 weeks); two in three people show spontaneous improvement
- Antidepressants (paroxetine and sertraline are licensed for PTSD)
- Eye movement desensitization and reprocessing (EMDR)
- Trauma-focused cognitive behavioural therapy (TF-CBT)
- Specialist services, depending on nature of trauma (Combat Stress, Rape Crisis, etc.)

Further reading

1. American Psychiatric Association. Diagnostic and Statistical Manual of Mental Disorders (DSM-5). 5th edition, 2013. Washington, DC: American Psychiatric Association
2. Blake DD, Weathers FW, Nagy LM, et al. The development of a clinician-administered PTSD scale. J Trauma Stress 1995;8:75–90
3. Weiss DS, Marmar CR. The Impact of Event Scale—Revised. In: Wilson JP, Keane TM (eds). Assessing Psychological Trauma and PTSD. 1997; pp. 399–411. New York, NY: Guilford Press

30.9 Compensation issues

- Suggestions are that financial compensation influences pain and treatment outcome via secondary gain, reward for the learnt pain behaviour, malingering, and compensation neurosis.

Primary and secondary gain

- Gains derived from the illness/symptom, which may act as a maintaining factor

Primary gain

- Subconscious internal psychological motivators for symptom presentation
- Produces positive internal motivation
- Reduction of internal distress/emotional conflict/anxiety as a result of the symptom/illness

Secondary gain

- Subconscious or conscious external motivator
- Interpersonal or social advantage
- Examples: increased care, disability benefits, reduction of responsibilities, etc.

Malingering

- Symptoms fabricated/exaggerated for secondary gain
- Rare
- DSM-IV diagnosis

Fictitious disorder

- Symptoms fabricated/exaggerated for primary gain

Compensation neurosis

- Compensation being sought for an injury/condition
- Financial compensation identified as the primary maintaining factor for symptoms
- Symptoms resolve on settlement
- Theory not supported by research evidence

Experience of pain and compensation

- Limited evidence that receiving financial compensation is associated with a greater experience of pain/disability
- Limited evidence to support that those going through litigation exaggerate pain

- Some evidence of worse prognosis for those who have received compensation, difficult to specify causal factors
    - Likely to be related to type of treatment/rehabilitation programme and nature of injury

Treatment outcome and compensation

- Perception that financial compensation has a negative effect on rehabilitation/treatment outcome
- Controversial, conflicting evidence
- Studies flawed (differing outcome measures, patients' conditions not comparable, types of compensation, disability not accounted for)
- Meta-analysis suggests no clear conclusion

Associated issues related to compensation and experience of pain/ treatment outcome

- Fears of financial difficulty
- Job satisfaction
- Anger at those perceived to be responsible for injury
- Lack of support/adaptations at work
- Employment status
- Trauma and PTSD
- Severity of pain
- Disability
- Levels of emotional distress
- Impact on life

Further reading

1. Rohling ML, Binder LM, Langhinrichsen-Rohling J. Money matters: a meta-analytic review of the association between financial compensation and the experience and treatment of chronic pain. Health 1996;14(6):537–47
2. Turk DC, Okifuji A. Perception of traumatic onset, compensation status, and physical findings: impact on pain severity, emotional distress, and disability in chronic pain patients. J Behav Med 1996;19(5):435–53

30.10 Cognitive behavioural therapy

Introduction

- Cognitions, emotions, physical sensations, and behaviours are linked
- Cognitive appraisals determine emotions and behaviours, the consequences of which reinforce thoughts/beliefs
- Patients identify how their thoughts, emotions, behaviours, and experience of pain are linked in maladaptive ways
- Patients are taught coping skills to modify these maladaptive responses
- Present focused and problem-specific approach

Aims of therapy

- Identify negative or maladaptive thoughts and behaviours
- Change these in order to improve physical sensations and emotional experience

Theoretical background/proposed mechanisms

Increase in more adaptive cognitions via

- Restructuring of maladaptive thoughts/beliefs
- Changes in attention focus (away from the pain)
- Development of more adaptive thoughts/beliefs

Increase in more adaptive behaviours via

- Habituation
- Extinction of maladaptive behaviours
- Behavioural activation
- Associative learning
- Reinforcement of more adaptive behaviours

Decrease in physiological arousal via

- Habituation
- Incompatible response training
- Changes in autonomic nervous system activity

Indications

- Chronic pain
- Insomnia
- Psychological disorders, including:
  - Anxiety disorders (panic disorder, agoraphobia, social phobia, specific phobia, and generalized anxiety disorder)
  - Depression
  - OCD
  - PTSD
  - Eating disorders
- Substance misuse
- Also indicated for chronic pain and other medical conditions in children and adolescents

Contraindications

- Patients with impaired cognitive functioning
- Patients who are actively psychotic or intoxicated
- Patients requiring emergency medical treatment
- Patients seeking a cure for pain
- Comorbid severe mood disorder may require medication, in addition to psychological therapy
- Patients should be on a stable dose if taking any antidepressants, mood stabilizers, or antipsychotic medication
- Actively suicidal patients should be monitored, and risk protocols adhered to

Complications/adverse effects

- Some emotional distress/anger, with exploration of difficult feelings/challenging beliefs
- Temporary increase in anxiety with exposure

Technique

Implementation of CBT

- Individually or in groups
- Couples/family sessions
- Pain management programmes
- Self-help resources, computerized CBT
- Sessions are goal-oriented and structured with an agreed agenda
- Therapy is time-limited
- Typically, 10–20 sessions, approximately 1 hour, once per week
- May require additional sessions in more complex cases

Therapeutic strategies

- Psychoeducation: to aid in the patient's understanding of chronic pain and adaptive strategies, to provide treatment rationale, and to introduce to CBT model
- Cognitive restructuring: to identify maladaptive thoughts/beliefs, to challenge these, and to enable the patient to produce more adaptive thoughts/beliefs
- Skills training:
  - Goal setting
  - Problem-solving
  - Attention diversion/distraction
  - Relaxation training
  - Behavioural techniques to reduce pain behaviours and increase adaptive behaviours (e.g. pacing)
  - Behavioural activation: to increase activities which provide pleasure/sense of mastery/achievement
  - Relapse prevention: to prepare for, and normalize setbacks, plans for coping with future pain/stressors
- Graded exposure: to reduce avoidance (of pain/stressors) and increase approach behaviour
- Homework: agreed tasks between sessions to facilitate the above and to practise adaptive coping skills

Common CBT goals

- Improvement of physical fitness/stamina
- Improvement of social skills, e.g. assertiveness
- Improvement of pain-coping skills, e.g. pacing

Special points

- CBT strategies should be modified/adapted for specific populations (e.g. older adults) to meet their individual needs

Effectiveness

- CBT is the most comprehensively researched psychotherapeutic treatment for pain
- Good evidence to support the use of CBT in chronic pain
- Level of evidence: 1+

Further reading

1. Butler AC, Chapman JE, Forman EM, et al. The empirical status of cognitive-behavioral therapy: a review of meta-analyses. Clin Psychol Rev 2006;26(1):17–31
2. Eccleston C, Palermo TM, Williams AC, et al. Psychological therapies for the management of chronic and recurrent pain in children and adolescents. Cochrane Database Syst Rev 2014;5:CD003968
3. Williams, A, Eccleston C, Morley S. Psychological therapies for the management of chronic pain (excluding headache) in adults. Cochrane Database Syst Rev 2012;11:CD007407

30.11 Acceptance and commitment therapy

Introduction

- Third-wave CBT
- Acceptance that pain is an inevitable part of life
- Suffering is caused by the response to pain, rather than the pain itself
- Suffering = resistance + pain
- Attempts to 'escape the pain' results in more suffering

Aim of therapy—pain acceptance

- To be willing to experience pain
- To engage in valued life activities, despite pain

Theoretical background/mechanisms

- Patient learns to observe the pain and their attempts to escape/avoid it
- Increased awareness of this process allows increased choice of avoidance or exposure behaviours

Indications

- Any issue where the only adaptive strategy is acceptance, e.g. chronic pain, childhood trauma
- Comorbid presentations may benefit from intensive ACT

Contraindications

- Patients with impaired cognitive functioning
- Patients who are actively psychotic or intoxicated
- Patients requiring emergency medical treatment
- Patients should be on a stable dose if taking any antidepressant, mood stabilizer, or antipsychotic medication
- Antisocial behaviours that can be controlled, e.g. aggression, criminal activity
- Actively suicidal patients should be monitored, and risk protocols adhered to

Complications/adverse reactions

- Some emotional distress/anger with exploration of difficult feelings/challenging beliefs
- Temporary increase in anxiety with exposure

Table 30.11.1 The Hexaflex

Mindfulness and acceptance processes	Commitment and behavioural change processes
1. Acceptance (of thoughts/sensations/urges)—reduction of maladaptive attempts to avoid pain 2. Defusion (observe thoughts without believing/acting upon them)—less investment in pain-related thinking 3. The observing self—increases present-moment self-awareness	4. Being present—focus on present moment despite pain 5. Values—identification of personal values and engagement value-related activities despite pain 6. Committed action—engagement in more helpful pain-coping strategies

Technique

- ACT can be implemented as individual therapy, couples therapy, group therapy, part of MDT pain management programmes, or self-help resources
- Can be delivered as brief (1–4 sessions), intensive, or longer term (10+ sessions) therapy
- Building skills/psychological flexibility in the six core processes shown in Table 30.11.1)
- Outcome measured with the CPAQ

Special points

- 'Clean pain' (unconditioned pain) is the experience of pain (sensory and affective)
- 'Dirty pain' (conditioned pain) is the associated response to the experience of pain—thoughts/judgements/expectations/beliefs, resistance to pain/emotional experience

Effectiveness

- Strong research base for ACT in chronic pain
- Effective within MDT, in both outpatient and residential programmes
- Acceptance of pain has been correlated with lower pain intensity, less pain avoidance, increased physical and social ability, improved work status, and less associated depression and anxiety
- Level of evidence: 1+

Further reading

1. Dahl J, Wilson K, Nilsson A. Acceptance and commitment therapy and the treatment of persons at risk for long-term disability resulting from stress and pain symptoms: a randomized control clinical trial. Behavior Therapy 2004;35:785–802
2. Eccelstone C. Psychology of chronic pain and evidence-based psychological interventions. In: Stannard CF, Kalso E, Ballantyne J (eds). Evidence-based Chronic Pain Management. 2010; pp. 59–67. Oxford: BMJ Books
3. McCracken LM, Vowles KE, Eccleston C. Acceptance of chronic pain: component analysis and a revised assessment method. Pain 2004;107:159–66

30.12 Mindfulness

Introduction

- Mindfulness-based approaches involve **meditation** and a way of living **focused upon present-moment** awareness, acceptance, and compassion
    - Develop attentional skills and acceptance
    - Reduce pain-related arousal and reactivity
- Focus upon accepting all experiences (neutral, unpleasant, or pleasant) to enable a choice of response to the pain

Aim

- To develop an accepting and kind relationship with the pain (primary suffering) in order to reduce secondary suffering (maladaptive reactions to the pain), and thereby improve QoL

Theoretical background/proposed mechanism

- To cultivate an attitude of acceptance/recognize the nature of experience as transient (reduction of hypervigilance and emotional reactivity, extinction through counter-conditioning)
- Distraction technique—shifts attention from pain
- Exposure to pain—habituation
- Higher activation levels in areas of the brain implicated in attention, cognitive control, somatic awareness, and stress regulation in pain-related regions (dorsal anterior cingulate cortex, insula, and thalamus)
- Lower activation in areas involved in appraisal, emotional regulation, stress, and memory (medial prefrontal cortex, orbitofrontal cortex, amygdala, and DLPFC)

Indications

- Chronic pain, chronic illness
- Stress and psychological distress
- Psychological disorders, including anxiety, depression, and OCD

Contraindications

- Dissociative tendencies/disorders, suicidal ideation
- Active addiction or <1-year recovery
- Psychosis, PTSD
- Patients who find it difficult to 'sit with' discomfort (physical, emotional, cognitive), those who habitually use avoidant coping strategies

Complications/adverse effects

- Rare cases of depersonalization, psychosis, increased anxiety and risk of seizures, loss of appetite, and insomnia have been reported
- Such adverse effects are more likely to occur with prolonged meditation

Technique

- Individually or in groups
- Patients are taught meditative practices to increase present-moment meta-awareness and to develop an accepting, non-judgemental, and kind attitude to all experiences (physical, emotional, and cognitive)
- Patients are encouraged to develop their own daily meditative practice

Special points

- Often included as a skill taught within psychological therapies such as mindfulness-based stress reduction (MBSR), mindfulness-based CBT (MCBT), ACT, and DBT
- The focus of mindfulness is not upon attempting to ignore/escape pain, but rather on cultivating an attitude of acceptance of it, thereby reducing secondary distress
- Although linked to certain religious philosophies in clinical practice, mindfulness is taught in a secular way

Effectiveness

- Reports suggest it can be a good alternative to CBT
- Growing evidence base
- Level of evidence 2++

Further reading

1. Carmody J, Baer RA. Relationships between mindfulness practice and levels of mindfulness, medical and psychological symptoms and wellbeing in a mindfulness-based stress reduction program. J Behav Med 2008;31(1):23–33
2. Zeidan F, Grant J, Brown CA, et al. Mindfulness meditation-related pain relief: evidence for unique brain mechanisms in the regulation of pain. Neurosci Lett 2012;520:165–73

30.13 Hypnotic therapy

Introduction

- Altered state of conscious awareness
- Patient becomes more open to 'suggestions', which can create changes in perception and behaviour
- Can be used alone or to enhance the effectiveness of other interventions
- Can develop skills in auto-hypnosis

Hypnotizability is dependent on:

- Motivation and beliefs
- Ability to achieve a state of hypnosis and experience a range of hypnotic phenomena
- Ability to learn/use self-hypnosis
- Being receptive/responsive to hypnotic suggestion

Theoretical background or proposed mechanisms

- Reduction of anxiety, increased relaxation
- Altered perception (reduction in hypervigilance for pain)
- Modification of maladaptive cognitions regarding pain
- Less dissonance in response to ideas/suggestions contrary to patient's maladaptive beliefs
- Information processing enhanced due to reduced preoccupation with pain
- Reduction of cortical activation associated with painful stimuli

Indications

- Post-operative pain
- Cancer pain

- IBS
- Labour pain
- Headaches
- Dental procedures
- Neuropathic pain
- MSK pain

Contraindications

- Patients with impaired cognitive functioning
- Patients who are intoxicated
- Patients requiring emergency medical treatment
- Psychosis, severe mood disorder, dissociative disorders, suicidal ideation
- Epilepsy, narcolepsy
- High/low BP and serious heart conditions
- Controversy over whether it should be provided in pregnancy (except during labour)

Complications/adverse effects

- Rare but can include headache, tiredness, anxiety, confusion, creation of false memories, and panic attacks

Technique

- Orient patient to hypnosis; assess beliefs related to hypnosis and hypnotizability
- Patient induced into a relaxed hypnotic state by practitioner using words and imagery
- Practitioner provides suggestions to modify patient's pain-related thoughts/images
- Build an adaptive repertoire of thoughts/images associated with pain relief
- Debrief patient and check for amnesia
- Set individual self-hypnosis exercise

Hypnobehavioural strategies

- Imagery and controlled breathing
- Relaxation, distraction
- Mental rehearsal of adaptive pain-coping behaviours
- Cognitive restructuring (via age regression, memory recall, memory reconstruction, positive self-suggestion, altering negative thoughts)
- Strategies for altering pain sensations (e.g. distraction, pain displacement, symptom substitution, hypno-analgesia, glove analgesia/anaesthesia, symptom reinterpretation/reframing, time distortion, pain relief imagery)

Special points

- Cannot hypnotize someone against their will
- One of the first mind–body approaches used for chronic pain
- Hypnotic state is difficult to measure objectively
- In research on efficacy, hypnosis may be viewed within the cognitive behavioural model rather than the hypnotic state theory
- Hypno-behavioural pain management psychotherapy
- Patients rated by practitioners as having 'high hypnotizability' report greater benefits from hypnosis

Effectiveness

- Established efficacy for chronic pain
- Hypnosis may help relieve pain in labour, but research conducted so far has not conclusively shown benefit
- Level of evidence: 1

Further reading

1. Ikins G, Johnson A, Fisher W. Cognitive hypnotherapy for pain management. Am J Clin Hypn 2012;54(4):294–310
2. Madden K, Middleton P, Cyna AM, Matthewson M, Jones L. Hypnosis for pain management during labour and childbirth. Cochrane Database Syst Rev 2012;11:CD009356

30.14 Neurolinguistic programming

Introduction

- Neurolinguistic programming (NLP) is a coaching method
- Often used in personal development and corporate settings
- It claims the following:
  - Individuals have unique internal mental maps
  - Connection between neurological processes and language and behavioural patterns learnt through experience (programming)
  - To achieve specific goals, these connections can be changed
  - Through 'modelling' skills of successful/exceptional people
- Seen as a pseudoscience, largely discredited scientifically

Aim of therapy

- To change conscious and subconscious beliefs about themselves, the pain/illness, and the world

Mechanism

- Uses techniques from hypnotherapy and psychotherapy
- Reports to 'reprogramme' limiting beliefs
- Behaviour modified through manipulating 'subjective representations' we hold about ourselves/the world
- Change internal representations and responses to stimuli in the world
- Enables patients to make adaptive lifestyle changes using an imitative method of learning (modelling)
- Placebo effect?

Indications

- Changing behavioural patterns
- Stress reduction
- Fears and phobia
- Coaching, personal performance

Contraindications

- Bipolar disorder, PDs, attachment and impulse control disorders
- Patients in recovery from substance misuse
- Patients with cognitive impairment
- Patients who struggle to understand/apply metaphors

Complications/adverse effects

- Often reported by practitioners as having no adverse effects
- However, some reports of adverse effects on mental health/well-being

Technique

- Can be implemented individually, in seminars, and as self-help resources
- Practitioners claim that problems can be 'reprogrammed' quickly, in some cases within <1 hour
- Identify negative attitudes and beliefs which have been 'programmed since birth'
- 'Reprogramme' beliefs via a wide variety of techniques, including:
  - Visualization/imagery
  - Mental rehearsal
- NLP for pain is useful when patients treat pain as a phobia. It helps increase self-efficacy and visualization, redirecting focus away from pain and 'remapping' beliefs

Special points

- Medical and psychological practitioners may employ aspects of NLP; however, it is **not** mainstream medical/psychological practice
- The field of NLP is self-regulated

Effectiveness

- There is limited evidence on the effectiveness of NLP in chronic pain
- Level of evidence: 3 and 4

Further reading

1. Bowers, L.A. An exploration of holistic and non-traditional methods including research in the use of neuro-linguistic programming in the adjunctive treatment of acute pain. Dissertation Abstracts International 1996;56(11-B):6379

30.15 Pain management programmes

Introduction

- Pain management programmes (PMPs) are an established part of care for patients suffering from chronic pain
- PMPs are one of the most important non-pharmacological ways of helping patients with chronic pain manage their condition

- They improve patients' understanding of chronic pain through a combination of psychological techniques and practical strategies designed to optimize physical functioning and QoL, and reduce emotional distress

Aims of PMPs

- To improve the patient's understanding of chronic pain
- To minimize the impact of pain on their everyday lives
- To optimize physical functioning and QoL
- To reduce emotional distress
- To promote a self-management approach to pain
- To provide coping skills and strategies for dealing with chronic pain, disability, distress, and life changes
- To reduce or modify the patient's future use of health care services
- To decrease the patient's reliance on medical management

Rationale for PMPs

- Based on the biopsychosocial approach to pain
- Addresses psychological and socio-cultural factors, in addition to biomedical/physiological aspects
- Takes into account the multi-dimensional nature of pain and the interplay of psychological and psychosocial factors
- Pain is influenced by not only its underlying pathophysiology, but also by the individual's cognitions and behaviour:
    - Psychological factors, such as mood, beliefs about pain, and coping style, play an important role in an individual's adjustment to living with chronic pain
    - Persistent pain can lead to unhelpful behaviours (over-dependency on family, friends, and the medical profession, avoidance of regular activities, e.g. work, social activities, hobbies), and negative beliefs about their experience of pain and negative thoughts about themselves
    - Negative cognitions, along with decreased activity, can then lead to depression and/or anxiety

Inclusion criteria

- Have had pain for >6 months. Pain is persistent, disabling, and unresponsive to other therapies
- Pain is causing significant disability/distress (e.g. widespread disruption of activity, habitual over-/underactivity leading to increased pain, poor progress in rehabilitation due to pain, high affective distress or clear signs or reports of emotional distress, high levels of reported or observed pain behaviour (guarding, fear avoidance, catastrophizing)
- The individual is receptive to adopting a self-management approach and is willing to participate in a group

Exclusion criteria

- Limited life expectancy/rapidly deteriorating disease/condition
- Suitable for further medical treatment
- Certain psychiatric problems that would interfere with group management

- Does not wish to take part in a group-based intervention for pain
- Unable to commit to a PMP

Method of PMPs

- Most PMPs apply a cognitive behavioural approach, a process of reconceptualization that maladaptive beliefs about the cause of pain can be modified
- PMPs with a cognitive behavioural approach can be delivered using the following therapeutic models:
  - CBT
  - ACT
- Other models are sometimes employed such as MBSR and compassion focused therapy (CFT)
- Graded activity which is guided by the individual in the form of goal setting
- Plan and practise activities to decrease fear and improve the ability to experience fear by a graded exposure technique
- Group format, usually between eight and 12 individuals
- Interdisciplinary team which can include medical staff, specialist nurses, physiotherapists, psychologists, occupational therapists, pharmacists, and past participants
- Recommended duration should be the equivalent of 12 half-day sessions (some patients may benefit from more intensive programmes, e.g. 15–20 full days)

Contents of PMPs

- Education on the nature, mechanisms, and factors influencing chronic pain
- Physical exercise
- Identifying and challenging unhelpful beliefs about pain
- Graded activation towards individual goals
- Graded exposure to perceived threatening situations to reduce avoidance
- Methods to enhance acceptance, mindfulness, and psychological flexibility
- Skills training and activity management (pacing, assertiveness, goal setting, managing setbacks/flare-ups, sleep)

Outcome measures

- Changes in function
- Psychological well-being
- Pain experience
- Health care use
- QoL
- Work status (where relevant)
- Social activities and social role performance

Effectiveness

- Effective in producing reduction in pain, improved mood, psychological coping, physical fitness, pain communication and behaviour, and social role functioning
- High level of evidence for interdisciplinary PMPs based on cognitive behavioural principles
- Level of evidence: 1++

Special points

- Introducing a self-management approach to patients can be very challenging as it is not a 'medical treatment'
- Patients' suitability for PMPs is an important factor for outcome. Suitability is based on the impact of pain
- Individual psychological and physiotherapy may also be required before, during, or after PMP

Further reading

1. The British Pain Society. Guidelines for pain management programmes for adults. 2013. https://www.britishpainsociety.org/static/uploads/resources/files/pmp2013_main_FINAL_v6.pdf
2. Dysvik E, Vinsnes AG, Eikeland OJ. The effectiveness of a multidisciplinary pain management programme managing chronic pain. Int J Nurs Pract 2004;10(5):224–34 https://pubmed.ncbi.nlm.nih.gov/15461692/
3. Royal College of Anaesthetists. Core standards for pain management services in the UK. Chapter 7, Section 7, 2015; pp. 119–35. London: Intercollegiate Colleges. https://fpm.ac.uk/sites/fpm/files/documents/2019-07/Core%20Standards%20for%20Pain%20Management%20Services.pdf
4. LeMarchand K, Raphael JH. An open prospective study of coping factor dimensions and psychophysical health in patients undergoing a cognitive-behavioural group pain management programme for chronic pain. J Pain 2008;1:pp. 307–16
5. Scottish Intercollegiate Guidelines Network. Management of chronic pain: a national clinical guideline. 2013. https://www.sign.ac.uk/assets/sign136.pdf

PHYSIOTHERAPY AND OCCUPATIONAL THERAPY

Physiotherapy and Occupational Therapy

Rebecca Elijah-Smith and Fiona Thomas

CONTENTS

31.1 Principles of physiotherapy

Definition based on the Chartered Society of Physiotherapy

- The physiotherapist uses exercise, manual therapy, education, and advice in order to help their patients restore movement and function when they are affected by an injury, illness, or disability
- The physiotherapist also helps to encourage development and facilitate recovery, enabling people to stay in work and helping them to remain independent for as long as possible
- They also help to maintain health for the wider population, including assisting their patients to manage pain and prevent disease

Role of physiotherapy

Physiotherapists use their knowledge and skills to help treat a variety of conditions:

- Neurological (e.g. post-stroke rehabilitation, MS, Parkinson's disease)
- Musculoskeletal or MSK (e.g. back pain, whiplash-associated disorder, sports injuries, OA)
- Cardiovascular (e.g. chronic heart disease, rehabilitation after MI)
- Respiratory (e.g. asthma, COPD, cystic fibrosis)

Role of musculoskeletal physiotherapists

- MSK physiotherapy can help with acute injuries such as sport injuries or whiplash. Physiotherapy can also help with the management of long-term conditions such as persistent lower back pain and Fibromyalgia Syndrome (FMS)
- An essential element in the rehabilitation of a patient is self-management. This is the patient's involvement in their own care through education, awareness, empowerment, and participation in their treatment
- Physiotherapy is an evidence-based profession and takes a holistic approach to health care

Musculoskeletal physiotherapy for chronic pain

- Over the past few years, physiotherapists have started to use psychological principles in the management of their patients with long-term pain
- More recent studies have also advocated the development of psychological skills within physiotherapy, and the term psychologically informed physiotherapists (PIPs) has now been widely adopted
- Studies include the STarT Back tool which enables the primary care clinician to stratify the management of their patient according to patient prognosis (low, medium, or high risk) and targets treatment accordingly
- The Back Skills Training Trial focuses on the management of chronic lower back pain using a cognitive behavioural intervention through a structured group-based programme

Skills of the chronic pain musculoskeletal physiotherapist

- The physiotherapist is a core member of the interdisciplinary team and this role continues to develop
- The pain physiotherapist or PIP will develop skills, which include:
  - Cognitive behavioural theoretical principles
  - Educational and teaching skills in order to be able to deliver appropriate information to a group of patients, but also to be able to educate their pain management colleagues in the area of physiotherapy management
  - Facilitating a team approach, including interdisciplinary teamworking
- In addition, the pain physiotherapist brings a variety of important skills to the pain team. These include manual therapy, electrotherapy, acupuncture, and therapeutic exercise knowledge
- The physiotherapist will be able to integrate these skills into treatments, such as individualized sessions or Self Management Programmes (SMP's), using cognitive behavioural principles

Effectiveness

- Level of evidence: 1A
- There is a recognized need for continuous research

Further reading

1. Lamb SE, Mistry DA, Lall RA, et al. Group cognitive behavioural interventions for low back pain in primary care: extended follow-up of the Back Skills Training Trial. Pain 2012;153(2):494–501
2. Hill JC, Whitehurst DGT, Lewis M, et al. Comparison of stratified primary care management for low back pain with current best practice (STarT Back): a randomized controlled trial. Lancet 2011;378(9802):1560–71
3. British Pain Society. Guidelines for pain management programmes for adults. 2013. https://www.britishpainsociety.org/static/uploads/resources/files/pmp2013_main_FINAL_v6.pdf

31.2 Principals of occupational therapy

Introduction

- Occupational therapy promotes the health and well-being of people through occupational participation and engagement

- Occupational therapists apply a client-centred, ecological approach to pain management, focusing on an individual's engagement in their daily life tasks
- Occupational therapists support clients over the age spectrum and across different clinical services such as acute care, rehabilitation, community, mental health, case management, and health promotion

Roleof the occupational therapist in pain management

- Intervention has a strong emphasis on self-management and functional engagement
- Provides pain management as part of a multidisciplinary team for patients with acute, chronic and cancer pain and when pain coexists with other comorbidities such as SCI, amputation, stroke, and mental health issues
- Assists individuals in identifying and addressing factors that limit their performance of self-care, productive roles, and leisure tasks. These factors may be a combination of individual, environmental, and/or people surrounding them
- Skilled in understanding the challenges that clients face on a daily basis, and the influence that the environment and social milieu have in supporting or hindering the client's ability to engage in meaningful activities

Occupational therapy assessment

- Assessing the person's functional life and how pain has impacted ADLs, rest, productivity, and leisure
- Utilizing client-centred tools such as the Canadian Occupational Performance Measure to explore occupational performance deficits in areas of self-care, productive roles, and leisure
- Optimization of client-centred care is undertaken by observation of performance in a variety of environments such as home, school/institution of education, work, community, and clinical-based settings

Occupational therapy treatment—general overview

- Functionally-focused treatments to enable occupational engagement—this involves working with the individual to address barriers to such engagement
- Treatments aimed at ameliorating the identified barriers through functional restoration or adaptive approaches targeting the individual and the environments in which they engage
- Group- or individually based and across the developmental life span

Occupational therapy treatment—specific strategies

- Provision of pain education, based on current neuroscience evidence, suitable for the person's level of health literacy and their cultural beliefs
- Collaborative functional goal setting and goal action planning
- Environmental modification (home, community, work, or school) to support function
- Consideration of assistive devices to support or enable an individual's level of function. This may also include prescription of equipment, construction of splints, and provision of support garments
- Sensory integration, processing, and modulation techniques to assist individuals in self-organizing their sensory system in order to optimize occupational performance. This may also include the use of graded motor imagery, sensory desensitization techniques, graded activity approaches, and development of improved interoceptive awareness
- Creation of daily routines to support the development of habits and roles that support independence

- Incorporation of psychological strategies that support functional independence such as CBT, ACT, cognitive restructuring, distraction, relaxation, and mindfulness techniques
- Use of biofeedback techniques to support improved awareness of activity performance. This may include use of mirrors, EMG biofeedback machines, HR monitors, activity monitors, and diaries
- Chronic disease self-management strategies such as:
    - Joint protection
    - Back care techniques and ergonomic principles
    - Sleep management
    - Energy conservation/fatigue management
    - Pacing education: strategies are developed, considering the individual's functional needs, capacities, and opportunities for support and assistance. Such techniques are then embedded in the individual's habits and routines to maximize compliance over time
    - Flare-up management
- Support for return to work and productive roles on the background of a persisting pain condition
- Support for return to school and study from preparatory through to university-level education
- Support for resuming independent community engagement, including driving public transport use, shopping, and financial management
- Enabling the individual to reconnect with others in their social network and intimate relationships
- Enabling the individual to locate appropriate, non-medical/health-based services within their local community that support self-management of their condition. Examples include local t'ai chi groups, linking into leisure interests, and finding social networks

Further reading

1. Carpenter L, Baker GA, Tyldesley B. The use of the Canadian occupational performance measure as an outcome of a pain management program. Can J Occup Ther 2001;68(1):16–22
2. Hill W. The role of occupational therapy in pain management. Anaesth Intensive Care Med 2016;17(9):451–3
3. Van Griensven H, Strong J, Unruh A. Pain: a textbook for health professionals. 2013. London: Churchill Livingstone

31.3 Graded exercise therapy and therapeutic exercise

Definition

Therapeutic exercise

- Comprises of a series of specific body movements, postures, or physical activities intended to provide the patient with the ability to:
    - Improve, restore, or enhance physical function
    - Prevent impairments
    - Prevent or reduce health-related risk factors such as diabetes
    - Optimize overall health and well-being and fitness

Graded exercise therapy (GET)

- GET is a method of delivering therapeutic exercise
- GET is a therapeutic exercise that starts very gradually and increases slowly over a period of time
- This approach is used widely in the treatment of long-term conditions such as fibromyalgia syndrome, chronic fatigue syndrome (CFS), and myalgic encephalomyelitis (ME), as well as many acute injuries
- Grade exercise programmes should be properly supervised by the physiotherapist and progressed according to the levels of discomfort and disability
- There are four main types of exercise:
  - *Passive exercise*—the joints and muscles are moved without effort from the patient, usually from an external force such as a machine or the therapist
  - *Isometric (static) exercise*—the joint does not move when the muscle is tensed, with very little changes in the length of the muscle
  - *Isotonic (dynamic) exercise*—the joint is moved by the patient against constant resistance either from the physiotherapist or an apparatus. It is progressive
  - *Isokinetic exercise*—this is a type of strength training which uses specialized equipment, or dynamometers, in order to maintain and control muscle contraction. The speed of the motion is always kept the same, even as the resistance alters

Pacing

- Pacing is a graded approach which aims to avoid the 'boom-bust' cycle of over-exercising when the pain is at a reasonable level. This inadvertently leads to a flare-up in pain levels and a period of relapse until the pain settles back down to a more manageable level and the cycle begins all over again
- NICE (2007) defines pacing as 'energy management, with the aim of maximising cognitive and physical activity, while avoiding setbacks/relapses due to overexertion.' It says, 'The keys to pacing are knowing when to stop and rest by listening to and understanding one's own body, taking a flexible approach and staying within one's limits; different people use different techniques to do this'
- Pacing is used widely in pain management in order to facilitate a patient's ability to participate in an exercise programme, be it home- or group-based, without causing an increase in their pain levels
- Adaptive pacing therapy involves both the patient and the health care professional initially working together in order to facilitate the patient in their activity and functional levels, with the intention to achieve self-management
- The Pain Toolkit describes pacing as one of the key tools to self-management of a chronic pain condition and activities must be balanced with periods of rest

Effectiveness

- Level of evidence: 1A
- Evidence supports the use of exercise for many long-term conditions, including fibromyalgia and lower back pain
- Currently there are insufficient data to be able to strongly state whether a specific type of exercise is more superior in the treatment of chronic pain

Further reading

1. Kisner C, Colby LA. Therapeutic Exercise—Foundations and Techniques. 6th edition, 2012. Philadelphia: FA Davis Company
2. Chartered Society of Physiotherapy. https://www.csp.org.uk
3. The Pain Toolkit. https://www.paintoolkit.org
4. National Institute for Health and Care Excellence. Chronic fatigue syndrome/myalgic encephalomyelitis (or encephalopathy): diagnosis and management. Clinical Guideline [CG53]. 2007. https://www.nice.org.uk/guidance/cg53

31.4 Functional restoration programme

Definition

- FRP is a combined physical and psychological treatment programme recommended for patients with persistent back pain
- It is offered either in groups or as one-to-one
- NICE guidelines state that a 'key focus is helping people with persistent non-specific low back pain to self-manage their condition'
- Patients who complete the programme should become experts at self-managing their condition, not require ongoing physical treatment, and be more likely to maintain a better health-related QoL

Inclusion criteria

- Adults (i.e. over 18-year olds) with persistent back pain of >12 weeks' duration
- Early management has not been effective, i.e. the patient has failed to respond to routine primary care managements such as GP advice, medications, and physiotherapy-based exercise regime
- The patient appears motivated in helping themselves to get better and has identified some clear goals
- The patient has modifiable psychosocial factors impacting on their ability to recover such as fear-avoidant pain behaviours, catastrophizing, etc.
- Work status—the patient is:
    - Either at work, paid or voluntary, but struggling to remain
    - Off work, but jobs remain open
    - Not employed, but actively seeking to improve function and QoL

Exclusion criteria

- Biomedical factors, including:
    - Serious spinal pathology such as tumours, infection, and cauda equina signs
    - Significant motor radiculopathy and signs of nerve root compromise requiring surgery
    - Rheumatological conditions
    - Other medical problems which would prevent involvement in physical exercise programme such as unstable heart conditions, significant respiratory problems, and poorly managed diabetes
- Communication barriers which would prevent the ability to follow the cognitive component of a programme

- Widespread multi-joint pain or fibromyalgia-type conditions
- Examples of other episodes of care:
    - No other open episodes of care for the same condition
    - No previous attendance to Pain Management/Self-Management Programmes

Treatment format and frequency

- Patients are asked to complete a biopsychosocial assessment prior to being accepted into the FRP
- Groups usually consist of up to 12 patients; classroom and gym-based
- Patients generally attend for around eight sessions. The frequency of the programmes can differ, but commonly groups run twice a week over a 4-week period, with the total programme time being around 12 hours
- Patients attending individual sessions with the physiotherapist typically attend five sessions

Group intervention

- The group intervention is generally provided by an interdisciplinary team which includes a doctor, a pain counsellor, and a physiotherapist

Group format

- The session includes education regarding the biology of pain, participation in physical exercise sessions in small groups, graded activity, management of flare-ups, and goal setting
- Patients are taught relaxation skills and introduced to the concepts of visualization or mental imagery and mindfulness to help with their rehabilitation
    - *Visualization*—our mind plays an important role in the creation of our experience and therefore, it may be possible to 'programme' our mind and body to act in a certain way to gain positive results such as pain relief
    - *Mindfulness*—is a way of paying attention to, and seeing clearly, what is happening in our lives. It will not eliminate life's pressures, but it can help us respond to them in a calmer manner that benefits our general health and well-being

Outcome measures

The Oswestry Low Back Pain Disability Questionnaire (Oswestry Disability Index (ODI))

- Is an important tool that researchers and disability evaluators use to measure a patient's permanent functional disability
- The test is considered the 'gold standard' of low back functional outcome tools

The Pain Self-Efficacy Questionnaire (PSEQ)

- A 10-item questionnaire, developed to assess the confidence people with ongoing pain have in performing activities while in pain
- For PSEQ scores of around 40 and above, there has been an increased association between patients returning to work and maintenance of functional gains

Medication reduction

- Is also a key goal to achieve in those patients who attend FRP
- Typical data demonstrate that approximately three-quarters of patients manage to reduce their analgesic medication following attendance to the programme

Effectiveness

- Level of evidence: 1A
- There is moderate-quality evidence that multidisciplinary interventions result in greater improvements in pain and daily function
- There is also moderate evidence to support return to work, compared to treatments aimed at physical factors alone

Further reading

1. National Institute for Health and Care Excellence. Low back pain in adults: early management. Clinical Guideline [CG88]. 2009. https://www.nice.org.uk/guidance/cg88
2. Burch V, Penman D. Mindfulness for Health: A Practical Guide to Relieving Pain, Reducing Stress and Restoring Wellbeing. 2013. London: Piatkus
3. Davenport L (ed). Transformative Imagery: Cultivating the Imagination for Healing, Change, and Growth. 2016. London: Jessica Kingsley
4. Rogers D, Gardner A, MacLean S, et al. A retrospective analysis of a functional restoration service for patients with persistent low back pain. Musculoskeletal Care 2014;12(4):239–43

31.5 Hydrotherapy

Definition

- Hydrotherapy is the use of water for treatment of many different conditions such as OA, RA, persistent lower back pain, and fibromyalgia syndrome. It is also used to treat patients post-surgery and post-trauma injuries such as fractures
- Aquatic exercise is defined by the Chartered Society of Physiotherapy (CSP) as a 'therapy programme designed by a qualified physiotherapist using the properties of water to improve function ideally in a suitably heated pool'
- Balneotherapy is use of hot water treatment to help reduce pain, with the addition of various other techniques such as various forms of salt or sulphur, mud packs, jet streams, etc.

Temperature of the pool

- The maximum temperature of the pool should not exceed 35°C, with a maximum of 60% humidity
- The external pool temperature should be between 25°C and 28°C
- Therapists should not spend >3 hours per day in the pool itself

Therapeutic effects of hydrotherapy

- The physiotherapist uses specific properties of water in order to develop a therapeutic graded exercise programme
- The thermal effects of water are considered to help relieve pain, facilitate movement, and enhance relaxation
- The simple act of body part submergence increases energy expenditure
- Exercise intensity can be increased with the use of equipment such as paddles and floats
- Specific properties of water include:
  - *Buoyancy*—with or without a buoyancy aid; can be used to assist or resist movements
  - *Resistance*—water viscosity also provides resistance against movements. Resistance can be increased or decreased by changing the speed or directional use

- *Flow*—the use of water jets to alter flow can modify the amount of resistance provided during treatment
- *Turbulence*—the more turbulence created using methods such as water jets or speed alteration, the greater the energy expenditure

Physiotherapy-prescribed exercise programmes

- Following assessment, the physiotherapist will instruct the patient on an appropriate treatment programme that the patient can perform independently
- Exercises should then be reviewed at regular intervals in order to modify the exercise programme, depending on the patient's condition and rate of progress required
- Frequently, a patient's hydrotherapy management will be integrated into an appropriate land-based exercise regime

Contraindications/precautions to hydrotherapy

- All patients should have an initial screening and a land-based physiotherapy assessment in order to determine their suitability for hydrotherapy before entering the water; this is to ensure patient suitability and safety maintenance
- The following areas should be assessed prior to therapy:
  - CVS (e.g. BP, cardiac problems)
  - Respiratory system (e.g. asthma, chest infections)
  - CNS (e.g. epilepsy, tonal changes)
  - GI tract (e.g. incontinence, infection)
  - Genitourinary tract (incontinence, infection, pregnancy)
  - Infectious conditions (e.g. methicillin-resistant *Staphylococcus aureus* (MRSA), herpes)
  - Skin conditions (e.g. surgical wounds, rashes, chemical sensitivity)
  - Eye and ear conditions (e.g. tubal implants, visual or hearing impairments)
  - Other conditions (e.g. fear of water, diabetes, mode of pool entry, psychiatric problems)

Effectiveness

- Level of evidence: 1A
- There is moderate-quality evidence that aquatic exercise may have an effect on patient-related outcomes in knee and hip arthritis
- There is low- to moderate-quality evidence that aquatic exercise is beneficial for improving wellness, symptoms, and fitness in adults with fibromyalgia

Further reading

1. Australian Physiotherapy Association. Australian guidelines for aquatic physiotherapists working in and/or managing hydrotherapy pools. 2nd edition, 2015. https://australian.physio/sites/default/files/tools/Aquatic_Physiotherapy_Guidelines.pdf
2. Bidonde J, Busch AJ, Webber SC, et al. Aquatic exercise training for fibromyalgia. Cochrane Database Syst Rev 2014;10:CD011336

31.6 Graded motor imagery and mirror box therapy

Definitions

- *Imagery* refers to the creation of an experience in the mind (auditory, visual, tactile, olfactory, and gustatory). It is a cognitive process used by humans

- *Motor imagery* (MI) is the mental representation of movement without any body movement. It is a highly complex cognitive process, which is self-generated using sensory and perceptual processes, facilitating the activation of specific motor actions to improve motor function
- Evidence suggests that MI has positive effects on motor performance in athletes, people who are healthy, and people with neurological conditions

Graded motor imagery (GMI)

- *GMI* is a sequential approach to MI, an individually tailored treatment process which has been used successfully for persistent and complex pain states
- It aims to give flexibility and creativity back to the brain via graded exposure and is commonly used in the treatment of CRPS
- It is composed of three separate phases:
  - The first phase consists of patients learning to recognize images of their left or right hands or feet which are shown to them in various positions
  - The second phase consists of patients practising these positions via MI of smooth and pain-free movements
  - In the third and final phase, they perform movements of both limbs using a mirror box to hide the affected limb

Mirror box therapy

- Mirror therapy means looking into a mirror to see the reflection of the limb or body part in front of it
- Brain activation during mirror therapy is less than during actual movement, but slightly more compared with imagining the same movement
- The patient places their affected limb inside the mirror box and works through a series of movements
- Looking at the mirror image of the unaffected limb gives the illusion of seeing the hidden affected limb
- In the initial phases of rehabilitation when the limb is at its most sensitive—the affected limb will be kept still inside the mirror box, while the unaffected limb outside the box will be performing tasks such as rotation, finger opposition, making a fist, wrist movements, etc.
- As treatment progresses, resistance can then be added, e.g. making a fist but adding in a squeeze in repetitions
- The affected limb will gradually start to join in the movements within the patient's pain limitations
- As the affected limb becomes less sensitive, the roles then reverse and the unaffected limb starts to copy the movements of the affected limb while it remains inside the box

Frequency of intervention

- For a general guide, studies have used a period of 2 weeks for each of the phases of GMI and have advised around 10 minutes for each waking hour
- In essence, there is no set frequency for mirror box therapy and treatment is focused very much on the individual's needs

Effectiveness

- Level of evidence: 1A
- Currently the quality of available evidence is variable
- There is a recognized need for further research

Further reading

1. Bowering KJ, O'Connell NE, Tabor A, et al. The effects of graded motor imagery and its components on chronic pain: a systematic review and meta-analysis. J Pain 2013;14(1):3–13
2. Dickstein R, Deutsch JE. Motor imagery in physical therapist practice. Phys Ther 2007;87:942–53
3. Moseley GL, Butler DS, Beames TB, et al. The Graded Motor Imagery Handbook. 2012. Adelaide: Noigroup Publications

31.7 Acupuncture and electro-acupuncture

Definition

- Acupuncture is the process of having fine needles inserted into certain sites in the body for therapeutic purposes. These sites are known as acupuncture points
- Derived from ancient Chinese medicine and forms part of traditional Chinese medicine (TCM)
- Practitioners of TCM believe that stimulating certain acupuncture points can help restore the balance between Yin and Yang that can become disturbed in illness or pain
- More often, scientific *evidence-based western medical acupuncture research* is combined with the principles of TCM as a means to help reduce pain and enhance other treatments such as exercise and functional-based activities
- The Bladder Meridian which is commonly used for lower back pain (see Figure 31.7.1)

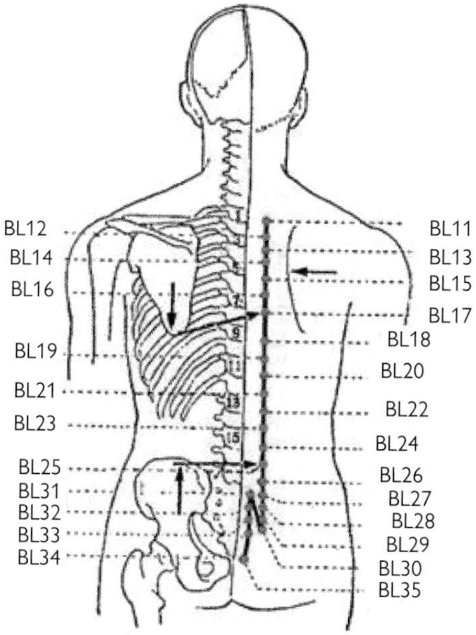

Figure 31.7.1 Bladder Meridian (commonly used for lower back pain)

Acupuncture practitioners

- Acupuncture practitioners are most often physiotherapists, GPs, and nurses who have attended appropriate accredited training courses
- Recognized professional bodies for trained acupuncturists include:
    - British Acupuncture Council (BAcC)
    - British Medical Acupuncture Society (BMAS)
    - Acupuncture Association of Chartered Physiotherapists (AACP)

Indications

- MSK conditions
- Spinal pain, joint pains
- Widespread body pains such as fibromyalgia syndrome
- Migraines and tension-type headaches
- Acupuncture should be used alongside other treatments such as exercise therapy, manual therapy, and education, as well as relaxation techniques, in order to enhance outcomes and facilitate self-management.

Theoretical mechanism

- Acupuncture stimulates the body to produce chemicals, which act to help relieve pain, reduce stress, and promote restful sleep, and to help produce a positive feeling of well-being. These chemicals include:
    - Endorphins: endogenous opioid neuropeptides found to be natural pain relievers and also to promote feelings of pleasure and euphoria
    - Oxytocin: hormone which has antidepressant-like effects
    - Melatonin: hormone that regulates sleep and wakefulness
    - Serotonin: monoamine NT which is thought to be a contributor to feelings of well-being and happiness
- Correlation has also been found between certain acupuncture points and myofascial trigger points

Contraindications

- Pregnancy—in the first and last 3 months and patients trying to conceive
- Pacemaker or any other electrical implant (no electro-acupuncture)
- Any damage to heart valves
- Risk of active infection or patients with a deficient or weak immune system, known skin infection, or poor skin condition in the area of treatment
- Known metal allergy
- Needle phobia
- Oedematous limb(s)

Precautions

- Fit, seizure, faint, or epilepsy
- Diabetes, low BP
- On anticoagulation or antiplatelet therapy, or a bleeding disorder, e.g. haemophilia
- Generally feeling unwell or with cold/flu symptoms

- Patients who are going to drive or operate machinery after treatment
- Malignancy

Number of sessions

- Most patients will receive between four and six sessions at weekly intervals
- Sometimes patients are offered top-up sessions
- If no noticeable benefits after the first 2–3 acupuncture sessions, then treatment should be stopped

Safety and side effects

- Mild and short-lived S/Es—fatigue, light-headedness/nausea/dizziness, bruising, localized bleeding, redness around the needle site, and mottling of the skin
- Rare S/Es—infection, allergic response to the metal
- Extremely rare—pneumothorax

Electro-acupuncture

- Insertion of needles that are coupled to electrodes attached to an electro-acupuncture machine
- These units deliver variable amplitudes and frequencies of electrical impulses
- Low-frequency electro-acupuncture contributes to the mechanism of delayed pain reduction by stimulating the production of endorphins
- High-frequency electro-acupuncture works via the serotonin route and is more quick-acting
- Electro-acupuncture may be more useful in persistent pain conditions

Further reading

1. British Acupuncture Council (BAcC). http://www.acupuncture.org.uk/
2. NHS. Acupuncture. 2019. http://www.nhs.uk/Conditions/acupuncture/Pages/Introduction.aspx
3. Acupuncture Association of Chartered Physiotherapists (AACP). https://www.aacp.org.uk/
4. White A. The safety of acupuncture—evidence from the UK. Acupuncture in Medicine 2006;24:53–7

31.8 Laser therapy

Definition

- LASER is an acronym for Light Amplification by Stimulated Emission of Radiation. Laser is therefore a form of light amplifier which provides enhancement of particular properties of light energy
- Therapy lasers can be categorized into a particular category of laser light known as 3A or 3B and are referred to as low-level laser therapy (LLLT)
- LLLT does not cause a detectable rise in temperature in the targeted tissues, nor does it cause any macroscopically visible changes in tissue structure. It is therefore considered to be a non-thermal modality
- LLLT is used as a therapeutic treatment to help reduce pain and disability associated with MSK and joint diseases, including lower back pain

Parameters

- Most LLLT devices generate light in the red visible and near infra-red bands of the electromagnetic spectrum, with typical wavelengths of 600–1000 nm
- The mean power of the therapeutic machines is typically low (1–100 mW), but the peak power could be much higher

Treatment devices

- The treatment device may be a single emitter or a cluster of several emitters
- The output may be pulsed or continuous
- Lower pulsing rates are more effective for acute conditions, while higher pulsing rates work better for more chronic conditions

Mode of action

- When LLLT is applied to the body tissues, it delivers energy at a level appropriate enough to disturb local electron orbits, which results in the production of heat
- This subtle change influences the cell membrane and can initiate a chemical change, disrupt chemical bonds, and produce free radicals
- LLLT is thought to affect fibroblast function and accelerate connective tissue repair
- There are also some reports that LLLT has anti-inflammatory effects as a consequence of its action in decreasing PG synthesis
- LLLT is mainly absorbed by superficial tissues, but it could possibly have a deeper effect. However, the exact mechanism for this action remains inconclusive; theories include chemical mediators or second messenger systems

Clinical application

- Laser therapy is generally used for the following conditions:
  - Wound healing
  - Inflammatory arthropathies
  - Soft tissue injuries
  - Pain conditions such as myofascial trigger point pain and fibromyalgia syndrome

Precautions/contraindications for laser therapy

- Precautions should be noted when treating the following:
  - Pregnancy (anywhere on the body)
  - Active implants, including pacemakers
  - Metal implants
  - Epilepsy
  - Local circulatory insufficiency/devitalized tissue
- Contraindications include:
  - Over the eyes and testis
  - Pregnancy (around the fetus)
  - Malignancy
  - Active epiphysis
  - Active bleeding tissue

Effectiveness

- Level of evidence: 1A
- Currently there are insufficient data to either support or refute the use of LLLT in the treatment of chronic pain conditions
- There is a recognized need for further research

Further reading

1. Montes-Molina R, Prieto-Baquero A, Martinez-Rodriguez ME, et al. Interferential laser therapy in the treatment of shoulder pain and disability from musculoskeletal pathologies: a randomised comparative study. Physiotherapy 2012;98:143–50
2. Yousefi-Nooraie R, Schonstein E, Heidari K, et al. Low level laser therapy for nonspecific low-back pain. Cochrane Database Syst Rev 2007;2:CD005107

EPIDEMIOLOGY AND STATISTICS

Epidemiology and Statistics

Sabina Bachtold, David Pang, and Alifia Tameem

CONTENTS

32.1 Epidemiology of chronic pain

Introduction

- Chronic pain is one of the most significant causes of long-term suffering and morbidity
- Despite its high prevalence, it remains under-recognized and poorly resourced, compared with other chronic medical conditions
- This is despite chronic pain being one of the most important causes of disability and work-related days off
- Precision in measurement of the prevalence and incidence of pain is hampered by many factors:
  - Pain is a subjective measure, and self-reported measures of pain are used to measure both intensity and occurrence
  - A level of pain that is significant to one individual cannot be reliably replicated on another
- Accurate measurement of prevalence and incidence of chronic pain and their causes is essential to direct healthcare policies and initiatives to improve the outcome of any interventions directed at relieving the morbidity of chronic pain
- In 2006, a large survey of 46 349 Europeans from multiple countries revealed that pain over 6 months was prevalent in 19% of all responders
- A recent meta-analysis estimated the prevalence of chronic pain in the UK as 43%
- The prevalence rises with age, and 10.4–14.3% of the population had pain that was moderate to severe
- It is likely that these numbers are an underestimation, yet most of chronic pain is managed in primary care or without help from health care professionals
- Multiple factors are associated with chronic pain, and many of our current therapies are directed at these factors, as well as at the pain itself

Clinical factors

- Chronic pain is now recognized as a disease in its own right, and not merely a symptom of another underlying problem
- One of the most important factors associated with chronicity is the severity and existence of multiple painful areas

- The association of chronic pain with other long-term diseases is well established and patients with severe chronic pain have a doubling of mortality from cardiorespiratory illness over a 10-year period

Psychological factors

- The relationship between mental well-being and chronic pain is likely to be bidirectional
- Mental health conditions and patient beliefs play an important part
- Poor prognostic indicators include anxiety, depression, catastrophizing, and avoidance beliefs
- Interventions directed at using active, rather than passive, coping strategies to target beliefs about chronic pain can be more effective
- Large public health interventions with the aim of changing attitudes and beliefs about chronic pain have shown mixed results

Social factors

- A higher prevalence of chronic pain is seen in:
    - Females
    - Increasing age
    - Low socioeconomic status
    - Unemployment
    - History of abuse
- Ageing of the population will have implications on pain management resources, as older age is associated with more chronic pain
- Many of the above factors cannot be altered, but recognizing their association with pain will assist in the provision of pain services

Genetics

- An increasing body of research has shown that genetic factors can play a significant role in chronic pain
- Children of parents with chronic pain show an association, and genetics play a part in determining pain thresholds

Specific pain conditions

Low back pain

- A point prevalence of 11.9% and a lifetime prevalence of 39.9% were measured in a large global study in 2012
- This increases with age, with implications for health care provision for an ageing population
- Most episodes of low back pain are self-limiting, but relapses are common
- There have been associations with smoking, job dissatisfaction, psychological comorbidity, low physical conditioning, and coexisting medical conditions

Neuropathic pain

- An estimate of the prevalence in the general population is 1.5%, but neuropathic pain varies with the underlying condition:
    - Most common are neuropathic low back/leg pain and diabetic neuropathy
    - Patients with neuropathic pain consume more health care resources and have a lower QoL, compared with matched controls

Chronic widespread pain and fibromyalgia

- This is the second most common rheumatic disorder after OA
- There is a female:male ratio of 2:1, and it is seen in both paediatric and adult populations

- No significant difference exists between different cultures, ethnic groups, or countries
- Genetic factors may play a role as first-degree relatives have a higher risk of developing fibromyalgia (odds ratio (OR) 8.5)

Further reading

1. Breivik H, Collett B, Ventafridda V, et al. Survey of chronic pain in Europe: prevalence, impact on daily life, and treatment. Eur J Pain 2006;10:287–333
2. Dionne CE, Dunn KM, Croft PR. Does back pain prevalence really decrease with increasing age? A systematic review. Age Ageing 2006;35:229–34
3. Fayaz A, Croft P, Langford RM, et al. Prevalence of chronic pain in the UK: a systematic review and meta-analysis of population studies. BMJ Open 2016;6:e010364
4. Torrance N, Smith BH, Bennett M, et al. The epidemiology of chronic pain of predominantly neuropathic origin. Results from a general population survey. J Pain 2006;7:281–9

32.2 Evidence-based medicine

Introduction

- Definition as '*the conscientious, explicit and judicious use of current best evidence in making decisions about the care of individual patients*'
- Integrates the clinician's expertise, the patient's values, and best research available to improve patient care

Levels of evidence

- Highest level of evidence must be sought unless the evidence is minimal and/or of low quality

GRADE methodology

- The GRADE (Grades of Recommendation, Assessment, Development, and Evaluation) working group has explained the quality of evidence which is used to develop good-quality EBM

SIGN methodology

- The Scottish Intercollegiate Guidelines Network (SIGN) follows the principles of GRADE methodology to assess the overall quality of evidence
- The working group were responsible for creating a grading system for recommendations, linked to the strength of evidence available. International and national guidelines for best practice use the SIGN methodology

Quality of evidence

- Based on robustness of the techniques used and depends on multiple factors:
  - Design of the study—minimal bias and maximum credit to the question posed
  - Quality of the study—poor randomization, non-blinding, and inappropriate statistics used would lead to poor-quality studies
  - Consistency—similarity of estimate of effect
  - Directness—properly matched patients to the interventions
- Follow a **typical** 'hierarchy of evidence' (see Table 32.2.1)

Table 32.2.1 Hierarchy of evidence

Levels	Evidence
1	At least one published systematic review of many well-designed randomized controlled trials (RCTs)
2	At least one published well-designed RCT of good size and appropriate setting clinically
3	Non-randomized, published, well-designed trials, cohort study, or case-controlled studies
4	Well-designed, non-experimental studies from multiple centres or research groups
5	Descriptive studies, expert opinions, consensus committee reports, anecdotal evidence from case reports

- Strength of recommendation essentially informs us whether an intervention should be applied or not. It depends on the quality of evidence described above, trade-offs (balance between risks and benefits), specific patient groups belonging to specific situations, and the amount of baseline risk in the specific population

Limitations/criticisms of EBM

- Publication bias can be responsible for unpublished negative trials, hence not a true reflection of EBM
- Research progress can be limited due to ethical and cost implications
- RCTs or meta-analyses cannot always answer all hypothetical questions
- A well-designed RCT can be expensive and sometimes unaffordable
- Pharmaceutical companies provide a lot of financial support, which can further introduce bias and conflict of interest
- Health economics has a role in the current climate and the best evidence for treatment may not necessarily be the 'best value for money'. This has implications for appropriate management of patients as per EBM
- Although guidelines and recommendations provide safe evidence-based pathways, they cannot always be applied to all clinical scenarios, especially in unique settings, and clinical acumen is still required

Further reading

1. Newport M, Smith A. Implementation of evidence-based practise in anaesthesia. BJA Educ 2015;15(6):311–15
2. Smith FG, Tong JL, Smith JE. Evidence-based medicine. Contin Educ Anaesth Crit Care Pain 2006;6(4):148–51

32.3 Statistics

Introduction

- It is a mathematical science which allows the data (numerical information) to be presented, analysed, and interpreted to draw conclusions

- Parameter—a characteristic of a population which can be measured
- Variable—a characteristic of a sample which can be measured, varies between individuals, and can be quantitative or qualitative
- Sample statistic—a mathematical calculation of the data variables of a given sample

Types of data

Numerical (quantitative) data

- Presented as tables, cumulative frequency curves, histograms, and plots (dot plots, x–y scatterplots)
- *Discrete data* have finite values (number of children)
- *Continuous data* can take any numerical value, including fractional values (weight, height)
- *Ratio data series* have zero as the baseline value (length, Kelvin temperature scale)
- *Interval data series* include zero as a point on a larger scale (Celsius temperature scales)

Categorical (qualitative) data

- Presented as tables (contingency table) or graphically as pie charts and bar charts
- *Nominal data* can only be named (ABO blood groups or different types of fruit)
- *Ordinal data* have an implicit order of magnitude (pain—nil/mild/moderate/severe or American Society of Anesthesiologists (ASA) score)

Describing data

Measures of central tendency

(See Fig. 32.3.1.)

- *Mean (average):*
  - The sum of data values divided by the total number of data points
  - Used to analyse interval data, especially when normally distributed
  - Uses all data but is readily influenced by outliers

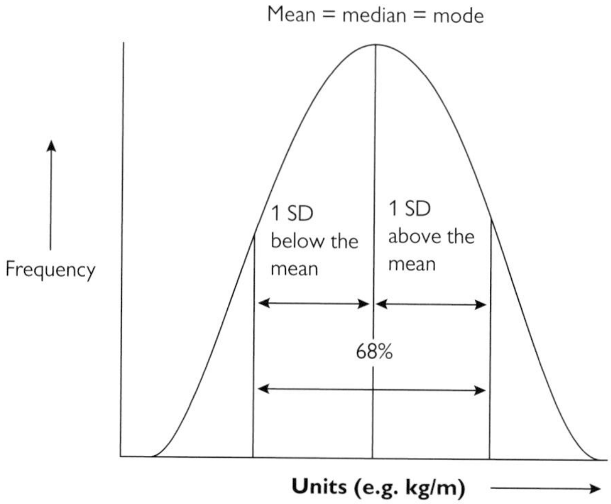

Figure 32.3.1 An example of Gaussian/normal distribution. One standard deviation (SD) refers to one SD above and below the mean; 2 SD = 96% of the population; 3 SD = 99.6%

- *Median:*
  - The middle value of a data series when arranged in a ranked order, with 50% of data points above and 50% below
  - It is not readily influenced by outliers but does not make use of all individual data values
  - It is a helpful measure of central tendency for ordinal and interval data
  - When the interval data set is not normally distributed, the median is preferred over the mean
- *Mode:*
  - The most frequently occurring value in a sample
  - It is not used much in statistical testing
  - It measures a frequently occurring value in a sample set, used mainly for categorical data

Measures of spread

- The Gaussian curve is the most useful bell-shaped graphical representation of interval data in statistics. If symmetrical, mean = median = mode, and the data is normally distributed
- Parametric, normally distributed data—mean and standard deviation are suitable
- Non-parametric data—median and interquartile range are appropriate
- Parametric skewed data—treat as non-parametric data or attempt to mathematically convert to normally distributed data
- When unsure whether the data are parametric, especially with small sample sizes, apply non-parametric analysis
- *Standard deviation (SD):*
  - A measure of the spread of data around a central point

$$SD = \sqrt{\frac{\Sigma(mean - x)^2}{n \text{ or } n-1}}$$

Where: mean − x = the difference from the sample mean for each value; n = number of observations or sample size; Σ = sum of. $n - 1$ is used if the number of observations is ≤ 30; n is used if >30 observations. 1 SD = 68% of the population; 2 SD = 95.7%; 3 SD = 99.7%

- *Variance = $(SD)^2$*
  - A measure of the spread of data around a central point
- *Confidence intervals (CI):*
  - The range of values that will contain the true population mean with a stated percentage confidence
  - 95% CI is the sample mean ± 1.96 SD (or SEM) and is the most frequently quoted
- *Standard error of the mean (SEM):*
  - SEM = SD/ $\sqrt{(n)}$
  - Measures how precisely the sample mean is estimated (how far from the population mean). It is not a measure of spread of the data
- *Percentile:*
  - The data are arranged in a ranked order and then divided into 100 points called percentiles
  - Each quarter (25%) is a quartile and the interval data are well represented by a box and whisker plot

- *Quartile:*
    - One of the three values that divide a given range of data into four equal parts—lower, middle, and upper quartile at 25th, 50th, and 75th percentile, respectively
- *Interquartile range (IQR):*
    - The data are ranked (i.e. put in order from lowest to highest) and divided into quarters
    - The IQR is the range between the lowest and the highest quarters (i.e. encompassing the middle half of the data)
    - If a dividing point is between two numbers, then an average is taken
- *Range:*
    - The simplest form of a measure between the lowest and highest value, minimal statistical value

Statistical tests

(See Table 32.3.1.)

Parametric tests

- Used for samples which contain data with a normal distribution

Non-parametric tests

- Do not rely on assumptions about the shape or parameters of the underlying population distribution

The null hypothesis (H_0)

- When performing a study, the first step is to pose a question, which is formulated as a hypothesis that must be proved or disproved
- This question represents the null hypothesis and it states that there is no difference between the sample groups

Table 32.3.1 Statistical tests

Sample group(s)	Parametric tests	Non-parametric tests	Categorical data tests
One group	One-sample t-test	Wilcoxon signed rank test	
Two groups	Unpaired normal distribution data: Student's unpaired two-sample t-test Paired normal distribution data: Student's paired two-sample t-test	Mann–Whitney U test (≈ unpaired t-test) Wilcoxon signed rank test (≈ paired t-test)	Unpaired data: Fischer exact test Paired data: McNemar's test
Three or more groups	ANOVA (analysis of variance)	Kruskal–Wallis Friedman	Pearson's chi-squared test (χ^2)

Power

- The ability of a statistical test to reveal a difference of a certain magnitude
- Power is $(1 - \beta) \times 100\%$ and acceptable power is 80–90% (β = probability of type II error)

Type I error

- There is no difference between the sample groups, but a statistical difference is found, as $P < 0.05$
- The null hypothesis is incorrectly rejected, leading to a false positive result
- The probability of making a type I error is called Alpha (α)

Type II error

- There is a difference between the sample groups, but a statistical difference is found, as $P > 0.05$
- The null hypothesis is incorrectly accepted, leading to a false negative result
- It is usually because of a small sample size
- The probability of making a type II error is called Beta (β)

P value

- The likelihood of the observed value being a result of chance alone
- Conventionally, a P (probability) value of <0.05 represents statistical significance, P <0.01 highly significant, and P >0.5 not significant
- It is important to distinguish statistical significance from clinical significance

Risk

- It is the probability or likelihood that an event may occur
- If RR >1, treatment group is better
- Absolute risk reduction (ARR) suggests that the incidence of effect is mainly due to the treatment
- Relative risk reduction (RRR) reflects the amount of risk that is removed by the treatment group

Relative risk (RR) = incidence in treatment group/incidence in control group
Absolute risk reduction (ARR) = incidence in treatment group − incidence in control group
Relative risk reduction (RRR) = absolute risk reduction/incidence in control group
Odds ratio (OR) = odds of outcome in treatment group/odds of outcome in control group

Number needed to treat (NNT)

- Number of patients who need to be treated to achieve an outcome in one patient
- NNT of 1 is the perfect outcome, but very difficult to achieve clinically
- The closer the treatment group to NNT of 1, the better the treatment

Number needed to harm (NNH)

- Number of patients who need to be treated (or exposed to a risk factor) in order for one person to have a particular adverse effect
- An NNH of 6 for minor adverse effects for amitriptyline means that for six patients treated with amitriptyline, one experiences minor adverse effects (e.g. drowsiness, dizziness, dry mouth, constipation)
- The lower the NNH, the more the risk of harm
- An NNH of 1 would mean that every patient treated is harmed

Table 32.3.2 Methods of data analysis

Test outcome	Positive	Negative
Positive (P <0.05)	True positive (TP)	False positive (FP) (type I error/α)
Negative (P >0.05)	False negative (FN) (type II error/β)	True negative (TN)

Outcome prediction

(See Table 32.3.2.)

Sensitivity

- The ability of a test to correctly identify a positive outcome when one exists

$$\text{Sensitivity (\%)} = TP/(TP + FN)$$

Where: TP = true positive; FN = false negative

Specificity

- The ability of a test to correctly identify a negative outcome where one exists

$$\text{Specificity (\%)} = TN/(TN + FP)$$

Where: TN = true negative; FP = false positive

Positive predictive value (PPV)

- The certainty with which a positive test result correctly predicts a positive value

$$\text{PPV (\%)} = TP/(TP + FP)$$

Negative predictive value (NPV)

- The certainty with which a negative test result correctly predicts a negative value

$$\text{NPV (\%)} = TN/(TN + FN)$$

Further reading

1. Campbell M. Medical Statistics. 2006. Chichester: Wiley
2. Lalkhen AG, McCluskey A. Statistics I–IV: introduction to clinical trials and systematic reviews. Contin Educ Anaesth Crit Care Pain 2007;(3–6):95–9
3. Lalkhen AG, McCluskey A. Statistics I–IV: introduction to clinical trials and systematic reviews. Contin Educ Anaesth Crit Care Pain 2007;(3–6):127–30
4. Lalkhen AG, McCluskey A. Statistics I–IV: introduction to clinical trials and systematic reviews. Contin Educ Anaesth Crit Care Pain 2007;(3–6):167–70
5. Lalkhen AG, McCluskey A. Statistics I–IV: introduction to clinical trials and systematic reviews. Contin Educ Anaesth Crit Care Pain 2007;(3–6):208–12

32.4 Clinical trials

Clinical trial design

- Define the problem that needs to be addressed by carefully observing clinical work
- Formulate a null hypothesis by choosing the correct research question
- Perform a literature search
- Obtain Ethics approval
- Types of Clinical Studies (see Table 32.4.1)
- Retrospective studies are helpful with rare disorders and are less expensive than prospective studies as they can utilize existing resources
- However, obtaining accurate and complete information without bias is difficult as there can be many confounding variables

Trial planning and design (statistician/methodology expert involved)

- Write a protocol detailing how the trial will be conducted
- Ideally it should be a double-blinded, randomized, case-controlled trial
- Estimate the number of patients required to perform the study and avoid a type II error (power calculation). An adequately powered study will ideally detect an effect in 80% of the times if it exists
- Risk assessment
- Sponsorship
- Ethics approval by completing the online research application form on the Integrated Research Application System (IRAS)
- Analysis of data to assess statistical and clinical significance. Traditionally, $P < 0.05$ has been used to determine statistical significance, as there would be a $<5\%$ chance that the null hypothesis has been wrongly rejected
- Over time, CIs are calculated to summarize the statistical significance
- Clinical significance is based on standards of care and expert opinions
- Reporting and dissemination of results—guidance provided by Consolidated Standards of Reporting Trials (CONSORT)
- Publication bias can occur when negative trials or statistically insignificant trials are not published. An inverted, symmetrical funnel plot of individual studies would suggest that all studies have been included, minimizing selection or publication bias

Table 32.4.1 Types of clinical studies

Retrospective	Prospective
• Cross-sectional studies or surveys (a random group or a well-defined population is studied) • Case-control studies (a specific condition is compared to the controls)	• Observational cohort studies (two or more groups are studied over a long period) • Randomized interventional control studies (evaluate the interventional arm of the study and reduce bias) • Non-randomized or cohort interventional controlled trials (evaluate interventions but can have an element of bias)

Table 32.4.2 Phases of clinical trials: preceded by *in vitro* and animal studies

Phase	Participants and purpose	Number of subjects
0	Optional exploratory trials (human micro-dosing) Does the drug behave in humans as was expected from preclinical studies?	10–15
1	Healthy volunteers/people with the disease Safety and dosage	20–50
2	People with the disease Efficacy and side effects	Several hundreds
3	People with the disease Efficacy and monitoring adverse reactions	300–3000
4	People with the disease Safety and efficacy (post-marketing surveillance)	Several thousands

Phases of clinical trials (see Table 32.4.2)

Types of trials

Case-control studies

- Observational study comparing patients; can be done rapidly for rare conditions

Case reports or series

- Reports of a patient or group of patients based on similar events
- They provide clinical management tools for rare conditions, but lack group comparisons and are not generalized to all patients

Cohort (longitudinal) studies

- Can be retrospective or prospective where people belong to the same group, but have an intervention and a control arm. It can be open to bias and the work is time-consuming since a large sample size is needed

Randomized controlled trial

Ideally, it should be:

- *Blinded:*
  - In double-blinded trials, neither the observer nor the subject are aware of the treatment and thus may not bias the result
- *Randomized:*
  - This avoids any bias in the allocation of treatments to patients. It guarantees that the probabilities obtained from statistical analysis will be valid
  - Randomization prevents the influence of confounding factors (e.g. when the effects of two processes are not separated)
- *Controlled:*
  - This provides a comparison to assess the effect of the test treatment
  - In many instances, the most appropriate control is a placebo, i.e. a tablet or medicine with no clinical effect

Systematic review

- It is an assessment, evaluation, and critical appraisal of various research studies and other relevant data available to address a specific issue
- It can be qualitative and offers a summary to guide clinical decision-making

Meta-analysis

- It is a quantitative measure where there is statistical integration of multiple similar research studies and can be graphically represented by Forest plots
- It is useful when a good-quality, large, prospective, randomized study is unavailable. A meta-analysis can produce NNT and/or NNH

Further reading

1. National Institute for Health Research. Clinical Trials Toolkit. Routemap. http://www.ct-toolkit.ac.uk/routemap/
2. US Department of Health and Human Services, Food and Drug Administration, Center for Drug Evaluation and Research (CDER). Guidance for industry, investigators, and reviewers. Exploratory IND Studies. 2006. https://www.fda.gov/regulatory-information/search-fda-guidance-documents/exploratory-ind-studies
3. Lalkhen AG, McCluskey A. Statistics V: introduction to clinical trials and systematic reviews. Contin Educ Anaesth Crit Care Pain 2018;8(4):143–6

Index

Note: Topics are listed in their expanded form. Abbreviations are listed on pages xxiii–xxviii

S

T